# THE ATHLETE'S SHOULDER

*Edited by*

## James R. Andrews, M.D.

Clinical Professor
Division of Sports Medicine
Department of Orthopaedics
University of Virginia School of Medicine
Charlottesville, Virginia
Medical Director
American Sports Medicine Institute
Orthopaedic Surgeon
Alabama Sports Medicine and Orthopaedic Center
Birmingham, Alabama
Orthopaedic Consultant, Toronto Bluejays Baseball Organization
Toronto, Ontario, Canada
Orthopaedic Consultant, University of Kentucky
Lexington, Kentucky

## Kevin E. Wilk, P.T.

National Director
Research and Clinical Education
Associate Clinical Director
HEALTHSOUTH Sports Medicine and Rehabilitation Center
Director
Rehabilitative Research
American Sports Medicine Institute
Birmingham, Alabama

Churchill Livingstone
New York, Edinburgh, London, Madrid, Melbourne, Tokyo

*# 2833 4281*

Library of Congress Cataloging-in-Publication Data

The Athlete's shoulder / edited by James R. Andrews, Kevin E. Wilk.
    p.   cm.
  Includes bibliographical references and index.
  ISBN 0-443-08847-0
  1. Shoulder—Wounds and injuries. 2. Sports—Accidents and
injuries. I. Andrews, James R. (James Rheuben), Date.
II. Wilk, Kevin E.
  [DNLM: 1. Shoulder—injuries. 2. Rotator Cuff—injuries. 3. Arm
Injuries—diagnosis. 4. Arm Injuries—therapy. 5. Athletic
Injuries. WE 810 A871 1993]
  RD557.5.A83 1993
  617.5'72044—dc20
  DNLM/DLC
  for Library of Congress         93-14313
                        CIP

Distributed in the United Kingdom by Churchill Livingstone, Robert Stevenson House, 1–3 Baxter's Place, Leith Walk, Edinburgh EH1 3AF, and by associated companies, branches, and representatives throughout the world.

Accurate indications, adverse reactions, and dosage schedules for drugs are provided in this book, but it is possible that they may change. The reader is urged to review the package information data of the manufacturers of the medications mentioned.

The Publishers have made every effort to trace the copyright holders for borrowed material. If they have inadvertently overlooked any, they will be pleased to make the necessary arrangements at the first opportunity.

Copy Editor: *Elizabeth Bowman-Schulman*
Production Supervisor: *Patricia McFadden*
Cover Design: *Paul Moran*

Printed in the United States of America

First published in 1994    7  6  5  4  3  2  1

*To my family*
*my wife, Debbie*
*my children, Justin, Summer, and Brittney*
*thank you for your love, support, and understanding*
*through all the years*

*To those students, fellows, physicians, therapists, and*
*trainers whose ideas, energy, and work have con-*
*tributed to our understanding of the shoulder*

*K.E.W.*

# Contributors

**James R. Andrews, M.D.**
Clinical Professor, Division of Sports Medicine, Department of Orthopaedics and Rehabilitation, University of Virginia School of Medicine, Charlottesville, Virginia; Medical Director, American Sports Medicine Institute; Orthopaedic Surgeon, Alabama Sports Medicine and Orthopaedic Center, Birmingham, Alabama; Orthopaedic Consultant, Toronto Bluejays Baseball Organization, Toronto, Ontario, Canada; Orthopaedic Consultant, University of Kentucky, Lexington, Kentucky

**Christopher A. Arrigo, M.S., P.T., A.T.C.**
Senior Physical Therapist, HEALTHSOUTH Sports Medicine and Rehabilitation Center, Birmingham, Alabama

**Champ L. Baker, M.D.**
Clinical Assistant Professor, Department of Orthopaedic Surgery, Tulane University School of Medicine, New Orleans, Louisiana; Staff Physician, Hughston Orthopaedic Clinic, P.C., Columbus, Georgia

**J. Gregory Bennett, M.S., P.T.**
Director of Physical Therapy, Dominion Physical Therapy, P.C., Alexandria / Herndon / Springfield / Woodbridge, Virginia

**Louis U. Bigliani, M.D.**
Associate Professor of Clinical Orthopedic Surgery, Columbia University College of Physicians and Surgeons; Chief, Shoulder Service, New York Orthopedic Hospital, Columbia-Presbyterian Medical Center, New York, New York

**T.A. Blackburn, M.Ed., P.T., A.T.C.**
Adjunct Assistant Professor, Sports Medicine, Columbus College; Director, Human Performance and Rehabilitation Center, Columbus, Georgia

**Joe P. Bramhall, M.D.**
Clinical Assistant Professor, Department of Surgery, Texas A&M University Health Science Center College of Medicine; Team Physician, Department of Athletics, Texas A&M University, College Station, Texas

**John W. Brautigam, P.T., A.T.C.**
Clinical Director, Morgantown Physical Therapy Associates, P.C., Morgantown, West Virginia

**Clive E. Brewster, M.S., P.T.**
Clinical Director, Department of Physical Therapy, Kerlan-Jobe Orthopaedic Clinic, Inglewood, California

**William G. Carson, Jr., M.D.**
Assistant Clinical Professor, Division of Orthopaedics, University of South Florida College of Medicine; Director, The Sports Medicine Clinic of Tampa, Tampa, Florida

**Richard B. Caspari, M.D.**
Clinical Professor, Division of Orthopedic Surgery, Virginia Commonwealth University Medical College of Virginia School of Medicine; Director, Orthopedic Research of Virginia, Richmond, Virginia

**Daniel Cipriani, M.Ed., P.T.**
Assistant Professor, Program in Physical Therapy, School of Allied Health, Medical College of Ohio; Physical Therapist, West Toledo Physical Therapy, Sylvania Therapy Services, Toledo, Ohio

**William G. Clancy, Jr., M.D.**
Clinical Professor, Division of Sports Medicine, Department of Orthopaedics and Rehabilitation, University of Virginia School of Medicine, Charlottesville, Virginia; Orthopaedic Surgeon, Alabama Sports Medicine and Orthopaedic Center, Birmingham, Alabama

**William M. Craven, M.D.**
Medical Director, Atlanta Orthopaedic Consultants, Atlanta, Georgia

**Elsie Culham, Ph.D., P.T.**
Assistant Professor, School of Rehabilitation Therapy, Queen's University Faculty of Medicine, Kingston, Ontario, Canada

**Steven A. Dickoff-Hoffman, P.T., M.S., A.T.C., S.C.S.**
Clinical Instructor, School of Physical Therapy, University of Pittsburgh, Pittsburgh, Pennsylvania; Clinical Instructor in Physical Therapy, State University of New York at Buffalo, Buffalo, New York; Clinical Instructor in Physical Therapy, West Virginia University, Morgantown, West Virginia; Rehabilitation Consultant to the Pittsburgh Pirates Baseball Club, Pittsburgh, Pennsylvania; Director of Sportsmedicine and Rehabilitation, HEALTH-SOUTH/North Hills Sportsmedicine Center, Pittsburgh, Pennsylvania

**Charles J. Dillman, Ph.D.**
Clinical Associate Professor, Department of Orthopaedics and Rehabilitation, University of Virginia School of Medicine, Charlottesville, Virginia; Executive Director, The Steadman Sports Medicine Foundation, Vail, Colorado; Consultant, American Sports Medicine Institute, Birmingham, Alabama

**Robert A. Donatelli, M.A., P.T., O.C.S.**
Instructor, Division of Physical Therapy, Department of Rehabilitation Medicine, Emory University School of Medicine; Assistant Regional Director, Physiotherapy Associates, Atlanta, Georgia

**Marsha Eifert-Mangine, M.Ed., P.T., A.T.C.**
Clinical Director, Kentucky Rehabilitation Services, Inc., Fort Mitchell, Kentucky

**Todd S. Ellenbecker, M.S., P.T., S.C.S.**
Clinical Director, Sports Medicine, HEALTHSOUTH Sports Medicine, Scottsdale, Arizona

**Robert P. Engle, P.T., A.T.C. (deceased)**
Formerly Adjunct Professor, Department of Physical Therapy, University of Delaware, Newark, Delaware; Clinical Professor, Department of Physical Therapy, Temple University School of Medicine, Philadelphia, Pennsylvania; Director, Knee Rehabilitation Institute, Berwyn, Pennsylvania; Director, Center for Sports Physical Therapy, Wyomissing and Berwyn, Pennsylvania

**Stephen Fealy, B.A.**
Medical Student, Columbia University College of Physicians and Surgeons, New York, New York

**Glenn S. Fleisig, M.S.**
Director of Research, American Sports Medicine Institute, Birmingham, Alabama

**Tandy R. Freeman, M.D.**
Staff, Texas Sports Medicine Group; Staff, Dallas Rehabilitation Institute; Provisional Staff, Medical Arts Hospital; Associate Staff, Presbyterian Hospital of Dallas, Dallas, Texas

**Vern Gambetta, M.A.**
Director of Conditioning, Chicago White Sox Baseball Club, Sarasota, Florida

**William B. Geissler, M.D.**
Assistant Professor, Division of Hand and Upper Extremity Surgery; Head, Section of Arthroscopic Surgery and Sports Medicine, Department of Orthopaedic Surgery, University of Mississippi School of Medicine and Medical Center, Jackson, Mississippi

**Bernard Ghelman, M.D.**
Professor, Department of Radiology, Hospital for Special Surgery, New York, New York

**Bruce Greenfield, M.M.Sc., P.T.**
Instructor, Division of Physical Therapy, Department of Rehabilitation Medicine, Emory University School of Medicine; Private Practice, Physiotherapy Associates, Atlanta, Georgia

**Eric J. Guidi, M.D.**
Attending Orthopedic Surgeon, Nirschl Orthopedic and Sports Medicine Clinic; Orthopedic Consultant, Virginia Sports Medicine Institute; Sports Medicine Fellow (1992–1993), Department of Orthopaedics, Arlington Hospital/Georgetown University School of Medicine, Arlington, Virginia

**Richard J. Hawkins, M.D. F.R.C.S.**
Clinical Professor, Department of Orthopaedics, University of Colorado School of Medicine, Denver, Colorado; Orthopaedic Consultant, Steadman Hawkins Clinic, Vail, Colorado

**Timothy Heckmann, P.T., A.T.C.**
Director of Rehabilitation, Cincinnati Sports Medicine and Orthopedic Center, Cincinnati, Ohio

**Kathryn P. Hemsley, M.Ed., A.T.C., L.P.T.**
Adjunct Faculty, Department of Physical Therapy, Beaver College, Glenside, Pennsylvania; Clinical Instructor, Temple University College of Allied Health Professions; Clinical Instructor, Department of Physical Therapy, Hahnemann University, Philadelphia, Pennsylvania; Senior Staff Therapist, Department of Orthopaedic Medicine, Temple University Hospital, Philadelphia, Pennsylvania; Staff Therapist, Bryn Mawr Rehabilitation Hospital, Malvern, Pennsylvania

**Frank W. Jobe, M.D.**
Associate Clinical Professor, Department of Orthopaedics, University of Southern California School of Medicine; Orthopaedic Consultant, Los Angeles Dodgers, Los Angeles, California; Associate, Kerlan-Jobe Orthopaedic Clinic, Inglewood, California

**Michael A. Keirns, Ph.D., P.T., A.T.C., C.S.C.S.**
Faculty, Department of Human Leisure and Sports, Metropolitan State College; Lecturer, Physical Therapy Curriculum, University of Colorado School of Medicine; Clinical Professor, Department of Biology, University of Denver; Director of Sports Medicine and Clinical Director, Therex Physical Therapy Sports Rehabilitation Center, Denver, Colorado

**Jeff G. Konin, M.Ed., A.T.C.**
Clinical Athletic Trainer, Pike Creek Sports Medicine Center; Coordinator, Clinical Research, All Sports Clinic of Delaware, Wilmington, Delaware

**Sanford S. Kunkel, M.D.**
Clinical Assistant Professor, Department of Orthopaedics, Indiana University School of Medicine; Director, Sports Medicine, Orthopaedics Indianapolis, Indianapolis, Indiana

**Seth P. Kupferman, M.D.**
Staff, South Carolina Sports Medicine and Orthopaedic Center, Charleston, South Carolina

**Lawrence J. Lemak, M.D.**
Clinical Assistant Professor, Division of Sports Medicine, Department of Orthopaedics and Rehabilitation, University of Virginia School of Medicine, Charlottesville, Virginia; Fellowship Director, American Sports Medicine Institute; Orthopaedic Surgeon, Alabama Sports Medicine and Orthopaedic Center, Birmingham, Alabama

**Stephen H. Liu, M.D.**
Assistant Professor, Sports Medicine Section, Department of Orthopaedic Surgery, University of California, Los Angeles, UCLA School of Medicine, Los Angeles, California

**Peter E. Loeb, M.D.**
Director, Sports Medicine, North Florida Sports Medicine and Orthopaedic Center, Tallahassee, Florida

**Terry R. Malone, Ed.D., P.T., A.T.C.**
Associate Professor and Director, Physical Therapy Division, University of Kentucky, Lexington, Kentucky

**Robert E. Mangine, M.Ed., P.T., A.T.C.**
Director, Kentucky Rehabilitation Services, Inc., Fort Mitchell, Kentucky

**Norman A. Marcus, M.D.**
Assistant Clinical Professor, Department of Orthopedics, Georgetown University School of Medicine; Assistant Clinical Professor, Department of Orthopaedic Surgery, George Washington University School of Medicine and Health Sciences, Washington, D.C.; Medical Staff, Department of Orthopaedic Surgery, Fairfax Hospital, Falls Church, Virginia; Private Practice, Associates in Orthopaedics, P.C., Springfield, Virginia

**Denise L. Massie, M.S., A.T.C.**
Instructor/Athletic Trainer, West Virginia University School of Physical Education; Coordinator, Education and Research, Morgantown Physical Therapy Associates, P.C., Morgantown, West Virginia

**T. Scott Maughon, M.D.**
Orthopaedic Teaching Staff, Department of Orthopaedics, Georgia Baptist Medical Center; Medical Director, The Sports Medicine and Orthopaedic Institute of Gwinnett, Lawrenceville, Georgia

**George M. McCluskey III, M.D.**
Clinical Assistant Professor, Department of Orthopaedic Surgery, Tulane University School of Medicine, New Orleans, Louisiana; Staff Orthopaedic Surgeon, Hughston Orthopaedic Clinic, P.C., Columbus, Georgia

**Frank C. McCue III, M.D.**
Alfred R. Shands Professor of Orthopaedic Surgery and Plastic Surgery of the Hand, Department of Orthopaedics and Rehabilitation, University of Virginia School of Medicine; Director, Division of Sports Medicine and Hand Surgery, Department of Orthopaedics and Rehabilitation, University of Virginia Health Sciences Center; Team Physician, Department of Athletics, University of Virginia, Charlottesville, Virginia

**Fred J. McGlynn, M.D.**
Associate Clinical Professor, Department of Orthopaedics, Virginia Commonwealth University Medical College of Virginia; Orthopaedic Surgeon, Tuckahoe Orthopaedic Associates, Richmond, Virginia

**Mark S. McMahon, M.D.**
Staff, Department of Orthopedic Surgery, Lenox Hill Hospital, New York, New York

**Diane R. Moynes, M.S., P.T.**
Director, Physical Therapy, Champion Rehabilitation, San Diego, California

**Timothy C. Murphy, M.A., P.T., A.T.C.**
President, Concorde Therapy Group, Canton, Ohio

**Stephen J. O'Brien, M.D.**
Associate Professor, Division of Orthopaedics, Department of Surgery, Cornell University Medical College; Associate Attending Orthopaedic Surgeon and Assistant Scientist, The Hospital for Special Surgery; Assistant Attending Orthopaedic Surgeon, New York Hospital; Chief Orthopaedic Consultant, St. John's University; Assistant Team Physician, The New York Football Giants; New York, New York

**Hugh M. O'Flynn, M.D.**
General Surgery Intern, The Cottage Hospital, Santa Barbara, California

**Judson W. Ott, M.D.**
Department of Orthopaedic Surgery and Sports Medicine, Medical Associates Clinic P.C., Dubuque, Iowa

**Michael J. Pagnani, M.D.**
Sports Medicine Fellow, The Hospital for Special Surgery, New York, New York

**Russell M. Paine, P.T.**
Director of Research and Education and Associate Clinical Director, Rehabilitation Services of Houston, Houston, Texas

**Robert A. Panariello, M.D., R.P.T., A.T.C.**
Physical Therapist, Professional Sports Care, Uniondale, New York; Physical Therapist, The Hospital for Special Surgery, New York, New York

**Christ J. Pavlatos, M.D.**
Orthopaedic Surgeon, Lake Forest Orthopaedics, Lake Forest, Illinois

**Malcolm Peat, Ph.D., P.T.**
Professor and Director, School of Rehabilitation Therapy, Queen's University Faculty of Medicine, Kingston, Ontario, Canada

**Victoria Rugo de Cartaya, P.T.**
Staff Physical Therapist, Physical Therapy Outpatient Department, Spaulding and Newton Wellesley Hospital Rehabilitation Center, Wellesley, Massachusetts

**Dorothy F. Scarpinato, M.D.**
Orthopaedic Surgeon, Department of Orthopaedic Surgery, Community Health Plan and Long Island Jewish Medical Center, New Hyde Park, New York

**Margaret Schenkman, Ph.D., P.T.**
Associate Professor, Graduate Program in Physical Therapy, and Senior Fellow, Center for the Study of Aging and Human Development, Duke University School of Medicine, Durham, North Carolina

**Clifford J. Schob, M.D.**
Teaching Staff, St. Joseph's Hospital, Patterson, New Jersey; Attending Staff, Overlook Hospital, Summit, New Jersey, and Union Hospital, Union, New Jersey

**Martin L. Schwartz, M.D.**
Clinical Instructor, Department of Radiology, University of Alabama School of Medicine, University of Alabama at Birmingham; Chairman, Department of Radiology, HEALTHSOUTH Sports Medicine and Rehabilitation Center, Birmingham, Alabama

**Judy L. Seto, M.A., P.T.**
Research Coordinator, Senior Physical Therapist, Department of Physical Therapy, Kerlan-Jobe Orthopaedic Clinic, Inglewood, California

**Clarence L. Shields, Jr., M.D.**
Associate Clinical Professor, Department of Orthopaedics, University of Southern California School of Medicine; Orthopaedic Consultant, Los Angeles Rams, Los Angeles, California; Associate, Kerlan-Jobe Orthopaedic Clinic, Inglewood, California

**James F. Silliman, M.D.**
Assistant Professor, Department of Orthopaedics, University of Texas Southwestern Medical School, Dallas, Texas

**Kevin P. Speer, M.D.**
Assistant Professor of Orthopaedic Surgery, Department of Surgery, Duke University School of Medicine/Duke University Medical Center, Durham, North Carolina

**Joseph S. Sutter, M.S., P.T.**
Private Practice, Tuckahoe Physical Therapy, Richmond, Virginia

**Jonathan B. Ticker, M.D.**
Senior Resident and Junior Annie C. Kane Fellow, Department of Orthopedic Surgery, New York Orthopedic Hospital, Columbia-Presbyterian Medical Center, New York, New York

**Laura A. Timmerman, M.D.**
Assistant Professor, Department of Orthopedic Surgery-Sports Medicine, University of California, Davis, School of Medicine, Sacramento, California

**Michael L. Voight, M.Ed., P.T., A.T.C., S.C.S.**
Instructor, Division of Physical Therapy, University of Miami School of Medicine; National Director, Sports Medicine, Sports Physical Therapy Inc., Miami, Florida

**Russell F. Warren, M.D.**
Professor of Orthopaedic Surgery, Department of Surgery, Cornell University Medical College; Director, Department of Sports Medicine, Hospital for Special Surgery, New York, New York

**Kevin E. Wilk, P.T.**
National Director, Research and Clinical Education, and Associate Clinical Director, HEALTHSOUTH Sports Medicine and Rehabilitation Center; Director, Rehabilitative Research, American Sports Medicine Institute, Birmingham, Alabama

**Bertram Zarins, M.D.**
Assistant Clinical Professor, Department of Orthopaedic Surgery, Harvard Medical School; Chief, Sports Medicine Unit, Massachusetts General Hospital, Boston, Massachusetts

**Joseph D. Zuckerman, M.D.**
Associate Professor, Department of Orthopaedic Surgery, New York University School of Medicine, New York, New York

# Preface

Over the past ten years an increased interest in the shoulder has led to a proliferation of knowledge, enlightening research, improved awareness, and enhanced critical thinking regarding our recognition and treatment of shoulder joint disorders.

The shoulder complex is a commonly injured region of the body, not only during sports but also as a result of work-related activities, overuse or disuse, and age-related degeneration. Therefore our goal was to make *The Athlete's Shoulder* a comprehensive textbook addressing not only sports-related shoulder disorders but also those occurring in the active orthopaedic patient. The text discusses many diverse topics such as instabilities, rotator cuff lesions, neurovascular syndromes, total joint replacement, biomechanics of sports, injuries in baseball, and so on. There are also several somewhat controversial topics including tensile rotator cuff failure, calcifying tendonitis, posterior instability, and traumatic rotator cuff tears in younger patients.

*The Athlete's Shoulder* is organized into four basic sections. The first, on the basic science of the shoulder complex, thoroughly discusses anatomy and biomechanics. This is followed by the examination section, which includes physical examination, imaging, and arthrography of the shoulder. The third section discusses the recognition and treatment of various pathologies. The last section discusses specific topics in rehabilitation. The concise chapters are intended to provide the reader with a reference that includes historical perspective, functional anatomy, evaluation, and treatment options. This text is not intended to be a cookbook, but rather a text that enhances the practitioner's expertise in the examination and treatment of shoulder injuries.

The way we think and look at the shoulder has changed throughout the years, and we hope this trend continues. The challenge has been to prepare a text that discusses current and advanced concepts in an area in which our knowledge is expanding daily. We hope that *The Athlete's Shoulder* stimulates interest, provokes thought, inspires additional research, and enhances our care of shoulder patients in the future.

We have learned a great deal from our earlier teachers—E.A. Codman, Charles Neer III—and from the current tutelage of Charles Rockwood, Frederick Matsen III, Richard Hawkins, Frank Jobe, Russell Warren, Louis Bigliani, and others.

We offer this textbook to clinicians, physicians, therapists, athletic trainers, and others involved in caring for shoulder patients. May it help you to discover more about the enormously fascinating shoulder joint, a truly complex functional structure that once you begin exploring becomes even more intriguing and complex in its interrelationships.

The contributors to this book represent the leaders in shoulder care, and we greatly appreciate their contributions. We would also like to thank Dale Baker and the staff of the American Sports Medicine Institute for their energy, assistance, and contributions to this book.

*The value of experience is not in seeing much, but rather in seeing wisely.*
*Sir William Osler*

*James R. Andrews, M.D.*
*Kevin E. Wilk, P.T.*

# Acknowledgments

**For their special help in preparing this text:**

Our office staff: Donna Metz, Jerry Conner, Regina Biddings, Glenn Dortch, Dennis Dismukes, and the entire staff at the American Sports Medicine Institute for their assistance in the manuscript preparation, and HEALTHSOUTH Rehabilitation Corporation for your support.

Churchill Livingstone staff, especially Robert A. Hurley for patience and assistance, Leslie Burgess for her belief in me many years ago, and Elizabeth Bowman for her assistance and devotion in this project.

The clinical staff: William Clancy and Lawrence Lemak, for allowing me the opportunity to be inquisitive and for providing me with guidance and direction.

My clinical staff at HEALTHSOUTH for allowing me to be a part of their lives and for asking me the questions from which I've learned so much. Also, for their assistance in text preparation and for their motivation.

**Special Shoulder Mentors:**

Thank you for your efforts in advancing shoulder care; you have taught us so much: Charles Neer III, Charles Rockwood, Frederick Matsen III, Richard Hawkins, Louis Bigliani, Russell Warren, David Altchek, Frank Jobe, Stephen O'Brien, the Sports Physical Therapy section, and my colleagues in The American Physical Therapy Association.

**Special Friends:**

American Sports Medicine fellows—being a part of your education has been a tremendous experience to me.

Alabama Orthopaedic & Sports Medicine Group—thanks for the accessibility of each of you and to your patients for their cooperation.

HEALTHSOUTH Rehabilitation Corporation—for encouragement, support, and the opportunity to accomplish a goal.

Northwestern University Physical Therapy Program, especially Sally Edelsberg, for providing me with an excellent foundation to build from, thanks for the opportunity.

William Clancy—thanks for challenging me to be better.

M.D.—thanks so much for your guidance, inspiration, and encouragement through the years.

Robert Mangine, Russell Paine, Steve Dickoff, Mike Voight, and George Davies for your friendship and encouragement.

Christopher Arrigo for your editorial comments, spiritual and emotional encouragement—thank you.

Donna Metz and Jerry Conner for typing the manuscripts from "those yellow sheets of paper,...again."

To my colleagues for asking the questions, providing information and ideas, and learning with me.

To my patients—thank you for the opportunity.

To my father, your illness introduced me to physical therapy. Your memory provides inspiration, compassion, and courage.

James R. Andrews—Thank you for your guidance, tutelage, and encouragement through the years.

Thank you to each of you for your inspiration, love, and support.

> *I expect to pass through this world but once. Any good therefore that I can do or any kindness that I can show for any fellow creature, let me do it now. Let me not defer or neglect it, for I shall not pass this way again.*
>
> *Ralph Waldo Emerson*

K.E.W.

# Contents

## IV. PATHOLOGY AND SURGERY

# 1

# Functional Anatomy of the Shoulder Complex

*MALCOLM PEAT*
*ELSIE CULHAM*

The overall function of the upper extremity is related to the shoulder complex, with the ultimate purpose of this mechanism being the placement and full use of the hand. The joint mechanisms of the limb permit the placement, functioning, and control of the hand directly in front of the body, where the functions can be observed.[1] Manipulation of the hand is controlled by the shoulder complex, which positions and directs the humerus; the elbow, which positions the hand in relation to the trunk; and the radioulnar joints, which determine the position of the palm.[2,3] Sports that involve throwing, using a racquet, swimming, etc., require excessive glenohumeral joint motion. For example, the excessive motion required to throw a baseball is accomplished through the integrated and synchronized motion of the various joints in the upper quadrant, most significantly the glenohumeral and scapulothoracic joints.

The shoulder complex provides the upper limb with a range of motion exceeding that of any other joint mechanism.[4] This range of motion is greater than that required for most daily functional activities. For example, use of the hand in limited activities of daily living is possible when the shoulder complex is immobilized with the humerus held by the side. Compensation for absent shoulder motion is provided by the cervical spine, elbow, wrist, and finger joint mechanisms.[5,6]

The shoulder complex consists of four joints that function in a precise, coordinated, synchronous manner. Position changes of the arm involve movements of the clavicle, scapula, and humerus. These movements are the direct result of the complex mechanism comprising the sternoclavicular, acromioclavicular, and glenohumeral joints and the scapulothoracic gliding mechanism.[4,7,8]

## STERNOCLAVICULAR JOINT

The sternoclavicular joint is the only joint connecting the shoulder complex to the axial skeleton.[9,10] Although the structure of this synovial joint is classified as plain, its function most closely resembles a ball-and-socket articulation.[4,11,12] The articular surfaces lack congruity. Approximately half of the large, rounded medial end of the clavicle protrudes above the shallow sternal socket. An intra-articular disc is attached to the upper portion of this nonarticular part of the clavicle. The articular surface is saddle-shaped, anteroposteriorly concave, and downwardly convex.[2,4]

The medial end of the clavicle is bound to the sternum and to the first rib and its costal cartilage. Ligaments strengthen the capsule anteriorly, posteriorly, superiorly, and inferiorly. The main structures stabilizing the joint, resisting the tendency for medial displacement of the clavicle, and limiting clavicular movement are the articular disc and the costoclavicular ligament[4,13] (Fig. 1-1).

The articular disc is fibrocartilaginous, strong, and almost circular and completely divides the joint cavity.[14] The disc is attached superiorly to the upper medial end of the clavicle and passes downward between the articular surfaces to the sternum and first costal cartilage.[4] This arrangement permits the disc to function as

1

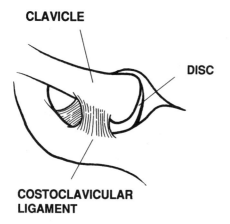

**CLAVICLE**

**DISC**

**COSTOCLAVICULAR LIGAMENT**

**Fig. 1-1.** Sternoclavicular joint showing major ligamentous structures influencing stability.

a hinge, a mechanism that contributes to the total range of joint movement. The areas of compression between the articular surfaces and intra-articular disc vary with movements of the clavicle. During elevation and depression, most motion occurs between the clavicle and the disc (Fig. 1-2). During protraction and retraction, the greatest movement occurs between the disc and the sternal articular surface.[2] The combination of taut ligaments and pressure on the disc and articular surfaces is important in maintaining stability in the plane of motion.

The disc also stabilizes the joint against forces applied to the shoulder that are transmitted medially through the clavicle to the sternum. Without this attachment, the clavicle would tend to override the sternum, resulting in medial dislocation. Forces acting on the clavicle are most likely to cause fracture of the bone medial to the attachment of the coracoclavicular ligament and rarely cause dislocation of the sternoclavicular joint.[5]

The costoclavicular ligament is a strong, bilaminar structure attached to the inferior surface of the medial end of the clavicle and the first rib. The anterior compo-

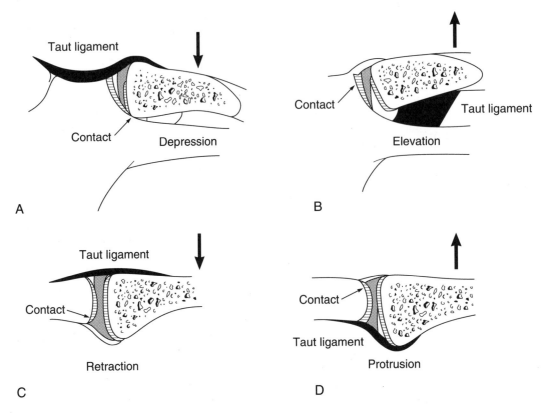

A    Taut ligament    Contact    Depression

B    Contact    Taut ligament    Elevation

C    Taut ligament    Contact    Retraction

D    Contact    Taut ligament    Protrusion

**Fig. 1-2.** Sternoclavicular joint illustrating compression of articular disc. (From Dempster,[2] with permission.)

nent of the ligament passes upward and laterally; the posterior part, upward and medially. The ligament is a major stabilizing structure and strongly binds the medial end of the clavicle to the first rib. The ligament becomes taut when the arm is elevated or the shoulder protracted.[4]

The joint capsule is supported by oblique anterior and posterior sternoclavicular ligaments. Both ligaments pass downward and medially from the sternal end of the clavicle to the anterior and posterior surfaces of the manubrium and limit anteroposterior movement of the clavicle. An interclavicular ligament runs across the superior aspect of the sternoclavicular joint, joining the medial ends of the clavicles. This ligament, having deep fibers attached to the upper margin of the manubrium, provides stability to the superior aspect of the joint.[4,9]

The sternoclavicular joint allows elevation and depression, protraction and retraction, and long-axis rotation of the clavicle. The axis for both angular movements lies close to the clavicular attachment of the costoclavicular ligament.[9]

## ACROMIOCLAVICULAR JOINT

The acromioclavicular joint is a synovial plane joint between the small, convex oval facet on the lateral end of the clavicle and a concave area on the anterior part of the medial border of the acromion process of the scapula.[4,9]

The joint line is oblique and slightly curved. The curvature of the joint permits the acromion, and thus the scapula, to glide forward or backward over the lateral end of the clavicle. This movement keeps the glenoid fossa continually facing the humeral head. The oblique nature of the joint is such that forces transmitted through the arm will tend to drive the acromion process under the lateral end of the clavicle with the clavicle overriding the acromion (Fig. 1-3). The joint also contains a fibrocartilaginous disc that is variable in size and does not completely separate the joint into two compartments.[9,14] The acromioclavicular joint is important because it contributes to total arm movement besides transmitting forces between the clavicle and the acromion.[4,15]

The acromioclavicular joint has a capsule and a superior acromioclavicular ligament that strengthen the up-

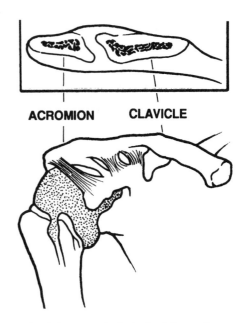

**Fig. 1-3.** Acromioclavicular joint surfaces.

per aspect of the joint.[4,11] The main ligamentous structure stabilizing the joint and binding the clavicle to the scapula is the coracoclavicular ligament. Although this ligament is placed medially and separate from the joint, it forms the most efficient means of preventing the clavicle from losing contact with the acromion.[4,5,8,9,15,16]

The coracoclavicular ligament consists of two parts: the trapezoid and the conoid. These two components, functionally and anatomically distinct, are united at their corresponding borders. Anteriorly, the space between the ligaments is filled with fat and, frequently, a bursa. A bursa also lies between the medial end of the coracoid process and the inferior surface of the clavicle. In up to 30 percent of subjects, these bony components may be opposed closely and may form a coracoclavicular joint.[2,16] The coracoclavicular ligament suspends the scapula from the clavicle and transmits the force of the upper fibers of the trapezius to the scapula.[2]

The trapezoid ligament, the anterolateral component of the coracoclavicular ligament, is broad, thin, and quadrilateral. It is attached from below to the superior surface of the coracoid process. The ligament passes laterally almost horizontally in the frontal plane to be attached to the trapezoid line on the inferior surface of the clavicle.[4,9] The primary function of this ligament is to prevent overriding of the clavicle on the acromion.[5,17]

The conoid ligament is located partly posterior and medial to the trapezoid ligament. It is thick and triangular, with its base attached from above to the conoid tubercle on the inferior surface of the clavicle. The apex, which is directed downward, is attached to the "knuckle" of the coracoid process (i.e., medial and posterior edge of the root of the process). The conoid ligament is oriented vertically and twisted on itself.[4,17] The ligament limits upward movement of the clavicle on the acromion. When the arm is elevated, the rotation of the scapula causes the coracoid process to move and increases the distance between the clavicle and the coracoid process. This movement increases the tension on the conoid ligament, resulting in dorsal (posterior) axial rotation of the clavicle. Viewed from above, the clavicle has a shape resembling a crank. The taut coracoclavicular ligament acts on the outer curvature of the crank-like clavicle and effects a rotation of the clavicle on its long axis.[11,18] This clavicular rotation allows the scapula to continue to rotate and increase the degree of arm elevation. During full elevation of the arm, the clavicle rotates 50 degrees axially.[11] When the clavicle is prevented from rotating, the arm can be abducted actively to only 120 degrees.[4,8]

Movement of the acromioclavicular joint is an important component of total arm movement. A principal role of the joint in the elevation of the arm is to permit continued lateral rotation of the scapula after about 100 degrees of abduction when sternoclavicular movement is restrained by the sternoclavicular joint ligaments. The acromioclavicular joint has three degrees of freedom. Movement can occur between the acromion and lateral end of the clavicle, about a vertical axis, around a frontal axis, and about a sagittal axis. Functionally, the two main movements at the acromioclavicular joint, however, are a gliding movement as the shoulder joint flexes and extends and an elevation and depression movement to conform with changes in the relationship between the scapula and the humerus during abduction.[5,9,16]

## GLENOHUMERAL JOINT

The glenohumeral joint is a multiaxial ball-and-socket synovial joint. This type of joint geometry permits a tremendous amount of motion; however, the inherent

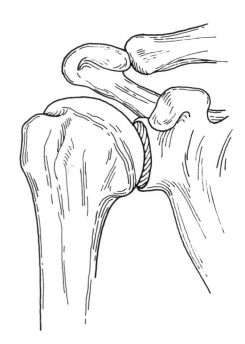

**Fig. 1-4.** Osseous structure of glenohumeral joint; large convex humeral head in relatively small glenoid fossa.

stability is minimal (Fig. 1-4). The articular surfaces, the head of the humerus, and the glenoid fossa of the scapula, although reciprocally curved, are oval and are not sections of true spheres.[4] As the head of the humerus is larger than the glenoid fossa, only part of the humeral head can be in articulation with glenoid fossa in any position of the joint. At any given time, only 25 to 30 percent of the humeral head is in contact with the glenoid fossa.[19–21] The surfaces are not congruent, and the joint is loose-packed. Full congruence and the close-packed position are obtained when the humerus is in full elevation.[22,23] The design characteristics of the joint are typical of an "incongruous" joint. The surfaces are asymmetric; the joint has a moveable axis of rotation; and muscles related to the joint are essential in maintaining stability of the articulation[9] (Table 1-1).

| Table 1-1. Factors Contributing to Glenohumeral Instability |
| --- |
| Shallow glenoid |
| Disproportionate size of the articular surfaces |
| Lack of congruency |
| Inadequate anterior soft tissue support |
| Repeated trauma/repetitive strain |
| Muscular weakness |
| Rotator cuff deficiency |

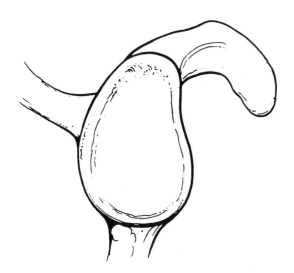

**Fig. 1-5.** Lateral view of glenoid fossa illustrating the pear-shaped appearance and inverted comma.

The humeral articular surface has a radius of curvature of 35 to 55 mm. The humeral head and neck make an angle of 130 to 150 degrees with the shaft and are retroverted about 20 to 30 degrees with respect to the transverse axis of the elbow.[24,25]

The glenoid fossa is somewhat pear-shaped and resembles an inverted comma (Fig. 1-5). The surface area is one-third to one-fourth, the vertical diameter 75 percent, and the transverse diameter 55 percent of that of the humeral head.[25] In 75 percent of subjects, the glenoid fossa is retrotilted an average of 7.4 degrees in relationship to the plane of the scapula.[26,27] It has been suggested that this relationship is important in maintaining horizontal stability of the joint and counteracting any tendency toward anterior displacement of the humeral head.[25–27] However, this concept has not been supported by subsequent studies.[27a,27b] The articular cartilage lining the glenoid fossa is thickest in the periphery and thinnest in the central region.

## GLENOID LABRUM

The glenoid labrum consists of fibrocartilage and fibrous tissue.[4,28] This rim of fibrocartilaginous tissue attaches around the margin of the glenoid fossa.[28] The inner surface of the labrum is covered with synovium; the outer surface attaches to the capsule and is continuous with the periosteum of the scapular neck. The shape of the labrum adapts to accommodate rotation of the humeral head, adding flexibility to the edges of the glenoid fossa. The tendons of the long head of the biceps brachii and triceps brachii muscles contribute to the structure and reinforcement of the labrum. The long head of the biceps brachii attaches to the superior region of the labrum. The width and thickness of the glenoid labrum varies. The anterior labrum appears thicker and at times larger than the posterior labrum.

The function of the labrum is controversial.[28] It is suggested that it protects the edges of the glenoid, assists in lubrication of the joint, and deepens the glenoid cavity, thus contributing to the stability of the joint.[4,5,9,29] Others state that the labrum does not increase the depth of the concave surface substantially and that the glenoid labrum is no more than a fold of capsule composed of dense fibrous connective tissue that stretches out anteriorly with external rotation and posteriorly with internal rotation of the humerus.[28] The main function of the labrum may be to serve as an attachment for the glenohumeral ligaments.[4,28] When that attachment is compromised, it represents a Bankart lesion in which the capsular-labral complex is torn from the glenoid rim (Fig. 1-6).

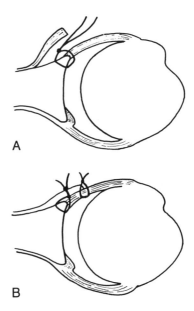

A

B

**Fig. 1-6.** Capsular-labral complex defect often described as a Bankart lesion. **(A)** Lateral capsular flap reattached to glenoid rim; **(B)** added strength from double-breasting the medial capsule, reinforcing the entire glenoid rim from 2:00 to 6:00.

# CAPSULE

The capsule surrounds the joint and is attached medially to the margin of the glenoid fossa beyond the labrum. Laterally, it is attached to the circumference of the anatomic neck, and the attachment descends about $1/2$ in. onto the shaft of the humerus. The capsule is loose-fitting, allowing the joint surfaces to be separated 2 to 3 mm by a distractive force.[4] Matsen[30] has shown 22 mm of inferior translation, 6-mm anterior and 7-mm posterior translation in normal subjects.

The capsule is relatively thin and, by itself, would contribute little to the stability of the joint. The integrity of the capsule and the maintenance of the normal glenohumeral relationship depend on the reinforcement of the capsule by ligaments and the attachment of the muscle tendons of the rotator cuff mechanism.[4,9,16]

The superior part of the capsule, together with the superior glenohumeral ligament, is important in strengthening the superior aspect of the joint and resisting the effect of gravity on the dependent limb.[4,31] Anteriorly, the capsule is strengthened by the anterior glenohumeral ligaments and the attachment of the subscapularis tendon.[32] Posteriorly, the capsule is strengthened by the attachment of the teres minor and infraspinatus tendons.[33] Inferiorly, the capsule is relatively thin and weak and contributes little to the stability of the joint. The inferior part of the capsule is subjected to considerable strain because it is stretched tightly across the head of the humerus when the arm is elevated.

The inferior part of the capsule, the weakest area, is lax and lies in folds when the arm is adducted. Kaltsas[34] compared the collagen structure of the shoulder joint capsule with that of the elbow and hip. When the joint capsules were subjected to a mechanical force, the shoulder joint capsule showed a greater capacity to stretch than to rupture. When the capsule was tested to failure, the structure ruptured anteroinferiorly.[34,35] Also, Reeves[35] demonstrated that the force required to cause glenohumeral joint dislocation is less below the age of 20 years and greater above 50 years of age.

Johnston[23] stated that, with the arm by the side, the capsular fibers are oriented with a forward and medial twist. This twist increases in abduction and decreases in flexion. The capsular tension in abduction compresses the humeral head into the glenoid fossa. As abduction progresses, the capsular tension exerts an external rotation moment. This external rotation "untwists" the capsule and allows further abduction. The external rotation of the humerus that occurs during coronal plane abduction thus may be assisted by the configuration of the joint capsule.[23]

The capsule is lined by a synovial membrane attached to the glenoid rim and anatomic neck inside the capsular attachments.[4] The tendon of the long head of the biceps brachii muscle passes from the supraglenoid tubercle over the superior aspect of the head of the humerus and lies within the capsule, emerging from the joint at the intertubercular groove. The tendon is covered by a synovial sheath to facilitate movement of the tendon within the joint. The structure is susceptible to injury at the point at which the tendon arches over the humeral head and the surface on which it glides changes from bony cortex to articular cartilage.[5]

# CORACOHUMERAL LIGAMENT

The coracohumeral ligament is an important ligamentous structure in the shoulder complex.[31] The ligament is attached to the base and lateral border of the coracoid process and passes obliquely downward and laterally to the humerus, blending with the supraspinatus muscle and the capsule (Fig. 1-7). Laterally, the ligament separates into two components that insert into the greater and lesser tuberosities, creating a tunnel through which the biceps tendon passes.[36] Inferiorly, the coracohumeral ligament blends with the superior glenohumeral ligament. The anterior border of the ligament is distinct medially and merges with the capsule laterally. The posterior border is indistinct and blends with the capsule.[4,9]

It has been suggested that the downward pull of gravity on an adducted arm is counteracted largely by the superior capsule, the coracohumeral ligament, and the inferior glenohumeral ligament (Table 1-2)[36,37]. As the arm is abducted the restraining force is shifted to the inferior structures and the primary restraining force is the inferior glenohumeral ligament.[37a] As the coracohumeral ligament is located anterior to the vertical axis about which the humerus rotates axially, the ligament checks lateral rotation during arm elevation between 0 and 60 degrees. When the humerus, in a position of neutral rotation, is elevated in the sagittal

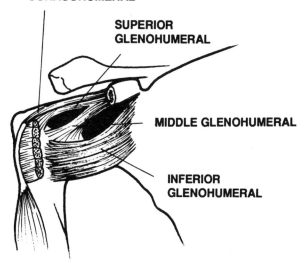

**CORACOHUMERAL**

**SUPERIOR GLENOHUMERAL**

**MIDDLE GLENOHUMERAL**

**INFERIOR GLENOHUMERAL**

**Fig. 1-7.** Coracohumeral and glenohumeral ligaments. Note the deficiencies between the glenohumeral ligaments and the Z arrangement of the three components of the ligament.

plane, the movement is limited to approximately 75 degrees by the coracohumeral ligament. For elevation to continue, the humerus is medially rotated and moved toward the scapular plane by the dynamic tension in this ligament.[22]

# GLENOHUMERAL LIGAMENTS

The three glenohumeral ligaments lie on the anterior and inferior aspect of the joint (Fig. 1-7 and 1-8). They are described as being thickened parts of the capsule.[4] The superior glenohumeral ligament passes laterally from the superior glenoid tubercle, the upper part of the glenoid labrum, and the base of the coracoid process to the humerus between the upper part of the lesser tuberosity and the anatomic neck.[36,37] The ligament lies anterior to and partly under the coracohumeral ligament. The superior glenohumeral ligament, together with the superior joint capsule and the rotator cuff muscles, assists in preventing downward displacement of the humeral head.[37,38]

The middle glenohumeral ligament has a wide attachment extending from the superior glenohumeral ligament along the anterior margin of the glenoid fossa down as far as the junction of the middle and inferior thirds of the glenoid rim.[37] From this attachment, the ligament passes laterally, gradually enlarges, and attaches to the anterior aspect of the anatomic neck and lesser tuberosity of the humerus. The ligament lies under the tendon of the subscapularis muscle and is intimately attached to it.[25,36] Note that the large variation in size of the middle glenohumeral ligament measures from 2 cm wide to being absent in some subjects. This structure exhibits the greatest amount of structural variation. The middle glenohumeral ligament and subscapularis tendon limit lateral rotation from 45 to 75 degrees of abduction and are important anterior stabilizers of the glenohumeral joint, particularly effective in the lower to middle ranges of abduction (Table 1-2).

### Table 1-2. Stability of the Glenohumeral Joint

| | |
|---|---|
| Dependent Position | Coracohumeral ligament |
| | Superior glenohumeral ligament |
| | Supraspinatus muscle |
| Elevation | |
| Lower range (0°–45°) | Anterior capsule |
| | Superior glenohumeral ligament |
| | Coracohumeral ligament |
| | Middle glenohumeral ligament |
| | Subscapularis, infraspinatus, and teres minor muscles |
| Middle range (45°–75°) | Middle glenohumeral ligament |
| | Supscapularis muscle (decreasing importance) |
| | Infraspinatus and teres minor muscles |
| | Inferior glenohumeral ligament (superior band) |
| Upper range (>75°) | Inferior glenohumeral ligament (axillary pouch) |
| Throughout elevation | Dynamic activity of rotator cuff |

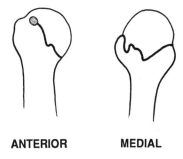

**ANTERIOR**     **MEDIAL**

**Fig. 1-8.** Attachments of the glenohumeral ligaments to the humerus.

The inferior glenohumeral ligament is the thickest of the glenohumeral structures and is the most important stabilizing structure of the shoulder in the overhead athlete. The ligament attaches to the anterior, inferior, and posterior margins of the glenoid labrum and passes laterally to the inferior aspects of the anatomic and surgical necks of the humerus.[4,25] The ligament can be divided into three distinct portions—the anterior band, the axillary pouch, and the posterior band[41] (Fig. 1-9). The inferior part is thinner and broader and is termed the axillary pouch. The anterior band strengthens the capsule anteriorly and supports the joint most

effectively in the upper ranges (>75 degrees) of abduction.[41] The anterior band of the inferior glenohumeral ligament provides a broad buttress-like support for the anterior and inferior aspects of the joint preventing subluxation in the upper part of the range[37] (Table 1-2).

O'Brien et al[41] demonstrated that with the arm abducted to 90 degrees and externally rotated, the anterior band of the inferior glenohumeral ligament complex wraps around the humeral head like a hammock to prevent anterior humeral head migration. This structure provides stability during the throwing motion, tennis serve motion, free-style stroke, or any arm position overhead.

Tightening of the inferior glenohumeral ligament during coronal plane abduction limits elevation to an average of 90 degrees. To continue to elevate, the humerus must move toward the scapular plane and laterally rotate. Gagey et al[22] stated that both movements occur because of dynamic tension in the inferior glenohumeral ligament.

The coracohumeral and glenohumeral ligaments viewed from the front form a **Z** pattern (Fig. 1-7). This arrangement creates potential areas of capsular weakness both above and below the middle glenohumeral ligament. The subscapularis bursa communicates with the joint cavity through the superior opening, or foramen of Weitbrecht, between the superior and middle glenohumeral ligaments. Ferrari[36] also reported the presence of an inferior subscapular bursa, between the middle and inferior glenohumeral ligaments. This bursa was present in all 14 specimens younger than 55 years of age and could be seen up to the age of 75 years. When the middle glenohumeral ligament is attenuated or absent, this anterior defect is enhanced and may contribute to anterior instability of the joint.[36]

## DYNAMIC STABILITY

The rotator cuff is the musculotendinous complex formed by the attachment to the capsule of the supraspinatus muscle superiorly, the subscapularis muscle anteriorly, and the teres minor and infraspinatus muscles posteriorly. These tendons blend intricately with the fibrous capsule. They provide active support for the joint and can be considered true dynamic ligaments and provide dynamic stability.[8] The capsule is less well-

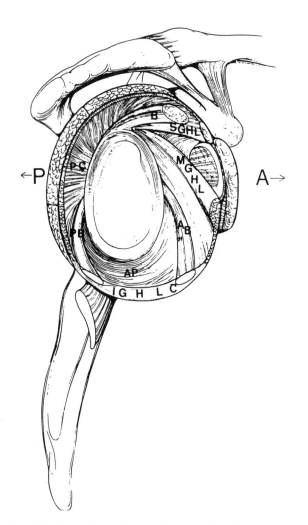

**Fig. 1-9.** Three distinct bands of anterior glenohumeral ligament; anterior band (*AB*), posterior band (*PB*), and axillary pouch (*AP*).

protected inferiorly because the tendon of the long head of the triceps brachii muscle is separated from the capsule by the axillary nerve and the posterior circumflex humeral artery.[4]

It is generally accepted that the deltoid and supraspinatus are the prime movers of glenohumeral abduction.[39,42,43] These muscles have been found to contribute equally to torque production in functional planes of motion.[43] With the arm at the side, the directional force of the deltoid muscle is almost vertical.[25,44] Thus, most of the deltoid force will cause upward translatory motion of the humeral head, which if unopposed would cause the humeral head to contact the coracoacromial arch, resulting in impingement of soft tissues.[45] The action lines of the infraspinatus, subscapularis, and teres minor muscles are such that each tends to have a rotatory component as well as a compressive force.[25,45] Each also has a downward translatory component that offsets the upward translation force of the deltoid.[10,44] Infraspinatus, teres minor, and subscapularis thus form a force couple with the deltoid and act to stabilize the humeral head on the glenoid fossa, allowing deltoid and supraspinatus to act as abductors of the humerus.[46] In studies on a mechanical model, Comtet et al[39] determined that the depressor forces are at their maximum between 60 and 80 degrees of elevation and disappear beyond 120 degrees. The supraspinatus has a small upward translatory component and thus does not help to offset the upward subluxation action of the deltoid.[24]

Lesions of the rotator cuff mechanism can occur as a response to repetitive activity over time or to overload activity that causes a spontaneous lesion.[47] Stress applied to a previously degenerated rotator cuff may cause the cuff to rupture. Often, this stress also tears the articular capsule, resulting in a communication between the joint cavity and the subacromial bursa. Rotator cuff tears result in considerably reduced force of elevation of the glenohumeral joint. In attempting to elevate the arm, the patient shrugs the shoulder. If the arm abducted passively to 90 degrees, the patient should be able to maintain the arm in the abducted position.[9]

The space between the supraspinatus and the superior border of subscapularis has been termed the rotator interval.[48] The floor of the interval is formed by the coracohumeral and superior glenohumeral ligaments and the capsule. The roof is covered by a thin elastic membrane. Lesions of the rotator interval may result

in increased anteroposterior instability with pain and inflammatory changes in the rotator cuff.[48] This lesion may resemble a rotator cuff tear or traumatic recurring subluxation.

The long head of biceps also contributes to the stability of the glenohumeral joint by preventing upward migration of the head of the humerus during powerful elbow flexion and forearm supination. Lesions of the long head of biceps therefore may produce instability and shoulder dysfunction.[49]

## CORACOACROMIAL ARCH

The coracoacromial ligament is triangular with the base attached to the lateral border of the coracoid process (Fig. 1-10). The ligament passes upward, laterally and slightly posteriorly, to the superior aspect of the acromion process.[4,50] Superiorly, the ligament is covered by the deltoid muscle. Posteriorly, the ligament is continuous with the fascia that covers the supraspinatus muscle. Anteriorly, the coracoacromial ligament has a sharp, well-defined, free border. Together with the acromion and the coracoid processes, the ligament forms an important protective arch over the glenohumeral joint.[9] The arch forms a secondary restraining socket for the humeral head, protecting the joint from

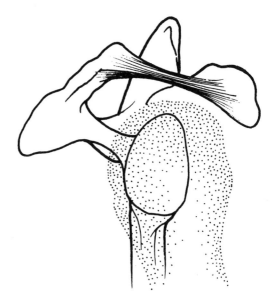

**Fig. 1-10.** Coracoacromial ligament and its relationship to the humeral head.

trauma from above and preventing upward dislocation of the humeral head. The supraspinatus muscle passes under the coracoacromial arch, lies between the deltoid muscle and the capsule of the glenohumeral joint, and blends with the capsule. The supraspinatus tendon is separated from the arch by the subacromial bursa[9] (Fig. 1-11). The space between the inferior acromion and the head of the humerus (subacromial distance) has been measured on radiographs and used as an indicator of proximal humeral subluxation.[51,52] The distance was found to be between 9 and 10 mm in 175 asymptomatic shoulders and was greater in men than in women.[51] A distance of less than 6 mm was considered pathologic and was thought to be indicative of supraspinatus tendon attenuation or rupture.[51]

During elevation with internal rotation of the arm in both abduction and flexion, the greater tuberosity (the supraspinatus tendon) of the humerus may apply pressure against the anterior edge and the inferior surface of the anterior third of the acromion and the coracoacromial ligament. This is, in part, because of the anterior orientation of the supraspinatus tendon. In some instances, the impingement also may occur against the acromioclavicular joint. This often occurs when the AC joint exhibits degenerative joint disease and/or spurring. Most upper-extremity functions are performed with the hand placed in front of the body, not lateral to it. When the arm is raised forward in flexion, the supraspinatus tendon passes under the anterior edge of the acromion and acromioclavicular joint. For this movement, the critical area for wear is centered on the supraspinatus tendon and also may involve the long head of the biceps brachii muscle.[53-57]

## BURSAE

Several bursae are found in the shoulder region.[4] Two bursae particularly important to the clinician are the subacromial and the subscapular bursae.[15] Other bursae located in relation to the glenohumeral joint structures are between the infraspinatus muscle and the capsule, on the superior surface of the acromion, between the coracoid process and the capsule, under the coracobrachialis muscle, between the teres major and the long head of the triceps brachii muscles, and in front of and behind the tendon of the latissimus dorsi muscle. Because bursae are located where motion is required between adjacent structures, they have a ma-

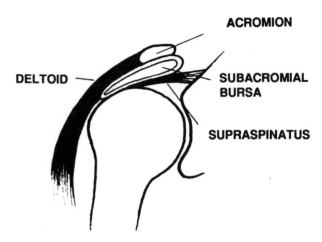

**Fig. 1-11.** Supraspinatus tendon and related structures.

jor function in the shoulder mechanism. The subacromial bursa (Fig. 1-11) is located between the deltoid muscle and the capsule, extending under the acromion and the coracoacromial ligament and between them and the supraspinatus muscle. The bursa adheres to the coracoacromial ligament and to the acromion above and to the rotator cuff below. The bursa does not frequently communicate with the joint; however, a communication may develop if the rotator cuff is ruptured.[50] The subacromial bursa is important for allowing gliding between the acromion and the deltoid muscle and the rotator cuff. It also reduces friction on the supraspinatus tendon as it passes under the coracoacromial arch.[9,50] Often, with repetitive overhead motion the bursae may become inflamed and thickened, which may decrease the critical space in the subacromial region.

The subscapular bursa lies between the subscapularis tendon and the neck of the scapula. It protects this tendon where it passes under the base of the coracoid process and over the neck of the scapula. The bursa communicates with the joint cavity between the superior and middle glenohumeral ligaments,[9,37] and in many cases also between the middle and inferior glenohumeral ligaments.[28,36]

## VASCULAR SUPPLY

The rotator cuff is a frequent site of pathologic conditions, usually degenerative and often in response to fatigue stress.[17] Because degeneration may occur even with normal activity levels, the nutritional status of the glenohumeral structures is of great importance. The blood supply to the rotator cuff comes from the posterior humeral circumflex and the suprascapular arteries.[4] These arteries supply principally the infraspinatus and teres minor muscle areas of the cuff. The anterior aspect of the capsular ligamentous cuff is supplied by the anterior humeral circumflex artery and occasionally by the thoracoacromial, suprahumeral, and subscapular arteries. Superiorly, the supraspinatus muscle is supplied by the thoracoacromial artery. The supraspinatus tendon has a region of relative avascularity 1 cm proximal to the humeral insertion and often including its insertion into the humerus.[58,59] Rothman and Parke[59] reported hypovascularity in the tendon in 63 percent of 72 shoulders studied. In a study by Rathbun and MacNab,[58] an avascular area was found in all specimens and was unrelated to age. Abduction of the arm resulted in relaxation of the tension on the supraspinatus muscle and complete filling of vessels throughout the tendon. In addition, as age increases, the area of avascularity also increases,[47] thus the potential for healing decreases with age. The other cuff tendons generally demonstrate good vascularity except for an occasional zone of hypovascularity in the superior portion of the insertion of the infraspinatus tendon.[58,59]

## ARTICULAR NEUROLOGY

Innervation of the shoulder region is derived from C5, C6, and C7; C4 also may add a minor contribution. The nerves supplying the ligaments, capsule, and synovial membrane are axillary, suprascapular, subscapular, and musculocutaneous nerves. Branches from the posterior cord of the brachial plexus also may supply the joint structures.

Occasionally, the shoulder may receive a greater supply from the axillary nerve than from the musculocutaneous nerve; the reverse may also be true. The complex, overlapping innervation pattern makes denervation of the joint difficult. The nerve supply follows the small blood vessels into periarticular structures.[4,5]

The skin on the anterior region of the shoulder complex is supplied by the supraclavicular nerves from C3 and C4 and by the terminal branches of the sensory component of the axillary nerve. The articular structures on the anterior aspect of the glenohumeral joint are supplied by the axillary nerve and, to a lesser degree, by the suprascapular nerves. The subscapular nerve and the posterior cord of the brachial plexus may also innervate the anterior aspect of the joint after piercing the subscapularis muscle.[4,5,9]

The supraclavicular nerves supply the skin on the superior and upper posterior aspects of the shoulder region. The lower, posterior, and lateral aspects of the shoulder are supplied by the posterior branch of the axillary nerve.

The periarticular structures on the superior aspect of the joint obtain part of their innervation from the suprascapular nerve. The axillary and musculocutaneous nerves and the lateral pectoral nerve may also contribute to the innervation of the superior aspect of the joint. Posteriorly, the main nerve supply is from the suprascapular nerve, which supplies the proximal part of the joint, and the axillary nerve, which supplies the distal region.[3–5,9]

The acromioclavicular joint is innervated by the lateral supraclavicular nerve from the cervical plexus (C4) and by the lateral pectoral and suprascapular nerves from the brachial plexus (C5 and C6). The sternoclavicular joint is innervated by branches from the medial supraclavicular nerve from the cervical plexus (C3 and C4) and subclavian nerve from the brachial plexus (C5 and C6).[4,9]

## SUMMARY

The shoulder complex is more mobile than any other joint mechanism of the body because of the combined movement at the glenohumeral and the scapulothoracic articulations. This wide range of motion permits positioning of the hand in space allowing performance of numerous gross and skilled functions. Shoulder complex stability is also required during dynamic activity, particularly when the distal extremity encounters resistance. The glenohumeral joint is inherently unstable because of the shallowness of the glenoid fossa as well as the disproportionate size and lack of congruency between the articular surfaces. During dynamic activities, stabilization of the humeral head on the glenoid fossa depends on an intact capsule and glenohumeral ligaments as well as on coordinated and synchronous activity in the deltoid and the rotator cuff muscles. Injury or disease of any of these structures can lead to instability and impingement of subacromial structures, resulting in pain and dysfunction in the shoulder region.

# REFERENCES

1. Kelley DL: Kinesiological Fundamentals of Motion Description. Prentice-Hall, Englewood Cliffs, NJ, 1971
2. Dempster WT: Mechanisms of shoulder movement. Arch Phys Med Rehabil 46:49, 1965
3. DePalma AF: Surgery of the Shoulder. 2nd Ed. JB Lippincott, Philadelphia, 1973
4. Warwick R, Williams P (eds): Gray's Anatomy. 35th Ed. Longman Group, London, 1973
5. Bateman JE: The Shoulder and Neck. WB Saunders, Philadelphia, 1971
6. Brantigan OC: Clinical Anatomy. McGraw-Hill, New York, 1963
7. Bechtol CO: Biomechanics of the shoulder. Clin Orthop 146:37, 1980
8. Inman VT, Saunders JB, Abbott LC: Observations on the function of the shoulder joint. J Bone Joint Surg 26:1, 1944
9. Moore KL: Clinically Oriented Anatomy. Williams & Wilkins, Baltimore, 1980
10. Perry J: Normal upper extremity kinesiology. Phys Ther 58:265, 1978
11. Abbott LC, Lucas DB: The function of the clavicle: its surgical significance. Ann Surg 140:583, 1954
12. Ljungren AE: Clavicular function. Acta Orthop Scand 50:261, 1979
13. Bearn JG: Direct observations on the function of the capsule of the sternoclavicular joint in clavicular support. J Anat 101:159, 1967
14. Moseley HF: The clavicle: its anatomy and function. Clin Orthop 58:17, 1968
15. Kent BE: Functional anatomy of the shoulder complex. Phys Ther 51:867, 1971
16. Frankel VH, Nordin M: Basic Biomechanics of the Skeletal System. Lea & Febiger, Philadelphia, 1980
17. Kessler RM, Hertling D: Management of Common Musculoskeletal Disorders: Physical Therapy Principles and Methods. Harper & Row, New York, 1983
18. Dvir Z, Berme N: The shoulder complex in elevation of the arm: mechanism approach. J Biomech 11:219, 1978
19. Bost FC, Inman VTG: The pathological changes in recurrent dislocations of the shoulder. J Bone Joint Surg 24:595, 1942
20. Codman EA: The Shoulder. Thomas Todd, Boston, 1934
21. Stindler A: Kinesiology of human body under normal and pathological conditions. Charles C Thomas, Springfield, IL, 1955
22. Gagey O, Bonfait H, Gillot C et al: Anatomic basis of ligamentous control of elevation of the shoulder (Reference position of the shoulder joint). Surg Radiol Anat 9:19, 1987
23. Johnston TB: The movements of the shoulder-joint: a plea for the use of the "plane of the scapula" as the plane of reference for movements occurring at the humeroscapular joint. Br J Surg 25:252, 1937
24. Norkin C, Levangie P: Joint Structure and Function: A Comprehensive Analysis. FA Davis, Philadelphia, 1983
25. Sarrafian SK: Gross and functional anatomy of the shoulder. Clin Orthop 173:11, 1983
26. Saha AK: Dynamic stability of the glenohumeral joint. Acta Orthop Scand 42:491, 1971
27. Saha AK: Mechanics of elevation of glenohumeral joint: its application in rehabilitation of flail shoulder in upper brachial plexus injuries and poliomyelitis and in replacement of the upper humerus by prosthesis. Acta Orthop Scand 44:668, 1973
27a. Cyprien JM, Vasey HM, Burdet A et al: Humeral retrotorsion and glenohumeral relationship in the normal shoulder and in recurrent anterior dislocation (scapulometry). Clin Orthop 175:8, 1983
27b. Randelli M, Gambrioli PL: Glenohumeral osteometry by computed tomography in normal and unstable shoulders. Clin Orthop 208:151, 1986
28. Moseley HF, Overgaard B: The anterior capsular mechanism in recurrent anterior dislocation of the shoulder: morphological and clinical studies with special reference to the glenoid labrum and the gleno-humeral ligaments. J Bone Joint Surg 44B:913, 1962
29. Perry J: Anatomy and biomechanics of the shoulder in throwing, swimming, gymnastics, and tennis. Clin Sports Med 2:247, 1983
30. Matsen FA, Harryman DT, Didles JA: Mechanics of glenohumeral instability. In Hawkins RJ (ed): Basic Science and Clinical Application in the Athlete's Shoulder. Clin Sports Med 10:783, 1991
31. Basmajian JV, Bazant FJ: Factors preventing downward dislocation of the adducted shoulder joint. J Bone Joint Surg 41A:1182, 1959
32. Ovesen J, Nielsen S: Anterior and posterior shoulder instability: a cadaver study. Acta Orthop Scand 57:324, 1986
33. Ovesen J, Nielsen S: Posterior instability of the shoulder: a cadaver study. Acta Orthop Scand 57:436, 1986
34. Kaltsas DS: Comparative study of the properties of the shoulder joint capsule with those of other joint capsules. Clin Orthop 173:20, 1983
35. Reeves B: Experiments on the tensile strength of the anterior capsular structures of the shoulder in man. J Bone Joint Surg 50B:858, 1968
36. Ferrari DA: Capsular ligaments of the shoulder: anatomi-

cal and functional study of the anterior superior capsule. Am J Sports Med 18:20, 1990

37. Turkel SJ, Panio MW, Marshall JL, Girgis FG: Stabilizing mechanisms preventing anterior dislocation of the glenohumeral joint. J Bone Joint Surg 63A:1208, 1981

37a. Bowen MK, Warren RF: Ligamentous control of shoulder stability based on selective cutting and static translation experiments. Clin Sports Med 10:757, 1991

38. Schwartz E, Warren RF, O'Brien SJ et al: Posterior shoulder instability. Orthop Clin North Am 18:409, 1987

39. Comtet JJ, Herberg G, Naasan IA: Biomechanical basis of transfers for shoulder paralysis. Hand Clin 5:1, 1989

40. Ovesen J, Nielsen S: Stability of the shoulder joint: cadaver study of stabilizing structures. Acta Orthop Scand 56:149, 1985

41. O'Brien SJ, Neeves MC, Arnoczky SN et al: The anatomy and histology of the inferior glenohumeral ligament complex of the shoulder. Am J Sports Med 18:451, 1990

42. deLuca CJ, Forrest WJ: Force analysis of individual muscles acting simultaneously on the shoulder joint during isometric abduction. J Biomech 6:385, 1973

43. Howell SM, Imobersteg AM, Seger DH, Marone PJ: Clarification of the role of the supraspinatus muscle in shoulder function. J Bone Joint Surg 68A:398, 1986

44. Lucas DB: Biomechanics of the shoulder joint. Arch Surg 107:425, 1973

45. Poppen NK, Walker PS: Forces at the glenohumeral joint in abduction. Clin Orthop 135:165, 1978

46. Saha AK: Mechanism of shoulder movements and a plea for the recognition of "zero position" of the glenohumeral joint. Clin Orthop 173:3, 1983

47. Brewer BJ: Aging of the rotator cuff. Am J Sports Med 7:102, 1979

48. Nobuhara K, Ikeda H: Rotator interval lesion. Clin Orthop 223:44, 1987

49. Kumar VP, Satku K, Balasubramaniam P: The role of the long head of biceps brachii in the stabilization of the head of the humerus. Clin Orthop 244:172, 1989

50. Rothman RH, Marvel JP, Heppenstall RB: Anatomic considerations in the glenohumeral joint. Orthop Clin North Am 6:341, 1975

51. Petersson CJ, Redlund-Johnell I: The subacromial space in normal shoulder radiographs. Acta Orthop Scand 55:57, 1984

52. Weiner DS, MacNab I: Superior migration of the humeral head: a radiological aid in the diagnosis of tears of the rotator cuff. J Bone Joint Surg 52B:524, 1970

53. Neer CS: Impingement lesions. Clin Orthop 173:70, 1983

54. Watson MS: Classification of the painful arc syndromes. In Bayley JI, Kessel L (eds): Shoulder Surgery. Springer-Verlag, New York, 1982

55. Neviaser TJ: The role of the biceps tendon in the impingement syndrome. Orthop Clin North Am 18:383, 1987

56. Post M, Cohen J: Impingement syndrome: a review of late stage II and early stage III lesions. Clin Orthop 207:126, 1986

57. Hawkins RJ, Abrams JS: Impingement syndrome in the absence of rotator cuff tear (states 1 and 2). Orthop Clin North Am 18:373, 1987

58. Rathbun JB, MacNab I: The microvascular pattern of the rotator cuff. J Bone Joint Surg 52B:540, 1970

59. Rothman RH, Parke WW: The vascular anatomy of the rotator cuff. Clin Orthop 41:176, 1965

# 2

# Kinesiology of the Shoulder Complex

*MARGARET SCHENKMAN*
*VICTORIA RUGO DE CARTAYA*

Normal function of the upper extremity requires smooth coordinated movement of the humerus, scapula, and clavicle.[1-3] These three bony segments with their ligaments and muscles function together as a unit for mobility and stability. The term *shoulder complex,* which refers to the humerus, clavicle, scapula, and their surrounding soft tissues, emphasizes their interdependent relationship.[4,5] A kinesiologic analysis of the shoulder complex includes an analysis of the coordinated movements of each segment of the shoulder complex and an analysis of the forces that produce those motions.[5]

Pathology and musculoskeletal impairments can significantly alter the coordinated shoulder complex motion. An understanding of the normal kinematics of the shoulder complex can allow the clinician to evaluate the effect of specific impairments on shoulder complex function and can provide a scientific basis for the most effective intervention.

In this chapter, movements of the humerus, clavicle, and scapula are analyzed kinematically with descriptions of shoulder complex motion and kinetically with explanation of the forces involved. First, motions of the three bony segments are considered with respect to the way in which structure determines function. Second, the coordinated motions of the shoulder complex are analyzed with emphasis on the mechanical constraints of their linked joints. Third, the internal and external forces that commonly act on the shoulder complex are discussed, with emphasis on the muscles as they function as primary movers, synergists, and stabilizers. Muscles intrinsic to the shoulder complex provide coordinated shoulder complex movements. Muscles extrinsic to the shoulder complex (from the neck and trunk) provide stability for intrinsic muscles of the shoulder complex. Thus, action of the postural muscles must be coordinated with action of the muscles of the shoulder complex itself for normal functional movement to occur. Fourth, the kinesiologic analysis of four specific functional tasks of the shoulder complex are provided as examples.

Structure dictates function whether in architecture, crystals, or the human body. Motions of body segments of the shoulder complex are determined by the shapes of bones, their articular surfaces, their ligaments, and the muscles.[5,6] The articular surfaces of bones define the direction of motion. Ligaments and muscles guide motion and provide constraints and power. Muscles provide forces that produce movement within the available range of motion or restrain movement produced by external forces. Thus, a kinesiologic analysis of the shoulder complex requires knowledge of the anatomy of the scapula, humerus, and clavicle as well as their muscles and soft tissues.

The anatomy of the shoulder complex has been reviewed in Chapter 1 and will not be presented in detail in this chapter. Specific aspects of shoulder complex anatomy will be reviewed as they contribute to the unique nature and problems of shoulder complex function. The shoulder complex is designed to allow exceptional mobility of the upper extremity in humans. This mobility is the result of the shallow glenoid fossa and freely moving scapula.[7] This complex is one of the least stable joint complexes of the human body. The entire complex, as well as the upper extremities, is attached to the thorax through a single bony articulation, the small and relatively unstable sternoclavicular joint.[8] The stability of the shoulder complex is provided predominantly by the muscles and ligaments that support the bony segments. This has important ramifications for the kinematics of the shoulder complex during functional movement. There is an essential need for coordinated muscle action of postural muscles in all upper extremity functions. The many degrees of freedom of the upper extremities place tremendous demand on coordinated muscle action to control the accurate position and orientation of the upper extremities for many fine motor skills. This demand is evident in the complex and changing interplay of muscles that act as prime movers, synergists, and stabilizers during shoulder complex motion. A further consequence of the many degrees of freedom is that there is no single kinematic organization for specific shoulder complex motions, nor are there unique groupings of muscles that function during tasks. Rather, the muscles and motions depend on the integrated result of body orientation, the individual's specific segmental alignment, and the balance of muscle length and strength for any given individual and task. It is therefore essential to understand the principles that dictate motion to be able to predict the actual movement and forces of the shoulder complex of individuals.

## MOTIONS OF THE SHOULDER COMPLEX

The entire shoulder complex moves with synchronization when the upper extremity is moved through space. This has been best studied for humeral elevation. The result of synchronized movement of the shoulder complex is that the upper extremity normally can be elevated 180 degrees either through abduction or through flexion. Much of the early literature related to humeral elevation does not distinguish abduction from flexion. The general term *elevation* is used in this chapter to indicate the coordinated motion of the three bones of the shoulder complex unless the authors specifically have identified the motion as abduction or flexion. The term *humeral elevation* is used to indicate elevation

of the humerus relative to the scapula. Motions of the individual segments must be described to appreciate the coordinated movements of the shoulder complex. The specific motions of the three bony segments of the shoulder complex are therefore analyzed first and then the coordinated motions of the shoulder complex are analyzed. Arthrokinematics are discussed in Chapter 1.

The humerus rotates around an axis that is generally located within the humeral head during elevation.[9] This axis, or instantaneous center of rotation, is not fixed but appears to vary during elevation of the humerus.[9] de Luca and Forrest[9] determined the instantaneous center showed that the axis was always medial and inferior to the greater and lesser tuberosities of the humerus but was not located within the head of the humerus at all times. The location of the instantaneous center of rotation is critical in determining the moment arm of muscles.

Elevation is limited by impingement of the surgical neck of the humerus against the acromion. The humerus only can be passively elevated a limited amount relative to the scapula when the clavicle and the scapula are not allowed to move.[10,11] It is at this point that the surgical neck reaches the acromion, preventing further humeral motion. Elevation of the humerus is also limited by the greater tubercle of the humerus. The humerus must be externally rotated to allow the greater tubercle to slide past the acromion. When the humerus remains internally rotated, it can only elevate about 60 degrees relative to the scapula.[10]

The clavicle elevates coordinately with the humerus as the arm is elevated as discussed by Inman and Saunders.[12] Clavicular elevation begins early in the range of humeral elevation and is nearly completed by the time the humerus has reached 90 degrees of elevation.[12] There are reportedly 4 degrees of clavicular elevation for every 10 degrees of humeral elevation.[12] The clavicle moves around two distinct axes during humeral elevation (Fig. 2-1). Clavicular elevation occurs around an anterior/posterior axis that is located near the sternal end of the clavicle.[7] Movement around this axis takes place during the initial 90 to 100 degrees of humeral elevation, at which time tension on the costoclavicular and coracoclavicular ligaments prevents further elevation.[13,14] The second axis of rotation is the longitudinal axis of the clavicle. Dvir and Berme[7] suggest that when the costoclavicular and coracoclavic-

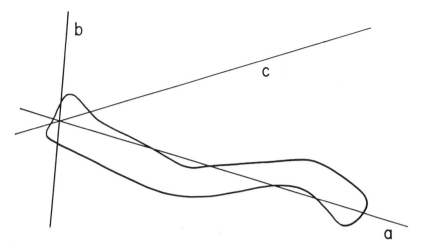

**Fig. 2-1.** Axes of motion of the clavicle. (*a*) Longitudinal axis of rotation; (*b*) vertical axis for protraction and retraction; (*c*) horizontal axis for elevation and depression. The sternal end of the scapula is on the left. (From Schenkman and Rugo de Cartaya,[5] with permission.)

ular ligaments become taut and check further elevation of the clavicle, they cause the clavicle to rotate backward around this axis. Because the clavicle is shaped like a crank shaft, the backward rotation elevates the acromial end of the clavicle. This backward rotation of the clavicle continues until the humerus reaches its maximum elevation.[7] Abbott and Lucas[13] noted that surgical excision of the clavicle does not prevent the full 180 degrees of upper extremity elevation but does result in both decreased strength and stability of the upper extremity.

Scapular upward and downward rotation occur in the plane of the scapula rather than in the coronal plane of the body.[7a] Dvir and Berme[7] have suggested that rotation occurs around two distinct axes (Fig. 2-2). One is along the spine of the scapula near the vertebral border. The second is near the acromial clavicular joint. By contrast Poppen and Walker[7a] suggested that motion occurs around a moving axis that begins more centrally in the scapula and migrates toward the glenoid fossa. For simplicity, we have used Dvir and Berme's[7] conceptualization.

The scapula rotates about 30 degrees around the first axis[3,7] so that the inferior angle of the scapula moves outward along the chest wall and the glenoid fossa is positioned superiorly (i.e., upward rotation of

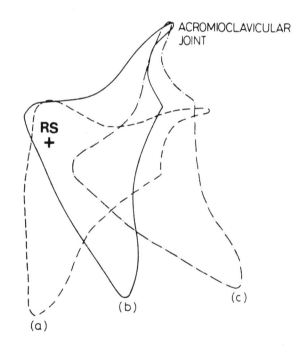

**Fig. 2-2.** Posterior view of the scapula. (*a*) Position at rest. (*b*) Position at 30 degrees scapular rotation. (*c*) Position at 60 degrees scapular rotation. The axis of motion is at RS from 0 to 30 degrees scapular rotation. The axis of motion is at the acromial end of the spine of the scapula. (From Dvir and Berme,[7] with permission.)

the scapula). After about 30 degrees of upward rotation, tension on the coracoclavicular and costoclavicular ligaments prevents further scapular rotation. As discussed above, the result of tension on these two ligaments is to force the clavicle into backward rotation. The clavicular rotation has the added consequence of causing the scapula to rotate around an axis located at its acromial end.[7,12] A further 30 degrees of upward rotation occurs around this axis.[7] In total, the scapula completes about 60 degrees of upward rotation during humeral elevation.

Scapular upward rotation is essential for complete elevation of the upper extremity. The upward rotation of the scapula positions the glenoid fossa superiorly. The humerus, which is seated in the glenoid fossa, is thereby moved into 60 degrees of elevation beyond the 120 degrees that occurs between the humerus and the scapula at the glenoid fossa. The combined motion of humerus, clavicle, and scapula is what permits elevation of the upper extremity of 180 degrees. Because upper extremity elevation depends on motion of the humerus, clavicle, and scapula, smooth coordinated limb movement requires synchronization of humeral, clavicular, and scapular motion. More than half a century ago, Codman[2] described this synchronized movement as scapulohumeral rhythm, noting that this synchronization takes place in a 1:2 ratio (1 degree of scapular upward rotation for every 2 degrees of humeral elevation).

It is now clear that this ratio is not constant throughout elevation of the humerus.[3,15,16] Inman et al[3] reported that during the first 30 degrees of abduction (or 60 degrees of forward flexion), the scapula seeks a position of stability, either remaining fixed, moving first laterally and then medially, or even oscillating.[3] This initial phase is called the setting phase to emphasize the setting action of muscles. Doody and co-workers[16] investigated the scapulohumeral rhythm of 25 women and reported similar findings to those of Inman, except that Doody et al showed that the scapular motion does not occur in a linear relationship with the humeral motion but rather varies markedly in different parts of the range.

Scapulohumeral rhythm may be further complicated by differences such as gender or morphologic differences and by the type of load being moved. For example, Doody and co-workers[16] noted differences in the final extent of abduction of the humerus of women as compared with men. Also, they noted that when the

women held a 4- or 6 lb weight, the scapula appeared to complete the setting phase more quickly so that its contribution to humeral elevation was initiated earlier in the range.

In summary, during upper extremity elevation, the humerus elevates and externally rotates. Concurrently, the scapula begins to rotate around an axis located in the scapular spine and near the vertebral border. About 30 degrees of scapular upward rotation occurs around this axis during the first 60 degrees of humeral rotation, with a result of 90 degrees of elevation of the upper extremity. Simultaneously, the clavicle elevates at its acromial end by rotating around an anteroposterior axis located near the sternal end. At about 90 degrees of upper extremity elevation, further rotation of the clavicle around this axis and of the scapula is checked by tension of two clavicular ligaments. The clavicle now begins to rotate posteriorly, positioning the acromial end in a superior position. This positions the scapula in a further 30 degrees of upward rotation. This scapular upward rotation occurs in synchrony with 60 degrees of humeral external rotation for a further 90 degrees of upper extremity elevation. In total, the upper extremity elevates approximately 180 degrees through this combined motion of humerus, clavicle, and scapula.

## MUSCLES OF THE SHOULDER COMPLEX

Anatomically, muscles of the shoulder complex can be divided into three groups depending on their attachment (Table 2-1). Functionally, muscles of the shoulder complex can be differentiated into those that act as movers of the shoulder complex, those that stabilize the complex in relation to the thorax as it is moved, and those that provide stability for the complex in regard to the remainder of the body. Mechanically, muscle actions can be differentiated into those that rotate the bony segment around an axis and those that translate the segment toward or away from the axis. Each of these distinctions is useful in categorizing muscles in preparation for an analysis of muscle action in combined shoulder motion.

### Anatomic Considerations

Anatomically, muscles of the shoulder complex can be divided into three groups: those that connect the

## Table 2-1. Muscles of the Shoulder Complex

Scapula to the humerus, radius, or ulna
  Deltoid
  Supraspinatus
  Infraspinatus
  Teres minor
  Subscapularis
  Teres major
  Coracobrachialis
  Biceps brachii
  Triceps brachii—long head
Scapula to trunk
  Serratus anterior
  Trapezius
  Rhomboids
  Pectoralis minor
  Levator scapulae
Humerus to trunk
  Latissimus dorsi
  Pectoralis major—sternal head

(Modified from Schenkman and Rugo de Cartaya,[5] with permission.)

scapula to the humerus, radius, or ulna; those that connect the scapula to the trunk; and those that connect the humerus to the trunk[5,11] (Table 2-1). These attachments have implications for mobility and stability functions of the shoulder complex. Those muscles that attach to the scapula (e.g., the rotator cuff muscles, rhomboids, and trapezius) have a less stable base from which to operate than do those muscles that connect the humerus to the thorax or pelvis (e.g., the latissimus dorsi and pectoralis muscle). Furthermore, those muscles that originate on the scapula and insert on the upper extremity are even less stable than those that originate on the scapula and insert on the thorax.

## Functional Considerations

In functional movement, muscles do not act in isolation. Rather muscles act in combination to produce desired motions. Thus muscle actions, like motions of the segments, are complex and require synchronized action of many muscles in different combinations. Several authors have provided definitions for the types of muscles that act together. We have summarized commonly used terminology modified from Schenkman and Rugo de Cartaya.[5] The definitions used in this chapter are as follows:

*Effort force* refers to force or forces causing the observed movement or, in the case of a maintained posture, the net force maintaining the posture.

*Mover* refers to a muscular force acting during concentric or activation as an effort force.

*Prime movers* are the main forces that produce motion at a joint. The function of a muscle as a prime mover depends on criteria such as physiologic cross section, moment arm, and muscle length. The middle deltoid and supraspinatus are prime movers for abduction of the humerus.[5]

*Secondary movers* produce only some of the desired motions or are recruited only when an action becomes forceful. Thus, a secondary mover has less moment capability than does a prime mover based on physiologic cross section, moment arm, muscle length, and forcefulness of the effort. The biceps brachii may be a secondary mover for humeral abduction when the humerus is externally rotated.

A *controller* is a muscular force acting as a resisting force during an eccentric activation. When the upper extremity is lowered with control against the force of gravity, the force of gravity moves the extremity and muscles such as the deltoids act as controllers, restraining the action of gravity on the extremity.[5] A prime controller serves as the most effective controller, based on the criteria of physiologic cross section, moment arm, muscle length, etc. A secondary controller is a muscle that serves as an assistant and less effective controller, based on the criteria of physiologic cross section, moment arm, muscle length, and forcefulness of the effort.

When analyzing muscle action during function, the movers of the extremity should be differentiated into primary and secondary movers or controllers, depending on whether the extremity is moved against the force of gravity or is controlled as it moves in the direction of the force of gravity.

*Synergists* are muscles that must act together to produce a desired effect. Two categories of synergists are the helping synergists and the neutralizing synergists. *Helping synergists* are pairs of muscles that have an action in common and an action that is opposite. That is, they act together to produce a desired movement in one plane and eliminate undesired movement in another plane or at another joint. When these pairs of muscles act coordinately, the common action is reinforced and the opposing action is canceled out. For example, from anatomic position, the anterior deltoid both flexes the humerus and abducts it; the posterior deltoid both extends the humerus and abducts it. When they act together, the anterior and posterior deltoid produce humeral abduction with the anterior and posterior fibers opposing each other's undesired action. *Neutralizing or stabilizing synergists* are muscles that prevent undesired motion produced by a mover or controller. Neutralizing synergists are of particular importance when multijoint muscles act. For example, the latissimus dorsi, which crosses many vertebral segments, could exert a rotational and extension force on the trunk during forceful internal rotation of the humerus. The abdominal musculature could provide a counteracting or neutralizing force to prevent these unwanted motions.

*Stabilizers* are muscles that steady or fixate the origin or the insertion of specific muscles so that the desired motion occurs.[5] It is essential for one attachment of any muscle to be firmly fixed for its force to be directed to the alternate attachment. This is especially important for muscles that cross more than one joint. This fixation may occur as a result of the weight of the relevant body segments or may require specific muscle action. For example, the rotator cuff muscles could potentially either rotate the humerus or upwardly rotate the scapula. The scapula is only connected to the thorax through muscular attachments. This nonbony connection of the scapula to the thorax demands that stabilizers fix its orientation relative to the thorax for the rotator cuff muscles to exert their intended force on the humerus. Dvir and Berme[7] suggested that with respect to the scapulothoracic connection, the serratus anterior moves the scapula; the main purpose of other muscles is to provide stability. Similarly, many of the muscles of the scapula and clavicle originate on the cervical spine or the occiput. The head and neck must be stabilized by muscle action to permit muscles such as the upper trapezius to exert their force on the scapula. The close interrelationship between the head/neck and shoulder complex is well known.[17]

Stabilizers play a second and equally essential role during any functional movement, counteracting the ever-changing center of mass of the body as the upper extremities are moved through space.[18] For example, when the upper extremity is held outstretched in front of the body, the mass of the arms could cause the person to fall forward. A counteracting force of posterior musculature of the trunk is necessary to stabilize the body to balance the mass held anteriorly. This necessity is especially apparent when limb movements become forceful such as in pitching a baseball or fencing.

Furthermore, muscles can work in normal or reverse action.[5] In *normal action,* muscles exert their force at the distal attachment. In *reverse action,* muscles exert their force at the proximal attachment. For example, the latissimus dorsi works in normal action to extend the humerus relative to the thorax; the same muscle works in reverse action to elevate the trunk relative to a fixed upper extremity. Actions of muscles of the shoulder complex are summarized in Table 2-2.

## Mechanical Considerations

In an excellent mechanical analysis of shoulder complex kinematics, Dvir and Berme[7] clearly identified the two competing mechanical demands for the shoulder complex. There is a requirement for stability between the scapula and the thorax. They suggest that this requirement is met through closed chain or closed link mechanisms. There is also a requirement for motion of the humerus and clavicle with respect to the thorax. This is an open-chain or open-link mechanism. These two mechanisms explain the two competing and simultaneous needs of the shoulder complex for stability and mobility. A vector representation of muscles that act on the shoulder complex aids in analyzing these requirements.

The motion that a muscle can produce depends on several factors. First, the force of motion produced depends on the distance of the muscle's line of pull with repsect to the joint axis of motion. The moment arm is an important determinant of muscle action. Second, the direction of motion produced is determined by the orientation of the muscle with respect to the moving lever. Muscles have an origin and a direction that are estimated as the average point of attachment of the muscle and the average line of pull of the muscle, respectively. The line of pull of the muscle is depicted as a vector. Figure 2-3 illustrates the vector representation of the deltoid and three of four rotator cuff muscles. Each of these muscles exert their force on the side of the joint axis that would allow them to pull the segment of interest in the appropriate direction. There is, however, another issue to consider: How much of the force of the muscle is directed toward moving the body segment in the desired direction? For example, only part of the force of the deltoid muscle rotates the humerus into elevation within the glenohumeral joint. The force vector of the deltoid muscle can be resolved into a rotational and translational component.[3,5,7] The

**Table 2-2. Major Muscle Actions of the Shoulder Complex**

| Muscle | Humerus | | | | | | | | Scapula | | | | | | |
|---|---|---|---|---|---|---|---|---|---|---|---|---|---|---|---|
| | Flex | Ext | IR | ER | Ab | Ad | H Ab | H Ad | Elev | Depr | DR | UR | Protr | Retr | Ant Tilt |
| Biceps brachii—short head | • | | | | | | | | | | | | | | |
| Biceps brachii—long head[a] | • | | | | • | | | | | | | | | | |
| Triceps brachii—long head | | • | | | | | • | | | | | | | | |
| Supraspinatus | | | | • | • | | | | | | | | | | |
| Deltoid | | | | | | | | | | | | | | | |
|  Anterior | • | | • | | | | | • | | | | | | | |
|  Middle | • | | | | • | | | | | | | | | | |
|  Posterior[b] | | • | | • | | • | • | | | | | | | | |
| Coracobrachialis | • | | | | | • | | | | | | | | | • |
| Latissimus dorsi | | • | • | | | • | | | | | • | | | | |
| Pectoralis major | | | | | | | | | | | | | | | |
|  Clavicular head | • | | • | | | | | • | | • | | | • | | |
|  Sternal head | | • | • | | | • | | • | | • | | | | | |
| Subscapularis | | | • | | | | | | | | | | | | |
| Teres major[c] | | • | • | | | • | | | | | | | | | |
| Infraspinatus | | | | • | | | | | | | | | | | |
| Teres minor | | | | • | | | | | | | | | | | |
| Pectoralis minor | | | | | | | | | | • | • | | • | | • |
| Rhomboids | | | | | | | | | • | | • | | | • | |
| Levator scapulae | | | | | | | | | • | | • | | | | |
| Trapezius | | | | | | | | | | | | | | | |
|  Upper | | | | | | | | | • | | | • | | • | |
|  Middle | | | | | | | | | | | | | | • | |
|  Lower[d] | | | | | | | | | | • | | • | | • | |
| Serratus anterior | | | | | | | | | | | | | | | |
|  Upper fibers | | | | | | | | | | | | • | • | | |
|  Lower fibers | | | | | | | | | | | | • | • | | |

*Abbreviations:* Flex, flexion; Ext, extension; IR, internal rotation; ER, external rotation; Ab, abduction; Ad, adduction; H Ab, horizontal abduction; H Ad, horizontal adduction; Elev, elevation; Depr, depression; DR, downward rotation; UR, upward rotation; Protr, protraction; Retr, retraction; Ant, anterior.

[a] Biceps brachii long head may abduct the humerus if the humerus is rotated externally.

[b] The joint angle will determine whether posterior deltoid can adduct the humerus.

[c] The joint angle will determine whether teres major abducts or adducts the limb.

[d] The joint angle will determine whether the lower trapezius upwardly or downwardly rotates the scapula. (Modified from Schenkman and Rugo de Cartaya,[5] with permission.)

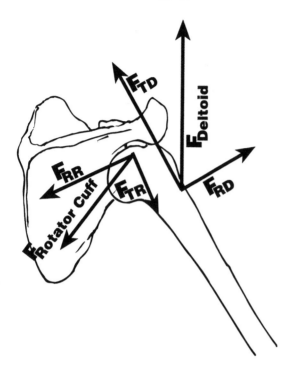

**Fig. 2-3.** Force couple of deltoid and rotator cuff muscles. Rotatory forces, acting on opposite sides of axis of motion, combine to produce upward rotation. Translatory forces cancel each other out. $F_{RR}$, rotatory force of rotator cuff; $F_{TR}$, translatory force of rotator cuff; $F_{RD}$, rotatory force of deltoid; $F_{TD}$, translatory force of deltoid. (Modified from Schenkman and Rugo de Cartaya,[5] with permission.)

cuff muscles illustrates the important role of force couples in shoulder complex motion. The rotatory component of the deltoid force is reinforced by the rotatory component of the rotator cuff muscles. (Fig. 2-3) When the force of the rotator cuff muscles is resolved into rotational and translational components, it is apparent that the translational component serves to glide the head of the humerus inferiorly while the translatory component of the deltoid muscle approximates the humeral head and the subacromial arch. Thus, the force couple of the deltoid and rotator cuff muscles serves two purposes: First, the rotational components of the muscle produce abduction. Second, the translational components act in opposite directions and thus eliminate the unwanted translation of the head of the humerus relative to the glenoid fossa. The rotator cuff muscles neutralize the force of deltoid that would cause jamming of the humeral head in the glenoid fossa by producing the inferior glide.

The scapular rotators provide a second example of force couple. The upper digitations of the serratus anterior, levator scapulae, upper trapezius, and lower trapezius have potential to act as upward rotators of the scapula,[20] and yet these muscles exert their force in three different directions relative to the scapula (Fig. 2-4). The serratus anterior pulls outward toward the axilla, the upper trapezius pulls upward toward the occiput, and the lower trapezius pulls downward toward the lumbar spine. The ability of these three muscles to each upwardly rotate the scapula depends on the location of the axis of rotation of the scapula.[5,7]

During the first 30 degrees of scapular upward rotation (the first 90 degrees of upper extremity elevation), the scapula rotates around an axis located on its spine and near the vertebral boarder. In this range of scapular motion, only the upper digitations of the serratus anterior and the upper trapezius can exert forces that upwardly rotate the scapula.[20] These two muscles therefore form a force couple, reinforcing each other's action on the scapula (Fig. 2-4A). According to Dvir and Berme's[7] analysis of the scapular axes of motion, the lower trapezius should not participate in scapular upward rotation at this point. During the second 30 degrees of scapular upward rotation (from about 90 to 180 degrees of upper extremity elevation), the axis of rotation (from about 90 to 180 degrees of upper extremity elevation), the axis of rotation of the scapula

rotational component of the deltoid muscle represents that component of the force of the deltoid muscle that causes rotation of the humerus. The translational component represents the part of the force of the deltoid that moves the humerus closer to the glenoid fossa. The ability of a muscle to act at a particular joint is dependent in part on the orientation of the fibers with respect to the joint axis of motion and the relative position with respect to the axis.

The translatory component of the deltoid force, if unopposed, would jam the head of the humerus into the glenoid fossa.[10,19] The use of a force couple prevents this unwanted aspect of the deltoid action.[7,19] A force couple can be described as two equal forces that act in opposite directions to rotate a segment around its axis of motion.[5] This occurs when the forces are applied on opposing sides of the joint axis of motion. The force couple of the deltoid muscle with the rotator

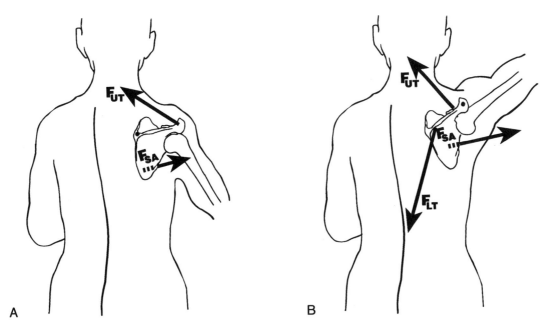

**Fig. 2-4.** Force couple of muscles acting at scapula. $F_{UT}$, force of upper trapezius; $F_{LT}$, force of lower trapezius; $F_{SA}$, force of serratus anterior. (**A**) Axis of scapular rotation from 0 to 30 degrees.; (**B**) axis of scapular rotation from 30 to 60 degrees. (Modified Schenkman and Rugo de Cartaya,[5] with permission.)

is now located near the acromioclavicular joint (Fig. 2-2). The lower trapezius now exerts a force that would turn the scapula around that axis of rotation into upward rotation (Fig. 2-4B). Thus, the lower trapezius participates as part of the force couple that upwardly rotates the scapula. The contribution of the lower trapezius may be of considerable importance during the latter portion of elevation, as it would appear that the upper trapezius may be actively insufficient to participate with adequate force.

Most authors do not differentiate between the role of the trapezius in the early and latter parts of the range of elevation. Basmajian,[20] however, showed that the lower trapezius and the lower fibers of the serratus anterior become increasingly active as the scapula becomes increasingly upwardly rotated. Inman et al[3] suggested that the lower trapezius is inactive until the humerus reaches about 90 degrees of abduction. These authors further noted that the lower trapezius is less active in flexion than in abduction, with the lower trapezius relaxing to allow flexion. They noted that the lower fibers of the serratus anterior become the more active component in flexion. The differences in activity

of the lower trapezius during the early and later part of the range of humeral elevation is easily observed both visually and by palpation. For some subjects, differential activity of the lower trapezius is more easily shown during eccentric action of that muscle. This occurs, for example, during controlled lowering of the upper extremity in the direction of the force of gravity.

## ANALYSIS OF SPECIFIC MOTIONS OF THE SHOULDER COMPLEX

Combined motions of the shoulder complex can be analyzed using the principles outlined in this chapter. In examining a particular motion, it is useful to first estimate the range of motion of each participating bony segment and to estimate the position of each joint axis of motion throughout the range. This will determine which muscles could potentially participate in producing the desired motion. The available range of motion of the different segments of the shoulder complex is summarized in Table 2-3. Second, it is necessary to determine whether the extremity is moving against

### Table 2-3. The Shoulder Complex—Range and Axis of Motion

| Joint and Motion | Range (degrees) | Axis of Motion |
|---|---|---|
| **Sternoclavicular** | | |
| 1. Rotation (counterclockwise) | 0–50 | Longitudinal axis of clavicle |
| 2. a. Elevation | 0–30 | Oblique axis through costoclavicular |
|    b. Depression | 0–5 | ligament |
| 3. a. Protraction | 0–15 | Vertical axis through costoclavicular ligament |
|    b. Retraction | 0–15 | |
| **Glenohumeral** | | |
| 1. a. Flexion | 0–180 | Coronal axis through glenohumeral joint |
|    b. Extension | 180–0 | |
|    c. Hyperextension | 0–55 | |
| 2. a. Abduction | 0–180 | Sagittal axis through glenohumeral joint |
|    b. Adduction | 180–0 | |
| 3. a. Horizontal abduction | 0–45 | Vertical axis through glenohumeral joint |
|    b. Horizontal adduction | 45–0 | |
| 4. a. Internal rotation | 0–70 | Vertical axis through shaft of humerus |
|    b. External rotation | 0–90 | |
| **Acromioclavicular** | | |
| 1. Winging of scapula | 0–50 | Vertical axis through acromioclavicular joint |
| 2. Abduction of scapula | 0–30 | Anterior-posterior axis |
| 3. Inferior angle of scapula tilts away from chest wall | 0–30 | Coronal axis |
| **Scapulothoracic** | | |
| 1. a. Upward rotation | 0–60 | From 0°–30° near vertebral border on spine of scapula |
|    b. Downward rotation | 60–0 | From 30°–60° near acromial end on spine of scapula |
| 2. a. Elevation | Translatory | No axis |
|    b. Depression | Translatory | No axis |
| 3. a. Protraction | Translatory | No axis |
|    b. Retraction | Translatory | No axis |

(Modified from Schenkman and Rugo de Cartaya,[5] with permission.)

gravity (requiring muscles to act concentrically as movers); is being controlled as it moves (requiring muscles to act eccentrically as controllers); or is being moved forcefully against resistance (requiring muscles to act concentrically to overcome the force of the externally applied resistance). A third step is to determine which parts of the motion occur as an open kinematic chain and which as a closed kinematic chain. This determination will indicate which attachment of participating muscles must be stabilized.

With this information, it is possible to interpret which muscles should serve as movers, synergists, and stabilizers for each motion. Considerable literature is available from electromyographic studies of the shoulder complex during upper extremity function that can be used in these interpretations. There are, however,

several notes of caution because the early studies often are very simple and limited to motions such as humeral abduction or flexion without attention to specific requirements of more functional movements. Also, it is apparent from the available information that changes of external load,[16,21–25] of limb orientation with respect to the body plane,[20,21,26] and of the limb position in the range of motion[27] all contribute to determining what muscles will be active at any given time.

More recently, several studies of the kinematics of arm movement during different sports activities including baseball pitching,[28] tennis,[29] and water polo[30] have been reported. There are also electromyographic studies of the muscles that are active in swimming[31] and pitching.[32–34] These and other studies provide the initial information from which to develop complete kinesiologic analyses of the nature described in this chapter. An individual's particular morphology will dictate which muscles actually participate in a particular activity and what roles they assume.

Schenkman and Rugo de Cartaya[5] used available information to interpret the different motions and muscles that contribute to movement of the shoulder complex in four different activities. They used a modification of a format of Riegger and Watkins[35] for completing these analyses. Using reported electromyographic results, Schenkman and Rugo de Cartaya[5] illustrated how the motions and muscles differ with respect to normal and reverse action and in roles as movers, synergists, and stabilizers. The motions that these authors analyzed included an unresisted upper extremity abduction (Table 2-4, Fig. 2-4), return of the upper extremity from full abduction to neutral (Table 2-5), adduction against resistance (Table 2-6, Fig. 2-5), and a sitting push-up (Table 2-7, Fig. 2-6).

## Upper Extremity Abduction Without Resistance

Unresisted upper extremity abduction from the anatomic position (Table 2-4, Fig. 2-4) illustrates the intricate interplay of muscles when the upper extremity is moved, as an open kinematic chain, against the force of gravity. This motion illustrates the importance of the changing axis of rotation of the scapula in determining the contribution of the lower trapezius to the force couple that causes its upward rotation. Also, this activity illustrates the multiple roles of the rotator cuff muscles. The infraspinatus, teres minor, and supraspinatus all act as external rotators of the humerus,[5] which prevents the tuberosities from impinging on the acromion. These same muscles contribute to the force couple that rotates the humerus into elevation. They also neutralize the action of the deltoid muscle that would jam the head of the humerus into the acromion. Finally, the rotator cuff muscles, in conjunction with other muscles of the scapula, assist in stabilizing the scapula against the thorax.[7] The teres major is not active during shoulder abduction. This muscle does become active during static positions of elevation, its activity increasing with increasing load. The middle trapezius and rhomboids serve to fix the scapula in the plane of motion during abduction but relax somewhat during flexion to allow

that motion to occur.[3] Thus, the role of stabilizers is both task- and motion-dependent.

Besides the requirements of muscles that act to move or stabilize the scapula for upper extremity abduction, there is a requirement for muscles to stabilize the origin of muscles within the cervical spine and to stabilize the thorax over the pelvic complex. These requirements become even more important as the movement becomes more forceful. There are increasing demands for stabilization of the shoulder complex itself. Furthermore, as the upper extremity moves away from the body, stabilization is required to counter the effect of the mass of the limb on the overall posture.

## Upper Extremity Adduction Without Resistance

Adduction of the humerus from 180 degrees to neutral (Table 2-5) illustrates the consequences of controlling motion of the upper extremity in the same direction as the force of gravity. In this situation, gravity acts as the effort force of the extremity. The same muscles that move the extremity against gravity now control the effect of gravity on the extremity. Thus, the prime movers and helping synergists become controllers. The requirement for neutralizing synergists and for stability remains the same. When muscles act to control motion due to the force of gravity of the extremity, they do not act with sufficient force to move the extremity against gravity.

## Upper Extremity Adduction Against Resistance

Adduction of the upper extremity against resistance (Table 2-6; Fig. 2-5) shows that forceful adduction is not accomplished by simply controlling motion due to the force of gravity acting on the upper extremity but requires the adductory muscles to act as movers. This activity is used therefore to illustrate the combination of muscles that adduct the humerus and simultaneously downwardly rotate the scapula. In particular, this activity illustrates the important role of the lower trapezius as a downward rotator of the scapula from 30 degrees to neutral.[5] This motion illustrates several other points as well. First, with respect to motion of the humerus, the major movers that adduct the humerus include the latissimus dorsi and the pectoralis ma-

## Table 2-4. Muscle Action Analysis for Upper Extremity Abduction, 0°–180°

| Joint and Motion | Range (degrees) | Axis | Prime Movers[a] | Secondary Movers | Helping Synergists | Neutralizers | Antagonists |
|---|---|---|---|---|---|---|---|
| **Glenohumeral** | | | | | | | |
| Abduction | 0–120 | Glenohumeral joint | Deltoid Supraspinatus | Biceps brachii (if humerus is rotated externally) | Anterior and posterior deltoid | Infraspinatus Subscapularis Teres minor: neutralize tendency of deltoid to compress humeral head | Glenohumeral adductors |
| External rotation | 0–70 | Long axis of humerus | Infraspinatus Teres minor Supraspinatus | Posterior deltoid | | | Internal rotators |
| **Scapular** | | | | | | | |
| Upward rotation | 0–30 | Spine of scapula near vertebral border | Upper trapezius Upper fibers of serratus anterior | | | | |
| | 30–60 | Near acromioclavicular joint | Upper and lower trapezius, all of serratus anterior | | Upper and lower trapezius | | Scapular downward rotators |
| **Clavicular** | | | | | | | |
| Elevation | 0–30 | Costoclavicular ligament | Upper trapezius | | | | |
| Backward rotation | 0–50 | Long axis of clavicle | Indirect muscle action producing tension on coracoclavicular and costoclavicular ligaments | | | | Clavicular depressors |

*Note:* Resistance to shoulder abduction is the mass of the upper extremity acting at the center of mass of the upper extremity.
[a] Prime movers act concentrically.
(Modified from Schenkman and Rugo de Cartaya,[5] with permission.)

**Table 2-5. Muscle Action Analysis for Unresisted Upper Extremity Adduction, 180°–0°**

| Joint and Motion | Range (degrees) | Axis | Primary Controllers[a] | Secondary Controllers[a] | Helping Synergists | Neutralizers | Antagonists |
|---|---|---|---|---|---|---|---|
| **Glenohumeral** | | | | | | | |
| Adduction | 120–0 | Glenohumeral joint | Deltoid Supraspinatus | Biceps brachii (if humerus is rotated externally) | Anterior and posterior deltoid | Infraspinatus Subscapularis and teres minor neutralize tendency of deltoid to compress humeral head | Humeral abductors |
| Internal rotation | 70–0 | Long axis of humerus | Infraspinatus Teres minor Supraspinauts | Posterior deltoid | | | |
| **Scapular** | | | | | | | |
| Downward rotation | 60–30 | Near acromioclavicular joint | Upper and lower trapezius Serratus anterior | | Upper and lower trapezius Upper trapezius and upper fibers Serratus anterior | Neck flexors | Scapular upward rotators |
| | 30–0 | Spine of scapula near vertebral border | Upper trapezius and upper fibers Serratus anterior | | Upper trapezius and upper fibers Serratus anterior | | |
| **Clavicular** | | | | | | | |
| Forward rotation | 50–0 | Long axis of clavicle | Indirectly produced by release of tension on coracoclavicular and costoclavicular ligaments | | | | Clavicular elevators |
| Depression | 30–0 | Sternal end of clavicle | Upper trapezius | | | | |

*Note:* Prime mover for upper extremity adduction from full abduction to neutral is the mass of the upper extremity acting at the center of mass of the upper extremity.

[a] Primary and secondary controllers act eccentrically.

(Modified from Schenkman and Rugo de Cartaya,[5] with permission.)

**Table 2-6. Muscle Action Analysis for Upper Extremity Adduction Against Resistance, 180°–0°**

| Joint and Motion | Range (degrees) | Axis | Prime Movers[a] | Secondary Movers[a] | Helping Synergists | Neutralizers | Antagonists |
|---|---|---|---|---|---|---|---|
| **Glenohumeral** | | | | | | | |
| Adduction | 180–90 | Glenohumeral joint | Latissimus dorsi Pectoralis major Sternal head Teres major | Triceps brachii Coracobrachialis | | | Glenohumeral abductors |
| | 90–0 | Glenohumeral joint | Latissimus dorsi Teres major | | | | |
| Internal rotation | 70–0 | Long axis of humerus | Latissimus dorsi Pectoralis major Subscapularis | Anterior deltoid | | | Glenohumeral external rotators |
| **Scapular** | | | | | | | |
| Downward rotation | 60–30 | Near acromioclavicular joint | Latissimus dorsi Rhomboid | Pectoralis minor Levator scapulae | Latissimus dorsi[b] and rhomboids | | Scapular upward rotators |
| | 30–0 | On spine of scapula near vertebral border | Rhomboid | Pectoralis minor Levator scapulae | | | |
| **Clavicular** | | | | | | | |
| Forward rotation | 50–0 | Long axis of clavicle | Subclavius | | | | |
| Depression | 30–0 | Sternal end of clavicle | | | | Intercostals and/or abdominus oblique may act to prevent elevation of the rib cage depending on force of activity | Clavicular elevators |

*Note:* Resistance to these muscles is applied on the humerus in an upward direction.

[a] Prime and secondary movers act concentrically.

[b] When latissimus dorsi attaches to the inferior angle of the scapula.

(Modified from Schenkman and Rugo de Cartaya,[5] with permission.)

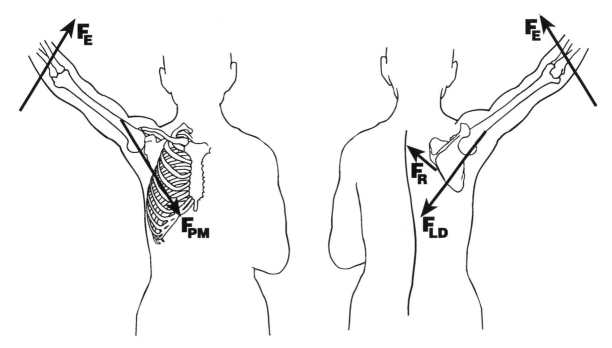

**Fig. 2-5.** Muscles acting during adduction against externally applied force. $F_{LD}$, latissimus dorsi; $F_{PM}$, pectoralis major; $F_R$, rhomboids; $F_E$, externally applied force. (Modified from Schenkman and Rugo de Cartaya,[5] with permission.)

jor,[20,24] both of which originate on the trunk and insert directly on the humerus. Because these muscles originate on the trunk rather than the scapula, the role of stabilizers is lessened compared with the role when muscles act on the humerus from the scapula. Second, the pectoralis major exerts a predominantly horizontal force with respect to the humerus, and the latissimus dorsi and teres major can potentially act as extensors of the humerus.[20,24] Thus, muscles such as the deltoids, supraspinatus, and biceps brachii must act as neutralizers of these unwanted motions to permit pure humeral adduction. Third, with respect to the scapula, this motion illustrates the role of muscles as helping synergists. The rhomboids and lower trapezius both retract the scapula; the rhomboids elevate it while the lower trapezius depresses it. Together, these muscles should retract the scapula without elevation or depression.

Forceful throwing, as in pitching, or hitting a ball with a racket, as in tennis and racquetball, requires the use of the upper extremity in an adduction direction and against resistance. Also, these particular types of activities require the use of the extremity in high-velocity situations, where the velocity particularly demands stabilization and instantaneous coordination of muscles.

## Upper Extremity in Closed Kinematic Chain Movements

The sitting push-up (Table 2-7; Fig. 2-6) illustrates the consequences of using the upper extremity in a closed kinematic chain. Because the hands are fixed with respect to the support surface, the muscles that would otherwise move the humerus with respect to the thorax now move the thorax with respect to the humerus. The muscles that are actively contracting cause the body to elevate relative to the stabilized humerus. This type of motion is essential in activities such as pole vaulting and vaulting in gymnastics. Prime movers for the sitting push-up include the latissimus dorsi, pectoralis major and minor, and to a lesser extent the lower trapezius.[11] Because these muscles act with the extremity as a closed kinetic chain, they exert their force at their origin rather than at their insertion. In other words, they work in reverse action. In contrast, muscles

**Table 2-7. Muscle Action Analysis for a Sitting Push-up**

| Joint and Motion | Range | Axis | Prime Movers[a] | Secondary Movers[a] | Helping Synergists | Neutralizers | Antagonists |
|---|---|---|---|---|---|---|---|
| **Scapular** depression (trunk is elevating on stabilized upper extremities) | Variable | No axis; translatory motion | Latissimus dorsi Pectoralis major sternal head Pectoralis minor Lower trapezius | | Latissimus dorsi and pectoralis major Pectoralis minor and lower trapezius | Infraspinatus and teres minor; neutralize internal rotation so the humerus remains neutral Abdominals neutralize any tendency of latissimus dorsi to anteriorly tilt the pelvis | Scapular elevators |

*Note:* Resistance is the mass of the body minus the upper extremities.

[a] Prime and secondary movers act bilaterally and in reverse action.

(Modified from Schenkman and Rugo de Cartaya,[5] with permission.)

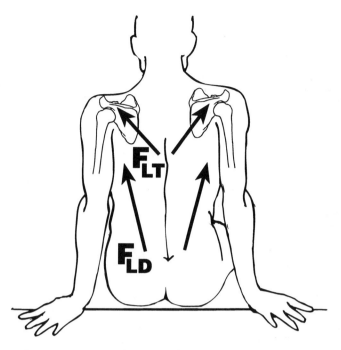

**Fig. 2-6.** Muscles acting during a sitting push-up. $F_{LD}$, latissimus dorsi; $F_{LT}$, lower trapezius. (Modified from Schenkman and Rugo de Cartaya,[5] with permission.)

that internally or externally rotate the humerus would work in normal action. Thus, some muscles that participate to complete the sitting push-up work in normal and some in reverse action, depending on how the specific body segments are moving relative to one another.

The thorax and pelvic complex must be stable for the latissimus dorsi and pectoralis muscles (that move the body relative to the humerus) to act effectively. Because these muscles work in reverse action, the stabilizers that act in synchrony with them are different from when they work in normal action.

## SUMMARY

The elements of a kinesiologic analysis of the shoulder complex have been presented in this chapter. The shoulder complex is composed of the humerus, scapula, and clavicle and their ligaments and muscles. These segments function as an integrated unit during all upper extremity function. Thus, a kinesiologic analysis

must include an identification and interpretation of their coordinated motion.

The elements for a kinesiologic analysis were identified: identification of the motion of individual segments with attention to both the range of motion that is completed and the joint axes of motion throughout that range; determination of the forces that produce and control motion; and determination of forces that provide stabilization for the movers and controllers, as well as muscles that provide stability for the total body during upper extremity motion. From these elements, it is possible to interpret the coordinated and integrated action of the both primary and secondary movements and muscle actions associated with even the simplest upper extremity maneuvers. Body position and support are important in any analysis.

Using this approach, four kinesiologic analyses were presented: unresisted upper extremity abduction, return from full abduction to neutral, resisted upper extremity adduction, and a sitting push-up. These four analyses were chosen to illustrate key issues of shoulder complex kinesiology including the effects of gravity on the extremity and on the muscles that move the extremity, the importance of normal versus reverse action of muscles in determining the secondary movers that work coordinately, and the importance of the changing joint axes of motion during the range of motion in determining muscle actions.

The kinesiologic analyses presented were developed from interpretations of electromyographic and kinematic literature. The same approach can be used to interpret any motion kinesiologically, to suggest preventative strategies to reduce the chance of injury in the athlete, and to make clinical judgments regarding rehabilitation of the shoulder complex once injury has occurred. During an evaluation, it is important to recognize that load, limb orientation with respect to the plane of the body, general body posture, muscle strength, ligament and joint integrity, bone integrity, and joint range of motion can all affect the muscles that will participate in any given activity.

In conclusion, it is essential to evaluate and treat the shoulder complex as a coordinated whole. This chapter was designed to provide the elements of a kinesiologic analysis that can be used to focus both evaluation and treatment.

# ACKNOWLEDGMENT

We thank Cheryl Riegger-Krugh, Sc.D., P.T. for her revisions of definitions of the roles of muscles in combined movement. We also gratefully acknowledge her thoughtful and comprehensive critique of this chapter.

# REFERENCES

1. Cathcart CW: Movements of the shoulder girdle involved in those of the arm and trunk. J Anat Physiol 18:211, 1884
2. Codman EA: The Shoulder. Thomas Todd, Boston, 1934
3. Inman VT, Saunders J, Abbott L: Observation on the function of the shoulder joint. J Bone Joint Surg 26:1, 1934
4. Engin E: On the biomechanics of the shoulder complex. J Biomech 13:537, 1980
5. Schenkman M, Rugo de Cartaya V: Kinesiology of the shoulder complex. J Orthop Sports Phys Ther 8:438, 1987
6. Dempster WT: Mechanisms of shoulder movement. Arch Phys Med Rehabil 46:49, 1965
7. Dvir Z, Berme N: The shoulder complex in elevation of the arm: a mechanism approach. J Biomech 11:219, 1978
7a. Poppen NK, Walker PS: Normal and abnormal motion of the shoulder. J Bone Joint Surg 58A:195, 1976
8. Serrafian JK: Gross and functional anatomy of the shoulder. Clin Orthop 173:11, 1987
9. de Luca C, Forrest WJ: Force analysis of individual muscles acting simultaneously in the shoulder joint during isometric abduction. J Biomech 6:385, 1973
10. Lucas DB: Biomechanics of the shoulder joint. Arch Surg 107:425, 1973
11. Perry J: Normal upper extremity kinesiology. Phys Ther 58:265, 1973
12. Inman VT, Saunders J: Observations on the function of the clavicle. CA Med 65:158, 1946
13. Abbott LR, Lucas DB: The function of the clavicle. Ann Surg 140:583, 1954
14. Kapandjii IA: The Physiology of the Joints. Vol. 1. The Upper Limb. Churchill Livingstone, Edinburgh, 1970
15. Saha AK: Dynamic stability of the glenohumeral joint. Acta Orthop Scand 42:491, 1971
16. Doody SC, Freedman L, Waterland JC: Shoulder movement during abduction in the scapular plane. Arch Phys Med Rehabil 51:595 1970
17. Braun BL, Amudsson LR: Quantitative assessment of head and shoulder posture. Arch Phys Med Rehabil 709:322, 1989
18. Schenkman M: Interrelationship between mechanical and neurologic factors in balance control. In Duncan PW (ed): Balance. Proceedings of the APTA Forum. American Physical Therapy Association, Washington, DC, 1990, pp 29–42
19. Bechtol CO: Biomechanics of the shoulder. Clinic Orthop 146:37, 1980
20. Basmajian JV: The surgical anatomy and function of the arm-trunk mechanism. Surg Clin North Am 43:1471, 1963
21. Jarvholm U, Palmerud G, Herberts P et al: Intramuscular pressure and electromyography in the supraspinatus muscle at shoulder abduction. Clin Orthop 245:102, 1989
22. Harms-Ringdahl K, Arborelius UP, Ekholm J et al: Shoulder externally rotating exercises with pully apparatus. Joint load and EMG. Scand J Rehabil Med 17:129, 1985
23. Sigholm G, Herberts P, Almstrom C, Kadefors R: Electromyographic analysis of shoulder muscle load. J Orthop Res 1:379, 1984
24. Basmajian JV: Muscles Alive. Their Function Revealed by Electromyography. 4th Ed. Williams & Wilkins, Baltimore, 1978
25. Scheving LE, Pauly JE: An electromyographic study of some muscles acting on the upper extremity of man. Anat Rec 135:237, 1959
26. Ringelberg JA: EMG and force production of some human shoulder muscles during isometric abduction. J Biomech 18:939, 1985
27. Turkel SJ, Panio MW, Marshall JL et al: Stabilizing mechanisms preventing anterior dislocation of the glenohumeral joint. J Bone Joint Surg 63A:1208, 1981

28. Pappas AM, Zawacki RM, Sullivan TJ: Biomechanics of baseball pitching. A preliminary report. Am J Sports Med 13:216, 1985

29. Elliot B, Marsh T: A biomechanical comparison of the topspin and backspin forehand approach shots in tennis. J Sports Sciences 7:215, 1989

30. Whiting WC, Puffer JC, Finerman GA et al: Three-dimensional cinematographic analysis of water polo throwing in elite performers. Am J Sports Med 13:95, 1985

31. Nuber GW, Jobe FW, Perry J et al: Fine wire electromyography analysis of muscles of the shoulder during swimming. Am J Sports Med 14:7, 1986

32. Jobe FW, Tibone JE, Perry J et al: An EMG analysis of the shoulder in throwing and pitching. A preliminary report. Am J Sports Med 11:3, 1983

33. Jobe FW, Moynes DR, Tibone JE, Perry J: An EMG analysis of the shoulder in pitching. A second report. Am J Sports Med 12:218, 1984

34. Gowan ID, Jobe FW, Tibone JE et al: A comparative electromyographic analysis of the shoulder during pitching. Professional versus amateur pitchers. Am J Sports Med 15:586, 1987

35. Riegger C, Watkins M: Applied Anatomy Laboratory Manual. 3rd Rev. Northeastern University Press, Boston, 1978

# 3

# The Subjective Evaluation of the Shoulder in the Athlete

*T. SCOTT MAUGHON*
*JAMES R. ANDREWS*

The successful treatment of any medical condition must first rely on an accurate and insightful history. To achieve this, the physician must elicit the facts in a direct, yet nonleading manner. Too often, the examiner is eager to make the diagnosis without first obtaining all the clues. In today's "high-tech" medical era, the clinician may tend to rely on investigative aids rather than the basic skills of the historical examination. There is no substitute for an accurate medical history. In this chapter, we discuss the method by which we obtain a thorough history for shoulder injuries in the athlete.

## INITIAL QUESTIONS

In the course of obtaining the history, the examiner must be careful not to focus too quickly on the shoulder joint. One should be aware of other pertinent facts such as the patient's general health status, previous injuries, previous conditions, and their individual treatments. If these steps are taken, the examiner can entertain a working diagnosis before starting the physical examination.

Our philosophy is simple. At the initial office visit, we routinely ask four questions: what, how, when, and where. The answers are placed on the front of the chart. At subsequent visits, the patient's initial problem can easily be found.

To elaborate on the four questions: What is the problematic area of anatomy? How did the problem occur? When did the problem develop? Where did the problem occur? Also, questions regarding the patient's age, handedness, occupation, marital status, domestic status (i.e., does the patient live alone?), leisure activities, and sports involvement are asked. Each of these questions may add additional insight to the problem.

Concurrent or underlying metabolic or genetic predispositions to illnesses may complicate the situation. Therefore, a general medical history should be obtained from each patient. If there is a problem, these areas may be pursued individually depending on their pertinence. For example, a person with adhesive capsulitis could be expected to have a more refractory course if the patient concomitantly is diabetic.[1] Another example would be the "voluntary dislocator" who has a history of psychiatric or emotional problems that could complicate the treatment.[2]

Once the problem and surrounding history have been identified, the next question that should be asked is "How long has this been bothering you?" (i.e., is this problem acute or chronic?). The most common presenting symptom with an acute injury is pain.[3-6] This may or may not be associated with instability. Chronic injuries may also present with the chief complaint being pain (i.e., a rotator cuff tear with night pain), but most chronic injuries present with other symptoms in addition, such as weakness, loss of motion, crepitus, deformity, catching, and inability to perform daily activities (Table 3-1).[4] Although a fall on the shoulder can cause a rotator cuff tear that may be tolerated initially, these problems commonly arise in an insidious manner rather than traumatically.[7]

**Table 3-1. Subjective Patient Information**

| Pathology | Subjective Comments |
| --- | --- |
| Impingement (stage I) | Intermittent mild pain with overhead activities. |
| Impingement (stage II) | Mild to moderate pain with overhead activities or strenuous activities. |
| Impingement (stage III) | Pain at rest or with activities. Night pain may occur. Weakness is noted. |
| Rotator cuff tears (full thickness) | Classic night pain. Weakness noted predominantly in abductors and external rotators. Loss of Motion. |
| Adhesive capsulitis (frozen shoulder) | Inability to perform activities of daily living owing to loss of motion. Loss of motion may be perceived as weakness. |
| Anterior instability | Apprehension to mechanical shifting limits activities. Slipping, popping, or sliding may present as subtle instability. Apprehension usually associated with horizontal abduction and external rotation. Anterior or posterior pain may be present. |
| Posterior instability | Slipping or popping out the back. This may be associated with forward flexion and internal rotation while the shoulder is under a compressive load. |
| Multi-directional instability | Looseness of shoulder in all directions. This may be most pronounced while carrying luggage or turning over while asleep. Pain may or may not be present. |

## PAIN

When the chief complaint is pain, it is important to know the age of the patient and the course and the nature of the pain. These questions alone will usually formulate the diagnosis, and the physical examination confirms the initial suspicion.

Often, the temptation is to focus directly on the shoulder for the underlying pathology, but we must rule out referred pain of cervical origin.[8] Radicular pain from the cervical spine is typically more dermatomal in distribution, and it may involve a "pins and needles" sensation. It also may radiate diffusely from the neck down over the top of the shoulder. This must be differentiated from the well-localized pain that the patient can pinpoint.

Next, one should ask about the character of the pain, the precipitating causes, and factors that aggravate and relieve the pain.

The character of the pain may be the most essential question. Describing the pain that typifies the problem can often lead to the diagnosis. Sharp pain may indicate an acute inflammatory process. A dull, aching pain or sense of heaviness may indicate chronic rotator cuff pathology or even a full-thickness tear.[7] Inability to take the arm across the side of the face or overhead after a blow to the shoulder may indicate acromioclavicular joint pathology.[9] Pain and apprehension associated with abduction and external rotation is classic for anterior instability.[10–12] Progressive pain or dull aching while pitching that is exacerbated with abduction and external rotation may indicate quadrilateral space syndrome or some vascular occlusion.[13] Pain associated with follow-through or cross-chest activities may correlate with posterior instability or be the manifestation of multidirectional instability.[5] A patient with advanced multidirectional instability may complain of pain associated with the shoulder "slipping" while sleeping or in association with positional changes. Joint noise associated with pain may suggest a loose body, a torn labrum, or subacromial bursitis.[5] Posterior pain that is deep and diffuse may be caused by entrapment of the suprascapular nerve, but this is usually a diagnosis of exclusion.[14,15]

Although pain about the shoulder may be nonspecific in origin, pain associated with apprehension is usually rather specific in making the diagnosis of instability. This is an aggravating factor that points the clinician toward the underlying process. The feeling of apprehension is due to the fear of impending instability if the position of subluxation or dislocation is attempted. The degree of instability is confirmed by physical examination.

## INSTABILITY

Once the suspicion of instability has occurred, it is important to determine the date of initial onset. By determining the frequency of instability episodes and the patient's age, the prognosis for recurrence can be given.[16] Often, patients who have instability will report a slipping out or a popping out sensation.

When instability is suspected, the primary direction should be ascertained. The most common pattern of dislocation is anterior and unilateral. This accounts for approximately 98 percent of all dislocations. Up to 60 percent of posterior dislocations are missed initially. This is believed to result from the physician's relying on the radiographs and not the clinical examination to make the diagnosis.[16] Anterior dislocations are classically known for the "apprehension" test.[16] The physician is able to reproduce the patient's symptoms by abducting and externally rotating the humerus. This allows translation of the humeral head anteriorly, thus creating the symptoms that cause the pain. The patient commonly will not allow the same degree of motion as is allowed in the contralateral extremity because of the pain and apprehension of possible dislocation. The anterior dislocation most often occurs because of an abducted arm with external rotation, and this motion is overstressed. Clients may report that when trying to throw or serve a tennis ball, they feel their shoulder popping out.

Posterior dislocations or subluxations are usually demonstrable by the patient. The patient may reproduce the feelings of subluxation by bringing the arm across the chest along with internal rotation. The clunk of reduction can be felt when the arm is brought toward the coronal plane of the body. The pathomechanics for posterior instability is much different from that of anterior; often it occurs from a fall onto an overstretched arm or from a pushing motion.

The posterior subluxator may be able to show the positional change that causes the painful subluxation; the voluntary dislocator has no difficulty and minimal pain associated with demonstrating the feat. One must be aware of the difference in the two types of patients. A further search into this subgroup of voluntary dislocators must be sought to expose any underlying personality disorders. Recognition of these patients with personality disorders is important because these patients may frustrate attempts at stabilization, whether operative or nonoperative.[2]

Multidirectional instability may present in a similar fashion to posterior instability. Patients may complain of "slipping" or a "loose feeling" in their shoulders. This feeling may be exacerbated by loading the shoulder inferiorly, as occurs with lifting a suitcase or carrying a heavy object. The patient with multidirectional instability may present the most clinical challenge. These patients are not always sure of their primary direction of instability. The physician must use all the clinical acumen available to diagnose accurately the primary direction.[17]

After the direction of instability is determined, the next question is how much disability is associated with the instability. The patient who dislocates once a month and requires relocation at the hospital is much more disabled than the patient who dislocates once every 3 years and spontaneously relocates. Further insight must be obtained by eliciting how the instability affects the patient's daily activities. If the patient is unable to perform certain activities because of fear of subluxation or frank dislocation, the patient may require more aggressive care.

## WEAKNESS

Weakness may also be the presenting complaint in the new patient with a shoulder problem. In the presence of pain, the diagnosis may be confusing. Weakness is related to a neurologic problem, rotator cuff deficiency, or occult subluxation. The most common cause of weakness is rotator cuff deficiency. Early pathology within the rotator cuff may exhibit minimal pain. As the problem progresses or in the face of a full-thickness tear, the shoulder may present with classic "night pain" or activity-induced pain, which may cause pain later that night.[7]

Neer[18] cited three stages of classic shoulder impingement. In stage 1 the patient is younger than 25 years of age and reports intermittent mild pain. Stage 2 develops in patients 25 to 40 years of age who have pain with shoulder activity. In stage 3, patients 40 years of age or older report pain with or without activity.

What appears to be weakness to the patient may be decreased motion related to adhesive capsulitis. This commonly occurs in the middle-aged homemaker after a minor insult. This usually comes on spontaneously and progresses from pain alone, to pain and stiffness, and then stiffness alone. This may be when the patient first presents to the physician. What the patient perceives as weakness is decreased motion secondary to adhesive capsulitis.

## DEFORMITY

Deformity as a primary presenting complaint is usually the result of an old or pre-existing problem that the patient suddenly notices. The prominence of the acromioclavicular joint after an old acromioclavicular separation, the prominence from residual callous after a clavicle fracture, and congenital abnormalities such as Sprengel's deformity or pseudoarthrosis of the clavicle may go unnoticed until the developmental awareness years. Although these are more atypical than the usual complaints, they must be considered.

## RELIEF

When all the inciting events have been isolated, it is time to ask the patient how relief of the symptoms is achieved. The physician must ask whether any over-the-counter or prescription drugs have been taken, and if so, whether they have had any effect. The physician must ask if rest, ice, or any other therapeutic modalities have given any relief. Some patients may have received injections from their primary care physicians. All these questions must be asked to perform an accurate and thorough history.

## SUMMARY

This chapter attempts to encompass the full historical examination of shoulder injuries. Although some pathologic entities have probably not been discussed, we hope this framework will allow the clinician to create an insightful preliminary diagnosis by performing an accurate historical examination.

If an accurate and thorough historical examination is performed, the physical examination should confirm the suspected diagnosis. Once this has been confirmed, the patient will be able to embark on a treatment course with the ultimate goal to return to his or her previous quality of life.

## REFERENCES

1. Bridgman JF: Periarthritis of the shoulder and diabetes mylitis. Ann Rheum Dis 31:69, 1972
2. Rowe CR, Pierce DS, Clark JG: Voluntary dislocation of the shoulder: a preliminary report of clinical, EMG, and psychiatric study of 26 patients. J Bone Joint Surg 55:445, 1973
3. Hawkins RJ, Hobeika P: Physical examination of the shoulder. Orthopedics 6:1270, 1983
4. Hawkins RJ: Clinical evaluation of shoulder problems. In Rockwood CA, Matsen FA (eds): The Shoulder. WB Saunders, Philadelphia, 1990
5. Jobe FW, Jobe CW: Painful athletic injuries of the shoulder. Clin Orthop 173:117, 1983
6. Jobe FW, Kvitne RS: Shoulder pain in the overhand or throwing athlete. The relationship of anterior instability and rotator cuff impingement. Orthop Rev 18:963, 1989
7. Cofield RH: Current concepts review, rotator cuff disease of the shoulder. J Bone Joint Surg 67A:974, 1985
8. Hawkins RJ: Cervical spine in the shoulder. Instr Course Lect 34:191, 1985
9. Allman FL: Fractures in ligamentous injuries of the clavicle and its articulations. J Bone Joint Surg 49A:774, 1967
10. Neer CS, Welsh RP: The shoulder in sports. Orthop Clin North Am 8:583, 1977
11. O'Brien SJ, Warren RF, Schwarz E: Anterior shoulder instability. Orthop Clin North Am 18:395, 1987
12. Rowe CR: Recurrent transient anterior subluxation of the shoulder, the "dead arm" syndrome. Clin Orthop 223:11, 1986
13. Redler MR, Ruland LJ, McCue FC: Quadrilateral space syndrome in a throwing athlete. Am J Sports Med 14:511, 1986
14. Post M, Mayer J: Suprascapular nerve entrapment, diagnosis and treatment. Clin Orthop 223:126, 1987
15. Rask MR: Suprascapular nerve entrapment. A report of two cases treated with suprascapular notch resection. Clin Orthop 123:73, 1977
16. Rockwood CA: Subluxations and dislocations about the shoulder. p. 722. In Green DP (ed): 2nd Ed. JB Lippincott, Philadelphia, 1984
17. Neer CS: Involuntary inferior and multidirectional instability of the shoulder: etiology, recognition, and treatment. Instr Course Lect 34:232, 1985
18. Neer CS: Impingement lesions. Clin Orthop 173:170, 1983

# 4

# Elements of a Standardized Shoulder Examination

*TERRY R. MALONE*

This chapter addresses the components of a standardized examination process for the shoulder. This process requires attention to detail, recognizing the function of the shoulder as that of multiple joints functioning in "complex" rather than individual actions at single joints. Most evaluation schemes have been derived through the particular emphases of the individual practitioner.[1-4] Most involve an anatomic inspection moving toward a functional examination through range of motion and neurologic assessment, followed by specific tests for particular structures. Fortunately, the contemporary clinician is able to increase this data base to include assessment of strength and the evaluation of function by multiple techniques. This chapter, a "primer" to the standardized shoulder evaluation, is not exhaustive but rather selective. Radiographic, magnetic resonance imaging, arthrotomography, and ultrasonography modes of assessment are discussed in other chapters.

The recommended schema for shoulder evaluation is presented, but the specific tests commonly used in the manual examination of the musculoskeletal complex are in Chapter 5. Additional portions of this chapter describe strength assessment (static and dynamic) and culminate in a discussion of functional assessments.

## EXAMINATION SCHEMA

Clinicians must develop an evaluation form or sequence to enable them to be effective and efficient. A written form is helpful to keep the clinician focused and to avoid becoming too "finding" oriented. We all tend to be more likely to jump to conclusions when an expected positive examination is confirmed by our hands. The following series of tenets may help in developing an evaluation form or sequence.

1. The evaluation should begin with the patient's subjective description of the chief complaint (i.e., why are you here in the clinic?; what was the onset of this problem—abrupt or insidious?; level of pain?; how long has it been hurting?; acute or chronic?; when does it hurt—do you have pain at night, do you have pain at rest?; what type of pain is present?; what has been the effect of rest, heat, ice, exercise, etc.?; have you tried an anti-inflammatory drug?; in both sport and work, what do you wish to do, and what are you unable to do?; have you had this problem before?; and is there a medical history of diabetes in your family?) and very important as you begin your objective evaluation, have the person point with one finger to the area of pain—this enables you to determine location and to begin the process of evaluation for referral of pain rather than structure only. These are examples of the types of questions that should be asked to get a "picture" of the condition before proceeding into an objective assessment.
2. Screen—Be certain to look at the cervical spine, as multiple "shoulder problems" are related to underlying nerve roots of segmental facilitation and are easily misinterpreted as a peripheral problem.
3. The general evaluation sequence (see Table 4-1).

Clinicians must develop a process that works for them and, in their particular setting, provides informa-

**Table 4-1. Objective Standardized Scheme**

Observation
Active motion
Palpation
Passive motion
Resisted motion
Joint play
Orthopaedic tests
Strength—isometric/dynamic assessment
Functional performance

tion to assess the patient on the initial visit but also allows them to assess the effectiveness of their treatment at ensuing clinical visits. This objective standardized scheme is described in Table 4-1. Most of Table 4-1 is described in Chapters 3, 5, 10, 15–17, 19, 31, and 32 of this text. We focus our attention on the difficult problems of strength assessment and functional performance.

## Strength Assessment

Unfortunately, our assessment of muscular output is typically performed noninvasively. Thus, although muscle tissue is generating tension through its attachments by tendon to the skeletal system, we are in turn not measuring the absolute tension generation capacity of the muscle. Rather, we are assessing changes in multiple components of the ability of the muscle to generate tension and alterations in the skeletal system and corresponding changes in length tension ratios, rotational orientation, compression, leverage, and angulation.[5,6]

Our operational definition of strength is delineated by the methodology of assessment and, thus, whether we are going to be looking at force, torque, power, and/or work values. Some individuals have gone so far

as to recommend isometric assessment as being the most appropriate to minimize some of the alterations previously described.[7] Unfortunately, the shoulder is a "dynamic" joint, as it completely depends on musculature for its stability and functional patterns. Although fraught with dangers, combining isometric assessment of individual muscle functions with dynamic assessment of movement patterns gives a clearer understanding of involved tissues and appropriate intervention.

## Muscle Actions

Characteristics of muscle action are presented in Table 4-2. The assessment of muscle action is best described as muscle activation with the external load determining the observed function. This means that an object will be controllably lowered, held in place, or raised by the applied muscular action. This avoids the problem of describing an eccentric activity as a muscle contraction when, in fact, the muscle fibers are controllably lengthening. It is important for the clinician to determine if the patient is describing difficulties with concentric or eccentric actions, as the inherent stability and functioning of the shoulder complex requires a controlled sequence of all three types of muscle activity or activation.

In general terms, eccentric contractions generate the highest tension per unit area of muscle, followed by isometric and concentric actions. Isometric assessment or action may present our best opportunity to assess tension capability of the active component of the musculature but may be of limited value in predicting functional capacity. Concentric actions can be performed isotonically or isokinetically but are frequently misinterpreted because of the inhibitory effects of effusion, pain, and altered recruitment.[6,8]

**Table 4-2. Characteristics of Muscle Actions**

| | Action | Level of Output/Unit Area | Metabolic Demands |
|---|---|---|---|
| Isometric | Tension-producing, no motion | Moderate | Intensity-related |
| Concentric | | | |
| Isotonic | Movement of a resistance (weight) through a range of motion | Low/moderate | High |
| Isokinetic | Machine-controlled speed of motion | Low/moderate | High |
| Eccentric | | | |
| Isotonic | Weight being lowered through a range of motion | Low | Low |
| Isokinetic | Machine-controlled speed of motion "driving" the muscle to a length while being activated | High | Low(?) |

## ISOMETRIC TECHNIQUES

### Manual Muscle Testing

Manual muscle testing is a frequently used system of manually applied loads against gravity or with gravity minimized to determine the voluntary response of the patient. Patients must be urged to be consistent in how they assess (make or break) and in position of evaluation (midrange or locked) to minimize differing results.[9]

The many problems of manual muscle testing include assessment of athletes who surpass normal and the tremendous difficulty in intertester reliability. Length of time allowed to generate tension as well as the ability to reproduce this on a repeated basis, coupled with the problems of multijoint muscle assessment, makes manual muscle testing useful in screening patients but of limited value in attempting to assess muscular output objectively in the "dynamic" shoulder.

### Hand-Held Dynamometry

Multiple hand-held dynamometers have been developed to enhance the objectivity of a manual examination, thus measuring manual muscle testing. These devices have been shown to be acceptable to clinical settings both in terms of reliability and validity[10] but again preclude the assessment of the dynamic shoulder.

### Cable Tensiometry

Cable tensiometers assess isometric output through a perpendicular tension assessment popularized by Clarke.[11] These devices have not gained wide acceptance in clinical settings and have been used primarily in a testing situation and have not carried over into the function or rehabilitation of patients.

## ISOTONIC ASSESSMENT

Isotonic weight lifting involves the movement of a weight through a range of motion both in raising (concentric) and lowering (eccentric). The multiple problems with this include the limitation by the neural drive provided through the central nervous system and the inhibition that may be provided through the peripheral system. This includes the person's ability to recruit muscle and also his or her ability to use it in different formats, including concentric and eccentric patterns. This also brings us to the difficulty of endurance and repeatability of actions. The isotonic movement is limited to the "weakest link" which is typically the maximal concentric pattern such as 90 degrees of abduction at the glenohumeral joint. Factors vital to isotonic assessment include lever arm length and speed of movement. The perpendicular distance from the axis of rotation dictates the force required for the movement, whereas the person's ability to move quickly and smoothly provides great input of the functional capability of the dynamic shoulder. A stronger individual has the ability to accelerate a particular weight in a more free and controlled pattern than the "weaker" individual, but this should also force us to look closely at substitution and requirement of synchronous action before automatically accepting the performance of the stronger individual as being adequate. Inherent in the isotonic assessment is fatigue and completion of range of motion during testing.

Isotonic measurements may reflect function, particularly in activities that require fairly slow movements. However, the average speed of isotonic assessment is approximately 60 degrees per second, and concentric assessment may not reflect eccentric performance.[6,7,12] Clinicians will continue to use isotonic assessment but should recognize that it primarily reflects concentric performance unless additional loading is provided during assessment. This author recommends such activity, particularly when assessing the supraspinatus and external rotators, because these are frequently functioning in an eccentric/stabilizing/reducing pattern.

## ISOKINETIC ASSESSMENT

Isokinetic exercise devices involve speed-controlled movements as the patient accelerates a lever arm to a predetermined maximal velocity and then moves through a range of motion and decelerates at the end of the range to the terminal position. These devices first emerged during the 1960s and now are nearly ubiquitous in orthopaedic and sports medicine practices. Isokinetic exercise has become extremely popular not only for assessment but also for rehabilitation with the concepts of recruitment, contraction synchrony, and multiple velocity exercise patterns.[13,14] One of the primary advantages of this type of assessment is the ability to evaluate individual muscle patterns in a dynamic orientation while providing some inherent stability to the testing positions. The information collected from these machines is on a machine-specific format; different machines handle the collected data through different software programs.[15]

A relatively new advancement in the isokinetic area involves the evaluation of eccentric actions. Isokinetic (speed-controlled) eccentric actions can be performed two ways: by overcoming a predetermined load and having the lever arm drive the extremity at the predetermined velocity; or by having the individual work against a "passively" moving lever arm at the predetermined velocity. The neurophysiology of these actions may be different from the eccentric activity seen with isotonic actions, and again these actions are very machine-specific in their interpretation. Clinicians have seen the different pattern of torque production with isokinetic concentric activity decreasing as speed increases versus a relative plateau seen in eccentric peak torque assessment.[6]

Although clinicians have grown accustomed to the interpretation of isokinetic exercise being very performance-oriented, minimal true patterns of function or performance are evaluated. Clinicians must recognize the limitations of isokinetic assessment with open and closed kinetic patterns and with functional levels in speed being somewhat inconsistent.

For isokinetic assessment to have meaning, a standardized protocol for the evaluation should be followed.[16] Evaluation via isokinetics should be accomplished only after the clinician has determined what he or she wishes to evaluate and the type of contraction that would be most appropriate, enabling meaningful information to be provided. Thus, the clinician must determine what plane of motion to evaluate and what would be the most appropriate testing position. This process is defined in detail in Chapter 43.

Assessment of strength is a multifaceted problem caused by our inability to take direct measurements and not have our assessment clouded by neural drive, inhibition, pain, changing lever arms, etc. Although our ability to measure output has improved substantially, we still have not developed techniques directly related to function. Because the shoulder joint is dynamic, we are forced to be cautious in our interpretation of muscular assessment. Clinicians are urged not to overly interpret and use single pieces of data that are frequently provided by our isokinetic devices.

## FUNCTIONAL ASSESSMENT

Performance evaluation is a critical part of the evaluation schema. It is not atypical for no problem to be determined through clinical evaluation until the high demands of dynamic shoulder function are requested. This is why many practitioners now use the terminology of clinical stability versus functional stability. Functional stability requires the neuromuscular integration and synchronous activity to enable the performance of high-demand dynamic movements.

The evaluation of performance should be directed toward the activities required of work or desired athletic pursuit and most likely is related to the reason the patient has come for evaluation. Thus, the evaluation of function should be patient-specific. As mentioned before, the clinician must attempt to determine not only location of pain but also the action of structures at that point in the functional pattern. An example of this will be elucidated in Chapter 32. "Concentric" pain usually indicates musculotendinous junction problems or impingement of either bony, labral, or soft tissues. Eccentric pain is typically related to tendinous lesions or high-demand decelerative efforts to provide dynamic stability.

Although this sounds fairly simplistic, the interpretation of functional activities can be extremely difficult and challenging for experienced as well as inexperienced clinicians.

## CONCLUSIONS

We must recognize the difficulty of assessing these multiple structures that function in a dynamic pattern about this soft tissue structure. Shoulder evaluation must be systematic and activity-specific. Unfortunately, not all problems are related to a single structure, which leads to difficulty in isolating our treatment sequence.

Clinicians have a tendency of wishing to apply a protocol of treatment that may not address all patterns or involved structures. The following case study exemplifies this problem.

A 15-year-old female swimmer with a 6-month history of bilateral shoulder pain (right greater than left) presented to our clinic with the previous diagnosis of impingement. Her previous treatment included strengthening (internal rotators and external rotators), anti-inflammatories, and rest. Continued problems led her to receive bilateral injections with corticosteroid with minimal response. Her radiographs had been negative and she had just been told that it is common for swimmers in her age group to continue to have such problems.

We observed a healthy 15-year-old swimmer whose right scapula was lower than the left; she had forward head posture and a very strong bilateral internal rotation bias. Her present swimming routine involved 3,000 to 5,000 m in the morning followed by 3,000 to 5,000 m in the afternoon, with most of these strokes being freestyle. Her routine included the use of hand paddles during the past 6 to 8 months, when she also developed her "impingement problems."

Range of motion evaluation, both active and passive, revealed an internal rotation limitation of approximately 10 degrees bilaterally, but she moves her scapulae and trunk to achieve the additional movement. Her instability assessment revealed a positive posterior apprehension test on the right as well as a similar apprehension relation on the right. She had some posterior labral tenderness on the right during testing and also exhibited positive impingement bilaterally. *Strength Assessment*—Her manual muscle test revealed weak external rotators with very strong internal rotators; her isokinetic assessment (prone data) revealed a 42 percent external rotation to internal rotation ratio. *Functional Assessment*—Her activities obviously revolved around swimming and her training techniques associated with this. She had been doing a strengthening routine but continued to emphasize internal rotators rather than attempting to correct the imbalance with her external rotators. It was important in testing of this individual to do the testing in a prone position to duplicate her functional positions.

Our assessment led to the recognition that she does have impingement but secondary to lack of humeral head control associated with instability, as well as an activity-related problem of swimming, particularly with the emphasis on the use of hand paddles.

As her external rotation strength was enhanced and her use of hand paddles eliminated, her symptoms began to rapidly resolve. She became essentially asymptomatic when a 50 percent external rotation to internal rotation ratio was achieved. Frequently a person who does have some instability and impingement overlap may do fairly well if dynamic control is enhanced.

As with most clinical activities, evaluation is the key. Proper rehabilitation and interventions can be provided only when specific structure is enhanced within an overall context. The goal of the clinical examination must be to establish the nature and severity of the injury or pathology and dysfunction and to address such in the most appropriate fashion.

# REFERENCES

1. Andrews JR, Gillogly S: Physical examination of the shoulder in throwing athletes. In Zarins B, Andrews JR, Carson WG (eds): Injuries to the Throwing Arm. WB Saunders, Philadelphia, 1985
2. Cyriax J: Textbook of Orthopaedic Medicine. 8th Ed. Bailliere Tindall, Philadelphia, 1982
3. Hoppenfeld S: Physical Examination of the Spine and Extremities. Appleton-Century-Crofts, East Norwalk, CT, 1976
4. Magee DJ: Orthopaedic Physical Assessment. WB Saunders, Philadelphia, 1987
5. Williams M, Lissner HR: Biomechanics of Human Movement. WB Saunders, Philadelphia, 1966
6. Malone TR: Muscle Injury and Rehabilitation. Sports Injury Management. Vol. 1, No. 3. Williams & Wilkins, Baltimore, 1988
7. Rothstein JM: Measurement in Physical Therapy. Churchill Livingstone, New York, 1985
8. DeAndrade J, Grant C: Joint distension and reflex inhibition in the knee. J Bone Joint Surg 47:313, 1965
9. Poland J, Hobart D, Payton O: The Musculoskeletal System. Medical Examination Publishers, Garden City, NY, 1981
10. Bohannon R: Test–retest reliability of hand-held dynamometry during a single session of strength assessment. Phys Ther 66:206, 1986
11. Clarke HH: Cable Tension Strength Test: A Manual. Stuart E Murphy, Springfield, MA, 1953
12. Sanders M, Sanders B: Mobility: active-resistive training. In Gould J, Davies G (eds): Orthopaedic and Sports Physical Therapy. CV Mosby, St. Louis, 1985

13. Davies G: A Compendium of Isokinetics in Clinical Usage. 2nd Ed. S&S Publishers, LaCrosse, WI, 1985
14. Lesmes GR, Costill DL, Coyle EF, Fink WJ: Muscle strength and power change during maximal isokinetic training. Med Sci Sports 10:266, 1978
15. Malone TR: Evaluation of Isokinetic Equipment. Sports Injury Management. Vol. 1, No. 1. Williams & Wilkins, Baltimore, 1988
16. Wilk KE, Arrigo CA, Andrews JR: Standardized isokinetic testing protocol for the throwing shoulder: the throwers' series. Isokin Exerc Sci 1:63, 1991

# 5

# Clinical Examination of the Shoulder Complex

*JAMES F. SILLIMAN*
*RICHARD J. HAWKINS*

Successful management of any clinical problem begins with an accurate history and physical examination. This chapter is dedicated to the physical examination of the athlete's shoulder. Overhead athletes who swim, throw, and serve present with special problems. The extreme forces that act on the shoulder girdle during these activities cannot be re-created in a typical examination. With new technology for assessment, such as motion analysis, we now know that these forces often exceed the physiologic limits of the capsuloligamentous restraints of the rotator cuff.[1] If the rate of injury (overuse) exceeds that of repair, impairment and dysfunction result.[2] Pain is the most common presenting symptom.[3] The emphasis of the etiology of this pain has evolved from biceps[3,4] and rotator cuff impingement tendinitis[5-9] to anterior instability, with obvious overlap between these etiologies in many athletes.

An accurate and thorough examination can only be performed in a relaxed environment. The patient should be clothed so the patient is relaxed, but the examiner should have adequate visibility of both shoulder girdles and the upper trunk. The examination is performed with the patient standing, sitting, supine, or prone as necessary. The history often biases the clinician to focus on a specific aspect of the examination; however, an organized screening examination should be performed in every patient. Because of the interaction of many factors contributing to the symptom complex in these athletes, it is essential to have a thorough understanding of the entire shoulder girdle, especially glenohumeral and scapulothoracic interplay.

We suggest an organized, thorough, and consistent format when examining an athlete's shoulder. Re-creation of the patient's symptoms with certain maneuvers may help the examiner to arrive at an accurate diagnosis. Great variability exists from patient to patient in range of motion, joint laxity, and strength. Often, certain sports require emphasis on different aspects of these facets. For example, gymnastics demands hypermobile or hyperlax joints, and weight lifting demands excess strength. The examination proceeds in the following sequence, remembering presentation can be in the acute setting immediately after an injury or more often in a chronic situation presenting to our clinic or office.

## INITIAL CURSORY IMPRESSION

On first visualizing the athlete, one forms an initial cursory impression encompassing many factors. For example, a large muscular individual with a mesomorph frame obviously suggests one in a strength-type of sport, such as weight lifting or football. A petite young woman might well suggest a gymnastics interest. In analyzing these patients, we may see those who have an acute injury presenting with significant pain, which influences our approach to the situation. The older athlete presenting to our office in a business suit presents a different impression from the 6 ft-10 in. basketball player who walks into our athletic clinic directly from practice.

## INSPECTION

Inspection should be performed from different perspectives (i.e., from the front, the side, the back, and the top), noting attitude (symmetry), muscles (wasting or hypertrophy), deformities (scars, lumps, bumps, etc.), any evidence of discoloration such as bruising, and finally swelling.

The way the athlete carries his or her upper trunk and shoulders provides clues as to diagnosis. For example, an athlete with a painful shoulder may show asymmetry between the trapezius contours when looking from the front and back. Dominance may lead to asymmetry between the size and contours of the different shoulder girdle muscles. The symmetry of the borders of the clavicle, acromioclavicular joint, and sternoclavicular joints should also be

noted. Deformities in these areas are often revealing. Scars should be inspected not only as evidence of previous surgical procedures but also for widening or spreading of the scars, which may denote a collagen abnormality as seen in patients with multidirectional instability.[10]

Evidence of wasting of different muscles or muscle groups may suggest certain diagnoses. Deltoid wasting may appear as prominence and "squaring" of the acromial borders. Supraspinatus and infraspinatus wasting can be related to rotator cuff tear[11] or rarely suprascapular nerve injury.[12] Occasionally, hypertrophy of a muscle such as the trapezius may be due to muscle spasm. A patient with a recent injury may have bruising with associated discoloration. Swelling and discoloration are uncommon in chronic complaints but often present with acute trauma.

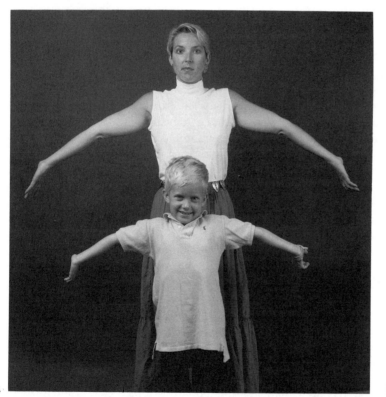
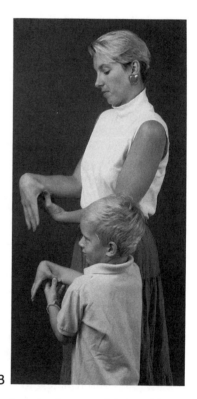

A                                                                    B

**Fig. 5-1(A&B).**  Ligamentous laxity and hypermobility can be appreciated from observing the patient's hyperextensible elbows or the thumb-to-forearm examination, as shown.

## OBSERVATION

Before focusing on range of motion about the shoulder, one might gain an appreciation for glenohumeral and scapulothoracic synchrony. Beginning at 30 degrees of abduction, every 30 degrees of glenohumeral abduction relates to 12 degrees of scapular rotation.[13–15] Dyskinesia or asynchrony of this coupled mechanism can be related to loss of range of motion or guarding. Weakness of the scapular stabilizers with resultant scapular winging can be part of the symptom complex of anterior shoulder pain, especially in the throwing athlete. It is common for the throwing athlete or for those patients with subtle forms of multidirectional and posterior instability to have scapular winging. This is usually not related to a neurologic deficit but rather to "dyskinesia" of the scapulothoracic articulation.

From behind the standing patient, observation of the scapulothoracic joint with forward flexion and abduction is performed. Scapular winging can be made more obvious by adding resistance to forward flexion of both arms simultaneously or observing a "wall push-up." A general appreciation for ligamentous laxity can be observed with extension of the elbow and thumb-to-forearm examination, to name two (Fig. 5-1).

## PALPATION

Thorough palpation of the shoulder girdle is now performed, noting warmth, tenderness, deformity, and crepitus. Starting from the back, palpation of the cervical spinous processes, scapular spine, medial border of the scapula, and scapular angle may reveal tender areas. Scapulothoracic bursitis at the inferior medial angle of the scapula may present in baseball pitchers.[16,17] Superior angle tenderness and snapping in the tennis serve are not uncommon presenting complaints. Posterior cuff and capsule should be palpated deep to the infraspinatus muscle belly. Posterior cuff is often tender not only with posterior instability but also with anterior instability. Posterior capsular ossification can lead to significant pain and dysfunction during the throwing motion.[18] Palpation of the rhomboids, latissimus, and supra- and infraspinatus can give an assessment of their tone. From the back, the location of the

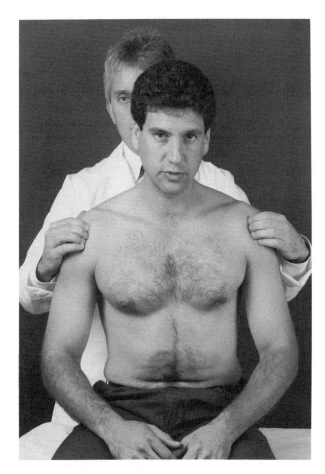

**Fig. 5-2.** From the back of the patient, bicipital groove anatomy and tendon can be appreciated by palpating simultaneously within the groove and noting whether this elicits pain from the patient.

bicipital tendons can be palpated simultaneously to ascertain tenderness (Fig. 5-2). Moving to the front of the standing or seated patient, palpation of the sternoclavicular joint statically and with arm rotation may reveal tenderness, crepitus, or even instability. The clavicle and acromioclavicular joint are also palpated in this fashion. A common injury in the collision athlete is to the acromioclavicular joint.[19] Acutely, athletes can present with a wide range of severity of injury and deformity to this joint, with varying degrees of prominence of the outer clavicle. The classification scheme of Rockwood and Green[20] is useful for appropriate management. Chronic injury to the acromioclavicular joint can lead to hypertrophy and pain with impingement or degenerative joint disease. The cross-arm test will be painful with acromioclavicular pathology.[21] The arm is forcibly adducted across the chest wall, causing pain. Injection of 5 ml 1 percent lidocaine directly into the joint with relief of the symptomatology in the cross-arm test can assist in the diagnosis of primary acromioclavicular pathology.

The subacromial arch is assessed initially with palpation of the greater tuberosity and the supraspinatus insertion. With circumduction of the arm, an appreciation of the crepitus is important, especially in rotator cuff disease and degenerative joint disease of the glenohumeral joint. A positive clunk test or labral grinding can point to labral pathology.[22] Palpable crepitus or grinding with the arm abducted to 90 degrees and the humeral head translated to the anterior rim of the glenoid with a posterior force (either prone or seated) and rotation of the arm is considered positive (Fig. 5-3).

## RANGE OF MOTION ASSESSMENT

The rhythm and synchrony of scapulothoracic and glenohumeral motion have been discussed. Athletes are often selectively or generally hypermobile in performing their different movements. For example, accomplished baseball pitchers show extremes of external rotation at times at the expense of internal rotation.[17] Gymnasts are hypermobile in many joints. The quality of the examination is often improved with use of a worksheet to record range of motion. Examination for different ranges in different circumstances can be performed standing, sitting, or supine, depending on clinician preference.

From behind the standing patient, active forward elevation is observed. The patient is allowed to flex his or her arm in the plane that is most comfortable, usually somewhere between the sagittal and scapular planes. Once the patient has achieved maximum active range, passive range is assessed by stressing the arm into

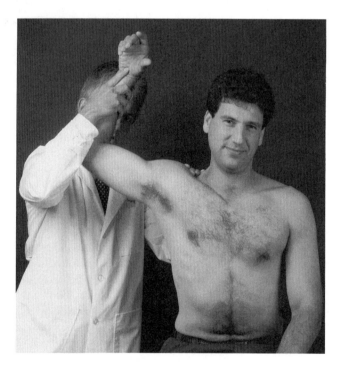

**Fig. 5-3.** The "crank" test is performed by placing the abducted arm to 90 degrees, translating the humeral head anteriorly by posterior force, and palpating and feeling for crepitus, or grinding, on the anterior rim of the glenoid.

forward elevation. This represents the classical "impingement sign," which is described later. The passive range is recorded bilaterally in degrees. External rotation is evaluated with the arm at the side and at 90 degrees of abduction in much the same manner. Internal rotation is measured by where the abducted thumb reaches in reference to spinal vertebrae (Fig. 5-4). These four motions (i.e., forward elevation, external rotation at neutral and 90 degrees, and internal rotation) should be the motions selected for documentation in the athlete according to the American Shoulder and Elbow Surgeons. Although strength is in the next section, it is assessed as range of motion testing is performed.

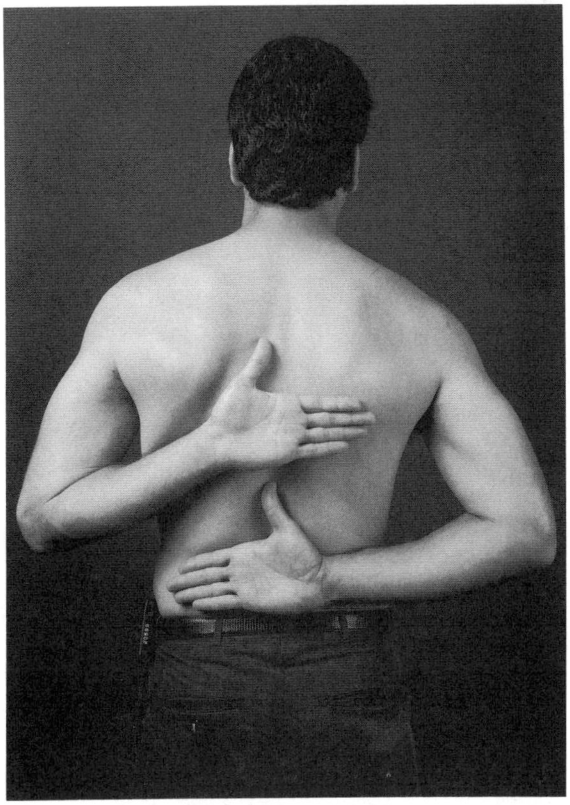

While performing range of motion, it seems timely to assess impingement signs. The three impingement signs assessed are in forced elevation, forced internal rotation, and the classical "painful arc."

From the front of the seated or standing patient,

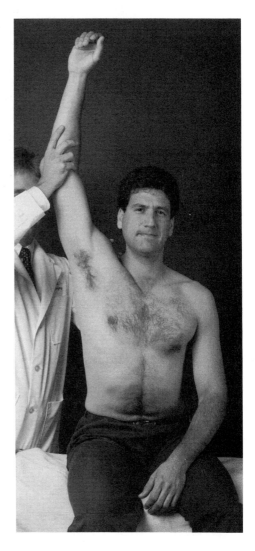

**Fig. 5-5.** Classical impingement sign. Forced forward flexion impinges the rotator cuff against the anterior edge of the acromion, producing pain. Pain expression is noted on the patient's face. This test can be repeated after injection of 10 ml 1 percent lidocaine into the subacromial space (the "injection test"). Abatement of pain after injection is further correlation of subacromial pathology.

**Fig. 5-4.** Internal rotation is measured by having the patient take the hitchhiking thumb as far up the spine as possible and recording the level at which the thumb reaches the most superior aspect of the spine (e.g., gluteal fold, belt line, L2, T6).

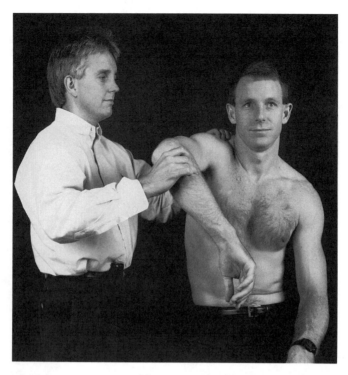

**Fig. 5-6.** Hawkins described the impingement test with the arm in forced internal rotation, forward flexed to 90 degrees to oppose the rotator cuff against a coracoacromial ligament. A pained expression is noted on the patient's face.

stressed passive forward elevation, which elicits pain as the rotator cuff opposes the anterior acromial arch, is a classic impingement sign[6,8] (Fig. 5-5). Pain with forced internal rotation in the arm that is forward flexed to 90 degrees in the sagittal plane opposes the rotator cuff on the coracoacromial ligament and is another impingement sign[5,23] (Fig. 5-6). A painful arc in the abducted position in the coronal plane is also an impingement sign. This pain is often increased with resistance. The stressed "cross-arm abduction test" can be performed, suggestive of acromioclavicular pathology as described earlier. Traumatic osteolysis of the distal clavicle seen in weight lifters can present with such a positive sign and frequently with signs of impingement.[3] These signs are all somewhat nonspecific. The yield from the impingement sign is improved by evaluation of an injection test. The subacromial space is injected with 10 ml 1 percent lidocaine, and the impingement tests are repeated. Abatement of pain postinjection suggests subacromial pathology.[24]

## STRENGTH ASSESSMENT

Strength assessment is easy to determine from behind the standing or sitting patient and can be performed in concert with range of motion. Unfortunately, the presence of pain may preclude a reliable assessment of strength. The routine strengths to be assessed in the athlete's shoulder consist of forward elevation, external rotation, and abduction.

Forward elevation strength (anterior deltoid) is assessed with resistance applied to the forward-flexed arm at approximately 70 to 80 degrees. Scapular winging may be present at this point. It aids in the assessment of cuff integrity. External rotation strength assesses the strength of the rotator cuff, which contributes 30 to 40 degrees of the power of elevation and 80 to 90 percent of the power of external rotation.[25] Abduction strength is also assessed in the coronal plane, and weakness may be suggestive of either deltoid or cuff deficiency.

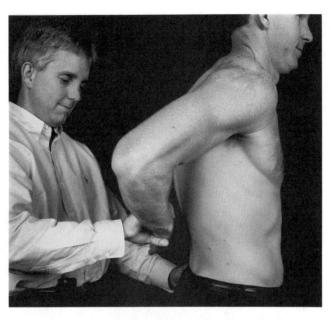

**Fig. 5-7.** Patient opposes the back of a hand to the lumbar spine and is asked to lift the hand from the spine against resistance. This test documents the strength and integrity of the subscapularis muscle and tendon complex.

Gerber popularized the "lift off" test to evaluate subscapularis strength and integrity. The patient is asked to lift the back of his or her hand away from the lumbar spine, and if performed appropriately, this suggests an intact subscapularis (Fig. 5-7). The assessment for the integrity of the subscapularis would be performed only in certain circumstances and not routinely.

The supraspinatus test, as described by Jobe and Jobe,[16] isolates and assesses the strength of the supraspinatus tendon (Fig. 5-8). The strength of elevation is assessed at 90 degrees of forward flexion in the scapular plane with the thumbs pointed to the floor. Downward pressure is resisted by the patient.[16,26] This test is supposedly specific for evaluation of the supraspinatus function and reasonably accurate in assessment of rotator cuff strength and integrity. Unfortunately, many patients have pain, precluding the reliability of such a test.

Although not assessing strength, perhaps it is appropriate at this point to comment on biceps tendon assessment. Biceps tendon involvement may be evaluated with the tests of Speed and Yergason.[26] Speed's test is performed with the shoulder in forward flexion, elbow extended, and hand supinated with applied resistance. Pain in this position from the area of the bicipital groove is suggested positive for bicipital tendinitis.[27] Resisted supination with the elbow flexed to 90 degrees is Yergason's test.[8] Once again, pain in the bicipital region with this maneuver is considered positive for biceps tendon involvement. These are not strength tests.

## GLENOHUMERAL STABILITY ASSESSMENT

Glenohumeral instability is assessed by provocative maneuvers such as an apprehension sign. It is also assessed by translation, anteriorly and posteriorly, of the humeral head in the glenoid fossa, as well as inferior translation with a sulcus sign. During these maneuvers, it is important to ask the patient if there is any reproduction of their symptom complex.

It is not uncommon for the throwing athlete to present with shoulder pain and have an underlying degree of subtle anterior instability. It is likewise not uncommon in the hyperlax and hypermobile patient to have an element of multidirectional instability.

Jobe[16] classifies pain and instability in the throwing athlete as follows:

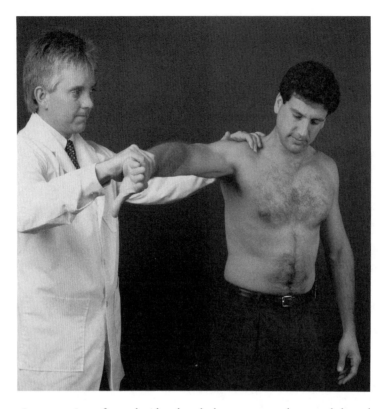

**Fig. 5-8.** The supraspinatus test is performed with a thumb-down posture, the arm abducted, and palpation over the superior aspect of the rotator cuff. The patient is asked to resist downward pressure on the abducted arm. This test is specific for the supraspinatus tendon. A test is considered positive when there is significant asymmetry and strength between the tested side and the contralateral side.

Grade I: pure impingement often seen in the older athlete

Grade II: impingement plus instability caused by labral and capsular trauma

Grade III: impingement plus instability caused by "loose" joints

Grade IV: primary instability

Many patients also present with arm weakness or heaviness, the so-called dead arm syndrome.[28-30] Therefore, it is imperative to consider the patient's pain symptoms during the examination as an important aspect of any provocative testing.

Initially, the patient should be as relaxed as possible. It is often prudent to begin the stability assessment with the contralateral or uninvolved shoulder to gain confidence in the patient during the examination. With this in mind, the stability assessment begins with the "load and shift" examination. When assessing the amount of translation, it is important to ensure that the humeral head is initially reduced concentrically into the glenoid fossa (i.e., "loaded"). In patients with significant laxity, the humeral head may have a resting position that is nonconcentric. Hence, at the commencement of any stress testing, the humeral head must be grasped and pushed into the glenoid fossa to assure its reduction in neutral position.[31] Once the humeral head is "loaded," directional stresses may be applied. To perform this maneuver, the examination initially involves assessment of the patient sitting and the examiner located just beside and behind the side to be examined. The examiner places the hand over the shoulder and scapula to steady the limb girdle and then with the opposite hand, grasps the humeral head.

As the head is "loaded," both anterior and posterior stresses are applied and the amount of translation is noted (Fig. 5-9). Next, the elbow is grasped and inferior traction applied. The area adjacent to the acromion is observed and dimpling of the skin may indicate a "sul-cus sign" (Fig. 5-10). If present, the sulcus sign should be reported in centimeters (i.e., the number of centimeters the humeral head is displaced from the inferior surface of the acromion).

Glenohumeral translation is also assessed with the patient supine. The arm is grasped in the position of approximately 20 degrees of abduction and forward flexion in neutral rotation. The humeral head is loaded, and then posterior and anterior stresses are applied. Inferior stress is applied again noting the sulcus sign. The accuracy of this test will depend not only on the examiner's skill but on the ability of the patient to relax. In some patients with associated tendinitis, it is too painful to grasp the humeral head between the thumb

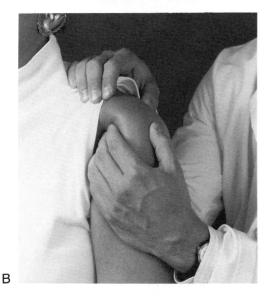

**Fig. 5-9.** The humeral head is "loaded." (**A**) Anterior translation is noted in its relationship to the glenoid rim (i.e., to the rim [grade I], over the rim [grade II]). (**B**) Posterior translation similarly graded.

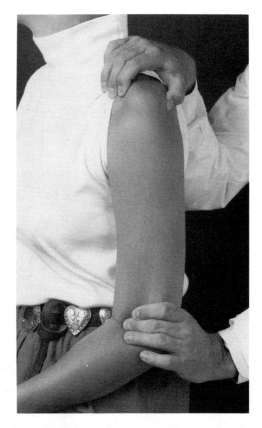

**Fig. 5-10.** "Sulcus sign." Distraction force is placed on the elbow and the space created between the undersurface of the acromion and the apex of the humeral head contour is noted. This sulcus sign should be recorded in centimeters (e.g., 1-cm, 2-cm sulcus).

and fingers. In this situation, grasping the upper arm distal to the shoulder may be the only method of assessing translation but is less reliable.

It is helpful to have a grading system of translations so that we are better able to communicate and relate that translation to any instability pattern that may or may not be present. It is impractical to use distances or percentages. Two important events may occur during this examination. First, the examiner feels the humeral head ride up to the face of the glenoid but not over the rim (grade I). Second, the head can be felt riding over the rim but reduces when the stress is released (grade II). In some situations, at least under anesthesia, once the stress is released, sometimes the head remains dislocated. For purposes of simplicity, this should probably not receive a separate grade. It is important during these maneuvers to ask the patient if this in any way reproduces their symptom complex. If so, it might be a significant clue toward diagnosis and direction of instability, especially for posterior instability.

Anterior and posterior drawer tests have also been described.[32] This is a variation of the glenohumeral translation test analogous to the Lachman test of the knee. This is performed with the patient in the supine position to make measurements more reliable. The affected shoulder is held in 80 to 120 degrees of abduction, 0 to 20 degrees of forward flexion, and 0 to 30 degrees of lateral rotation. While pressing the scapular spine forward with counterpressure on the coracoid process, the relative movement between the fixed scapula and the moveable humerus can be appreciated (Fig. 5-11). Occasionally, a positive grind test can be felt during this maneuver, noting labral pathology. The posterior drawer test is performed with the elbow at 120 degrees of flexion and the shoulder in 80 to 120 degrees of abduction and 20 to 30 degrees of forward flexion. Again, the scapula is stabilized, and a posterior directed force is placed on the humeral head with the thumb.

Significant expansion of the base of knowledge of the athlete's shoulder has come from recent advances in arthroscopy.[33] During arthroscopy, particularly under general anesthesia, an appreciation of glenohumeral translation can be obtained. This is sometimes important in completing the examination of the athlete who has a confusing diagnosis and gets to the stage of surgical reconstruction.[34]

The next phase of stability assessment is to attempt reproduction of the symptom complex by eliciting apprehension with certain provocative positions of impending subluxation or dislocation. This is especially

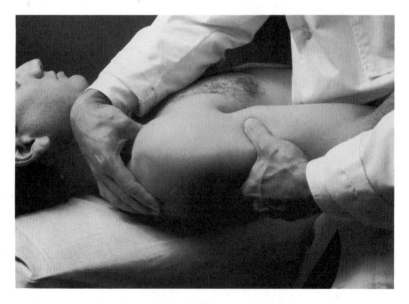

**Fig. 5-11.** Anterior drawer test. Affected shoulder is held in 80 to 120 degrees of abduction, 0 to 20 degrees of forward flexion, and 0 to 30 degrees of lateral rotation. While pressing the scapular spine forward with counterpressure on the coracoid process, relative movement between the fixed scapula and the moveable humerus can be appreciated.

applicable for anterior instability. The "apprehension test" is an evaluation of the patient's sense of pending anterior subluxation or dislocation with the arm in stressed external rotation abduction.[30,35] The role of pain needs to be interpreted because frequently a patient may not be apprehensive in this position but only painful. The usual position of the arm when subluxation or dislocation occurs is abduction in external rotation. The apprehension test for anterior instability can be performed with the patient either in the supine or seated position, although maximum muscle relaxation is best achieved with the patient supine. With the patient sitting, the examiner stands behind the shoulder to be examined. To assess the patient's left shoulder, the examiner raises the arm to 90 degrees of abduction and begins to externally rotate the humerus. The right hand of the examiner is placed over the humeral head with the thumb pushing from posterior for extra leverage, and with the fingers anterior to control for any sudden instability episode that may occur. With increasing external rotation and controlled general forward pressure exerted against the humeral head, an impending feeling of anterior instability may be produced (i.e., an apprehension sign). This may be referred to as a "crank test." An apprehensive look may appear on the patient's face as he or she contracts his or her muscles to prevent dislocation or if the stress is continued he or she may volunteer that the shoulder will "come out." Pain alone is not a positive apprehension sign, although it is often present.

This test can be repeated with the patient supine. The shoulder to be examined is positioned so that the scapula is supported by the edge of the examining table and the proximal humerus then is stressed in varying degrees of abduction and external rotation, again attempting to reproduce impending instability. In the supine position, the body acts as a counterweight. The edge of the table serves as the fulcrum and the arm as the lever. When the apprehensive position is located, note is taken of the amount of external rotation. With the arm in this position, a posterior stress may be exerted on the proximal humerus and the apprehension may disappear, allowing external rotation before emergence of the apprehension sign. The "relocation test" occurs and has two possible explanations; at the apprehensive point, the humeral head is subluxed slightly and pushing it posteriorly causes reduction or the posteriorly directed pressures act as a supportive buttress anteriorly to give the patient more

confidence, preventing apprehension. The relocation test was originally described in the presence of pain only and not with apprehension. A positive relocation test in such a situation is suggestive of anterior instability. The positive relocation test allows greater external rotation in the abducted position with less pain. If the arm is suddenly released when stressed with external rotation and abduction, the patient has substantial increase in pain, and this may be referred to as a "release test" (Fig. 5-12). This may be caused by the humeral head jumping forward on release of the posteriorly applied stress. One can also augment the pain with external rotation and abduction by pulling forward on the back of the arm ("augmentation test"). These findings may be present but are not necessarily related nor represent the classic "apprehension sign." Their value, however, is in the differentiation of impingement or anterior subluxation as the source of pain.

Posterior instability is a subluxation rather than a dislocation and, if recurrent, can usually be demon-

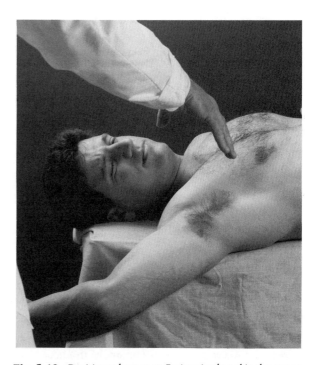

**Fig. 5-12.** Positive release test. Patient is placed in the apprehensive position of abduction and external rotation. A relocation maneuver is performed by pressing the anterior aspect of the humerus posteriorly; external rotation is then taken further and suddenly released. Exacerbation of the patient's pain and apprehension is a positive examination.

strated by the patient either with the arm positioned in forward elevation or selective muscular control in different positions of elevation with applied internal rotation. Having ascertained the compromising maneuver, the examiner may attempt to reproduce the instability by manually duplicating the stresses. Because this is usually a painless subluxation that easily reduces, posterior apprehension is not commonly present and, therefore, not a reliable sign. With posterior stresses, patients who are painful may resist, and this is sometimes erroneously interpreted as apprehension. In posterior instability, the patient who cannot demonstrate the instability may present a diagnostic challenge. It is perhaps in these patients that posterior translation of the humeral head on the glenoid with reproduction of the symptom complex may provide the only clue to their diagnosis. Patients with inferior instability may say that the distal traction on the arm reproduces their symptom complex, suggesting underlying multidirectional instability.[36,37]

## NEUROLOGIC EXAMINATION

The interplay of referred pain in cervical spine disease is not as common in the athlete. It is, however, common in many athletes who throw, swim, and serve to present with dysesthesias into their extremities. For example, this is a common presentation with instability patterns. The timing of performing a neurologic examination in our format may vary. It is frequently helpful to do the examination during range of motion because we do strength testing almost synonymously with that, and it seems appropriate to complete the sensory and reflex examination at that time.

Normally, a dermatomal sensory examination is performed in the usual manner. Deep tendon reflexes at the elbow and wrist are noted. Evaluation of muscle mass and tone was performed during the palpation part of the examination as was the strength assessment performed during that segment of the examination. The addition of evaluation of wrist extension, finger abduction and adduction, thumb abduction, and elbow extension can give a quick assessment of the health of the cervical roots.

Cervical spine radiculopathy can mimic intrinsic shoulder disease (e.g., C5 radiculopathy can mimic a rotator cuff tear).[38–40] Spurling's test is helpful to distinguish cervical disease (Fig. 5-13). The neck is

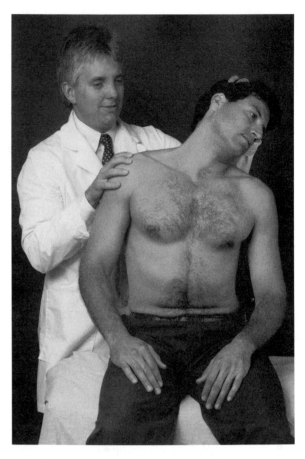

**Fig. 5-13.** Spurling's test. Neck is extended, right and left lateral rotation are performed, and radicular pain is evaluated. Addition of compression can illicit subtle pathology.

flexed and rotated to one side with corresponding compression to elicit pain.[41] In the absence of tenderness of the posterior cervical spinous processes to palpation and in the presence of a negative Spurling's test, cervical spine pathology and radiculopathy can usually be excluded.

## VASCULAR EXAMINATION

The vascular examination consists of palpation of the pulses at the wrist and elbow, along with an assessment of vascular changes from dystrophy such as swelling, discoloration, and lack of sweating. There are also tests to examine for thoracic outlet syndrome. Adson's maneuver is performed with shoulders extended, breath held, neck extended, and chin turned to the same side. The arm is in a slightly abducted and extended position. Diminution of a palpable pulse at the wrist is considered positive for thoracic outlet syndrome. Other thoracic outlet tests are less reliable, perhaps the most helpful being provocative testing. This is performed with the arms elevated forward with repetitive opening and closing of the fist to reproduce the symptoms distal to the forearm. This often causes an aching fatigue, suggestive of thoracic outlet.

## SUMMARY

Athletes often present a diagnostic dilemma. If the examiner systematically approaches the history to classify the patient into specific symptom patterns and gives a thorough physical examination, paying particular attention to how the assessment relates to the patient's symptomatology, accurate diagnoses can be made in most patients with athletic injuries of the shoulder. Management techniques are obviously predicated on an accurate diagnosis. Many times patients are able to relate the exact mechanism of injury and actually have a clear understanding of their symptom pattern. However, with increasing demands from an athletic population, many patients present with unclear histories of their symptoms. If care is taken during the examination to be thorough and organized, the correct diagnosis can be achieved.

## REFERENCES

1. Glousman R, Jobe F, Tibone J et al: Dynamic electromyographic analysis of the throwing shoulder with glenohumeral instability. J Bone Joint Surg 70A:220, 1988
2. Jobe FW, Bradley JP: Rotator cuff injuries in baseball: prevention and rehabilitation. Sports Med 6:377, 1988
3. Butters KP, Rockwood CA Jr: Office evaluation and management of the shoulder impingement syndrome. Orthop Clin North Am 19:755, 1988
4. Nirschl RP: Shoulder tendinitis. In: Upper Extremity Injuries in Athletes. American Academy of Orthopaedic Surgeons Symposium, Washington, D.C. CV Mosby, St. Louis, 1986
5. Hawkins RJ, Hobeika P: Impingement syndrome in the athletic shoulder. Clin Sports Med 2:391, 1983
6. Neer CS II: Impingement lesions. Clin Orthop 173:70, 1983
7. Neer CS II: Anterior acromioplasty for the chronic impingement syndrome in the shoulder. J Bone Joint Surg 54A:41, 1972
8. Neer CS II, Welsh RP: The shoulder in sports. Orthop Clin North Am 8:583, 1977
9. Perry J: Anatomy and biomechanics of the shoulder in throwing, swimming, gymnastics and tennis. Clin Sports Med 2:247, 1983
10. Hawkins RJ, Bell RH: Collagen analysis in patients with multidirectional instability. ASES Specialty Day, Anaheim, CA, 1991
11. Hawkins RJ, Hobeika P: Physical examination of the shoulder. Orthopedics 10:1270, 1983
12. Drez D Jr: Suprascapular neuropathy in the differential diagnosis of rotator cuff injuries. Am J Sports Med 4:43, 1976
13. Codman EA: Normal motions of the shoulder joint. P. 32. In: The Shoulder. Thomas Todd, Boston, 1934
14. Freeman L, Monroe RR: Abduction of the arm in the scapular plane: scapular and glenohumeral movement. J Bone Joint Surg 48A:1503, 1966
15. Poppen NK, Walker PS: Normal and abnormal motion of the shoulder. J Bone Joint Surg 58A:195, 1976
16. Jobe FW, Jobe CM: Painful athletic injuries of the shoulder. Clin Orthop 173:117, 1983
17. Sisto DJ, Jobe FW: The operative treatment of scapulothoracic bursitis in professional pitchers. Am J Sports Med 14:192, 1986
18. Lombardo SJ, Jobe FW, Kerlan RK et al: Posterior shoulder lesions in throwing athletes. Am J Sports Med 5:106, 1977
19. Hoyt WA Jr: Etiology of shoulder injuries in athletes. J Bone Joint Surg 49A:755, 1967
20. Rockwood CA, Green DP: Fractures in Adults. JB Lippincott, Philadelphia, 1984
21. Shields CL, Glousman RE: Open management of rotator cuff tears. p. 223. In Grana (ed): Advances in Sports Medicine and Fitness. Vol. 2. Year Book Medical Publishers, Chicago, 1989
22. Hurley JA, Anderson TE: Shoulder arthroscopy: its role in evaluating shoulder disorders in the athlete. Am J Sports Med 18:480, 1990
23. Hawkins RJ, Kennedy JC: Impingement syndrome in athletes. Am J Sports Med 8:151, 1980
24. Scheib JS: Diagnosis and rehabilitation of the shoulder impingement syndrome in the overhead and throwing athlete. Rheum Dis Clin North Am 16:971, 1990
25. Colachis SC Jr, Strohm BR: Effect of suprascapular and axillary nerve blocks and muscle force in upper extremity. Arch Phys Med Rehabil 52:22, 1971
26. Yergason RM: Supraspinatus sign. J Bone Joint Surg 13:60, 1931
27. Crenshaw AII, Kilgore WE: Surgical treatment of bicipital tenosynovitis. J Bone Joint Surg 48A:1496, 1966

28. Hastings DE, Coughlin LP: Recurrent subluxation of the glenohumeral joint. Am J Sports Med 9:352, 1981
29. Protzman RR: Anterior instability of the shoulder. J Bone Joint Surg 62A:909, 1980
30. Rowe CR, Zarins B: Recurrent transient subluxation of the shoulder. J Bone Joint Surg 63A:863, 1981
31. Hawkins RJ, Schutte JP, Huckell GH, Abrams J: The assessment of glenohumeral translation using manual and fluoroscopic techniques. Orthop Trans 12:727, 1988
32. Gerber C, Ganz R: Clinical assessment of instability of the shoulder with special reference to anterior and posterior drawer tests. J Bone Joint Surg 66B:551, 1984
33. Pappas AM, Goss TP, Kleinman PK: Symptomatic shoulder instability due to lesions of the glenoid labrum. Am J Sports Med 11:279, 1983
34. Cofield RH, Irving JF: Evaluation and classification of shoulder instability with special reference to examination under anesthesia. Clin Orthop 223:32, 1987
35. Zarins B, Rowe CR: Current concepts in the diagnosis and treatment of shoulder instability in athletes. Med Sci Sports Exerc 16:444, 1984
36. Neer CS II: Involuntary inferior and multidirectional instability of the shoulder: etiology, recognition and treatment. Instr. Course Lect 34:232, 1985
37. Neer CS II, Foster CR: Inferior capsular shift for involuntary inferior and multidirectional instability of the shoulder. J Bone Joint Surg 62A:897, 1980
38. Bateman JE: Neurologic painful conditions affecting the shoulder. Clin Orthop 173:44, 1983
39. Bennett RM: The painful shoulder. A four-article symposium. Postgrad Med 73:153, 1983
40. Bowling RW, Rockar PA Jr, Erhard R: Examination of the shoulder complex. Phys Ther 66:1866, 1986
41. Spurling RG, Scoville WB: Lateral rupture of the cervical intervertebral discs. Surg Gynecol Obstet 78:350, 1944

# 6

# Diagnostic Imaging of the Shoulder Complex

*MARTIN L. SCHWARTZ*

Evaluation of shoulder pathology has become much easier over the past several years, partly because of advances in imaging techniques. Diagnosis had been based on physical examination, plain x-ray studies, and possibly arthrography, but since computed tomography (CT) and magnetic resonance imaging (MRI) have been introduced, the sensitivity and specificity of different conditions have improved dramatically. It is no longer necessary for orthopaedic surgeons to perform surgery without some idea of what they will encounter in the shoulder joint. Different imaging modalities are available to the radiologist for accurate diagnosis in the athletic shoulder.

## IMAGING TECHNIQUES

After a thorough clinical examination of the shoulder, the first diagnostic test obtained should be plain radiographs. There should be a minimum of three views including anteroposterior internal and external rotation and an axillary film (Fig. 6-1). Additional views may be obtained depending on the specific pathology involved. We routinely obtain five radiographs for our overhead athletes. This series of radiographs, called the "throwers' series," includes a west point, axillary, stryker notch, and internal/external rotation views, and occasionally an acromial profile view. These basic views should enable the clinician to grossly evaluate skeletal structures and to exclude most fractures and dislocations that commonly occur. It must be stressed that plain radiographs of the shoulder are of little benefit for the evaluation of most soft tissue pathology, with

the exception of calcific tendonitis. Calcification in the region of the rotator cuff or biceps tendon can often be visible on plain films. If the plain radiographs are normal, the next diagnostic imaging test required will vary according to the specific condition that the physician needs to exclude based on the mechanism of injury and the physical examination.

Arthrography is excellent for the diagnosis of rotator cuff tears and as a prelude to CT for labral evaluation. Double-contrast arthrography is preferred at our hospital because most of our patients do have a follow-up CT scan. We perform the examination using sterile technique and fluoroscopic guidance with the patient in the supine position and the shoulder in external rotation. A 22-gauge spinal needle is placed in the joint and 6 ml of contrast plus 12 cc of air are injected with direct visualization. Five radiographs are obtained after controlled exercise by the technologist. Included in the study are internal and external rotation views, an axillary view, and weight-bearing views (Fig. 6-2). Single-contrast techniques are rarely used and are only beneficial for diagnosing rotator cuff tears and adhesive capsulitis. Arthrography is an invasive procedure requiring the injection of contrast into the joint, and there is the remote possibility of infection, hematoma, or contrast reaction.

CT is an excellent imaging modality for evaluation of complex fractures; however, like plain radiographs, it gives little information regarding the soft tissues (Fig. 6-3). CT-arthrography gives information about the skeletal structures, rotator cuff, glenoid labrum, and other soft tissues. Regardless of whether intra-articular contrast is injected, we perform the CT scan with the patient supine. Three-millimeter contiguous axial slices are

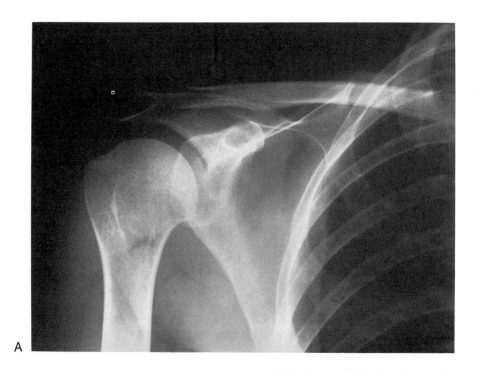

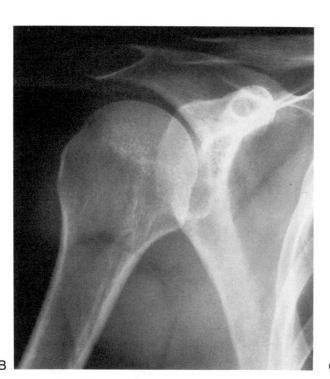

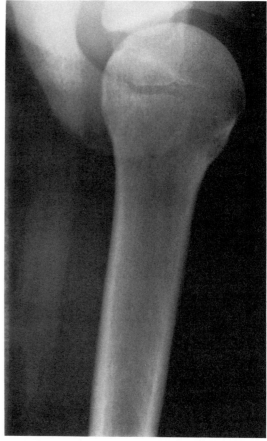

**Fig. 6-1.** Anteroposterior internal (**A**) and external (**B**) rotation and axillary view (**C**) in a normal patient.

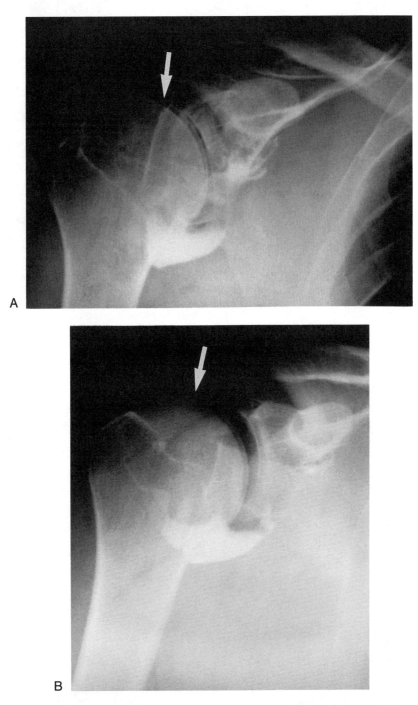

**Fig. 6-2.** Normal double-contrast arthrogram. Anteroposterior internal (**A**) and external (**B**) rotation. Note that contrast and air are contained underneath rotator cuff tendon (*arrows*).

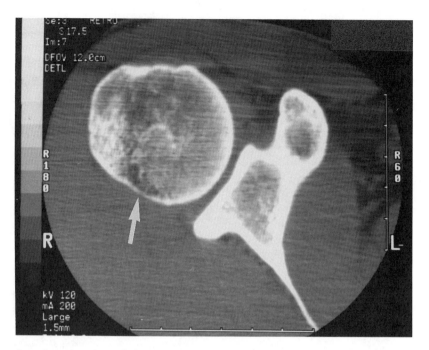

**Fig. 6-3.** Normal axial CT slice through the right shoulder joint. Humeral head (*arrow*) is normal and is normally located in the joint.

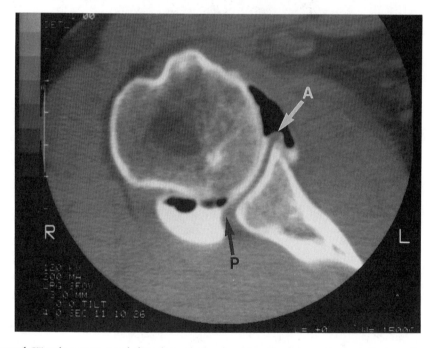

**Fig. 6-4.** Normal CT-arthrogram. Axial slice through the shoulder after intra-articular injection of contrast and air. Anterior (*A*) and posterior (*P*) glenoid labrum are well demonstrated and show no abnormality. Capsular structures are also normal.

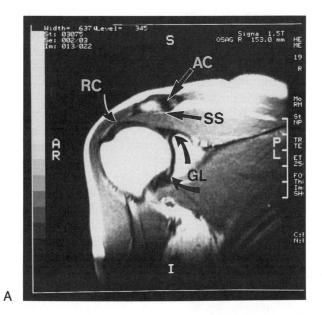

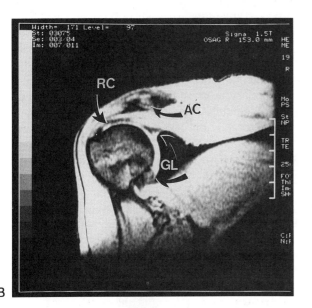

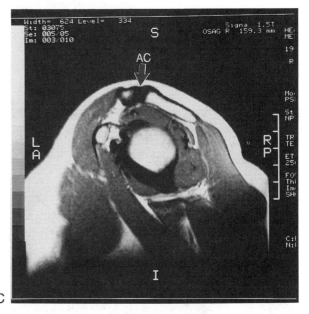

**Fig. 6-5.** (**A**) Proton density (TR 3000, TE 20) (**B**) MPGR (TR 417, TE 12), coronal oblique; and (**C**) T$_1$-weighted (TR 1300, TE 20) sagittal oblique MRI in asymptomatic patient. Rotator cuff tendon (*RC*) is seen as well as many muscles composing the rotator cuff. The acromioclavicular joint (*AC*) and subacromial space (*SS*) are also nicely shown. Note that the glenoid labrum (*GL*) is not optimally visualized.

obtained targeting the shoulder joint, and filming is performed using modified bone windows (Fig. 6-4).

MRI is a common procedure at our institution for most pathologic conditions. Although there are still some limitations to its diagnostic use, MRI gives a global view of the shoulder joint and is becoming more sensitive and specific as imaging sequences are refined. We perform the examination on a 1.5 Tesla Signa (General Electric, Milwaukee, WI) system and use a dedicated shoulder coil. Routine sequences include partial saturation sagittal oblique images, double-echo and multiplanar gradient recall (MPGR) coronal oblique images, and MPGR axial images (Fig. 6-5). Some researchers advocate the use of MRI-arthrography with gadolinium,[1] although the diagnostic advantage over routine MRI remains to be proved.

We have performed more than 350 MR examinations with intra-articular saline injection and have found that it greatly enhances visualization of the glenoid labrum as well as documenting subtle rotator cuff tears (Fig. 6-6). Joint injection for MRI requires close approximation of a fluoroscopy suite to the scanner site for logistical reasons.

Other diagnostic tools are available, including tomography, nuclear imaging, ultrasound, and venogra-phy/arteriography. Each of these procedures has limited clinical use, and they will be discussed in the next section when applicable. Often, combinations of imaging techniques may be needed, especially in complex pathologic conditions.

## IMAGING OF SPECIFIC PATHOLOGIC CONDITIONS

### Fracture/Dislocation

In 1970, Neer[2] published his classic paper of acute proximal humeral fractures and showed that the prognosis depended not only on the number of fracture fragments but also on the amount of displacement and angulation. Minimally displaced fractures could be treated without surgery; however, significant separation of fragments or rotation required surgery to prevent chronic changes and loss of function.

After careful examination, if a fracture or dislocation is suspected, plain radiographs should be obtained (Figs. 6-7, 6-8, and 6-9). Most fractures will be obvious on the films, and no further imaging is required. Occasionally, complex humeral fractures will not be well demonstrated because the patient is unable to cooperate with positioning or there is superimposition of fracture fragments. CT would be helpful in these circumstances, possibly avoiding unnecessary surgery[3] (Fig. 6-10).

Dislocations, particularly posterior in position, are problematic for plain film analysis. Subtle dislocations can be missed if only anteroposterior internal and external views are obtained. For this reason, we include an axillary view as part of our routine series. CT can be useful for the evaluation of the changes associated with chronic dislocation, especially in the humeral head and glenoid.[4]

CT-arthrography can also be useful in chronic dislocation for diagnosis of rotator cuff and labral tears. Little additional information is gained from MRI in patients with acute fracture/dislocation. MRI will nicely show the chronic soft tissue and skeletal abnormalities seen on other modalities and can show additional soft tissue findings such as joint effusion.

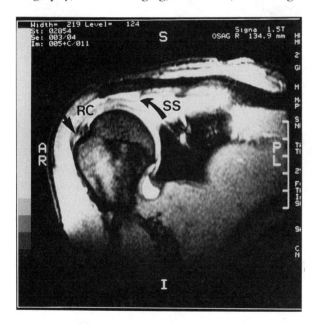

**Fig. 6-6.** MPGR (TR 466, TE 12) coronal oblique MRI showing marked increased signal in the rotator cuff tendon (*rc*) with fluid in the subacromial space (*ss*) indicating a complete tear of the tendon.

### Impingement Syndrome

The impingement syndrome is a significant cause of shoulder dysfunction. The patient has severe pain dur-

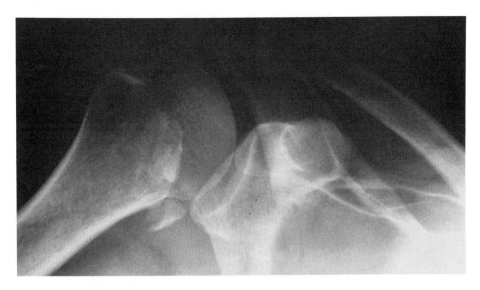

**Fig. 6-7.** Anteroposterior radiograph showing fracture of the humeral head with a displaced fragment.

ing abduction and external rotation of the arm. Entrapment of soft tissue structures under the coracoacromial arc is responsible for the syndrome. Chronically, rotator cuff tendonitis develops, possibly progressing to fibrosis and rupture.

Diagnosis of the impingement syndrome generally had been determined clinically before the develop-ment of MRI. Plain radiographs suggest this condition, showing subacromial proliferation of bone, inferior spurring of the acromioclavicular joint, and degenerative changes in the humeral head.[5] If performed properly, MRI can now give a definitive noninvasive demonstration of this syndrome.[6] Partial saturation coronal oblique or $T_1$-weighted sagittal oblique images show

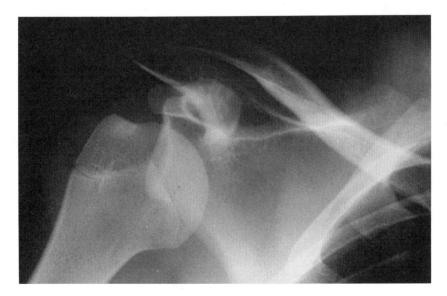

**Fig. 6-8.** Anterior dislocation of the humeral head on plain radiograph. Note that humeral head is inferior to and overriding the scapular glenoid.

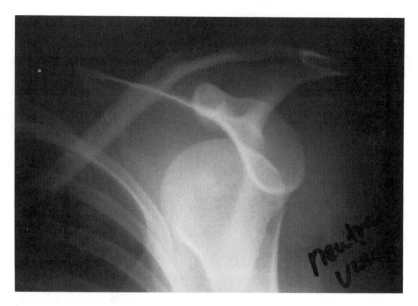

**Fig. 6-9.** Anterior/inferior dislocation of the left humeral head.

impingement of the acromion on the supraspinatus tendon (Fig. 6-11). The normal fat plane in this region is obliterated, usually by an inferior acromial spur. Also, there is almost always abnormal signal in the rotator cuff indicating either tendonitis or partial-thickness tear. Chronic cases manifest themselves with complete rotator cuff tear. Arthrography had been used in the past to confirm the MRI findings; however, with recent advances and refinement of scanning techniques, this is no longer necessary.

## Adhesive Capsulitis

As with the impingement syndrome, diagnosis of adhesive capsulitis is usually based on clinical examination. Often, patients presenting with this condition have undergone previous surgery, have had multiple injections into the joint, or are chronic dislocaters. Arthrography is the only imaging test available to confirm the physical findings. The total volume of the joint space is reduced, often limiting the quantity of contrast and/or air that can be injected. Postarthrography radiographs demonstrate an irregular axillary recess with the previously mentioned reduction in volume (Fig. 6-12). This condition is often associated with other joint pathology such as rotator cuff tear, labral tear, tendonitis, or previous fracture/dislocation.

## Rotator Cuff Tear

Abnormalities of the rotator cuff of the shoulder are common orthopaedic problems. The preoperative difference between individuals with complete tears and those with partial tears or tendonitis is important because treatment and prognosis are different. Usually, complete tears are managed surgically, whereas partial tears and tendonitis are managed conservatively.

Suspected rotator cuff tears have traditionally been diagnosed by arthrography. Complete tears can reliably be shown by communication between the glenohumeral joint and the subacromial bursa (Fig. 6-13). Partial tears can also be shown, although less consistently. Arthrography is invasive and cannot be used to visualize soft tissues of the shoulder. Ultrasound visualization of the rotator cuff has been inconsistent in the literature, with some authors showing great success in demonstrating both complete and incomplete tears, whereas others have not been able to duplicate those results.[7-9]

MRI has become the imaging method of choice at our institution for the diagnosis of rotator cuff tears. The procedure is noninvasive and has become as good as arthrography for diagnosing complete tears.[10] MRI has been shown to be superior to arthrography for demonstrating partial tears and tendonitis.[11-13] This

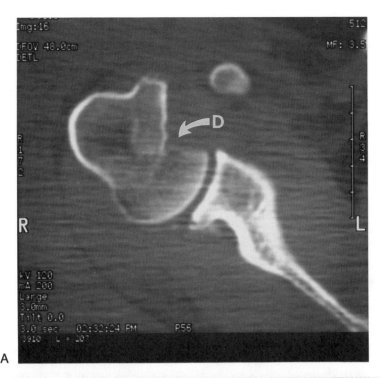

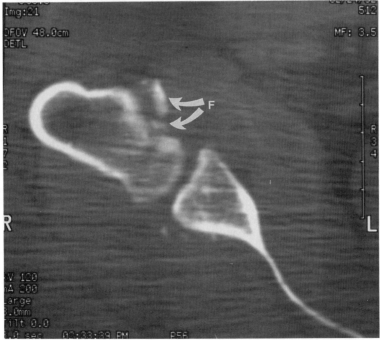

**Fig. 6-10.** Axial CT scan of the same patient in Fig. 6-7. A large defect (*D*) is present in the anteromedial aspect of the humeral head with at least two fracture fragments (*F*) adjacent to the bone defect.

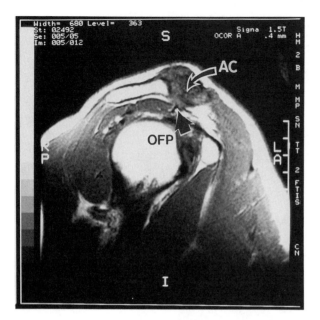

**Fig. 6-11.** $T_1$-weighted (TR 900, TE 18) sagittal oblique MRI scan showing marked degenerative change in the acromioclavicular joint (*AC*) with moderate impingement. The fat plane between the acromioclavicular joint and the supraspinatus muscle has been obliterated (*OFP*).

technique can also show other soft tissue structures that are not seen on other diagnostic tests.

Classic findings of a complete tear on MRI are marked increased signal on the T2-weighted images in the cuff with fluid in the subacromial space (Fig. 6-14). Some degree of impingement may or may not be seen. Partial tears show increased signal in the cuff, although not as severe as complete tears. No significant fluid is present in the subacromial space with partial tears. The subdeltoid fat plane is obliterated in complete tears and preserved in cases of partial tear. Tendonitis is difficult to differentiate from a partial tear, as the MRI findings are similar in both conditions.

## Calcific Tendonitis

Many individuals suffer from shoulder disorders even if they are not involved in competitive athletics. The athlete, however, can be affected by calcific tendonitis at an earlier age because of repetitive microtrauma. Calcific tendonitis usually presents with chronic pain similar to rotator cuff tear, but the pain is not as severe or debilitating. Unlike rotator cuff tear, people suffering from calcific tendonitis can generally overcome the pain and can continue to function reasonably well.

Plain radiographs will usually show calcification in the region of the rotator cuff[14] (Fig. 6-15). Radiographs should be analyzed using a bright light, because the calcifications may be faint on the viewbox. If the calcifications are small enough, they will not be visible on the films. Ultrasound may show some shadowing in the region of the rotator cuff, but this is an unreliable finding. The only other diagnostic technique is MRI, in which areas of decreased signal will be seen in the tendon. This region of diminished signal remains constant on all sequences. Inflammatory changes may be seen in the soft tissues adjacent to the tendinous structures. All other imaging techniques are unreliable in this clinical setting.

## Glenoid Labrum Tear

Disability caused by recurrent subluxation of the humerus is a common clinical problem that is thought to be due to a lax capsular mechanism. Recently, it has been shown that arthroscopic surgical repair of the anterior glenoid labrum is providing clinical improvement. Because of this, the identification of labral tears has become important. The only imaging techniques available to visualize the labrum are CT-arthrography and MRI.[15] CT-arthrography is currently the gold standard for visualization of the glenoid labrum (Fig. 6-16). Wilson et al[16] showed 100 percent sensitivity and 97 percent specificity in the diagnosis of anterior tears. Also, CT-arthrography gives detailed information about the skeletal structures in the shoulder joint.

Continued refinement of MRI of the shoulder makes this imaging modality useful now and probably the procedure of choice for labral abnormalities in the future.[17] Anterior and superior tears are relatively easy to identify, and adding more sophisticated sequences can enhance diagnostic accuracy. Posterior and inferior tears are less reliably seen using MRI. The axial images are the most important for analysis of the anterior labrum. Oblique coronal images show the superior and inferior labrum to best advantage.

The most common appearance of a torn anterior labrum on MRI is visible linear increased signal cutting

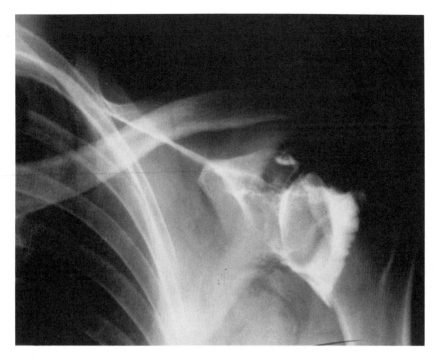

**Fig. 6-12.** Double-contrast arthrogram shows reduction in size of the axillary recess with marked contour irregularity. The radiographic findings are consistent with adhesive capsulitis.

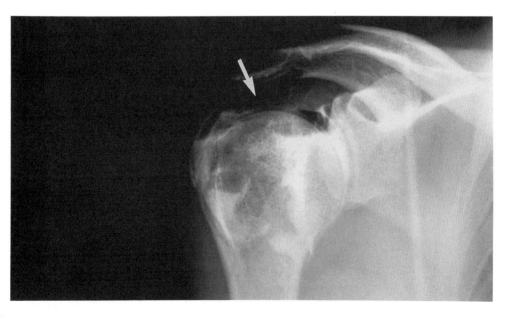

**Fig. 6-13.** Complete rotator cuff tear. Double-contrast arthrogram shows air and contrast in the subacromial space (*arrow*), indicating leakage through the rotator cuff tendon.

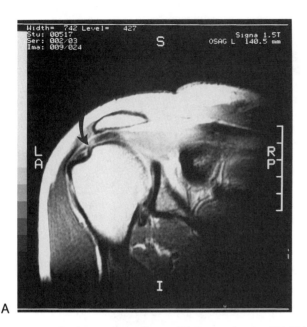
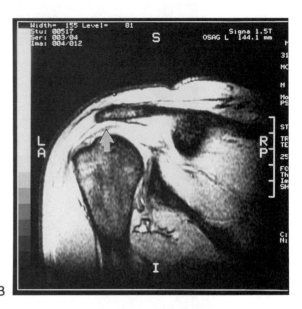

A        B

**Fig. 6-14.** Rotator cuff tear. (**A**) Proton density (TR 2000, TE 15) and (**B**) MPGR (TR 550, TE 15) coronal oblique images with (**A**) increased signal (*arrow*) in the rotator cuff and (**B**) fluid in the subacromial space (*arrow*). Mild impingement is also present.

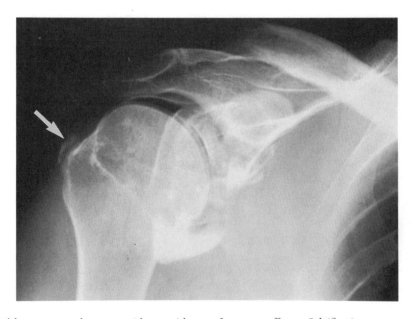

**Fig. 6-15.** Double-contrast arthrogram without evidence of rotator cuff tear. Calcification present in the region of the distal rotator cuff (*arrow*) is consistent with the diagnosis of calcific tendonitis.

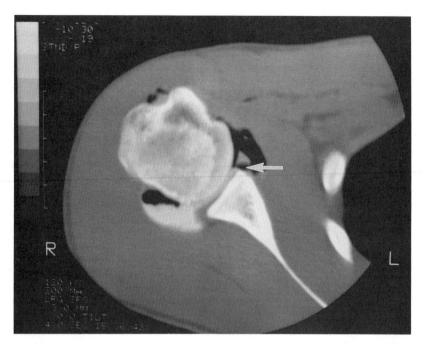

**Fig. 6-16.** Anterior labral tear and avulsion. CT-arthrogram with air between anterior labral fragments (*arrow*). The posterior labrum is normal.

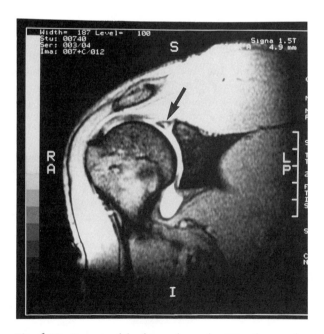

**Fig. 6-17.** Superior labral tear shown by MR-arthrography. MPGR (TR 467, TE 12) coronal oblique image after intra-articular saline injection shows increased signal in the superior labrum (*arrow*).

through the substance of the labrum. Other abnormalities associated with anterior labral tears are a severely truncated or absent labrum. The most common finding of a superior tear is the absence of the superior labrum.[18,19] With increasing sophistication of MRI, all labral tears should be identified in the future. As stated previously, MR-arthrography using gadolinium or saline may facilitate the transition from CT-arthrography to MRI for the diagnosis of labral abnormalities (Fig. 6-17).

## Acromioclavicular Joint Abnormalities

All patients with suspected cases of acromioclavicular joint pathology, whether acute or chronic, should be evaluated initially with plain radiographs. In the acute setting, plain films will show fractures and dislocations.

Weight-bearing views on the affected side can help to diagnose subtle acromioclavicular joint separations, as well as help to classify the severity of the separation. Comparative view of the uninjured joint can show laxity in the joint as opposed to acute dislocation, particularly in younger individuals. CT and MRI are of little use acutely, except for complex fractures and when associated soft tissue injuries are anticipated.

Radiographs can show degenerative changes in the acromioclavicular joint such as spurring and narrowing. Impingement syndrome can be suspected from plain films, although the diagnosis needs to be confirmed either with surgery or MRI. Also, associated rotator cuff tears can be seen with MRI. Arthrography and CT-arthrography are of little clinical use for isolated chronic pathology affecting the acromioclavicular joint.

## SUMMARY

Radiographic imaging of the athletic shoulder is complex and needs to be tailored to the specific pathology that is suspected. Procedures that can be used range from plain radiographs to MR-arthrography. As imaging becomes technically more sophisticated, diagnosis will become highly sensitive and specific. Clinicians will be able to diagnose most shoulder pathology with only a handful of imaging techniques.

## REFERENCES

1. Flannigan B, Kursunoglu-Brahme S, Snyder S et al: MR arthrography of the shoulder: comparison with conventional MR imaging. AJR 155:829, 1990
2. Neer CS: Displaced proximal humeral fractures. Part I: classification and evaluation. J Bone Joint Surg 52A:1077, 1970
3. Kilcoyne RF, Shuman WP, Matsen FA III et al: The Neer classification of displaced proximal humeral fractures: spectrum of findings on plain radiographs and CT scans. AJR 154:1029, 1990
4. Newberg AH: Computed tomography of joint injuries. Radiol Clin North Am 28:445, 1990
5. Kilcoyne RF, Reddy PK, Lyons F, Rockwood CA Jr: Optimal plain film imaging of the shoulder impingement syndrome. AJR 153:795, 1989
6. Kursunoglu-Brahme S, Resnick D: Magnetic resonance imaging of the shoulder. Radiol Clin North Am 28:941, 1990
7. Soble MG, Kaye AD, Guay RC: Rotator cuff tear: clinical experience with sonographic detection. Radiology 173:319, 1989
8. Brandt TD, Cardone BW, Grant TH et al: Rotator cuff sonography: a reassessment. Radiology 173:323, 1989
9. Vick CW, Bell SA: Rotator cuff tears: diagnosis with sonography. AJR 154:121, 1990
10. Farley TE, Neumann CH, Steinbach LS et al: Full thickness tears of the rotator cuff of the shoulder: diagnosis with MR imaging. AJR 158:347, 1992
11. Zlatkin MB, Iannotti JP, Roberts MC et al: Rotator cuff tears: diagnostic performance of MR imaging. Radiology 172:223, 1989
12. Rafii M, Firooznia H, Sherman O et al: Rotator cuff lesions: signal patterns at MR imaging. Radiology 177:817, 1990
13. Kjellin I, Ho CP, Cervilla V et al: Alterations in the supraspinatus tendon at MR imaging: correlation with histopathologic findings in cadavers. Radiology 181:837, 1991
14. Burk DL Jr, Karasick D, Mitchell DG, Rifkin MD: MR imaging of the shoulder: correlation with plain radiography. AJR 154:121, 1990
15. Coumas JM, Waite RJ, Goss TP et al: CT and MR evaluation of the labral capsular ligamentous complex of the shoulder. AJR 158:591, 1992
16. Wilson AJ, Totty WG, Murphy WA, Hardy DC: Shoulder joint: arthrographic CT and long-term follow up, with surgical correlation. Radiology 173:329, 1989
17. Neumann CH, Petersen SA, Jahnke AH: MR imaging of the labral-capsular complex: normal variations. AJR 157:1015, 1991
18. Legan JM, Burkhard TK, Goff WB II et al: Tears of the glenoid labrum: MR imaging of 88 arthroscopically confirmed cases. Radiology 179:241, 1991
19. McCauly TR, Pope CF, Jokl P: Normal and abnormal glenoid labrum: assessment with multiplanar gradient-echo MR imaging. Radiology 183:35, 1992

# 7

# Computed Tomography–Arthrography of the Shoulder

*KEVIN P. SPEER*
*BERNARD GHELMAN*
*RUSSELL F. WARREN*

Injury to the shoulder in the athletic patient always has involved a spectrum of pathology to include both hard and soft tissue. Imaging of the hard tissue (bone) component has been relatively straightforward with conventional radiographs or more sophisticated techniques such as tomography or computed tomography (CT); this also applies for the visualization of calcium deposition in soft tissues as well. However, the imaging of the soft tissue component of injury always has required the addition of intra-articular contrast agents to these conventional radiographic techniques. Single-contrast arthrography was first performed in 1939 and proved to be very helpful in the diagnosis of rotator cuff tears.[1] The labrum was usually unable to be imaged, though, because of overlying contrast material.[2] Double-contrast arthrography was first introduced by Goldman and Ghelman in 1978.[3] This was soon established as the standard for imaging full-thickness rotator cuff tears. The double-contrast technique has the advantage of coating the disrupted tendons and outlining them with air, which shows the quality of the remaining tissue. However, the identification of the labrum (especially the anterior labrum[4]) with this technique is often impossible because of pooling of contrast material.[5,6]

Polytomography of the shoulder after double-contrast arthrography has been used to overcome the problem of overlapping pools of contrast material.[7,8]

Criteria developed for detecting labral abnormalities using polytomography have been shown to be very accurate. However, proper execution of polytomography requires considerable experience, particularly in regard to the oblique patient positioning; also, the patient must be able to maintain the appropriate position for the duration of the study, which can be difficult for those with shoulder pain. Polytomography also involves a large radiation dose, some five to ten times that required for a conventional CT scan.[9]

Combining CT with double-contrast arthrography (CT-arthrography) first was suggested in 1981.[10] CT-arthrography of the glenohumeral joint provides axial images and the potential for reformatting in the coronal and sagittal planes. Several reports have described the features and advantages of this technique.[4,6,11–26] Excellent visualization of the soft tissues can also be achieved with CT-arthrography without positive contrast material (injection of air only) in patients who are allergic to contrast agents.[4,13]

Before the application of magnetic resonance imaging (MRI) to the shoulder, CT-arthrography was considered the imaging standard for labral and capsular injury to the shoulder. In this chapter, we review the techniques, interpretations, and diagnostic pitfalls associated with CT-arthrography and critically evaluate its accuracy against an open surgery or arthroscopy standard. We also compare and contrast the results of CT-arthrography with that of MRI for hard and soft tissue injuries about the shoulder to provide a basis for the proper use of both.

## CT-ARTHROGRAPHY TECHNIQUE

The importance of understanding the technical aspects of how an image is created cannot be underemphasized. The physician ordering the CT-arthrography must have at least a working knowledge of how the radiologist can manipulate the parameters of the imaging protocol to generate the optimum visualization of the structures in question. To this end, it is also of critical importance for the ordering physician to communicate to the radiologist precisely what he or she wants imaged or what questions he or she wants answered.

The procedure begins with the injection of 1 to 5 ml positive contrast material (and usually 0.3 ml 1:1,000 epinephrine solution) into the glenohumeral joint under fluoroscopic control. This is immediately followed by the injection of 10 to 25 cc of room air into the joint. The literature is mixed on the necessity of exercising the shoulder after the injections; proponents argue that

is allows even dispersion of the contrast agent on all intra-articular structures, whereas critics insist that it promotes extravasation of the air into the extra-articular tissues. With proper air injection technique alone, we have found that the contrast material will predictably be evenly dispersed. Next, standard radiographs are obtained according to the methods of Goldman and Ghelman.[3] However, many argue that this double-contrast shoulder arthrogram is unnecessary because the CT-arthrography is just as accurate in diagnosing rotator cuff tears.[12] We still rely on the double-contrast arthrogram exclusively to evaluate a possible rotator cuff tear, having found CT-arthrography difficult to interpret for this injury.

The patient is then placed supine in the CT gantry with the arm at the side and the shoulder in neutral rotation. Saline bags can be placed anterior to the shoulder and neck to decrease artifacts.[6,14] The shoulder can be variably rotated to allow better visualization of certain structures; internal rotation relaxes the anterior capsule, which then allows better anterior distension, which can assist in visualizing the anterior capsule and labrum (Fig. 7-1). The converse of this applies for external rotation and visualizing the posterior structures. One study, though, found no difference in the imaging results with neutral versus internal rotation.[27]

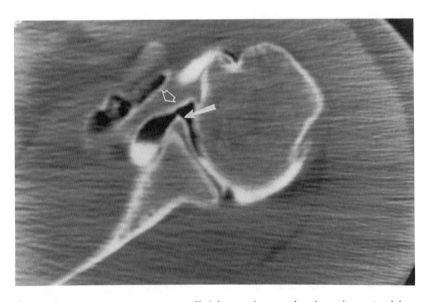

**Fig. 7-1.** Normal CT arthrogram. *Arrow* points to well-delineated triangular-shaped anterior labrum. *Open arrow* indicates subscapularis tendon. Note that the posterior labrum is not well visualized with this supine image.

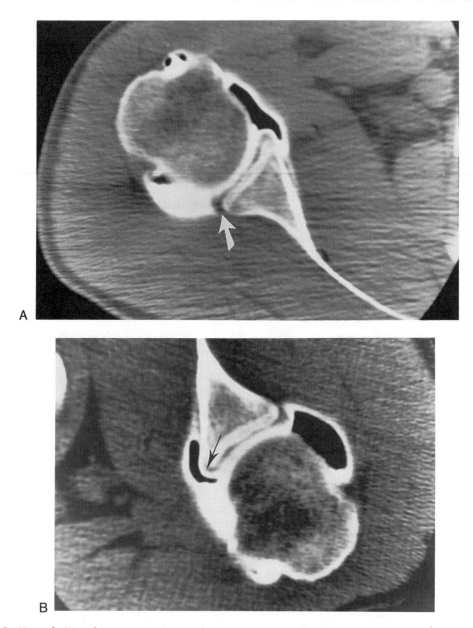

**Fig. 7-2.** Normal CT arthrogram, supine and prone images. Difficulty in delineating the posterior labrum (**A**; *arrow*) is eliminated with prone positioning (**B**; *arrow*).

We currently use the prone position on occasion to assist in imaging the posterior labrum and capsule (Fig. 7-2). Supine positioning can cause puddling of the contrast material about the posterior labrum, thus obscuring the view; with prone positioning, any excessive contrast material collects about the anterior labrum and recess. The addition of prone imaging to the overall protocol is usually influenced by the clinician who has a definite suspicion of posterior labrum-capsule injury.

CT is performed superior to the humeral head to the axial recess with slice thicknesses ranging from 3 to 5 mm and interslice gaps of 3 to 5 mm. Clearly, a variable amount of information is available to the image interpreter because of the potential wide ranges of slice thicknesses and gaps used. Bone and soft tissue windows are commonly used. Technical factors may contribute to an unsatisfactory examination. These include extra-articular injection of the contrast media, more than 10 to 15 minute delay in obtaining the CT scan, and the presence of a joint effusion.[20] Exercise after the injection also can lead to an unsatisfactory examination because of the extravasation of air and positive contrast material; this is of particular concern when labral and capsular pathology is in question. Obviously, the imaging of full-thickness cuff tears is enhanced by the exercise.

# CLINICAL RESULTS

The literature is replete with studies proclaiming the accuracy of CT-arthrography as a diagnostic imaging modality. However, most studies present surgical confirmation for only a fraction of the total cases presented. In this section, we present the results of studies assessing the accuracy of CT-arthrography against a surgical standard in which at least 50 percent of the total cases had the imaging results compared with the findings of open surgery or arthroscopy.

## Rotator Cuff

The criterion used for rotator cuff tears is the presence of air or contrast material within the subacromial bursa or within the supraspinatus tendon. A review of the literature reveals few studies with any more than a handful of cases with confirmed rotator cuff injury, so no hard conclusions can be formed. In general, CT-arthrography is poor for partial-thickness rotator cuff injury.[28] Its accuracy for full-thickness tears most likely approaches that of double-contrast shoulder arthrography. Wilson et al[12] found CT-arthrography to be superior to conventional arthrography. Nine full-thickness rotator cuff tears were identified with CT-arthrography, of which only seven were seen with conventional arthrography. Wilson et al found no rotator cuff tears on conventional arthrography that could not be found with CT. Hayes et al[28] found a 94 percent accuracy for full-thickness rotator cuff tears. In the largest series to date, Resch et al.[29] surveyed 185 patients who underwent CT-arthrography with subsequent surgery. They found the sensitivity for full-thickness tears was 88 percent, as compared with 91 percent sensitivity for conventional double-contrast arthrography. They also noted that it was not possible to determine the extent and location of the tear in conventional axial scans. In our experience, CT-arthrography has proved to be difficult in the diagnosis of rotator cuff tears. We have had excellent experience with double-contrast arthrography and continue to use this modality along with MRI exclusively for rotator cuff tears.

## Glenoid Labrum

Labra are classified as abnormal based on morphologic criteria: attenuation or absence, deformity, tear in substance, detachment from glenoid margin, and enlargement (Fig. 7-3). Detached labra can also include a fragment of the underlying glenoid margin (Fig. 7-4). An enlarged labrum is thought to represent degenerative changes and may reflect synovial hypertrophy, inflammation, or hydropic changes.

Singson et al[23] imaged 52 shoulders with subsequently surgically proven anterior labral abnormalities. Overall, CT-arthrography had no false-positive findings and only two false-negatives. In a prospective study, Callaghan et al[21] found a sensitivity/specificity/accuracy for anterior labral injury of 90/73/83 percent and for posterior labral injury of 100/100/100 percent, respectively. They also found an accuracy of 96.6 percent for injuries to the bicipital-labral complex. Resch et al[29] surveyed 205 patients and found an overall sensitivity for lesions of the labrum of 93 percent and a specificity of 96 percent. They found most of the false-negatives were due to basal labral disruptions, in which the labrum had retained its continuity and returned to its original position. Wilson et al[12] studied 40 surgically confirmed cases and found a sensitivity of 100 percent and a specificity of 97 percent for labral injury. Nottage et al[17] reviewed 30 patients who underwent both CT-arthrography and arthroscopy and found one false-positive study and two false-negative studies. The false-negative studies both represented isolated low anterior labral detachments.

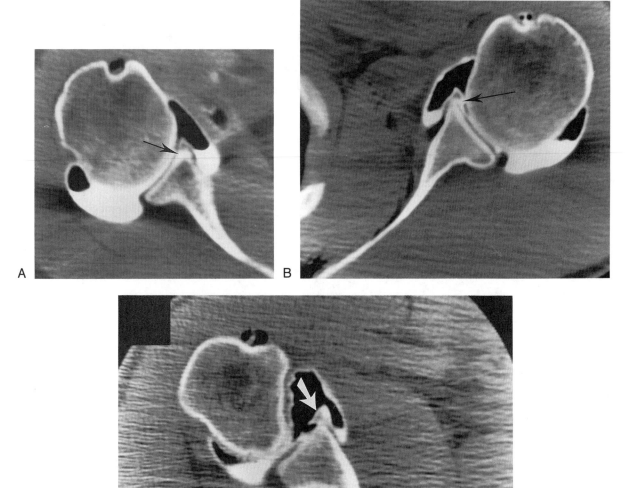

**Fig. 7-3.** Variable appearance of anterior labrum in patients with anterior instability. (**A**) Essentially normal morphology of anterior labrum with contrast agent seen within the anterior labrum (*arrow*), indicating injury. (**B**) Morphologically deformed anterior labrum (*arrow*) also with evidence of contrast agent within the labrum indicating injury. (**C**) Classic Bankart lesion (*arrow*) in patient after anterior glenohumeral dislocation.

It has been suggested that different types of labral lesions can be imaged with varying degrees of accuracy.[13] It may be that the clinical setting in which the labral injury occurs can be used as a predictor for the subsequent accuracy of the imaging test for the labral injury. Kneisl et al[18] evaluated this theory in patients with clear-cut instability and in patients without instability who presented only with pain. From a group of 55 patients, they found a sensitivity of double-contrast arthrotomography of 91 percent in the instability group and a sensitivity of only 63 percent in the pain group. These findings were corroborated by Matsui and

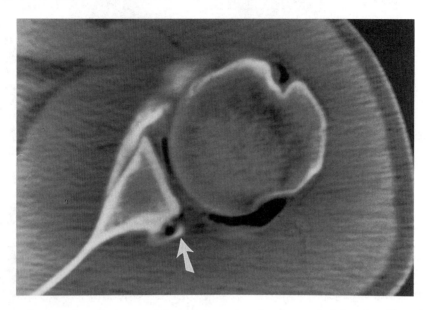

**Fig. 7-4.** Supine CT arthrogram in patient following posterior glenohumeral dislocation. There is deformity at posterior edge of the labrum including both soft tissue and bone (*arrow*).

Ogawa[13] using pneumoarthro-CT. For frank detachments or defects in the labrum, they found a sensitivity of 100 percent. These are the labral findings most commonly seen in the setting of instability. For labral lesions consisting of cracks only, the overall sensitivity was only 30 percent. A crack was defined as a fissure between the glenoid rim and the labrum but without complete exfoliation.

## Shoulder Capsule

An almost constant finding of CT arthrography in anterior glenohumeral instability is a disturbance of the capsular attachments to the glenoid rim. This finding is one for which CT-arthrography is particularly accurate because of the joint insufflation and axial plane imaging.[25,26] This capsular lesion is invariably found at a location on the glenoid margin consistent with the determined direction of instability. The capsular reflection can appear distorted with either loss or thickening of the intervening soft tissue layer over the scapula.[25] These medialized scapular neck insertions have been corroborated by surgical findings in several studies.[12,23,25,26] These capsular abnormalities are usually associated with lesions of the fibrocartilaginous labrum.

The real issue of the capsule insertion site is what is normal and what is abnormal. Variations have been reported to exist in the insertion sites of the anterior capsule onto the glenoid.[30] In type 1 insertion, the capsule inserts onto the glenoid rim in close proximity to the glenoid labrum. In types 2 and 3, the capsular insertion is farther away from the glenoid rim and may reach the scapular neck. Presumably, the more medial the capsular insertion, the less passive restraint to anterior dislocation.[12,23,25,26,30] Other anatomic variations observed include the development of the glenohumeral ligaments (especially the middle glenohumeral ligament) and the number and size of joint bursae.[26]

Wilson et al[12] found that in 101 shoulders that had undergone CT-arthrography, 83 percent had a capsular attachment that was medial to the articular margin at one of the three recorded levels. In a subgroup of 34 patients with surgical confirmation, 80 percent of the type 1 capsules were found to be abnormal, 82 percent of the type 2 capsules, and 100 percent of the type 3 capsules. All the type 3 capsules had labral tears. Singson et al[23] reported that capsular abnormalities were more common in recurrent dislocation (83 percent) as opposed to recurrent subluxation (61 percent).

The issue of capsular insertion variability and its impact on the interpretation of the CT-arthrography remains confusing. No definitive anatomic study has been performed to corroborate or refute the findings of CT-arthrography. In our clinical practice, we invariably see the anterior capsule attach to or about the anterior labrum during shoulder arthroscopy for conditions other than anterior instability. We remain unconvinced that medial scapula neck attachment exists in the normal undisturbed glenohumeral joint. The artifact seen with CT-arthrography may reflect a capsular redundancy that is rotation-dependent and can be eliminated by the addition of external rotation to the imaging protocol.

Capsular-synovial folds are occasionally present in the shoulder and seem to be analogous to the plicae

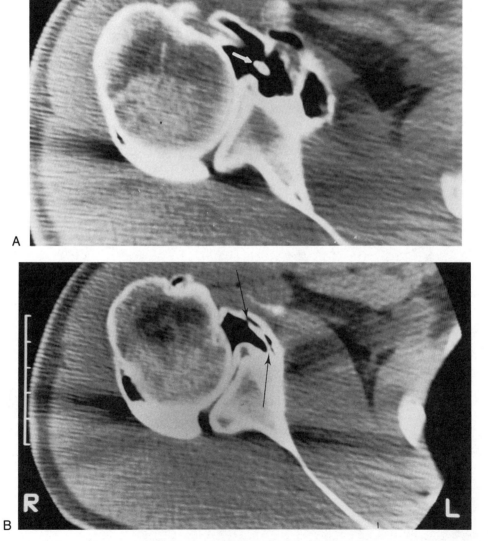

**Fig. 7-5.** Assessment of serial CT arthrogram images is necessary to evaluate fully the possible presence of an intraarticular loose body. (**A**) Image shows what appears to be an intra-articular loose body (*arrow*) in anterior inferior joint recess. (**B**) Image shows that the structure is nothing other than a synovial fold with a clear extension into the glenoid capsular margin (*arrows*).

seen in the knee. Whether these folds can be a source of clinical symptoms is in doubt. However, these folds can present interpretive difficulties in that they can resemble loose bodies on individual images. It is essential to assess serial images when evaluating the shoulder for a possible loose body to ensure that the structure in question has no attachment to the capsule (Fig. 7-5).

## Bone and Articular Cartilage

CT in the axial plane is superb for delineating injury to humeral head bone or glenoid bone (Fig. 7-4). An overall accuracy of 100 percent in delineating Hill-Sachs or glenoid margin injuries has been reported in several studies.[12,13,29] One study found that only 50 percent of the Hill-Sachs lesions seen with CT-

arthrography were visualized with plain radiographs alone.[12] Callaghan et al[21] found only a 50 percent sensitivity for Hill-Sachs lesion when compared with the findings of arthroscopy. This discrepancy may be accounted for by the known poor resolution of CT-arthrography for chondral lesions. The loss of sensitivity may have been due to chondral lesions only.

The imaging of humeral head articular cartilage has generally been regarded as poor by CT-arthrography. Wilson et al[12] found that the humeral head cartilage was visible on only 60 percent of imaging studies. However, the imaging of glenoid cartilage has generally been much better. Cartilage visibility has been found in more than 95 percent of images and focal thinning or full-thickness loss can be readily appreciated.[12] Our experience has been much more favorable for chondral imaging. Technically, it is important to

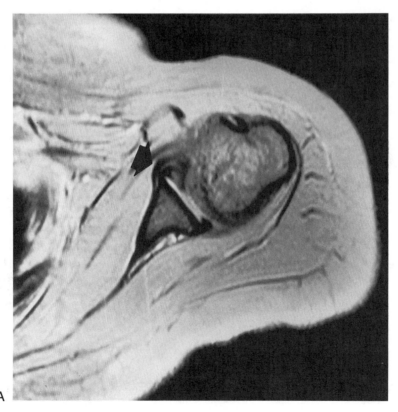

A

**Fig. 7-6.** Joint insufflation gives CT arthrography a great advantage over plain MRI for the delineation of anterior capsular-labral injury. Relaxed position of anterior capsule potentially can hide anterior injury. (**A**) MRI (TR 450 ms, TE 13 ms) shows relaxed inferior glenohumeral ligament (*arrow*) in this neutrally rotated shoulder. Anterior capsuloligamentous structures are normal. (*Figure continues.*)

minimize the amount of positive contrast material used; we routinely use no more than 3 to 5 ml. At present, we believe that a properly performed CT-arthrogram can show chondral lesions better than can a spin-echo MRI. We fully anticipate that the advancement of MRI chondral imaging protocols to include volumetric imaging will supplant CT-arthrography as the imaging modality of choice for chondral injury.

## COMPARISON OF CT-ARTHROGRAPHY AND MRI

Since the application of MRI to shoulder disorders in the mid-1980s, many investigators have speculated that it would eventually replace CT-arthrography as an imaging modality. MRI has many inherent advantages over CT-arthrography including noninvasiveness, no ionizing radiation, direct imaging capability, and superior tissue resolution. We believe that CT-arthrography still has an important role in the assessment of shoulder disorders in the athletic patient and may have an increasing role in the future as ongoing concerns of MRI cost and availability come to light.

MRI is clearly superior to CT-arthrography in the imaging of full-thickness rotator cuff tears and also sheds light on the degree of retraction, quality of the tendon ends and muscle belly, and actual size of the tear.[31-33,41] MRI also has the added capability of imaging partial thickness tears,[34] but CT-arthrography has little use for this injury.[28]

MRI can image metaphyseal bone better than CT-arthrography because it can delineate "bruising," whereas CT-arthrography must rely on some degree of

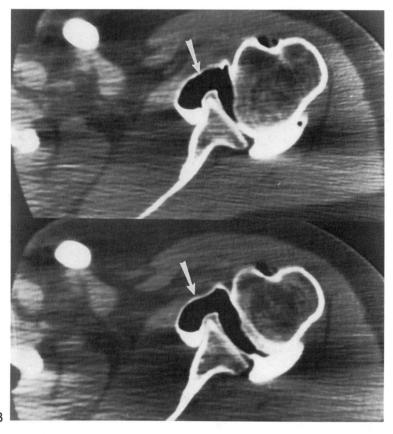

B

**Fig. 7-6** *(Continued )*. (**B**) CT arthrogram of same shoulder and image at same level showing distention of these previously relaxed anterior capsular structures (*arrows*). Visualization of anterior capsular-labral complex is greatly enhanced after joint insufflation.

architectural distortion.[32,35] Thus, Hill-Sachs osseous contusions invisible on CT-arthrography are visualized readily with MRI. Chondral imaging by MRI offers no clear advantages over CT. Spin-echo MRI has great difficulty imaging articular cartilage lesions in the shoulder. MR-arthrography has been shown to image cartilage defects better than that with MR alone.[33,36]

There is great variability in the accuracy of MRI in the detection and characterization of labral injuries.[35,37,38] It is likely that MRI will be at least as good and probably better than CT-arthrography for the imaging of labral lesions. One study has documented that MRI is significantly better than CT for the evaluation of labral structures.[39]

The characterization of capsular injury and its detachment from the glenoid remains a great problem for MRI.[40] The anterior capsule is relaxed with the arm at the side and the shoulder in neutral rotation. Significant detachments can appear normal because of the lack of tension on these tissues. CT-arthrography has an advantage in this area in that the insufflation technique tenses the capsule and readily illustrates any detachments or stripping (Fig. 7-6). Resch et al[29] found that the anterior soft tissue structures within the joint were better delineated with CT-arthrography than with MRI without contrast medium. Studies contrasting plain MRI with MR-arthrography have consistently found that the addition of intra-articular contrast agents (gadolinium) to insufflate the joint improves the diagnostic accuracy for the detection of labral and capsular abnormalities.[33,36] We have had some limited experience with MRI external rotation axial views to tense the anterior structures and highlight anterior capsular abnormalities. Early results show this to be a promising adjunct in the detection of anterior capsule/labral injury.

## SUMMARY

CT-arthrography remains a very reliable imaging modality with well-established advantages and disadvantages. It is doubtful that MRI will replace CT-arthrography as an imaging modality in the injured athletic shoulder. With an understanding of the techniques, interpretations, and pitfalls of CT-arthrography, the clinician can put this imaging modality in proper perspective with the other available radiographic imaging techniques. In this way, this test can best be used to assist the clinician in the evaluation and treatment of injuries to the athletic shoulder.

## REFERENCES

1. Linblom K, Palmer I: Arthrography and roentgenography in ruptures of tendons of the shoulder joint. Acta Radiol 20:548, 1939
2. Braustein EM, O'Connor G: Double-contrast arthrotomography of the shoulder. J Bone Joint Surg 64A:192, 1982
3. Goldman AB, Ghelman B: The double contrast arthrogram. Radiology 127:655, 1978
4. Deutsch AL, Resnick D, Mink JH et al: Computed and conventional arthrotomography of the glenohumeral joint: normal anatomy and clinical experience. Radiology 153:603, 1984
5. Mink JH, Richardson A, Grant TT: Evaluation of glenoid labrum by double-contrast shoulder arthrography. AJR 133:883, 1979
6. Shuman WP, Kilcoyne RF, Matsen FA et al: Double-contrast computed tomography of the glenoid labrum. AJR 141:581, 1983
7. McGlynn FJ, El-Khoury G, Albright JP: Arthrotomography of the glenoid labrum in shoulder instability. J Bone Joint Surg 64A:506, 1982
8. El Khoury GY, Kathol MH, Chandler JB et al: Shoulder instability: impact of glenohumeral arthrotomography on treatment. Radiology 160:669, 1986
9. Baird RA, Schobert WE, Pais MJ: Radiographic identification of loose bodies in the traumatized hip joint. Radiology 145:661, 1982
10. Tirman RM, Nelson CS, Tirman WS: Arthrography of the shoulder joint: state of the art. CRC Crit Rev Diagn Imaging 17:19, 1981
11. Cook JV, Tayar R: Double-contrast computed tomographic arthrography of the shoulder joint. Br J Radiol 62:1043, 1989
12. Wilson AJ, Totty WG, Murphy WA, Hardy DC: Shoulder joint: arthrographic CT and long-term follow-up, with surgical correlation. Radiology 173:329, 1989
13. Matsui K, Ogawa K: Pneumoarthro-computed tomography of the shoulder joint for anterior and multidirectional instability. p. 14. In Post M, Morrey BF, Hawkins RJ (eds): Surgery of the Shoulder. Mosby Year Book, St Louis, 1990
14. Haynor DR, Shuman WP: Double contrast CT arthrography of the glenoid labrum and shoulder girdle. Radiographics 4:411, 1984

15. Kinnard P, Tricoire J, Levesque R et al: Assessment of the unstable shoulder by computed arthrography. Am J Sports Med 11:157, 1983
16. Ribbans WJ, Mitchell R, Taylor GJ: Computerized arthrotomography of primary anterior dislocation of the shoulder. J Bone Joint Surg 72B:181, 1990
17. Nottage WM, Duge WD, Fields WA: Computed arthrotomography of the glenohumeral joint to evaluate anterior instability: correlation with arthroscopic findings. Arthroscopy 3:273, 1987
18. Kneisl JS, Sweeney HJ, Paige ML: Correlation of pathology observed in double contrast arthrotomography and arthroscopy of the shoulder. Arthroscopy 4:21, 1988
19. Rafii M, Firooznia H, Golimbu C et al: CT arthrography of capsular structures of the shoulder. AJR 146:361, 1986
20. Rafii M, Firooznia H, Bonamo JJ et al: Athlete shoulder injuries: CT arthrographic findings. Radiology 162:559, 1987
21. Callaghan JJ, McNiesh LM, DeHaven JP et al: A prospective comparison study of double contrast computed tomography arthrography and arthroscopy of the shoulder. Am J Sports Med 16:13, 1988
22. McNiesh LM, Callaghan JJ: CT arthrography of the shoulder: variations of the glenoid labrum. AJR 149:963, 1987
23. Singson RD, Feldman F, Bigliani L: CT arthrographic patterns in recurrent glenohumeral instability. AJR 149:749, 1987
24. Singson RD, Feldman F, Bigliani LU et al: Recurrent shoulder dislocation after surgical repair: double contrast CT arthrography. Radiology 164:425, 1987
25. Rafii M, Firooznia H, Golimbu C et al: CT arthrography of capsular structures of the shoulder. AJR 146:361, 1986
26. Rafii M, Minkoff J, Bonamo J et al: Computed tomography arthrography of shoulder instabilities in athletes. Am J Sports Med 16:352, 1988
27. Pennes DR, Jonsson K, Buckwalter K et al: Computed arthrotomography of the shoulder: comparison of examinations made with internal and external rotation of the humerus. AJR 153:1017, 1989
28. Hayes MG, Magarey M, White J: The shoulder complex: correlation of clinical examination, computed arthrotomography, magnetic resonance imaging, and arthroscopic evaluation. p. 18. In Post M, Morrey BF, Hawkins RJ (eds): Surgery of the Shoulder. Mosby Year Book, St Louis, 1990
29. Resch H, Furtschegger A, zur Nedden D et al: The value of different screening methods in the diagnosis of shoulder lesions: ultrasonography, arthrography, CT, MR imaging, arthroscopy, bursoscopy. p. 22. In Post M, Morrey BF, Hawkins RJ (eds.): Surgery of the Shoulder. Mosby Year Book, St Louis, 1990
30. Rothman RH, Marvel JP, Heppenstall RB: Anatomic considerations in the glenohumeral joint. Orthop Clin North Am 6:341, 1975
31. Zlatkin MB: Rotator cuff disease. p. 55. In Zlatkin MB (ed): MRI of the Shoulder. 1st Ed. Raven Press, New York, 1991
32. Meyer SJF, Dalinka MK: Magnetic resonance imaging of the shoulder. Orthop Clin North Am 21:497, 1990
33. Flannigan B, Kursunoglu-Brahme S, Snyder S et al: MR arthrography of the shoulder: comparison with conventional MR imaging. AJR 155:829
34. Seeger LL, Gold RH, Bassett LW et al: Shoulder impingement syndrome: MR findings in 53 shoulders. AJR 150:343, 1988
35. Zlatkin MB: Shoulder instability. p. 99. In Zlatkin MB (ed): MRI of the Shoulder. 1st Ed. Raven Press, New York, 1991
36. Shobert W, Nottage W, Stauffer A: Saline MRI of the shoulder. Presented at Annual AOSSM meeting, Orlando, FL, 1991
37. Legan JM, Burkhard TK, Goff WF et al: Tears of the glenoid labrum: MR imaging of 88 arthroscopically confirmed cases. Radiology 179:241, 1991
38. Garneau RA, Renfrew DL, Moore TE: Glenoid labrum: evaluation with MR imaging. Radiology 179:519, 1991
39. Neumann CH, Petersen SA, Jahnke AH et al: MRI in the evaluation of patients with suspected instability of the shoulder joint including a comparison with CT-arthrography. ROFO 154:593, 1991
40. Kieft GJ, Bloem JL, Rozing PM et al: MR imaging of recurrent anterior dislocation of the shoulder: comparison with CT arthrography. AJR 150:1083, 1988
41. Rafii M, Firooznia H, Sherman O et al: Rotator cuff lesions: signal patterns at MR imaging. Radiology 177:817, 1990

# 8

# Arthroscopic Techniques of the Shoulder

*WILLIAM B. GEISSLER*
*RICHARD B. CASPARI*

The techniques of diagnostic and surgical shoulder arthroscopy have become a valuable adjunct in the management of shoulder disorders. A thorough understanding of the anatomy of the shoulder girdle is mandatory as the complexity of arthroscopic shoulder procedures continues to expand. Precise placement of arthroscopic portals is imperative in the shoulder because of the proximity of many neurovascular structures and the muscles that are perforated. This chapter reviews the operative technique and anatomy pertaining to establishing the various portals for arthroscopic surgery of the shoulder.

## OPERATIVE TECHNIQUE

The importance of the operating room setup cannot be overemphasized for a successful and efficient arthroscopic shoulder procedure. The procedure may be performed under general endotracheal anesthesia or interscalene block. Most surgeons prefer general endotracheal anesthesia, particularly if the lateral decubitus position is used. Intubation in this position is difficult if the patient becomes uncomfortable and may require repreparing and draping. Interscalene blocks are more frequently used when the patient is placed in the beach chair position. This allows the patient to help position him- or herself for the procedure, and the anesthesiologist has more optimal access to the patient's airway if the need should arise.

Vital information is gained from the examination of the shoulder under anesthesia, and this opportunity should not be missed. The shoulder girdle muscles are relaxed, allowing the examiner to freely translocate the humeral head on the glenoid and measure any existing instability. The evaluation also should include range of motion of both shoulders, noting any limitations in passive motion suggesting adhesive capsulitis. Occasionally, increased external rotation in abduction is observed, reflecting anterior capsular laxity and possible anterior instability. In cases of shoulder subluxation, the information obtained from the clinical examination is correlated with the arthroscopic findings to confirm the diagnosis.[1] After the clinical examination, the patient is placed in either the lateral decubitus or beach chair position, depending on the surgeon's preference. In the lateral decubitus position, the patient is placed on his or her side with the affected shoulder up. The patient is supported by an inflatable bean bag or kidney rests, or both. It is important to tilt the patient back 30 degrees to allow easier access to the front of the shoulder.[2] The patient is further stabilized with tape running from the side rails across the pelvis. After the anesthesiologist has checked the position of the head and down ear, the head is covered and lightly taped to prevent any displacement during the procedure (Fig. 8-1). A skin traction device is applied to the forearm after the patient has been prepared and draped, and the arm is suspended by an overhead rope and pulley traction apparatus. The arm is placed in

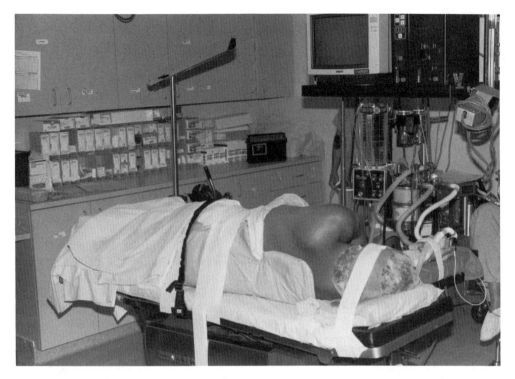

**Fig. 8-1.** The patient is placed in the lateral decubitus position and slanted back 30 degrees for easier access to the front of the shoulder.

approximately 30 to 40 degrees of abduction and 20 degrees of forward flexion. The arm is suspended by 10, 15 or rarely 20 lb of traction. This provides distraction and inferior subluxation of the humerus. This displacement allows the surgeon to see and work in the anteroinferior area of the glenoid where most pathology related to anterior instability is present. In the beach chair position, the patient is placed as if sitting in a chair.[3] Temporary traction may be applied by a surgical assistant if required during the procedure.

In the lateral decubitus position, the monitor, light, and power equipment source is placed opposite the patient's shoulder in front of the surgeon. The scrub nurse and Mayo stand are situated at the head of the operating table (Fig. 8-2). Using this format, the surgeon has easy access to the whole shoulder without having to move any equipment or personnel.[4] The scrub nurse is in the ideal position to pass instruments and to assist the surgeon when an extra hand is needed. The standard-sized instruments that are used in the knee may be used in the shoulder.

## EXTERNAL ANATOMY

Knowledge of the external anatomy and palpable landmarks of the shoulder is essential to precise portal placement. The palpable bony landmarks include the clavicle and coracoid anteriorly, the acromion laterally, and the scapular spine posteriorly. The coracoid is located just inferior to the palpable acromioclavicular joint. It is important to note the location of the coracoid when making an anterior portal because the neurovascular bundle runs medial to it. The posterior lateral corner of the acromion is almost always palpable, no matter how large or obese the patient is. This is an important landmark, as the placement of the initial posterior portal is based on its location.

The shoulder is surrounded by a thick soft tissue envelope that can make palpation of landmarks difficult, particularly in obese or well-muscled individuals. It is often helpful to draw the bony landmarks on the shoulder skin to help maintain proper orientation. These should be palpated and drawn before the intro-

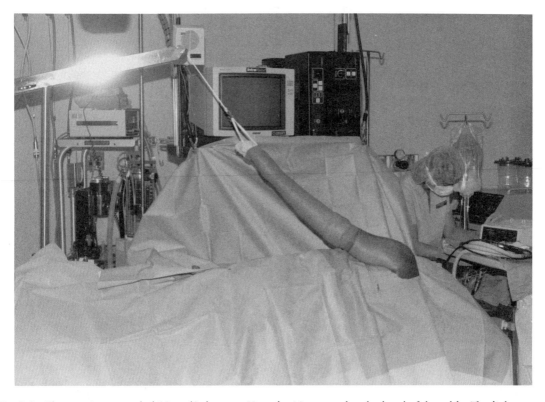

**Fig. 8-2.** The arm is suspended 30 to 40 degrees. Note the Mayo stand at the head of the table. The light source and camera cords are passed under the arm and the shaver above.

duction of irrigation fluid, which may extravasate and further obliterate identification of these landmarks (Fig. 8-3).

## PORTALS AND ANATOMY

Establishing a portal in the shoulder involves perforation of several layers of tissue. Also, in some patients the shoulder joint lies a considerable distance from the skin. It is important to maintain a portal in the shoulder once it has been established, as the chance of reintroducing an instrument or cannula exactly through the same hole in the tissue is remote.[5] Attempts to re-establish a previous portal not only leads to unnecessary soft tissue damage but also promotes extravasation of irrigation fluid into the soft tissues obliterating bony landmarks. For this reason, interchangeable cannula systems are used that allow the passage of the arthro-scope and motorized instruments through the same cannula.

Langer's lines are observed during skin incisions for portal placement. The anterior and posterior portal skin incisions are vertical, aiming at the axillary fold. The lateral portal incision is horizontal, and the superior portal incision is established in the anteroposterior direction. When making an incision for a portal, only the skin is cut, avoiding deep plunges with the knife.

### Posterior Portal

The posterior portal is the most frequently used portal for shoulder arthroscopy. It allows almost complete visualization of the entire glenohumeral joint. Precise positioning of the posterior portal is important, because improper placement can make viewing of the joint difficult and will displace the normal position of the anterior portal if the inside-out technique is used.

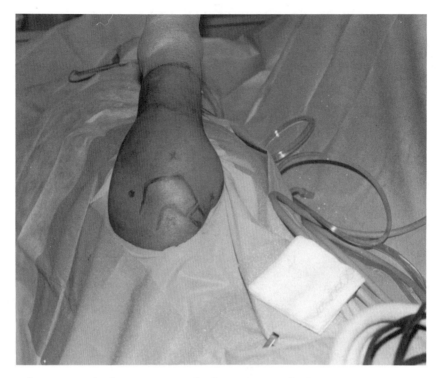

**Fig. 8-3.** External anatomy and relative positions of arthroscopic portals. *"X"* anteriorly marks coracoid process. Note position of posterior portal medial to posterolateral edge of the acromion.

The posterior portal is located approximately 2 cm distal and 1 cm medial to the posterolateral corner of the acromion. This portion of the acromion is almost always palpable regardless of the size of the individual. It is important to avoid the tendency to stray laterally down the arm and stay 1 cm medial to the edge of the acromion when making this portal. The portal is located in the usually palpable "soft spot" of the shoulder. The glenohumeral joint may be insufflated with irrigation solution before insertion of the cannula, depending on the surgeon's preference. After the skin is incised, a sharp cannula is inserted and directed toward the coracoid on the opposite side of the shoulder. The cannula passes through the deltoid muscle and a portion of the subdeltoid bursa. It then perforates the muscular belly of the infraspinatus or passes between the interval of this muscle and the teres minor. The cannula finally pierces the capsule and synovium to enter the joint.

The posterior portal is relatively safe when placed in the correct position. The axillary nerve passes below the teres minor through the quadrilateral space to innervate it and the deltoid. The nerve becomes at risk if the cannula is advanced too far inferiorly, passing below rather than above the teres minor. The suprascapular nerve passes around the scapular spine after it has innervated the supraspinatus to supply the infraspinatus muscle. The nerve passes 2 cm medial to the posterior edge of the glenoid. It becomes at risk if the cannula is advanced too far medially along the glenoid neck.

## Anterior Portal

The anterior portal is used mainly to pass instrumentation into the joint. The anterior glenoid neck and labrum, articular surface of the rotator cuff, and the intra-articular portion of the biceps tendon are easily accessible through this portal. The arthroscope may be placed through the anterior portal to further evaluate pathology of the glenohumeral joint if not properly seen from the posterior portal. This is particularly helpful when judging the effectiveness of the anterior inferior glenohumeral ligament from a different perspective in patients with a history of shoulder subluxation.

The anterior portal may be made in one of two ways. The preferred method is to pass the arthroscope from the posterior portal across the joint to the desired location on the anterior capsule. The desired location on the capsule lies within a triangle bounded by three easily identifiable landmarks. The triangle is formed by the biceps tendon superiorly, the intra-articular portion of the subscapularis inferiorly, and the anterior glenoid medially. The arthroscope is advanced against the anterior capsule and withdrawn from its sheath. A sharp obturator is placed in the sheath, and this is passed through the capsule to tent the skin anteriorly. A small skin incision is made, and a cannula is placed over the obturator as it exits the skin. Most cannulas are slightly larger than the arthroscopic sheath and snugly slide over it. The cannula then follows the obturator as it is withdrawn posteriorly to enter the joint. The obturator is removed, and the arthroscope is replaced back into its sheath. Using this method, the cannula passes through the rotator cuff interval between the subscapularis inferiorly and the supraspinatus superiorly. It then pierces the anterior deltoid to exit the skin. Once this portal has been established, it should never be lost because of the risk of extravastion of fluid into the soft tissues.

The anterior portal may also be established directly by passing a spinal needle from the anterior shoulder into the joint. If the position of the needle is satisfactory intra-articularly, a cannula is passed through a small skin incision, reproducing the tract of the needle into the joint. This method is more difficult because of the thick soft tissue envelope of the shoulder and following the exact path of the spinal needle with a cannula is not easy. Occasionally, this method is required when the arthroscope sheath cannot be advanced across the joint secondary to improper placement of the original posterior portal or severe adhesive capsulitis.

The anterior portal is relatively safe if properly placed and close attention is paid to the palpable external landmarks. Whether the inside-out or direct method of portal placement is used, the position of the portal must always be lateral to the palpable coracoid. The conjoined tendon inserts on the coracoid. The musculocutaneous nerve runs along the medial border of the conjoined tendon approximately 3 to 7 cm inferior to the coracoid. Any portal placed medial to the

coracoid places this nerve at unnecessary risk. The anterior portal should also not be placed below the subscapularis tendon. The axillary nerve passes below the subscapularis to innervate the deltoid and will be at jeopardy if the portal is placed too inferior.

## Supraspinatus Fossa Portal

The supraspinatus fossa portal is used primarily as an inflow portal.[6] Inflow may be provided by an accessory anterior or posterior portal, but additional cannulas in these positions often result in overcrowding and become a nuisance. A cannula inserted through the supraspinatus portal to supply irrigation is placed down the posterior gutter of the shoulder out of the way of the arthroscope and other instruments. The arthroscope and mechanical shavers are rarely used through this portal because the surrounding bony structures inhibit manipulation of these instruments. The use of this portal may be avoided if an infusion pump is used to supply irrigation fluid through the arthroscope sheath or if the procedure is a limited diagnostic arthroscopy not requiring a large amount of fluid.

The supraspinatus fossa is located by palpating the soft spot bounded anteriorly by the clavicle, laterally by the acromion, and posteriorly by the scapular spine. A spinal needle is passed at a 30-degree angle from the horizontal and aimed slightly posterior through the soft spot. It should enter the joint just above the superior portion of the glenoid neck, posterior to the biceps tendon. A puncture wound is made, and a cannula is advanced along the identical tract of the spinal needle into the joint. The cannula is tucked down the posterior recess of the glenohumeral joint to supply irrigation fluid and still be out of the way of the other instruments. The cannula passes through the trapezius muscle, which covers the supraspinatus fossa. It then pierces the muscle belly of the supraspinatus medial to the tendonous portion to enter the joint without injury to the rotator cuff. The cannula may pass through the tendonous portion of the supraspinatus, causing injury to the rotator cuff, if the arm is placed in excessive abduction.[7]

The supraspinatus fossa portal is relatively safe, as the only major nerve in the area is the suprascapular nerve. This nerve enters the fossa through the suprascapular notch medial to the coracoid. The nerve passes along the floor of the supraspinatus fossa to supply the supraspinatus muscle. It then travels around the lateral aspect of the scapular spine to exit the fossa. The nerve lies approximately 3 cm medial to the suprascapular portal.[8]

## Subacromial Portals

A thorough arthroscopic examination of the shoulder includes both the glenohumeral joint and subacromial space. The subacromial portals are useful to examine the superior surface of the rotator cuff for full- or partial-thickness tears and the undersurface of the acromion for signs of impingement. Arthroscopic subacromial decompression, distal clavicle resection, and debridement of the rotator cuff are possible procedures that can be performed through these portals.

A considerable amount of irrigation fluid may be extravasated into the soft tissues after arthroscopy of the subacromial space. For this reason, the subacromial space is usually approached after the examination of the glenohumeral joint. The arthroscope sheath with a sharp obturator is placed through the original skin incision for the posterior glenohumeral portal and tracked subcutaneously toward the posterior edge of the acromion. It is then advanced under the acromion into the subacromial space, aiming for the anterolateral corner of the acromion. The undersurface of the acromion should be palpated with the arthroscope sheath to confirm its postion in the subacromial space. The sharp obturator is replaced with the arthroscope, and inflow is provided through the scope sheath with an infusion pump or through a separate anterior portal. A second portal for inflow is usually required if an irrigation pump is not used, because bleeding into the subacromial space can be profuse and a high flow rate may be required. To establish the anterior inflow portal, the arthroscope sheath and obturator are advanced past the anterior acromion and out the previous

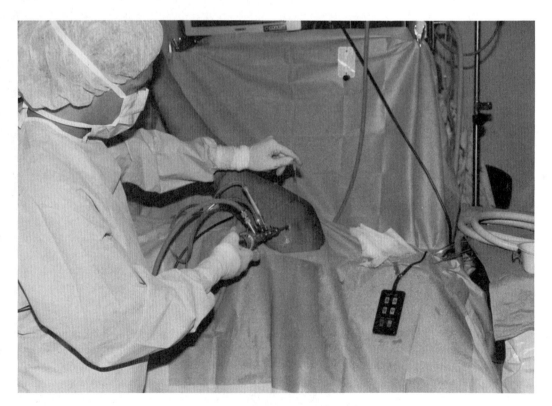

**Fig. 8-4.** Ideal position of lateral subacromial portal is initially determined with a spinal needle. Position of the needle in the subacromial space is viewed arthroscopically and is modified accordingly.

skin incision for the anterior glenohumeral portal. A cannula is placed over the arthroscope sheath and is guided into the subacromial space as the sheath is retracted. A working portal is frequently made lateral to the acromion to pass instrumentation or the arthroscope. The position of this portal is approximately 3 cm distal to the anterolateral corner of the acromion (Fig. 8-4). An incision is made just through the skin to avoid any possible injury to the underlying deltoid muscle or the axillary nerve. A blunt obturator is passed obliquely and can be seen to enter the subacromial space with the arthroscope. The position of this portal places the instrumentation parallel to the anterior acromion and in ideal position to resect the coracoacromial ligament if required. The position of the axillary nerve should always be kept in mind when making this portal because it runs 5 cm distal to the lateral edge of the acromion under the deltoid to supply this muscle.

## SUMMARY

A knowledge of shoulder arthroscopy is imperative as it continues to evolve and become popular in the diagnosis and management of shoulder disorders. Arthroscopy of the shoulder has helped advance the understanding of various maladies of the shoulder such as the complex relationship between impingement and instability in the throwing athlete. As with any surgical technique, a thorough knowledge of the anatomy of the shoulder girdle relative to portal placement is essential before undertaking this rewarding procedure.

## REFERENCES

1. McGlynn FJ, Caspari RB: Arthroscopic findings in the subluxating shoulder. Clin Orthop 183:173, 1984
2. Caspari RB: Shoulder arthroscopy: a review of the present state of the art. Contemp Orthop 4:523, 1982
3. Skyhar MJ, Altchek DW, Warren RF et al: Shoulder arthroscopy with the patient in the beach-chair position. Arthroscopy 4:256, 1988
4. Caspari RB: Instrumentation and operating room organization for arthroscopy of the shoulder. p. 155. In McGinty JB (ed): Arthroscopic Surgery Update, Techniques in Orthopaedics. Aspen Systems Corp., Rockville, MD, 1985
5. Andrews JR, Carson WG: Shoulder joint arthroscopy. Orthopedics 6:1157, 1983
6. Neviaser TJ: Arthroscopy of the shoulder. Orthop Clin North Am 18:361, 1987
7. Souryal TO, Baker CL: Supraclavicular fossa portal anatomy. Arthroscopy 6:297, 1990
8. Caspari RB: Anatomy and portals for arthroscopic surgery of the shoulder. p. 15. In Jackson DW (ed): Shoulder Surgery in the Athlete, Techniques in Orthopaedics. Aspen Systems Corp., Rockville, MD, 1985

# 9

# Normal Arthroscopic Anatomy of the Shoulder

## WILLIAM G. CARSON, JR.

Diagnostic and operative arthroscopy of the shoulder have been well established for the treatment of various shoulder disorders.[1-18] The diagnostic and surgical techniques as well as the arthroscopic anatomy of the shoulder have been well described.[3,5,7,9,14,19-27] Surgical techniques include glenoid labrum resections,[2,11,15] certain rotator cuff debridements, or impingement releases,[1,28-33] for the debridement of a degenerative shoulder[17] or for the resection of a degenerative acromioclavicular joint.[16,18] More recently, arthroscopic techniques have been developed for arthroscopic Bankart repairs[34,35] or for arthroscopic staple capsulorrhaphy of the shoulder for recurrent anterior instability.[36-40]

A knowledge of the normal anatomy of the shoulder as viewed arthroscopically is an essential prerequisite for those orthopaedic surgeons performing any of the above-described surgical procedures. This chapter describes this normal arthroscopic anatomy of the shoulder.

The arthroscopic anatomy and various relationships or diagrams illustrated below are representative of those seen with the patient in the lateral decubitus position with the shoulder superior. The arm is abducted approximately 70 degrees and forward flexed 15 degrees[3-5,23] Most of the photographs and illustrations represent a posterior portal, which is the preferred approach for diagnostic arthroscopy of the shoulder. This posterior portal is located approximately 3 cm inferior to and slightly medial to the posterolateral corner of the acromion (Fig. 9-1). This point corresponds to the "soft spot" on the posterior aspect of the shoulder that comprises the relative interval between the infraspinatus and teres minor muscles (Fig. 9-2).

## BICEPS TENDON

The long head of the biceps tendon is usually the first structure identified after the arthroscope has been inserted into the shoulder through a posterior portal. This gives one proper orientation, and with the patient positioned in the lateral decubitus position, the long head of the biceps tendon is oriented approximately 10 to 15 degrees away from an imaginary vertical line. It attaches to the supraglenoid tubercle at the posterosuperior aspect of the glenoid and in this area is related to and appears to be continuous with the glenoid labrum (Fig. 9-3). The patient's arm can be externally rotated to facilitate visualization of the biceps tendon, which can be followed anteriorly to portions of the bicipital groove. The normal biceps tendon should appear glistening and smooth and free of any adhesions, fraying, synovitis, or partial tearing.

## HUMERAL HEAD AND GLENOID

After inspection of the biceps tendon is complete and proper orientation is once again obtained, the articular surfaces of the humeral head (superiorly) and the glenoid (inferiorly) are examined. Both of these articular surfaces are covered by hyaline cartilage. With the patient positioned in the lateral decubitus position, one can see approximately one-third of the articular surface

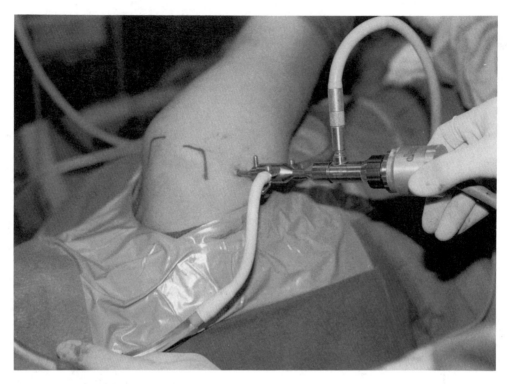

**Fig. 9-1.** Example of arthroscope in place through a posterior portal in a right shoulder.

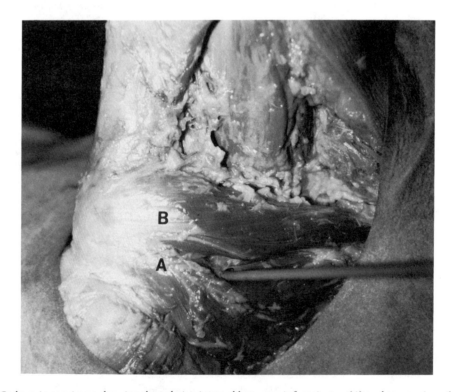

**Fig. 9-2.** Cadaveric specimen showing the relative interval between infraspinatus (*A*) and teres minor (*B*) muscles that the arthroscope traverses when establishing a posterior portal.

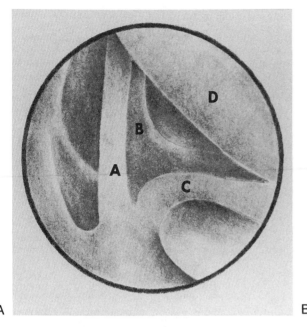

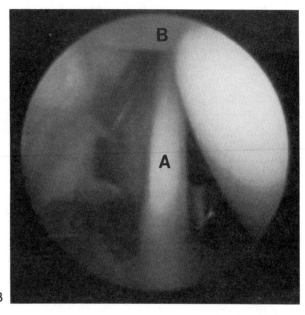

A

B

**Fig. 9-3.** (**A**) Arthroscopic view of a right shoulder with the patient in lateral decubitus position with the arm abducted 70 degrees. Structures that can be identified are long head of biceps tendon (*A*), superior glenohumeral ligament (*B*), anterior portion of glenoid labrum (*C*), and humeral head (*D*). (**B**) Biceps tendon is oriented in a vertical direction (*A*). The supraspinatus portion of the rotator cuff (*B*) is just superior and is intimately related to the biceps tendon in this view.

of the humeral head, which is oriented in 30 degrees of retroversion. Examination of the entire articular surface of the humeral head is facilitated by rotating the arthroscope superiorly and moving the humeral head into internal and external rotation. Anteriorly, the articular surface of the humeral head extends to the level of the humeral neck and near the insertion of the subscapularis. However, posteriorly there can be variations in the humeral head's articular surface extension to the soft tissues. Posteriorly, the rotator cuff attaches lateral to the actual extent of the articular cartilage, and thus a "bare area" of bone can be visualized. This bare area is located, for the most part, straight posteriorly and should not be confused with the Hill-Sachs lesion located more posterolaterally. The size of the normal bare area can vary; however, in most cases this normal area is smooth and rounded without evidence of fraying or degeneration indicative of possible trauma. Also, many times the bare area is characterized by different blood vessels that can be seen coursing through the area.

The glenoid is a bean- or pear-shaped cavity approximately one-fourth the size of the humeral head. Its surface is longer in the superior-to-inferior dimension than it is in the anterior-to-posterior dimension. The articular surface clinically appears to be thicker near its periphery than it is in its central portions.

## GLENOID LABRUM

The glenoid labrum is a wedge-shaped structure that borders the glenoid cavity and appears to provide inherent stability to the glenohumeral joint, thus restricting anterior and posterior excursion of the humerus[41,42] (Fig. 9-3). The glenoid labrum consists of hyaline cartilage, fibrocartilage, and fibrous tissue.[41–47] This fibrocartilagenous rim of tissue surrounds the glenoid circumferentially and portions of the labrum appear to overlap the articular surface of the glenoid or articular surface. This overlap portion of the glenoid labrum appears to deepen the glenoid, providing some inherent stability to the glenohumeral joint primarily by restricting anterior excursion. The glenoid surface of the labrum is continuous with the hyaline cartilage of the glenoid cavity, whereas the capsular surface blends with the joint capsule and glenohumeral ligaments. There can be variations in the width or thickness of the glenoid labrum, particularly at the different locations of the glenoid as it relates to the glenoid rim. Thus, clinically the anterior glenoid appears to be thicker at times than the posterior aspect of the glenoid labrum. At times, particularly anteriorly, the glenoid labrum can appear to be quite large and almost appear to be hypermobile and at times appears to be analogous to a meniscus that one sees arthroscopically in the knee joint. At other times, the glenoid labrum can be smaller and appears to be more firmly attached to the edge of the glenoid and to blend more with the actual hyaline cartilage surface.

The normal glenoid labrum should appear to be smooth and should lack any fraying, partial tearing, or excessive hypermobility. The usual inspection of the glenoid begins at the insertion of the biceps tendon, which appears to insert through the superior portion of the labrum into the supraglenoid tubercle. With additional traction placed on the arm with the traction apparatus, portions of the inferior glenoid rim can be visualized. Slight retraction and posterior rotation of the arthroscope will allow examination of the posterior rim of the glenoid labrum from a posterior arthroscopic portal. The arthroscope can be changed to an anterior portal for better visualization of the more posterior portions of the glenoid rim at times.

## GLENOHUMERAL LIGAMENTS

The superior, middle, and inferior glenohumeral ligaments are the terms used to describe the different thickenings of the anterior and inferior capsule of the shoulder joint. These glenohumeral ligaments are not free-standing distinct ligaments that one sees, for example, in the ankle or the knee joint, and the glenohumeral ligaments represent simply the different portions or thickenings of the capsule of the shoulder. There can be much variation in the thickness or the presence of the superior, middle, and inferior glenohumeral ligaments.

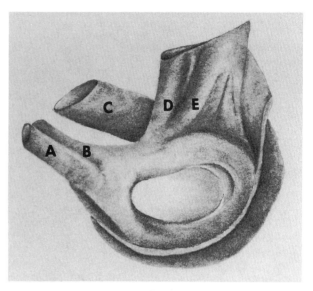

**Fig. 9-4.** Intra-articular structures that can be visualized arthroscopically in a right shoulder include long head of biceps tendon (*A*), superior glenohumeral ligament (*B*), subscapularis tendon (*C*), middle glenohumeral ligament (*D*), and inferior glenohumeral ligament (*E*).

The superior, middle, and inferior glenohumeral ligaments stabilize the anterior and inferior portions of the shoulder capsule.[43,46,48-51] When viewed arthroscopically the glenohumeral ligaments are displaced anteriorly because of fluid distention within the shoulder joint. In actuality, these ligaments normally lie closer to the glenoid labrum (Fig. 9-4). Occasionally, they will be seen to have distinct labral origins rather than their usual capsular origins originating off the edge of the glenoid labrum.

The superior glenohumeral ligament together with the coracohumeral ligament stabilizes the shoulder joint when the arm is in the abducted dependent position.[46,48] This ligament has two proximal attachments: one to the superior aspect of the labrum conjoined with the biceps tendon and one to the base of the coracoid.[51] This ligament courses laterally to insert on the anterior aspect of the anatomic neck of the humerus. The superior glenohumeral ligament can occasionally be seen near the insertion of the biceps tendon into the superior aspect of the glenoid; however, it may be hidden behind the biceps tendon or may appear to be absent.

The middle glenohumeral ligament stabilizes the glenohumeral joint when the shoulder is abducted 45 degrees.[51] Although the attachments of this ligament are wide, they may be difficult to visualize arthroscopically. However, the middle portion of the ligament can usually be seen just posterior to the subscapularis tendon with which it occasionally appears to fuse. The middle glenohumeral ligament extends from just beneath the superior glenohumeral ligament along the anterior border of the glenoid to the junction of the middle and inferior one-third of the glenoid rim. It blends with the capsule of the anteroinferior aspect of the shoulder joint and inserts near the lesser tuberosity over the anterior aspect of the anatomic neck of the humerus.

The inferior glenohumeral ligament stabilizes the glenohumeral joint when the arm is abducted to approximately 90 degrees.[51] This triangular ligament arises from the anteroinferior margin of the glenoid and inserts into the inferior aspect of the surgical neck of the humerus. It can be seen arthroscopically when the arm is in abduction.

## SUBSCAPULARIS TENDON AND RECESS

With the arm in the abducted position, the posterosuperior aspect of the subscapularis tendon can be seen over the anterior aspect of the shoulder between the superior and middle glenohumeral ligaments (Fig. 9-5). At times, however, the subscapularis tendon may be obscured by or appear to blend with the middle glenohumeral ligament. When viewed in most anatomy textbooks or when viewed grossly at the time of "open" or arthrotomy surgery to the shoulder, the subscapularis muscle and tendon usually appear to be a broad flat structure extending from the more medial aspects of the anterior aspect of the scapula to insert onto the lesser tuberosity of the humerus. However, at the time of arthroscopic surgery with the patient's arm abducted approximately 70 degrees and when viewed from a posterior arthroscopic portal, one only sees the posterosuperior edge of the tendon, which now appears to be a distinct rope-like banded structure quite different from that normally seen in anatomy textbooks (Fig. 9-6).

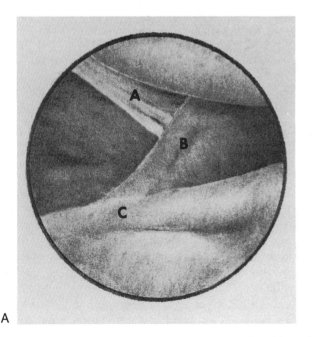

A

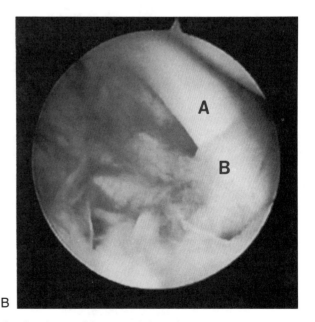

B

**Fig. 9-5. (A)** Example of subscapularis tendon (*A*), middle glenohumeral ligament (*B*), and anterior aspect of glenoid labrum (*C*) in a right shoulder. (**B**) Arthroscopic view of subscapularis tendon (*A*) and middle glenohumeral ligament (*B*) in a right shoulder.

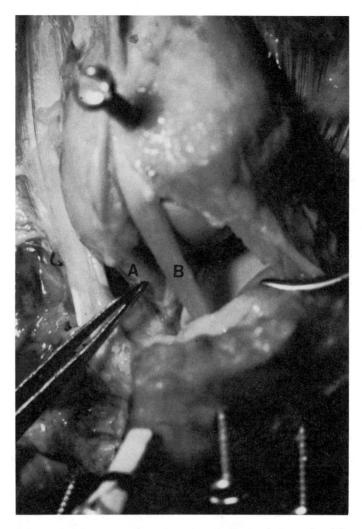

**Fig. 9-6.** Cadaveric specimen showing posterosuperior edge of subscapularis tendon (*A*) and biceps tendon (*B*) when viewed from a posterior arthroscopic portal.

The subscapularis recess is found over the anterior aspect of the shoulder in the area of the middle glenohumeral ligament. There can be much variation in the appearance of the relationship of the middle glenohumeral ligament to the recess, which at times can appear to be absent.

## ROTATOR CUFF

Arthroscopic evaluation of the rotator cuff begins by identifying the biceps tendon and obtaining proper orientation. The supraspinatus portion of the rotator cuff can be seen just superior to the biceps tendon (Fig. 9-7A). To visualize the more posterior portions of the rotator cuff, the arthroscope is retracted and directed superiorly and slightly posteriorly to reveal the insertion of the tendinous portion of the infraspinatus and teres minor into the humeral head (Fig. 9-7B). Arthroscopically, as one visualizes the more posterior portions of the rotator cuff inserting into the humeral head and moves toward the glenoid surface, the posterior portions of the rotator cuff appear to blend with the posterior capsule.

The rotator cuff should be one continuous structure and be free of any partial tears, complete tears, or

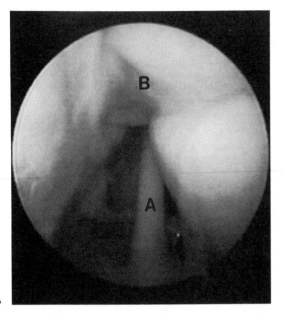

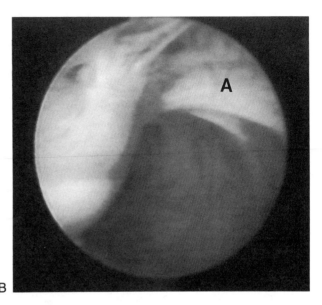

**Fig. 9-7. (A)** Arthroscopic view of biceps tendon (*A*) and supraspinatus portion of rotator cuff (*B*) in a right shoulder. **(B)** Arthroscopic view of the more posterior portions of rotator cuff (infraspinatus and teres minor) in a right shoulder (*A*).

fraying. The attachment of the rotator cuff should be firm, and no bone should be visualized beneath the insertion site.

## SUPERIOR RECESS

The superior recess is located superior to and slightly anterior to the superior aspect of the glenoid and to the insertion of the biceps tendon (Fig. 9-8).

## SUBACROMIAL SPACE

The subacromial space or "subacromial bursa" is that area inferior to the distal clavicle, acromioclavicular joint, and acromion and superior to the humeral head and rotator cuff. This subacromial space is bordered superiorly by the subacromial arch, consisting of the undersurface of the acromion, the outer end of the clavicle, the acromioclavicular joint, and the coracoacromial ligament, which forms a fibrous roof. The base of the subacromial space is the greater tuberosity of the humerus and the insertion of the rotator cuff. The

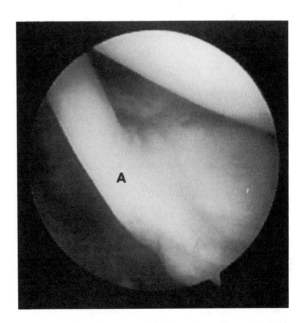

**Fig. 9-8.** The superior recess is located just above the biceps tendon insertion or to left of the biceps tendon (*A*) in this arthroscopic view of a right shoulder.

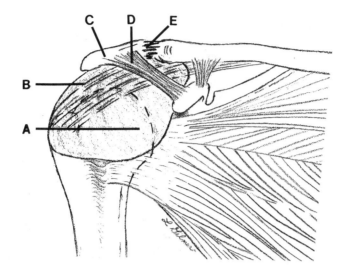

**Fig. 9-9.** Subacromial space structures: (*A*) bursa, (*B*) rotator cuff, (*C*) acromion, (*D*) coracoacromial ligament, (*E*) acromioclavicular joint.

subacromial bursa forms the actual "joint" cavity (Fig. 9-9). The subacromial bursa attaches superiorly to the undersurface of the acromion and below to the greater tuberosity at the insertion of the rotator cuff tendons.[52]

Arthroscopic visualization of the subacromial bursa is difficult at times, and many authors feel that visualization of this subacromial bursa should always be difficult if the patient has an impingement syndrome[29] or other pathology in the subacromial space. If one visualizes a normal-appearing bursa, most likely the patient's problems are not related to the subacromial space or to an impingement problem.

Structures that should be visualized in the subacromial space are the inferior surface of the acromion, the acromioclavicular joint, the superior portion of the coracoacromial ligament, the superior surface of the rotator cuff, and the bursa itself.

On entering the subacromial bursa through a posterior portal, one often encounters a bursal curtain or sheet that can make visualization difficult (Fig. 9-10). The arthroscope has to be passed well anterior to this bursa shelf for one to visualize the actual subacromial space itself. Once in the subacromial space, one should be able to identify the inferior surface of the acromion, which is covered by periosteum and extended fibers from the coracoacromial ligament and therefore has a "softer" appearance as compared with a bony appear-

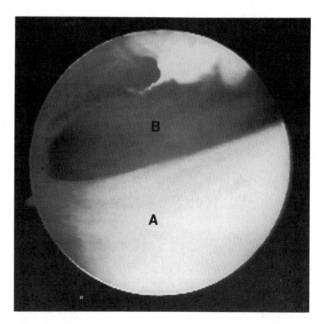

**Fig. 9-10.** Arthroscopic view of bursal "shelf" or curtain (*A*) normally seen on visualization of subacromial space (*B*) in a right shoulder.

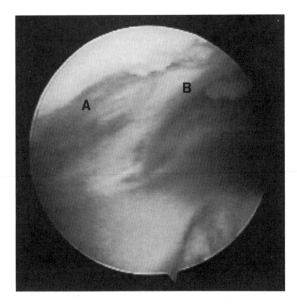

**Fig. 9-11.** Arthroscopic subacromial space visualization of inferior surface of acromion (*A*) and superior edge of coracoacromial ligament (*B*) in a right shoulder.

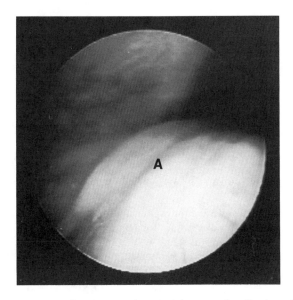

**Fig. 9-12.** Arthroscopic subacromial space visualization of superior surface of rotator cuff (*A*) in a right shoulder.

ance. Also, one should be able to visualize clearly the superior portion of the coracoacromial ligament (Fig. 9-11). The superior surface of the rotator cuff should be inspected carefully for any evidence of partial tearing or full-thickness tears and should have a smooth homogenous appearance (Fig. 9-12).

Portions of the inferior surface of the acromioclavicular joint can usually be visualized arthroscopically; however, it may be obscured by a large fat pad covering the inferior surface of this joint.

The subacromial bursa is a reasonably large space, and in the absence of any pathologic processes, most of the above-described structures can be viewed arthroscopically. In the presence of pathologic processes such as subacromial bursitis or inflammation or with partial or complete rotator cuff tears, the subacromial space at times can be nearly obliterated by hypertrophic bursal tissue so that visualization is nearly impossible until one creates a space with the motorized instrumentation performed arthroscopically.

## CONCLUSIONS

Diagnostic and operative arthroscopy of the shoulder is a reasonably demanding surgical procedure, and attention to detail is required to perform a safe, reproducible, and systematic arthroscopic evaluation. The above-described structures should be visualized on each arthroscopic evaluation of the shoulder and should be performed in a systematic fashion to ensure an accurate and reproducible examination.

## REFERENCES

1. Andrews JR, Broussard TS, Carson WG: Arthroscopy of the shoulder in the management of partial tears of the rotator cuff: a preliminary report. Arthroscopy 1:117, 1985
2. Andrews JR, Carson WG, McLeod WD: Glenoid labrum tears related to the long head of the biceps. Am J Sports Med 13:337, 1985
3. Andrews JR, Carson WG: Shoulder joint arthroscopy. Orthopedics 6:1157, 1983
4. Andrews JR, Carson WG: Operative arthroscopy of the shoulder in the throwing athlete. p. 84. In Zarins B, Andrews JR, Carson WG (eds): Injuries to the Throwing Arm. WB Saunders, Philadelphia, 1985

5. Andrews JR, Carson WG: Arthroscopic surgery of the shoulder. p. 231. In Parisien JS (ed): Arthroscopic Surgery. McGraw-Hill, New York, 1987

6. Gross RM, Fitzgibbons TC: Shoulder arthroscopy: a modified approach. Arthroscopy 1:156, 1985

7 Neviarser TJ: Arthroscopy of the shoulder. Orthop Clin North Am 18:361, 1987

8. Ogilvie-Harris DJ, Wiley AM: Arthroscopic surgery of the shoulder. J Bone Joint Surg 68B:201, 1986

9. Johnson LL: Shoulder arthroscopy. p. 1301. In Johnson, LL (ed): Arthroscopic Surgery. CV Mosby, St Louis, 1986

10. McFlynn FJ, Caspari RB: Arthroscopic findings in the subluxing shoulder. Clin Orthop 183:173, 1984

11. Snyder SJ, Kargel RP, DelPizzo W et al: SLAP lesions of the shoulder. Arthroscopy 6:274, 1990

12. Wheeler JH, Ryan JB, Arciero RA, Moliman RN: Arthroscopic versus nonoperative treatment of acute shoulder dislocations in young athletes. Arthroscopy 5:213, 1989

13. Buss DD, Warren RF, Galinat BJ: Indications for shoulder arthroscopy. p. 465. In McGinty JB (ed): Operative Arthroscopy. Raven Press, New York, 1991

14. Andrews JR, Heckman MM: Shoulder arthroscopy, operating room set-up. p. 473. In McGinty JB (ed): Operative Arthroscopy. Raven Press, New York, 1991

15. Snyder SJ, Ramer RD, Walbert E: Labral lesions. p. 491. In McGinty JB (ed): Operative Arthroscopy. Raven Press, New York, 1991

16. Meyers JF: Arthroscopic debridement of the acromioclavicular joint and distal clavicle resection. p. 557. In McGinty JB (ed): Operative Arthroscopy. Raven Press, New York, 1991

17. Matthews LS, Wolock BS, Martin DF: Arthroscopic management of degenerative arthritis of the shoulder. p. 567. In McGinty JB (ed): Operative Arthroscopy. Raven Press, New York, 1991

18. Gartsman GM, Combs AH, Davis PF, Tullos HS: Arthroscopic acromioclavicular joint resection. An anatomical study. Am J Sports Med 19:2, 1991

19. Andrews JR, Carson WG, Ortega K: Arthroscopy of the shoulder: technique and normal anatomy. Am J Sports Med 12:1, 1984

20. Matthews LS, Zarins B, Michael RH, Helfet DL: Anterior portal selection for shoulder arthroscopy. Arthroscopy 1:33, 1985

21. Carson WG: Arthroscopy of the shoulder: normal anatomy. p. 83. In Zarins B, Andrews JR, Carson WG (eds): Injuries to the Throwing Arm. WB Saunders, Philadelphia, 1985

22. Wolf EM: Anterior portals for shoulder arthroscopy. Arthroscopy 5:201, 1989

23. Andrews JR, Carson WG: Arthroscopic anatomy of the shoulder. Shoulder surgery in the athlete. p. 25. In Jackson DW (ed): Techniques in Orthopaedics. Aspen System Corp. Rockville, MD, 1985

24. Blanchut PA, Day B: Arthroscopic anatomy of the shoulder. Arthroscopy 5:1, 1989

25. Matthews LS, Fadale PD: Subacromial anatomy for the arthroscopist. Arthroscopy 5:36, 1989

26. Arnoczky SP, Altchek DW, O'Brien SJ: Anatomy of the shoulder. p. 425. In McGinty JB (ed): Operative Arthroscopy. Raven Press, New York, 1991

27. Souryal TO, Baker CL: Anatomy of the supraclavicular fossa portal in shoulder arthroscopy. Arthroscopy 6:297, 1990

28. Ellman H: Arthroscopic subacromial decompression. Analysis of one- to three-year results. Arthroscopy 3:173, 1987

29. Ellman H: Arthroscopic acromioplasty. p. 543. In McGinty JB (ed): Operative Arthroscopy. Raven Press, New York, 1991

30. Snyder SJ, Pachelli AF, DelPizzo W et al: Partial thickness rotator cuff tears: results of arthroscopic treatment. Arthroscopy 7:1, 1991

31. Levy HJ, Uribe JW, Delaney LG: Arthroscopic assisted rotator cuff repair: preliminary result. Arthroscopy 6:55, 1990

32. Paulos LE, Franklin JL, Beck CL: Arthroscopic management of rotator cuff tears. p. 529. In McGinty JB (ed): Operative Arthroscopy. Raven Press, New York, 1991

33. Levy JH, Gardner RD, Lemak LJ: Arthroscopic subacromial decompression in the treatment of full thickness rotator cuff tears. Arthroscopy 7:8, 1991

34. Caspari RB, Savoie FH: Arthroscopic reconstructions of the shoulder: the Bankart repair. p. 507. In McGinty JB (ed): Operative Arthroscopy. Raven Press, New York, 1991

35. Morgan CD, Bodenstab AB: Arthroscopic Bankart suture repair: technique and early results. Arthroscopy 3:111, 1987

36. Hawkins RB: Arthroscopic stapling repair for shoulder instability: a retrospective study of 50 cases. Arthroscopy 5:122, 1989

37. Detrisac DA: Arthroscopic shoulder staple capsulorrhaphy for traumatic anterior instability. p. 517. In McGinty JB (ed): Operative Arthroscopy. Raven Press, New York, 1991

38. Matthews LS, Vetter WL, Oweida SJ et al: Arthroscopic staple capsulorrhaphy for recurrent anterior shoulder instability. Arthroscopy 4:106, 1988

39. Wiley AM: Arthroscopy for shoulder instability and a technique for arthroscopic repair. Arthroscopy 4:25, 1988

40. Matthews LS, Helfet DL, Spearman J, Oweida S: Arthroscopic staple capsulorrhaphy for anterior instability of the shoulder. Arthroscopy 2:116, 1986

41. Bankart ASB: The pathology and treatment of recurrent dislocation of the shoulder joint. Br J Surg 26:23, 1938

42. DePalma AF: Surgery of the shoulder. JB Lippincott, Philadelphia, 1973

43. Bost FC, Inman VT: The pathological changes in recurrent dislocation of the shoulder. A report of Bankart's operative procedure. J Bone Joint Surg 24A:595, 1942

44. Dutoit GT, Roux D: Recurrent dislocation of the shoulder. A twenty-four year study of the Johannesburg stapling operation. J Bone Joint Surg 38A:1, 1956

45. Warwick R, Williams P (eds): Gray's Anatomy of the Human Body. WB Saunders, Philadelphia, 1973

46. Mosely JF, Overgaard B: The anterior capsular mechanism in recurrent anterior dislocation of the shoulder. J Bone Joint Surg 44B:913, 1962

47. Rowe CR, Patell D, Southmayd WW: The Bankart procedure. a long-term, end-results study. J Bone Joint Surg 60A:1, 1978

48. Basmajian JV, Bazant FJ: Factors preventing downward dislocation of the adducted shoulder. J Bone Joint Surg 41A:1182, 1959

49. Rowe DR, Zarins B: Recurrent transient subluxation of the shoulder. J Bone Joint Surg 63A:863, 1981

50. Schlemm F: Ueber die verstarkungsbander am schultergelenk. Arch Anat 45, 1853

51. Turkel SJ, Panio MW, Marshall JL et al: Stabilizing mechanism preventing anterior dislocation of the glenohumeral joint. J Bone Joint Surg 63A:1208, 1981

52. Ellman H: Arthroscopic subacromial decompression. p. 243. In Parisien JS (ed): Arthroscopic Surgery. McGraw-Hill, New York, 1988

# 10

# Operative Arthroscopy of the Shoulder

JOE P. BRAMHALL
DOROTHY F. SCARPINATO
JAMES R. ANDREWS

The understanding of the management of the athlete's shoulder has been difficult and controversial. With the different technologic advances and the convergence of ideas from orthopaedic surgeons who perform shoulder surgery, a better understanding of the pathology and treatment is evolving.

The most important aspect of diagnosis in the overhead athlete is still the history and physical examination. The exact mechanism of injury, the activity that reproduces symptoms, the location and duration of pain, and aggravation factors are a necessary part of history taking. The physical examination cannot be overemphasized. Identifying areas of tenderness, limitations of range of motion, and other physical findings such as rotator cuff dysfunction and/or laxity is essential.

The initial management in most cases is conservative. Along with active rest and a well-designed rehabilitation program, the athlete will often recover and return to competition. In certain instances, the diagnosis cannot be arrived at by physical examination, and ancillary tests such as computed tomography-arthrography, magnetic resonance imaging, ultrasound, and isokinetic testing are necessary. In some instances, because of overlapping findings of different disorders, arthroscopy becomes important in providing information leading to the appropriate diagnosis and treatment.

Surgical treatment, in general, should be as conservative as possible. Operative arthroscopy has its role, especially after conservative treatment fails. In other

more severe cases, open operative intervention has a place in the treatment armamentarium.

This chapter addresses special considerations for the indications and contradictions for arthroscopic examination of the athlete's shoulder and use in treatment of the throwing athlete's shoulder. The actual recognition and treatment of each of these pathologies are addressed in other chapters.

## PRIMARY COMPRESSIVE CUFF DISEASE

Primary compressive cuff disease can be a primary cause for cuff disease when associated with a type III hooked acromion,[1] degenerative spurs, os acromiale, or in some cases a congenitally thick coracoacromial ligament. It can also be caused by a prominence of a degenerated acromioclavicular joint. Compressive cuff disease results in an outside-in type of rotator cuff tear.

Overhead sports movements that require using the arm in a 90 degree or greater horizontally abducted position with rotation into internal and horizontal adduction are likely to produce impingement symptoms. This is reproducible on physical examination by forceful forward flexion (positive impingement sign).[2] Pain relief by injecting 1 percent lidocaine into the subacromial space helps confirm the diagnosis. Most patients respond to a conservative program of active rest, nonsteroidal anti-inflammatory medication, and progressive rotator cuff strengthening and stretching exercises.[3]

If the athlete's symptoms are not relieved by nonoperative measures, surgical treatment may be warranted. Arthroscopy of the subacromial space may reveal bursitis that can be easily debrided with a motorized resector. An acromioplasty is performed using a motorized burr, removing approximately 8 mm of the anterior acromion extending medially to the acromioclavicular joint and beveled posteriorly for about 2 cm. This is a technically demanding procedure, and care should be taken to control bleeding.

If there is partial tearing of the superior surface of the rotator cuff, this is debrided to healthy, bleeding tissue. At this time, the humeral head is rotated to assess the adequacy of the amount of space available between the acromion and the rotator cuff.

Arthroscopic decompression of the subacromial space has minimal morbidity because the insertion of the deltoid is not violated.[4] It also allows for early rehabilitation, which in turn allows for the earlier return to competition.

## SECONDARY COMPRESSIVE CUFF DISEASE

Impingement may be secondary to another underlying problem, such as glenohumeral instability.[4] The correct diagnosis is mandatory, as treatment includes alleviating the primary problem. The patient may present only with a complaint of pain; therefore, a thorough history and physical examination must be performed. Emphasis should be placed on comparing range of motion and anterior/posterior translation of the humeral head to the opposite shoulder. Generalized ligamentous laxity should be noted. A special test that is helpful to determine anterior capsular laxity is the so-called Lachman's test of the shoulder. It is likened to the Lachman's test of the knee for anterior cruciate ligament laxity. With the patient supine and the shoulder abducted 90 degrees and externally rotated about 45 degrees, an anterior force is applied to the humeral head to assess the anterior translation of the glenohumeral joint and the end point of the anterior capsule.

If anterior laxity is evident, the compressive cuff disease may certainly be secondary to anterior shoulder laxity. If only mild instability is present, treatment options in this situation include rehabilitation with an emphasis on dynamic stabilization by muscular strengthening. If this fails, arthroscopic or open stabilization may be warranted.

Primary rotator cuff failure from tensile overload may also cause secondary impingement. This failure occurs because of repetitive tensile overloading of the cuff, as is seen in the deceleration phase of throwing. These forces encountered in athletic activity may ultimately exceed the ability of both the dynamic stabilizers of the rotator cuff as well as the anterior static stabilizers to compensate, which may lead to a secondary impingement phenomenon of the rotator cuff.[4] Again, rehabilitation may be the first line of treatment; if this fails, arthroscopic debridement of the tensile tear is performed along with anterior stabilization and/or decompression of the coracoacromial arch as necessary.

## TENSILE LESIONS

The tensile lesions usually seen in the athlete's shoulder occur as undersurface rotator cuff tears and/or biceps-labral complex tears. The mechanism of injury in a primary tensile rotator cuff tear is deceleration of the rotator cuff as it resists horizontal adduction and internal rotation, anterior translation, and distraction forces seen during the deceleration phase of throwing. This results in eccentric tensile overload failure. Partial tears usually ensue secondary to repetitive microtrauma.[3] These are found in the region of the undersurface of the supraspinatus tendon and may extend posterior to the area of the infraspinatus tendon. These tears may also be found isolated to the infraspinatus tendon and the posterior cuff capsule.

It is not uncommon, especially in throwing athletes, for the athlete to experience pain only during the pitching motion. On physical examination, tenderness may be elicited over the supraspinatus and/or infraspinatus tendons. Obvious weakness is present; it is usually found by testing for external rotation weakness from the abducted position. Computed tomography-arthrography or magnetic resonance imaging may reveal a partial undersurface tear of the rotator cuff. Initially, the athlete is started on a rehabilitation program with emphasis on strengthening the rotator cuff.

If there is no improvement over 2 to 3 months, arthroscopy may be performed, which will reveal a partial tearing of the undersurface of the rotator cuff at or near its insertion into the humeral head. Arthroscopic debridement with a motorized shaver is performed to healthy, bleeding tissue.[3,5]

Next, inspection of the subacromial space is performed. Frequently, there are no signs of impingement intraoperatively, but in chronic cases, secondary impingement may be present with further tearing of the outer surface of the rotator cuff. In these cases, subacromial decompression with an acromioplasty should be performed (Fig. 10-1).

Andrews et al[5] reported on 34 athletes with partial tears who underwent arthroscopic debridement. Seventy-six percent had excellent results; 9 percent had good results; and all were able to return to their previous athletic activities. Fifteen percent were rated as poor results and were not able to return to competitive throwing.

Debridement of partial rotator cuff tears appear to reduce the pain in the athlete's shoulder sufficiently to enable him or her to engage in a program of progressive strengthening exercises[3] and to make a gradual return to competitive throwing, which usually takes 6 months or more.

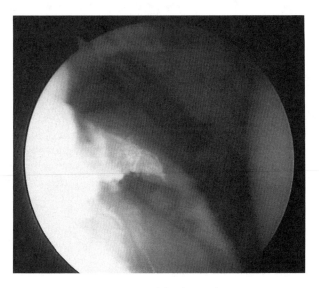

**Fig. 10-2.** Biceps—labral complex tear.

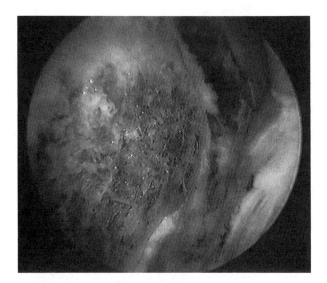

**Fig. 10-1.** Acromioplasty postarthroscopic subacromial decompression.

Biceps-labral complex tears are thought to occur during the deceleration and follow-through phase of throwing. Large forces are placed on the proximal attachment of the biceps tendon at or near 90 degrees of abduction, as the humerus internally rotates at the same time as deceleration of elbow extension is occurring.[6,7] There may also be some type of concurrent entrapment of the biceps-labral complex associated with glenohumeral laxity.

Physical examination may reveal a popping or catching when the arm is in full abduction and external rotation, brought out by circumducting the humeral head on the glenoid—"the clunk test." This test is performed with the patient in the supine position.[7] The examiner's hand lies posterior to the humeral head, applying an anterior directed force, while the opposite hand rests on the distal humerus, rotating the humerus. The patient's arm is brought into the full overhead abducted position, assessing for a clunk or grind in the shoulder suggesting a labral tear.

At arthroscopy, a tear of the labrum in the anterosuperior quadrant at the insertion of the long head of the biceps is evident (Fig. 10-2). A partial tear of the biceps tendon near its origin may also be evident. Andrews et al[6] suggested a mechanism for the anterosuperior glenoid labral tear. In 73 shoulder arthroscopies performed in pitchers and throwing athletes with labral tears, 83 percent had glenoid labral tearing at the biceps-labral complex anterosuperiorly. Electrical stimulation of the biceps in five patients at arthroscopy produced tension in the biceps tendon and lifting up of the superior labrum off the glenoid. Andrews et al hypothesized that this eccentric contraction may cause tearing of the anterosuperior labrum. Treatment for this lesion usually entails limited arthroscopic debridement of the labral tear, as well as the biceps tendon if it is partially torn.[3] Infrequently, the tear may propagate into the superior attachment of the middle and inferior glenohumeral ligaments, with subsequent instability present. If this is the case, the lesion should be repaired. Arthroscopic debridement is followed by rehabilitation.

# GLENOHUMERAL LAXITY

Most of the time, the diagnosis of shoulder laxity can be made on the basis of the history and physical findings. The athlete may have a history of documented anterior dislocation with subsequent redislocations, or the athlete may only present with the complaint of pain, clicking, or the so-called dead arm syndrome.[8] In this syndrome, the athlete feels a sudden sharp or paralyzing pain when the shoulder is forcibly, externally rotated in the abducted overhead position.

The most reliable finding on physical examination is the apprehension test, in which the abducted arm is rotated externally while forward pressure is exerted on the humeral head. This pushes the humeral head forward against the anterior capsule. If the patient experiences pain and apprehension, this suggests anterior instability.

Approximately one-half of the patients with shoulder subluxation are unaware of it.[8] Therefore, physical examination, radiography, and arthroscopy become important aids in the diagnosis.[8–11]

After the patient is administered general anesthesia, the shoulder is examined and compared with the contralateral shoulder. Range of motion, anterior/posterior translation, and the clunk test are assessed. Next, diagnostic arthroscopy is performed to assess redundancy of the anterior capsule and glenohumeral ligaments.[10,12] The glenoid labrum is evaluated and probed, looking for tears and detachment. A detachment of the inferior glenohumeral ligament/labral complex from the lower half of the glenoid margin is most often associated with anterior instability.[9–11] Under direct visualization using the arthroscope, the humeral head is "pushed" anterior, posterior, and inferior, and the amount of translation or subluxation is noted. This is helpful in deciding the main direction of instability, although it may be difficult to measure humeral head luxation with arthroscopy. If the labrum is torn and degenerating, conservative debridement is performed with the understanding that it may increase the laxity or instability.

A decision must be made regarding the treatment plan. Athletes with mild instability may be tried with strengthening exercises first[11]; if this fails, further intervention may be warranted. Those athletes with moderate to severe instability may certainly require an arthroscopic or open stabilization procedure.

If there is an early true Bankart lesion, arthroscopic repair may be performed as described by Caspari,[13] Johnson,[14] and Morgan and Bodenstab.[15] Postoperatively, the shoulder is immobilized in the adducted and internally rotated position in a shoulder immobilizer for 4 weeks to assure soft tissue healing.

At the American Academy of Orthopaedic Surgeons meeting in 1989, Caspari[13] reported a 4 percent resubluxation rate for the arthroscopic Bankart repair, with 90 percent good or excellent results. Regardless of this early enthusiasm for the arthroscopic repair of the unstable shoulder, most surgeons still do not recommend this procedure for those athletes going back to contact sports.

To date, limited experience exists regarding arthroscopic treatment of posterior instability. Treatment considerations are the same as for anterior instability.[16] Most athletes will respond to an aggressive exercise program, especially those with generalized ligamentous laxity. Arthroscopy should be considered in those who fail an adequate trial of conservative therapy. Again, a thorough examination under general anesthesia is mandatory. Arthroscopic debridement of labral lesions may decrease the athlete's pain sufficiently enough to allow him or her to return to competition. Most reverse Bankart lesions require open stabilization procedures.

## GLENOID LABRAL TEARS

Not all labral tears are associated with instability.[9] A tear of the upper half of the labrum may occur with throwing and racquet sports or with some other type of deceleration injury. The mechanism of labral tearing can be caused by repetitive overhead activity as in throwing, tennis, swimming, etc.[17] It may also be caused by forceful entrapment associated with an avulsion sprain of the biceps-labrum complex between the humeral head and the glenoid rim, such as a player diving to catch a baseball on the outstretched arm (Fig. 10-3). A significant percentage of labral tears in the throwing athlete involve the anterosuperior portion near the insertion of the long head of the biceps tendon and are not associated with instability.[18] Pappas et al[19] noted a functional instability from the torn hypermobile labrum. There was no increase in glenohumeral translation, yet the patient felt insecure about the shoulder. They theorized that there was clicking, catching, or locking in the joint secondary to the intermittent interposition of a partially attached fragment or bucket-handle tear between the glenoid and humeral head (Fig. 10-4). One must always be cautious that these functional tears may represent occult laxity and may lead to overt instability.

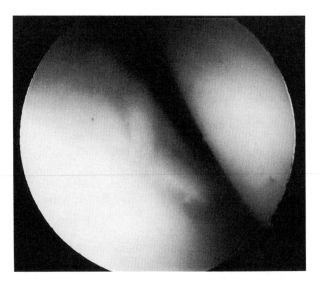

**Fig. 10-4.** Anterior glenoid labral tear.

Arthroscopy is indicated in the athlete with shoulder pain and symptoms of catching, etc., who on physical examination may demonstrate a positive clunk test.[17]

Andrews and Carson[20] reported on arthroscopy in 73 athletes with labral tears and found 83 percent with anterosuperior tears. After arthroscopic debridement, 88 percent had good to excellent results at 13.5 months follow-up.

## THROWERS' EXOSTOSIS

The finding of a posterior glenoid exostosis in throwers with shoulder pain was first described in 1941 by Bennett, who studied a group of professional baseball players.[3] The exostosis is located at approximately the 8 o'clock position on a right glenoid and is probably a secondary reaction associated with repeated microtrauma and tearing of the posterior and inferior capsule off of its glenoid insertion.[3] For many years, it was thought that the exostosis was calcification in the long head of the triceps tendon insertion.

Although there have been no published results of arthroscopic resection of this lesion, it has been performed on many pitchers, with relief of their symptoms allowing them to return to competitive pitching.

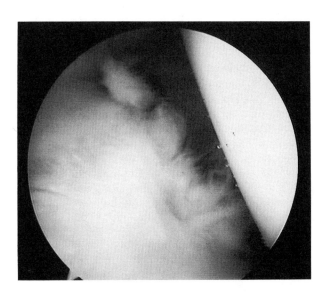

**Fig. 10-3.** Anterior glenoid labral tear.

## ACROMIOCLAVICULAR JOINT INJURIES

Athletes who lift weights as part of their training program and weight lifters are prone to acromioclavicular joint injuries. These include osteolysis of the distal clavicle secondary to longitudinal shear or compressive forces across the joint and partial or complete acromioclavicular separations secondary to post-traumatic injury to the joint. The athlete usually complains of a dull ache or pain over the acromioclavicular joint. Conservative treatment is tried first, consisting of nonsteroidal anti-inflammatory medication, physical therapy, modification of physical activity, and finally, steroid injection into the joint. If this fails, arthroscopic debridement of the acromioclavicular joint may be performed with decompression on the acromion and the clavicular side of the joint.

## CONCLUSIONS AND SUMMARY

The athlete with shoulder pathology should be treated both conservatively and aggressively at the same time. More often than not, the diagnosis is established with the history and physical examination. Ancillary tests are important and may be needed to confirm or substantiate the clinical impressions. Depending on the pathology and time constraints of the athlete, most are placed on a rehabilitation program first. Three months of conservative treatment is generally needed before surgery is indicated. Diagnostic and operative arthroscopy certainly has its role in the treatment armamentarium. Caution must be exercised here; treatment must be aggressive enough to return the athlete to competition in the shortest period of time but also conservative enough so that it does not compromise the athlete's subsequent performance. There are many factors to consider in the treatment process, thus making the definitive decision a difficult one.

This chapter briefly describes the different lesions one may encounter in the athlete's shoulder and their arthroscopic management. These lesions are not mutually exclusive but may occur together or secondary to another underlying problem that must be identified. The following chapters discuss each one of these pathologies in detail and explain different treatment options.

## REFERENCES

1. Bigliani LU, Morrison DS, April EW: The morphology of the acromion and its relationship to rotator cuff tears. Orthop Trans 10:216, 1986
2. Hawkins RJ, Kennedy JC: Impingement syndrome in athletes. Am J Sports Med 8:151, 1980
3. Andrews JR, Angelo RL: Shoulder arthroscopy for the throwing athlete. p. 79. In Paulos LE, Tibone JE (eds): Operative Techniques in Shoulder Surgery. Aspen Publishers, Rockville, MD, 1991
4. Jobe FW, Glousman RE: Rotator cuff dysfunction and associated glenohumeral instability in the throwing athlete. p. 85. In Paulos LE, Tibone JE (eds): Operative Techniques in Shoulder Surgery. Aspen Publishers, Rockville, MD, 1991
5. Andrews JR, Broussard TS, Carson WG: Arthroscopy of the shoulder in the management of partial tears of the rotator cuff: a preliminary report. Arthroscopy 1:117, 1985
6. Andrews JR, Carson WG, McLeod WD: Glenoid labrum tears related to the long head of the biceps. Am J Sports Med 13:337, 1985
7. Andrews JR, Carson WG, Ortega K: Arthroscopy of the shoulder: technique and normal anatomy. Am J Sports Med 12:1, 1984
8. Zarins B, Rowe CR: Current concepts in the diagnosis and treatment of shoulder instability in athletes. Med Sci Sports Exerc 16:444, 1984
9. Ellman H: Shoulder arthroscopy: current indications and techniques. Orthopedics 11:45, 1988
10. McGlynn FJ, Caspari RB: Arthroscopic Findings in the Subluxating Shoulder. Aspen Publishers, Rockville, MD, 1991
11. O'Brien SJ, Warren RF, Schwartz E: Anterior shoulder instability. Orthop Clin North Am 18:395, 1987
12. Yahiro MA, Matthews LS: Arthroscopic stabilization procedures for recurrent anterior shoulder instability. Orthop Rev 18:1161, 1989
13. Caspari RB: Arthroscopic reconstruction for anterior shoulder instability. p. 57. In Paulos LE, Tibone JE (eds): Operative Techniques in Shoulder Surgery. Aspen Publishers, Rockville, MD, 1991
14. Johnson LL: Shoulder arthroscopy. In Johnson LL (ed): Arthroscopic Surgery, Principles and Practice. CV Mosby, St. Louis, 1986
15. Morgan CD, Bodenstab AB: Arthroscopic Bankart suture repair: technique and early results. Arthroscopy 3:111, 1987
16. Schwartz E, Warren RF, O'Brien SJ, Fronek J: Posterior shoulder instability. Orthop Clin North Am 18:409, 1987

17. Andrews JR, Kupferman SP, Dillman CJ: Labral tears in throwing and racquet sports. Clin Sports Med 10:901, 1991

18. Andrews JR, Gidumal RH: Shoulder arthroscopy in the throwing athlete; perspectives and prognosis. Arthroscopy 6:565, 1987

19. Pappas AM, Goss TP, Kleinman PK: Symptomatic shoulder instability due to lesions of the glenoid labrum. Am J Sports Med 11:279, 1983

20. Andrews JR, Carson WG: The arthroscopic treatment of glenoid labrum tears in the throwing athlete. Orthop Trans 8:44, 1984

# 11

# Tensile Failure of the Rotator Cuff

## SETH P. KUPFERMAN

Rotator cuff injury in the athlete can arise from several different etiologies. Pathomechanics can include acute trauma, impingement, glenohumeral instability, or repetitive tensile loading of the rotator cuff. This latter mechanism, which can lead to the injury complex known as primary tensile failure of the rotator cuff,[1] is most typically seen in the throwing athlete.

The repetitive throwing motion is a dynamic activity that places extraordinary stresses on the athlete's shoulder,[2-4] the capsuloligamentous complex, and in particular, the rotator cuff. Remarkably high forces are generated by the cuff musculature, specifically during the deceleration phase of throwing to slow the rapidly moving shoulder.[2,5] These forces, applied repetitively with the throwing motion, are thought to underlie primarily the mechanism for tensile rotator cuff failure.[1]

## FORCES AND MUSCLE ACTIVITY

In a further attempt to better understand and to measure more precisely the forces acting on the shoulder during throwing, laboratory studies have been undertaken. One approach to collecting this data is with a "throwing laboratory," in which subjects wearing reflective markers throw a baseball while being filmed with multiple high-speed video cameras (Fig. 11-1). This computer-digitized high-speed videography allows the rapid collection of data that can then be used to calculate velocities and forces acting about the shoulder during the different phases of throwing (Fig. 11-2).

For example, healthy conditioned throwing athletes during the acceleration phase of throwing have shoulder angular velocities exceeding 1,100 degrees/s (CJ Dillman, unpublished data) (Fig. 11-3). Shoulder rotation from external to internally rotated positions has been calculated to be in excess of 7,000 degrees/s (CJ Dillman, unpublished data) (Fig. 11-4). Last, during the deceleration phase of throwing, the distraction force acting on the glenohumeral joint is approximately 90 percent of body weight (CJ Dillman, unpublished data) (Fig. 11-5). A thorough description of the forces incurred during throwing can be found in Chapter 31.

Electromyographic data collected at the time of deceleration and follow-through phases have revealed intense firing of the rotator cuff musculature.[5,6] This substantiates the role of the supraspinatus, infraspinatus, and teres minor eccentrically contracting to decelerate the rapid internal rotation and horizontal adduction of the throwing shoulder.

It is this rather significant tensile load generated to counter the extraordinary internal rotation, adduction, and distraction forces that may lead to intrinsic tissue injury or tensile failure. This repetitive microtrauma may ultimately manifest as partial or undersurface tearing of the supraspinatus and/or infraspinatus tendons[1,2,7] (Fig. 11-6).

## TENSILE FAILURE

Undersurface rotator cuff tearing that occurs from repetitive tensile loading has been referred to as primary tensile failure.[1] The tissue damage appears to be a direct consequence of repetitive eccentric contraction of the rotator cuff muscles during deceleration of the throwing shoulder.

Whenever considering shoulder pain in a throwing athlete, a high index of suspicion must be maintained

113

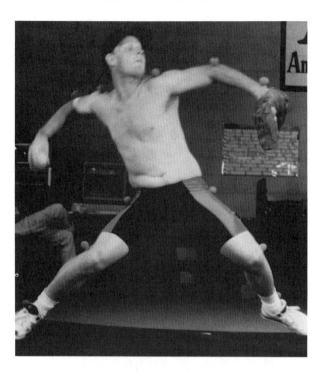

**Fig. 11-1.** Throwing laboratory subject wears reflective markers enabling computer-digitized high-speed videography.

for concurrent operating pathomechanics. In particular, the clinician needs to actively seek evidence for occult glenohumeral instability in this population.[4,8,9] Skilled overhead athletes will not uncommonly have physiologically increased ligamentous laxity in general and increased external rotation in their dominant shoulder. However, pathologic subtle anterior glenohumeral instability, posterior subluxability, or even multidirectional instability may also be present.[4,8,9]

Jobe et al[8,9] suggested that anterior glenohumeral instability may lead secondarily to rotator cuff impingement in the throwing athlete. They suggested that repetitive throwing may cause progressive injury or attenuation of the static stabilizers of the shoulder joint, leading to increased glenohumeral translation. Consequently, increased rotator cuff activity is required to counteract this increased humeral translation or subluxation. In time, these dynamic stabilizers may fatigue, allowing the rotator cuff to impinge on the coracoacromial arch with resultant rotator cuff injury.

Similarly, secondary tensile failure of the rotator cuff can occur in the presence of glenohumeral instability.[1] In the face of uni- or multidirectional instability, repeated throwing activity will continue to place extraordinary demands on the rotator cuff musculature to stabilize the lax shoulder dynamically. Thus, this increased activity required of the rotator cuff in the presence of the unstable shoulder may in itself result secondarily in intrinsic injury or tensile cuff failure, even in the absence of true impingement.

It is important to distinguish tensile failure of the rotator cuff, which occurs from repeated intrinsic loading, from rotator cuff injury that results from impingement. The pathomechanics of primary impingement is due to a repeated compressive mechanism of the rotator cuff under the coracoacromial arch[1,8,9] and is not from the repeated microtrauma of forceful eccentric muscle contraction.

## DIAGNOSIS

Differential diagnosis of the painful shoulder in the athlete can be difficult. A careful and complete history that details the precise occurrence and precipitation of symptoms is necessary. Pain that is isolated to the very early acceleration phase of throwing, when anterior translation forces are high, would suggest glenohumeral instability.[8] Pain related to certain precipitating activities might suggest a diagnosis of tendonitis or impingement. The pain of a rotator cuff tear is classically described as persisting even at rest or as night pain. These distinctions are not always clear, however, especially when glenohumeral instability coexists with a rotator cuff tear or impingement.

A thorough physical examination is crucial. Inspection for asymmetry and atrophy and documentation of motion are initial steps. Tenderness over the supraspinatus insertion or over the subacromial bursa would direct attention to impingement of the rotator cuff. Marked improvement in symptoms with local anesthetic infiltration of the bursa would support the subacromial space as the primary area of pathology. A positive clunk test[10] would suggest a labral tear that may or may not be associated with glenohumeral instability.[4] A positive apprehension test is further support for anterior glenohumeral instability. Maneuvers such

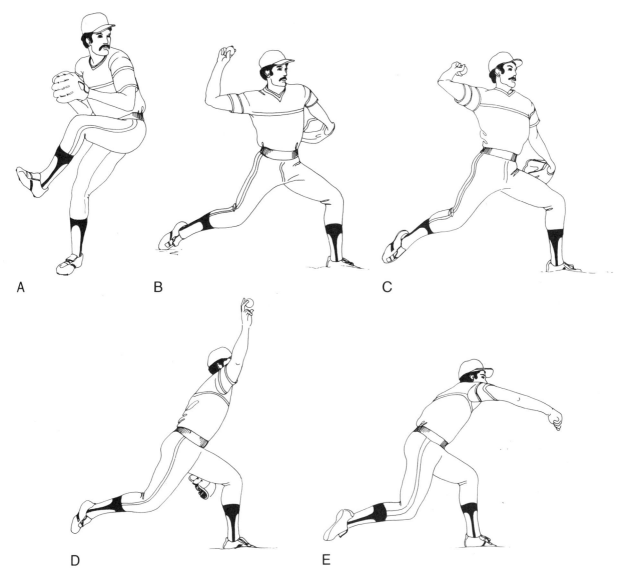

**Fig. 11-2.** (**A**) Wind-up phase of pitching motion; (**B**) cocking phase; (**C**) acceleration phase; (**D**) release and deceleration phase; (**E**) follow-through phase. (From McLeod,[19] with permission.)

as the relocation test,[8,9] whereby the apprehension test is repeated with a posteriorly directed force applied to the humeral head, are even more helpful. Athletes with isolated anterior glenohumeral instability would improve with such testing, whereas those with pain from impingement and rotator cuff injury would likely remain symptomatic.

Further objective evidence of instability is assessed by examining for abnormal glenohumeral translation with provocative testing. At times, such assessments are best made with the patient under general anesthesia. These findings are often subtle and can be difficult to appreciate, even by the most experienced examiner.

Roentgenographic studies complete the evaluation, even though they are frequently unrevealing. Os acromiale, subacromial spurs, and markedly curved or

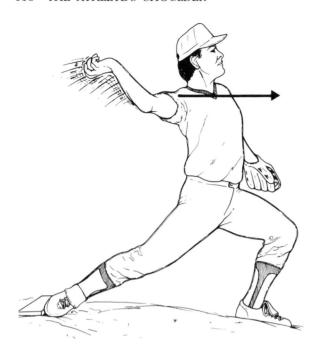

**Fig. 11-3.** During acceleration phase of throwing, shoulder angular velocity may exceed 1,100 degrees/s. (Modified from Andrews et al.,[4] with permission.)

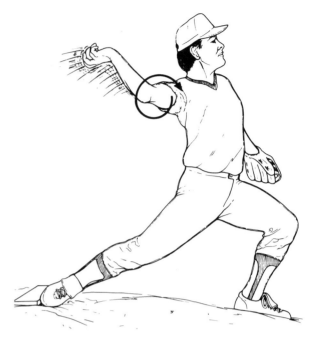

**Fig. 11-4.** During acceleration phase of throwing, shoulder rotation from external to internal rotated positions have been calculated to exceed 7,000 degrees/s. (Modified from Andrews et al.,[4] with permission.)

hook-shaped acromions[11] may play a role in rotator cuff impingement. The rare finding of a bony Bankart lesion would support a diagnosis of instability. Hill-Sachs lesions, or posterolateral defects of the humeral head, may be noted radiographically.[12] Arthrograms of the shoulder are useful for complete tears of the rotator cuff but are less revealing for partial undersurface tears as seen with tensile injuries. Computed tomography-arthrography at times can identify subtle abnormalities in the glenoid labrum. Magnetic resonance imaging is assuming an ever-important role in assessing complete and partial injuries to the rotator cuff. Improvement in equipment and increasing experience in interpretation is generating greater confidence in magnetic resonance assessment of partial tears to the rotator cuff (Fig. 11-7).

Also, arthroscopy of the shoulder can provide helpful information. It permits the inspection of the glenohumeral joint for pathology, suggestive of instability such as Hill-Sachs lesions, labral tears, and deficient glenohumeral ligaments.[2,4,7,13] It also permits the direct inspection of the undersurface of the rotator cuff for partial tears, as well as the evaluation of the subacro-

mial space for superior surface injury and evidence of impingement.[2,7,14]

## TREATMENT OPTIONS

For the throwing athlete with suspected partial rotator cuff tears, the initial approach and management includes modification of activities, anti-inflammatories, and rehabilitation. The latter program would include use of modalities, progressive range of motion, and a strengthening program addressing the rotator cuff and the scapula stabilizers. The emphasis is placed on posterior shoulder muscular strengthening (i.e., posterior deltoid, infraspinatus, teres minor), particularly with eccentric muscular strengthening. Additionally, the anterior muscles should be strengthened to enhance dynamic shoulder stability. Scapular strengthening is also employed to provide a stable proximal base of attachment for the shoulder muscles (see Ch. 32).

For the individual who remains refractory to these conservative measures, arthroscopy and other surgical intervention may prove helpful. For the subset of pa-

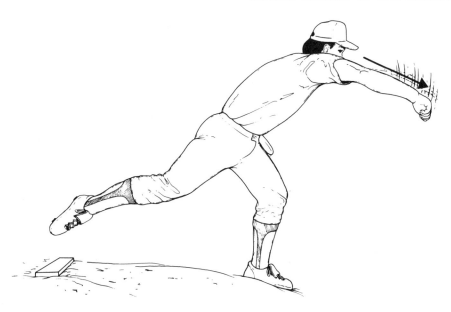

**Fig. 11-5.** During deceleration phase of throwing, distraction force acting on glenohumeral joint is approximately 90 percent of body weight. (Modified from Andrews et al.,[4] with permission.)

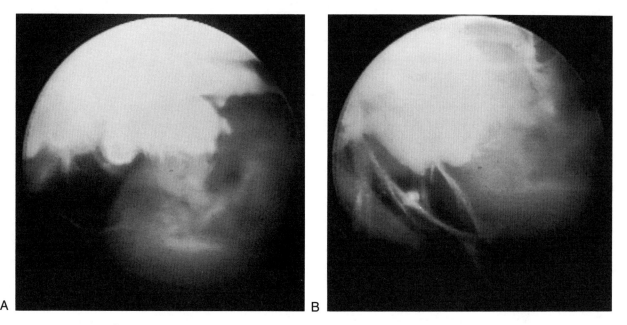

**Fig. 11-6.** (**A** & **B**) Arthroscopic views of undersurface partial-thickness tears of supraspinatus.

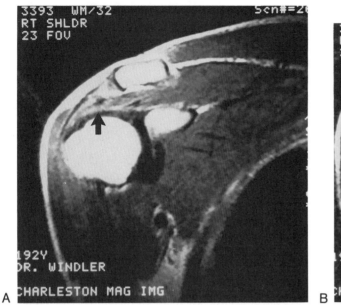
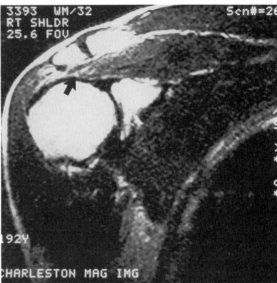

**Fig. 11-7.** Magnetic resonance image of partial-thickness supraspinatus tear. True coronal T1 (SE: TR = 530, TE = 32) and T2 (SE: TR = 1800, TE = 80) images revealing increased signal intensity (*arrows*) of supraspinatus tendon indicative of partial-thickness tear.

tients with tensile rotator cuff failure as a consequence of glenohumeral instability, it is imperative that the shoulder instability be addressed. These unstable shoulders that have not responded to physical therapy can now be approached with surgical options to include different open surgical reconstructions or arthroscopic stabilization techniques.[7,15–17] An advantage of the latter, particularly in the dominant extremity of a throwing athlete, includes the ability to better preserve shoulder range of motion. Its long-term effectiveness, however, particularly in the contact athlete, remains to be established.

For the athlete with primary tensile rotator cuff failure with partial tearing, one approach has been rotator cuff debridement, typically performed arthroscopically.[2,14] The hope is that bleeding cuff tissue may stimulate the healing response (Fig. 11-8). In a full-thickness tear of the rotator cuff, the best approach remains formal rotator cuff repair. It, however, remains difficult for the competitive throwing athlete to resume the same level of activity after open repair of the rotator cuff.[18]

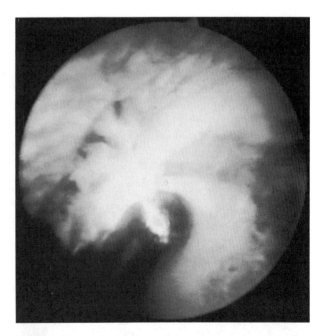

**Fig. 11-8.** Bleeding rotator cuff surface after arthroscopic debridement of partial-thickness undersurface supraspinatus tear.

## SUMMARY/CONCLUSION

Extraordinary stresses are placed on the athlete's shoulder during the throwing motion. Electromyelographic studies and high-speed three-dimensional videography have furthered our understanding of throwing mechanics and helped to define the significant tensile forces acting on the rotator cuff musculature during deceleration and follow-through phases of throwing. Tensile rotator cuff failure may result primarily from these repeated stresses or may relate to subtle recurrent glenohumeral instability.

Rehabilitation remains central to the treatment of these athletes. In a select group, arthroscopy of the shoulder and/or open shoulder surgery may prove useful for these rotator cuff injuries.

More work remains to be done. Further definition of the forces and individual muscle activity about the shoulder is needed. More understanding is required about how the biomechanics of "proper" throwing mechanics differs from "improper" mechanics and how this relates to rotator cuff failure. Finally, long-term controlled studies are needed to assess whether rotator cuff debridement techniques and arthroscopic methods of shoulder stabilization are permitting these athletes to return to their previous levels of competition.

## REFERENCES

1. Andrews JR: The athlete's shoulder: biomechanics, diagnosis and treatment. Presented as Joseph B. Wolffe Memorial Lecture, American College of Sports Medicine Annual Meeting, Salt Lake City, Utah, May 22, 1990
2. Andrews JR, Angelo RL: Shoulder arthroscopy for the throwing athlete. Techniques Orthop 3:75, 1988
3. Andrews JR, Gidamal RH: Shoulder arthroscopy in the throwing athlete: perspectives and prognosis. Arthroscopy 6:565, 1987
4. Andrews JR, Kupferman SP, Dillman CJ: Labral tears in throwing and racquet sports. Clin Sports Med 10:901, 1991
5. Jobe FW, Tibone JE, Perry J et al: An EMG analysis of the shoulder in throwing and pitching: a preliminary report. Am J Sports Med 11:3, 1983
6. Jobe FW, Moynes DR, Tibone JE et al: AMG analysis of the shoulder in pitching: a second report. Am J Sports Med 12:218, 1984
7. Scarpinato DF, Bramhall JP, Andrews JR: Arthroscopic management of the throwing athlete's shoulder: indications, techniques, and results. Clin Sports Med 10:901, 1991
8. Jobe FW, Kvitne RS: Shoulder pain in the overhead or throwing athlete. The relationship of anterior instability and rotator cuff impingement. Orthop Rev 28:963, 1989
9. Jobe FW, Tibone JE, Jobe CM et al: The shoulder in sports. p. 961. In Rockwood CA, Matsen FA (eds): The Shoulder. WB Saunders, Philadelphia, 1990
10. Andrews JR, Gillogly S: Physical examination of the shoulder in throwing athletes. p. 51. In Zarins B, Andrews J, Carson W (eds): Injuries to the Throwing Arm. WB Saunders, Philadelphia, 1985
11. Bigliani LU, Morrison DS, April EW: The morphology of the acromion and its relationship to rotator cuff tears. Orthop Trans 10:216, 1986
12. Hill HA, Sachs MD: The grooved defect of the humeral head. A frequently unrecognized complication of dislocations of the shoulder joint. Radiology 35:690, 1940
13. McGlynn FJ, Caspari RB: Arthroscopic findings in the subluxating shoulder. Clin Othrop 183:173, 1984
14. Andrews JR, Broussard TS, Carson WG: Arthroscopy of the shoulder in the management of partial tears of the rotator cuff: a preliminary report. Arthroscopy 1:117, 1985
15. Morgan CD, Bodenstab AB: Arthroscopic Bankart suture repair; technique and early results. Arthroscopy 3:111, 1987
16. Rowe CR, Patel D, Southmoyd WW: The Bankart procedure: a long-term end-result study. J Bone Joint Surg 60A:1, 1978
17. Yahiro MA, Matthews LS: Arthroscopic stabilization procedure for recurrent anterior shoulder instability. Orthop Rev 28:1161, 1989
18. Tibone JE, Elrod B, Jobe FW et al: Surgical treatment of tears of the rotator cuff in athletes. J Bone Joint Surg 68A:887, 1986
19. McLeod W: The pitching mechanism. p. 22. In Zarins R, Andrews JR, Carson W (eds): Injuries to the Throwing Arm. WB Saunders, Philadelphia, 1985

# 12

# Impingement Pathology of the Rotator Cuff

*JONATHAN B. TICKER*
*LOUIS U. BIGLIANI*

In this chapter, the anatomy of the subacromial space and its relationship to the pathology of impingement of the rotator cuff and biceps tendons are outlined. Anatomic variations and pathologic changes in the acromion and adjacent structures of the coracoacromial arch and their effect on the soft tissues of the subacromial space are discussed. An understanding of the effects that these structures have in the pathophysiology of rotator cuff disease is necessary when considering therapeutic options for impingement lesions.

The etiology of rotator cuff pathology has been the source of much controversy. Although rotator cuff tears were first described in 1834 by Smith,[1] disagreement remains as to which factors are principally responsible for this disease. Extrinsic factors relating impingement pathology to mechanical wear of the rotator cuff under the coracoacromial arch have been described as the primary etiology. Furthermore, intrinsic factors, including degenerative tendonopathy and aging of the cuff tendons and vascular insufficiency of the supraspinatus tendon, have also been supported.

Abnormal pathology of the acromion and its role in the impingement syndrome were described by Neer in 1972.[2] He isolated the undersurface of the anterior third of the acromion rather than its lateral or posterior aspect as the area responsible for mechanical wear on the structures of the subacromial space. Furthermore, Neer implicated the coracoacromial ligament and the acromioclavicular joint as structures that also contribute to impingement on the rotator cuff. The region primarily affected, referred to as the critical area, centers on the supraspinatus tendon, approximately 1 cm proximal to its insertion.

The pathology may involve one or more of the rotator cuff tendons and the long head of the biceps, and Neer[3] outlined three progressive stages. Initially, in stage I, there is edema and hemorrhage of the subacromial bursa, and it is reversible with conservative treatment. With continued insult to these soft tissues, the changes of stage II develop, including fibrosis and tendonitis. Without intervention at this point, either rest and conservative modalities or operative treatment, progression to stage III may result. This can present as incomplete tears or complete rupture of the rotator cuff and biceps tendons, with associated pathologic changes in the acromion and the acromioclavicular joint. In the general population, most individuals will not progress to stage III until about 40 years of age. However, in the athletic population, especially in those sports that require overhead motion, an individual may progress through each stage more rapidly. As a result, such patients will present with pathology at an earlier age.

The acromion, coracoacromial ligament, and coracoid are the components of the coracoacromial arch (Fig. 12-1). The coracoacromial arch superiorly and the proximal humerus inferiorly serve as rigid boundaries for the soft tissue contents of the subacromial space. These include the subacromial bursa, the tendons of the rotator cuff, and the long head of the biceps. It is this unique anatomic arrangement that exposes the soft tissues to wear and degeneration as the arm

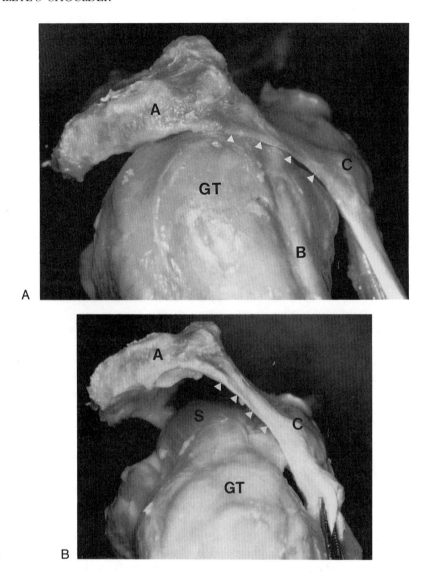

**Fig. 12-1.** **(A)** Human cadaver specimen showing the relationship between the coracoacromial arch and tendons of the rotator cuff and long head of the biceps. **(B)** With the humerus displaced inferiorly, the position of the supraspinatus tendon directly below the coracoacromial arch can be appreciated. (*A*, acromion; *B*, tendon of long head of biceps; *C*, coracoid; *GT*, greater tuberosity; *S*, supraspinatus tendon and muscle. *White arrowheads* define leading edge of coracoacromial ligament.)

is elevated during range of motion of the shoulder. Furthermore, this impingement may be accelerated by any architectural changes in the acromion or the acromioclavicular joint that reduce the volume of the subacromial space.

## NORMAL ANATOMY

The development and function of the acromion is unique in humans. Studies of human embryos have shown that the acromion is identifiable by 5 or 6 weeks[4,5] and is composed of cartilage at birth.[6,7] The centers of ossification in the acromion, most often two, are the last to present in the scapula, appearing during puberty or adolescence,[8] and usually fuse between 18 and 25 years of age.[7] One variation that has been well outlined is failure of these ossification centers to fuse to each other or to the spine of the scapula and is referred to as an unfused acromial epiphysis, or os acromiale. There are four different types of unfused acromial epiphyses: pre, meso, meta, and basi, progressing from anterior to posterior and reflecting greater involvement of the acromion (Fig. 12-2). This anomaly may be present in up to 8 percent of cases[9,10] and is often bilateral.[10]

The acromion is positioned above the superior aspect of the shoulder as the lateral extension of the spine of the scapula. It is defined posteriorly at the acromial angle, where the acromion and crest of the spine of the scapula converge. This posterior extent and the lateral border of the acromion are easily defined with palpation. Anteriorly, at its tip, is the attachment of the coracoacromial ligament, and this is where spur formation may be found. The acromioclavicular joint involves the medial aspect acromion and the lateral aspect of the clavicle and is the only diarthrodial articulation of the acromion. The opposing articular surfaces of the acromioclavicular joint may vary in their angulation when viewed anteriorly. Although these surfaces are separated by an intra-articular disc in the early stages of life,[11,12] degeneration of the acromioclavicular joint occurs with age, and the formation of inferior osteophytes on the acromial or clavicular side increases in frequency with advancing years.[11-13]

The coracoacromial ligament, as noted above, is located superior to the subacromial space. This structure is a broad fan-shaped ligament between the anterior aspect of the acromion and the lateral tip of the coracoid (two regions of the same bone, the scapula). Early anatomists thought that this ligament may function to inhibit superior migration of the humeral head.[14] Its role in the coracoacromial arch is still unclear.

The tendons of the rotator cuff, which pass through the subacromial space, include the supraspinatus, infraspinatus, and teres minor muscles, which insert into the greater tuberosity. The subscapularis muscle inserts into the lesser tuberosity of the humerus and courses below the coracoid, thus creating the rotator interval between the subscapularis and supraspinatus tendons at the base of the coracoid. All four rotator cuff tendons interlace with each other over the humeral head before their insertions. This continuity allows a unique functional interaction of the rotator cuff muscles and the ability to contribute to all motions of the glenohumeral joint. Subjacent to the anterior aspect of the supraspinatus lies the tendon of the long head of the biceps, which courses between the lesser and greater tuberosity in the bicipital groove.

The vascular supply to the cuff muscles and tendons is generous, involving the suprascapular, anterior and posterior humeral circumflex, thoracoacromial, and subscapular arteries. However, many investigators have described a region of hypovascularity in the supraspinatus tendon corresponding to the critical area, where rotator cuff pathology usually initiates.[15-18] The significance of this has not been fully defined.

## VARIATIONS IN ARCHITECTURE ASSOCIATED WITH ROTATOR CUFF PATHOLOGY

Native anatomy of the architecture described above can differ substantially. As Neer noted in his original paper on this subject,[2] individual variation in the shape

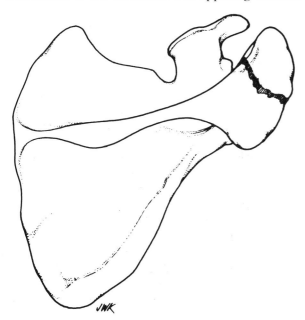

**Fig. 12-2.** Meso-acromion, as illustrated here, is the most common form of unfused acromial epiphysis.

or slope of the acromion may affect the progression of impingement lesions. This aspect of the impingement syndrome has stimulated new areas of research[19] and has motivated other investigators to examine the relationship of acromial morphology and rotator cuff pathology.

In 1986, Bigliani et al[20] studied the shape of the acromion in 140 cadaver shoulders to determine its relationship to full-thickness tears of the rotator cuff. The overall incidence of full-thickness tears in this elderly population was 34 percent. Three types of acromions were identified: type I (flat) occurred in 17 percent, type II (curved) occurred in 43 percent, and type III (hooked) occurred in 39 percent (Fig. 12-3). The type III acromion was present in 70 percent of the rotator cuff tears, whereas only 3 percent of type I acromions were associated with a tear. Also, anterior acromial spurs were noted in 14 percent of the series overall but in 70 percent of patients with rotator cuff tears. It is important, however, to distinguish between spurs, which are probably acquired, and variations in the native architecture of the acromion.

To examine the differences in acromial morphology in a clinical population, these investigators evaluated the supraspinatus outlet view in 200 consecutive patients with different shoulder problems.[21] The incidence of acromial types correlated closely with the anatomic study: 18 percent type I, 41 percent type II, and 41 percent type III. In those patients with a positive arthrogram, 80 percent had a type III acromion. In another group of 50 patients who underwent open subacromial decompression, 6 percent had a type I, 28 percent had a type II, and 66 percent had a type III acromion. Seventy percent of this symptomatic group had a full-thickness rotator cuff tear. These findings established a correlation between the type III acromion and rotator cuff tears and confirmed the importance of the supraspinatus outlet radiographic view for evaluating the acromion.

Other investigators have evaluated the slope of the acromion. Aoki and co-workers[22] developed a technique for measuring the acromial slope using the supraspinatus outlet view of the scapula. Their investigations of bleached skeleton shoulders revealed that a flatter acromial slope may be associated with the presence of a spur and narrowing of the supraspinatus outlet. They then studied this in normal and symptom-

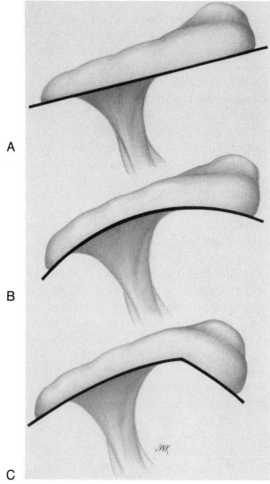

**Fig. 12-3.** Three types of acromion. **(A)** Type I, flat; **(B)** type II, curved; **(C)** type III, hooked. There is an increased incidence of rotator cuff tears with type III. (From Bigliani,[59] with permission.)

atic individuals with stage II impingement. When comparing these two populations, patients with stage II impingement had a statistically significant flatter acromial slope.[23]

Besides acromial morphology, other factors have been associated with impingement of the rotator cuff. Many authors have described the occurrence of inferiorly protruding osteophytes from the anterior aspect of the acromion and the inferior aspect of the acromioclavicular joint, which may compromise the integrity of the rotator cuff tendons when they pass below these structures.[2,20,24] Also, several series involving overhead athletes have suggested that the coracoacromial ligament is a primary source of pathology in this population. Developmental problems, such as failure of fusion of the acromial epiphyses, may alter the structure of the undersurface of the acromion and decrease the volume of the subacromial space.[10,25,26] In fact, this factor was outlined by Smith in 1834.[1] Finally, impingement by the coracoid on the subscapularis has been described.[27,28] Although this may lead to bursal and rotator cuff lesions, coracoid impingement should be distinguished from the much more common form of subacromial, or outlet, impingement that typically initiates in the supraspinatus tendon.

## IMPINGEMENT IN THE ATHLETIC SHOULDER: PATHOPHYSIOLOGY AND CLINICAL CORRELATION

Reports concerning injuries of the rotator cuff in athletes have increased tremendously during the past 20 years.[29-47] There is a greater awareness about overuse syndromes and the impact that repetitive motions have on the rotator cuff, particularly those motions occurring above the horizontal plane. As a result, impingement and its pathophysiology have been well described in this population. Although acute traumatic episodes do occur,[41] microtrauma to the subacromial bursa and rotator cuff tendons abutting the coracoacromial arch during repeated overhead motion will more commonly cause pain and a decrease or complete loss in function, depending on the extent of injury.[31,35,36,43-45,47-49] Furthermore, involvement of the biceps tendon and its association with impingement of the supraspinatus tendon have been well defined.[3,31,35,36,39,42-50]

Function of the rotator cuff muscles and motion of the shoulder in overhead sports have been well outlined.[34,39,40,44,45,51-54] The rotator cuff muscles serve dynamically to compress the humeral head into the glenoid, providing stability during motion of the glenohumeral joint. Also the supraspinatus assists the deltoid with abduction, the subscapularis acts as an internal rotator, and the infraspinatus and teres minor contribute to external rotation. The complex shoulder motions and the muscles involved in athletics have also

been described in detail.[40,52-55] In general, many motions in sports require maximal abduction with external rotation, such as throwing or pitching in baseball, serving or overhead returns in tennis, and freestyle and butterfly strokes in swimming. This subjects the subacromial bursa and rotator cuff tendons to wear under the anterior acromion and coracoacromial ligament as the arm accelerates forward. Impingement also may be seen if the rotator cuff muscles are weak and fail to stabilize the humeral head in the glenoid for proper mechanics. As a result, the action of the deltoid muscle will not be counterbalanced, and the humeral head may translate superiorly into the coracoacromial arch.

When treating an athlete with impingement syndrome, the anatomy of the coracoacromial arch must be carefully considered as part of the evaluation. For example, the patient in Figure 12-4 is a professional

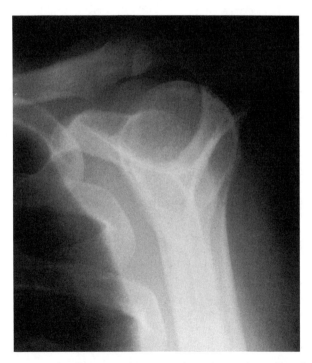

**Fig. 12-4.** This supraspinatus outlet radiograph, or lateral of the scapula, shows a type III acromion in a symptomatic professional tennis player with a full-thickness rotator cuff tear. This morphologic finding was treated with an anterior acromioplasty and rotator cuff repair. This athlete returned to tennis at the preinjury level.

tennis player who presented with a history and physical examination consistent with rotator cuff pathology. On the supraspinatus outlet radiograph, a type III hooked acromion was detected. This morphologic variation resulted in mechanical impingement of the contents of the subacromial space. A full-thickness rotator cuff tear of the supraspinatus and infraspinatus tendon was found. This patient was treated with an open procedure consisting of (1) an anterior acromioplasty to remove the offending structure and increase the volume of the subacromial space and (2) repair of the torn rotator cuff tendons. Another anatomic variation that must be considered in the athlete or any patient population is an unfused acromial epiphysis. Furthermore, in an elderly athlete, pathologic changes such as osteophyte formation of the anterior acromion and undersurface of the acromioclavicular joint are more often associated with rotator cuff pathology.

The role of the coracoacromial ligament in impingement[56] has been given more attention in the athlete.[15,36,37,43,48,53] Most overhead motions in sports incorporate abduction and external rotation with forward flexion and internal rotation. With repetition of these motions, pain and decreased function may result from mechanical wear on the bursa and rotator cuff as they pass below the leading edge of the coracoacromial ligament and anterior acromion. Surgical resection of the coracoacromial ligament without acromioplasty has uniformly provided the patients with pain relief but has not allowed most of those athletes to return to their previous level of function.[36,43,46] In particular, this has been noted in pitchers.[46] This should not imply that the addition of an anterior acromioplasty will lead to improved outcome in these patients. Tibone et al[47] studied 45 athletes with incomplete or complete rotator cuff tears. They found that 80 percent of patients with incomplete tears treated with an anterior acromioplasty had improved pain relief, but an overall good result was seen in only 50 percent.

In the athletic population, anterior instability follows impingement pathology as the second most common shoulder problem.[48] Interestingly, recent reports have concentrated on the role of instability in impingement and suggest that instability and impingement are intimately related in the athletic individual with anterior shoulder pain.[39] Instability may lead to subluxation of the humeral head, causing a mechanical impingement secondarily. Whether or not impingement is the primary or secondary etiology for rotator cuff pathology in a particular individual with shoulder pain, early intervention with a specifically designed rehabilitation program can alleviate symptoms and restore function.[32,38,39,52,57,58]

## GOALS OF REHABILITATION

The goal of a treatment protocol in an athlete or any patient with subacromial impingement should be to maintain or increase range of motion without causing further impingement and to initiate strengthening exercises only when pain has subsided. Pain is usually secondary to inflammation of the subacromial bursa and rotator cuff tendons.

The appropriate modalities and gentle range of motion exercises below the horizontal plane are the initial measures. Exercises above the horizontal plane should be performed later and done with the arm in external rotation, as this will facilitate clearance for the greater tuberosity beneath the acromion. Repetitive stretching exercises in abduction and internal rotation should be avoided. Strengthening exercises are started gradually, first concentrating on the external rotators and the deltoid and then the internal rotators and scapula muscles. With impingement lesions, inflammation causing pain is the primary source of weakness. Overly aggressive strengthening may cause inflammation to the supraspinatus tendon and bursa and retard the healing process.

## SUMMARY

Variations in the architecture of the coracoacromial arch can lead to a clinically symptomatic rotator cuff lesion. Differences in the shape and slope of the acromion and the presence of anterior acromial spurs or inferior protruding acromioclavicular osteophytes may decrease the volume of the subacromial space, leading to impingement. When planning surgical procedures in this setting, an important goal is increasing the space beneath the coracoacromial arch to reduce wear on the rotator cuff.

# REFERENCES

1. Smith JG: Pathological appearances of seven cases of injury of the shoulder joint; with remarks. London Med Gaz 14:280, 1834
2. Neer CS: Anterior acromioplasty for the chronic impingement syndrome in the shoulder. A preliminary report. J Bone Joint Surg 54A:41, 1972
3. Neer CS: Impingement lesions. Clin Orthop 173:70, 1983
4. Bardeen CR, Lewis WH: The development of the limbs, body-wall, and back. Am J Anat 1:1, 1901
5. Lewis WH: The development of the arm in man. Am J Anat 1:145, 1902
6. Gardner E, Gray DJ: Prenatal development of the human shoulder and the acromioclavicular joint. Am J Anat 92:219, 1953
7. Trotter M, Peterson RR: Osteology. p. 133. In Anson BJ (ed): Morris' Human Anatomy: A Complete Systematic Treatise. 12th Ed. McGraw-Hill, New York, 1966
8. Gardner E, Gray DJ, O'Rahilly R: Bones of the upper limb. p. 107. In: Anatomy: A Regional Study of Human Structure. WB Saunders, Philadelphia, 1960
9. Grant JCB: The upper limb. p. 72. In: A Method of Anatomy. 2nd Ed. Williams & Wilkins, Baltimore, 1940
10. Lieberson E: Os acromiale: a contested anomaly. J Bone Joint Surg 19:683, 1937
11. DePalma AF: Surgical anatomy of acromioclavicular and sternoclavicular joints. Surg Clin North Am 43:1541, 1963
12. Moseley HF: The clavicle and its articulations. p. 176. In: Shoulder Lesions. 2nd Ed. Hoeber, New York, 1953
13. Petersson CJ: Degeneration of the acromioclavicular joint: a morphological study. Acta Orthop Scand 54:434, 1983
14. Cheselden W: The Anatomy of the Human Body. 11th Ed. London, 1778
15. Lindblom K: On pathogenesis of ruptures of the tendon aponeurosis of the shoulder joint. Acta Radiol 20:563, 1939
16. Moseley HF, Goldie I: The arterial pattern of the rotator cuff of the shoulder. J Bone Joint Surg 45B:780, 1963
17. Rathbun JB, Macnab I: The microvascular pattern of the rotator cuff. J Bone Joint Surg 52B:540, 1970
18. Rothman RH, Parke WW: The vascular anatomy of the rotator cuff. Clin Orthop 41:176, 1965
19. Bigliani LU, Ticker JB, Flatow EL et al: The relationship of acromial architecture to rotator cuff disease. Clin Sports Med 10:823, 1991
20. Bigliani LU, Morrison DS, April EW: The morphology of the acromion and its relationship to rotator cuff tears. Orthop Trans 10:228, 1986
21. Morrison DS, Bigliani LU: The clinical significance of variations in acromial morphology. Orthop Trans 11:234, 1987
22. Aoki M, Ishii I, Usui M: The slope of the acromion and rotator cuff impingement. Orthop Trans 10:228, 1986
23. Aoki M, Ishii I, Usui M: Clinical application for measuring the slope of the acromion. p. 200. In Post M, Hawkins RJ, Morrey BF (eds): Surgery of the Shoulder. Mosby Year Book, St Louis, 1990, p 200
24. Petersson CJ, Gentz CF: Ruptures of the supraspinatus tendon: the significance of distally pointing acromioclavicular osteophytes. Clin Orthop 174:143, 1983
25. Bigliani LU, Norris TR, Fischer J, Neer CS: The relationship between the unfused acromial epiphysis and subacromial lesions. Orthop Trans 7:138, 1983
26. Mudge MK, Wook VE, Frykman GK: Rotator cuff tears associated with os acromiale. J Bone Joint Surg 66A:427, 1984
27. Dines DM, Warren RE, Inglis AE, Pavlov H: The coracoid impingement. Orthop Trans 10:229, 1986
28. Gerber C, Terrier F, Ganz R: The role of the coracoid process in the chronic impingement syndrome. J Bone Joint Surg 67B:703, 1985
29. Bateman JE: Cuff tears in athletes. Orthop Clin North Am 1:721, 1973
30. Bigliani LU, D'Alessandro DF, Duralde XA, McIlveen SJ: Anterior acromioplasty for subacromial impingement in patients younger than 40 years of age. Clin Orthop 246:111, 1989
31. Cofield RH, Simonet WT: The shoulder in sports. Mayo Clin Proc 59:157, 1984
32. Fowler P: Swimmer problems. Am J Sports Med 7:141, 1979
33. Fu FH, Harner CD, Klein AH: Shoulder impingement syndrome: a critical review. Clin Orthop 269:162, 1991
34. Gainor BJ, Piotrowski G, Puhl J et al: The throw: biomechanics and acute injury. Am J Sports Med 8:114, 1980
35. Hawkins RJ, Kennedy JC: Impingement syndrome in athletes. Am J Sports Med 8:151, 1980
36. Jackson DW: Chronic rotator cuff impingement in the throwing athlete. Am J Sports Med 4:231, 1976
37. Jackson DW: Problems among the inexperienced and experienced athlete. Am J Sports Med 7:142, 1979
38. Jobe FW: Thrower problems. Am J Sports Med 7:139, 1979
39. Jobe FW: Impingement problems in the athlete. ICLS 38:205, 1989
40. Jobe FW, Tibone JE, Perry J, Moynes D: An EMG analysis of the shoulder in throwing and pitching: a preliminary report. Am J Sports Med 11:3, 1983
41. Neer CS, Welsh RP: The shoulder in sports. Orthop Clin North Am 8:583, 1977

42. Neviaser RJ: Lesions of the biceps and tendonitis of the shoulder. Orthop Clin North Am 11:343, 1980

43. Penny JN, Welsh RP: Shoulder impingement syndromes in athletes and their surgical management. Am J Sports Med 9:11, 1981

44. Priest JD, Nagel DA: Tennis shoulder. Am J Sports Med 4:28, 1976

45. Richardson AB, Jobe FW, Collins HR: The shoulder in competitive swimming. Am J Sports Med 8:159, 1980

46. Tibone JE, Jobe FW, Kerlan RK et al: Shoulder impingement syndrome in athletes treated by an anterior acromioplasty. Clin Orthop 198:134, 1985

47. Tibone JE, Elrod B, Jobe FW et al: Surgical treatment of tears of the rotator cuff in athletes. J Bone Joint Surg 68A:887, 1986

48. Jobe FW, Jobe CM: Painful athletic injuries of the shoulder. Clin Orthop 173:117, 1983

49. Norwood LA, Del Pizzo W, Jobe FW, Kerlan RK: Anterior shoulder pain in baseball pitchers. Orthop Trans 2:20, 1978

50. Neer CS, Bigliani LU, Hawkins RJ: Rupture of the long head of the biceps related to subacromial impingement. Orthop Trans 1:111, 1977

51. Glousman R, Jobe F, Tibone J et al: Dynamic electromyographic analysis of the throwing shoulder with glenohumeral instability. J Bone Joint Surg 70A:220, 1988

52. Pappas AM, Zawacki RM, McCarthy CF: Rehabilitation of the pitching shoulder. Am J Sports Med 13:223, 1985

53. Perry J: Anatomy and biomechanics of the shoulder in throwing, swimming, gymnastics, and tennis. Clin Sports Med 2:247, 1983

54. Tullos HS, King JW: Throwing mechanism in sports. Orthop Clin North Am 1:709, 1973

55. Pink M, Jobe FW, Perry J: Electromyographic analysis of the shoulder during the golf swing. Am J Sports Med 18:137, 1990

56. Pujadas GW: Coraco-acromial ligament syndrome. J Bone Joint Surg 52A:1261, 1970

57. Connolly P, Wolfe I, Bigliani LU: Rehabilitation of the shoulder. p. 792. In Dee R, Mango E, Hurst LC (eds): Principles of Orthopaedic Practice. McGraw-Hill, New York, 1988

58. Jobe FW, Moynes DR: Delineation of diagnostic criteria and a rehabilitation program for rotator cuff injuries. Am J Sports Med 10:336, 1982

59. Bigliani LU: Impingement syndrome: aetiology and overview. p. 237. In Watson MS (ed): Surgical Disorders of the Shoulder. Churchill, Livingstone, Edinburgh, 1991

# 13

# Traumatic Avulsion Tears of the Rotator Cuff

*WILLIAM M. CRAVEN*

Traumatic avulsive tears of the shoulder rotator cuff tendon represent a challenge to both the patient and physician. These tears are challenging from a diagnostic, treatment, and rehabilitative standpoint.

An avulsive tear of the rotator cuff with subsequent significant functional limitations can have significant psychological and financial impact on the patient and health care delivery system. The torn rotator cuff can present a devastating dilemma to the athlete, resulting in diminished performance with the possibility of ending an amateur or professional career.[1-3]

Traumatic avulsive tears of the rotator cuff, previously commonly seen in the older patient, are becoming more common in a younger age group (younger than 40 years old).[1,4-6] These tears, however, are rare in normal healthy tissue tendon and require significant trauma, such as a shoulder dislocation, to occur.[1]

Why then are physicians seeing an increased incidence of traumatic avulsive tears?

A more likely scenario for a traumatic avulsive tear is the occurrence of significant trauma to an athlete who has participated for several years in overhead sports activities and has had recurrent episodes of shoulder problems (bursitis, tendonitis, impingement, or a "sore shoulder"). These recurrent episodes have been treated conservatively with ice, rest, nonsteroidal anti-inflammatory drugs, and steroid injections, resulting in relief of symptoms and an early return to sports-related activities. But, as will be noted later, these recurrent episodes alter the musculotendinous structure of the rotator cuff, resulting in decreased tensile strength and elasticity.[7-10]

With the increase in the length of the playing seasons, athletes starting formal participation at younger ages, and increased participation in overhead activity sports (e.g., weight lifting, shoulder strengthening machines, racquet sports, and throwing), a whole new population of athletes is evolving who are exposing their shoulders to increased micro- and macrotraumatic stress patterns.

The classic tear of the rotator cuff is in an individual older than the age of 40 years.[7,8,11-16]

But, with the above-mentioned factors, we must add to this older-than-40-years group, the group of younger athletes who have played sports since an early age (9 or 10 years old), competed in longer seasons, used "advanced" weight training machines and systems that stress the shoulder, and experienced repeated episodes of "sore shoulders."

This group has experienced a phenomenon we will label as *athletically accelerated aging* of tissue of the rotator cuff musculotendinous unit.

This patient group now has a rotator cuff that experiences frequent and long-term microtrauma, resulting in changes in the structure of the tendon and making it more susceptible to further injury such as a traumatic avulsive tears—interstitial, partial, and complete.[1-5,17]

To-develop the concept of traumatic avulsive tears of the rotator cuff from athletically advanced aging, this chapter reviews the classic work of the early investigators of rotator cuff tears, reviews basic anatomy, and discusses the demands on the shoulder and how these factors contribute to this pathology. Important emphasis is placed on the role of recurrent microtrauma and the resultant pathologic changes that occur in the rotator cuff–musculotendinous unit.

# HISTORY

Many orthopaedists of the past two centuries have been intrigued by and contributed to our understanding of rotator cuff tears.[7,8,12,18] The early comprehensive works by Codman,[7,11,12,18,19] Meyer,[20] DePalma,[13,21–23] and many others gave clear insight into the problems associated with the evaluation and treatment of rotator cuff pathology.[14,15]

Later physicians, such as Neer,[14,15] Neviaser,[16,24,25] Hawkins,[5,26,27] Rockwood,[9] and others, continued to advance the understanding of difficult tears of the rotator cuff. These studies more clearly delineated the pathology involved and outlined surgical approaches.

The past 20 years have seen a significant increase in the number of clinical and basic science studies producing information regarding a special population of patients with rotator cuff pathology—the athlete.

Andrews,[19,28] Jobe,[2,3] Hawkins,[5,26] and others have taken this unique group of patients and developed a diagnostic test, rehabilitative protocol, and surgical techniques that treat rotator cuff tears. Most in this group have increased episodes of traumatic events (micro and macro) through athletic participation when compared with previous population groups.

# ANATOMY/FUNCTION

The anatomy and function of the rotator cuff have been examined extensively.[7,9,12,18,21] With the development and advances in diagnostic tests, such as computed tomography–arthrography, magnetic resonance imaging, electromyogram/nerve conduction study, and computerized video analysis, new volumns of information concerning the function of the rotator cuff have been generated.

Anatomically, the rotator cuff can be thought of as a unit comprising four muscles (subscapularis, supraspinatus, infraspinatus, and teres minor); all originate from the scapula and insert into the tuberosities of the humerus. The shoulder capsule, which adds stability, blends with the tendon near its insertion.

The vascular supply of the rotator cuff has been studied extensively.[8,29,30] The primary blood supply of the rotator cuff is provided by the anterior humeral circumflex artery and subscapular and suprascapular arteries. The unique blood supply contributes to the development of problems in the rotator cuff. Extensive

work has been undertaken to enhance our understanding of the role blood supply plays in rotator cuff function.

The work of Uhthoff et al[10] reported areas of hypovascularity at an area near the tendon insertion. The now classic injection studies by Rathbun and Macnab[30] further elucidated the reason for the degeneration of the tendon in the "critical zone" of Codman.[11] These findings correspond to the thought that people have been exposed to shoulder problems since they became bipedal and started to reach for the stars overhead.

The importance of the bony and ligamentous structures surrounding the rotator cuff must be appreciated to understand the development of shoulder pathology. The shoulder consists of three diarthrodial joints (glenohumeral, acromioclavicular, and sternoclavicular). The glenohumeral joint has little bony stability and relies on ligaments and muscles for essentially all stability.

Neer[15] analyzed this unique structure and developed the concept of impingement, which clarified the role of the shoulder bony ligamentous arch in the development of shoulder problems.

This unique mobility of the shoulder is a blessing for function but a curse for healthy tissue, because it allows exposure to injury from trauma unlike other more stable joints. Jobe and Bradley,[3] by combining concepts of instability and impingement, showed how structure, instability, and athletic demand can lead to clinical patterns resulting in pathologic shoulder entities.

The rotator cuff muscle complex has multiple functions: It stabilizes the shoulder, steers the head of the humerus during movement, provides power in all directions, and produces, in conjunction with the deltoid, torque about the shoulder. The rotator cuff works synergistically with the deltoid, biceps, trapezius, pectoralis, and latissimus dorsi—for both power and stability.

# PATHOLOGY

Neviaser[16,24] noted five mechanisms for rotator cuff tears; four involved significant single episodes of trauma. Yet acute traumatic avulsive tears of the rotator cuff, resulting from single events, are rare when compared with chronic tears with no known single event of trauma. Reeves[31] and Mosely[32] noted a low incidence of rotator cuff tears after shoulder dislocations.

A review of the literature pertaining to rotator cuff tears concludes that age is the most important factor in the etiology of tears.[4,11,12,16,18,21,25,33] The vast majority of tears start after age 40 years, and the incidence increases with each subsequent decade.[1,8,11,15,18,34] Studies by DePalma,[21] Neer,[16] Pettersson,[35] and Codman[18] all reported that the vast majority of rotator cuff tears were in patients older than 40 years. Neer found only eight patients of 233 with rotator cuff tears who were younger than 40 years.[14,15] Additional factors include recurrent microtrauma, steroid injections, subacromial impingement, and previous partial tears.[8,11,16,18] De-Palma[23] noted that massive energy injuries to the shoulder typically resulted in ligamentous injuries and fractures rather than acute avulsive complete tears of the rotator cuff. The rotator cuff tendon in a young person's shoulder, with no history of shoulder injury, is extremely strong and difficult to rupture despite significant trauma. The research undertaken by McMasters[36] showed that healthy tendon rarely tears in the midsubstance despite large forces. Tears were usually located at the musculotendinous junction or the bony insertion.

Studies of shoulder dislocations that resulted from large forces show a low incidence of acute avulsive tears of the rotator cuff. DePalma's[21] review of 56 cases of recurrent dislocations of patients aged 19 to 33 years found five tears (two supraspinatus and three subscapularis tears). Reeves[31] showed two of 27 patients in their 30s sustained rotator cuff tears after dislocations.

The work by Meyer[20,37] suggested that tears of the rotator cuff resulted from attrition. The research of Uhthoff et al[10] and Pettersson[35] concerning age-related degeneration of the rotator cuff tendon agreed with this concept of accumulated attrition from microtrauma built up over decades.

These studies elucidated a picture of tendon changes on the cellular level, including calcium deposits, fibrinoid thickening, cell degeneration, necrosis, and scar formation. The studies showed a healed tendon with decreased tensile strength and decreased elasticity. Other changes noted included microscopic tears, granularity, and loss of normal-appearing collagen fibers.[9]

Neer's[15] observations combined age groups and pathology to form a system of classification with distinct groups and presented a clinical continuum of age and pathology as the reason for development of shoulder problems.

Rockwood and Matsen[9] suggested a combination of traumatic and degenerative theories to explain rotator cuff tears. A combination of microtears, impingement, inflammation, injections, and age combine to lead to a tendon that becomes susceptible to traumatic avulsive tears.

Nixon and DiStefano[38] noted in their studies of vigorous athletes with partial ruptures that the histologic pattern in these tears was similar to tears of the Achilles tendons, suprapatellar tendons, and infrapatellar tendons. The pattern was one of the chronic changes including edema, interstitial hypercellularity and a healing pattern of disorganized tendon.

The research of Codman and Akerson[7] and Lindblom's[39] investigative work showed histologic patterns consistent with a loss of normal tendon structure and a resultant "sclerotic tissue." The healing process of a tendon after an acute inflammatory period results in changed structure and, therefore, a change in function. A healed tendon has some loss of tensile strength and elasticity.

The existence of partial tears of the rotator cuff has been noted for years. Cadaveric studies by Cotton and Rideout[40] showed the existence of "slight tears in the deep surface of the supraspinatus."

More recent investigations have revealed the large incidence of partial tears of the rotator cuff in young patients. Andrews and Carson[1] reported on 36 patients from a group of 106 arthroscopically evaluated shoulders. All 36 patients were competitive athletes, average age was 22 years, and all had been treated conservatively for shoulder pain. Sixty-one percent of the patients examined preoperatively had tenderness over the supraspinatus. This group was found to have partial tears of the rotator cuff. The tendon usually was torn near its insertion into the humerus.

Tibone et al[6] reported on a group of 45 athletes with partial or complete tears of the rotator cuff treated with anterior acromioplasty and repair of the tear. They noted that tears are usually not appreciated in the younger patient and believed that the partial tears resulted from chronic overuse activities. The area of the tear also corresponded to the "critical zone" described by Rathbun and Macnab[30] and Codman[8] typically seen in the older population group.

## TREATMENT

As with any injury, a careful history and an extensive physical examination should be obtained in the evaluation of a possible traumatic avulsive tear of the rotator cuff.

As part of the history, the mechanism of injury should be determined. As noted before, the commonly proposed causes of rotator cuff failure include attrition, ischemia, impingement, and trauma.

The mechanism of injury for traumatic avulsive tears can be divided into two major groups: group 1—single episodes of significant trauma on a shoulder with a healthy rotator cuff or a cuff with chronic attritional changes; and group 2—episodes of trauma that are usual for a particular sport or event but are experienced by an athletically accelerated aged rotator cuff.

Group 1 traumatic events usually involve a shoulder dislocation or violent fall.[11,12,18,35,36] The shoulder is most commonly in an abducted and externally rotated position, and the trauma results in an anterior dislocation and subsequent tear of the rotator cuff. A fall on the flexed and abducted arm is more consistent with the less common posterior shoulder dislocation.[9]

Group 2 traumatic avulsive tears can occur with any trauma that is typical for a particular sport. This type of trauma can be significant or minor and can be enough to injure an already chronically damaged musculotendinous unit.

The diagnosis of traumatic avulsive tears of the rotator cuff is made in a systematic manner. A complete history and comprehensive physical examination are obtained. Special attention is noted for areas of tenderness, limitations of range of motion, and loss of strength, especially for abduction, external rotation, and supraspinatus strength.[41]

In certain instances, additional information is obtained with the use of radiographs, magnetic resonance imaging, and computed tomography–arthrography.

If surgical intervention for diagnosis and treatment is necessary, it should be as conservative as possible.[28] The technique for arthroscopy has been previously described by Andrews et al.[1,42] If additional open surgery is required after arthroscopy, it can be performed at the same operative setting and typically performed through a small lateral incision. The type surgery must be tailored to the injury, the athlete, and the surgeon's skill and experience.

## CONCLUSION

The diagnosis of traumatic avulsive tears of the rotator cuff is often missed or identified late. The concept that rotator cuff tears primarily occur in those older than 40 years is no longer valid in view of today's large group of young active patients who vigorously participate in overhead sports activities. This is especially true for tears in the shoulder of young athletes. Their symptoms and clinical examination often do not mirror the usual picture of the older patient.

The diagnosis of traumatic avulsive tear should be entertained in any young athlete with shoulder disability that does not significantly improve with conservative treatment in 2 to 4 weeks. An appropriate workup should be performed in these cases.

A larger consideration, which evolves from the concept of athletically accelerated aging, is the prevention of this condition. Efforts should be made to avoid the evolution of a tendon with decreased strength and elasticity and more susceptible to injury.

Recommendations would center around a program of comprehensive prevention and treatment for athletes who put high demands on their shoulders.

1. Increased training and awareness of the problem through education of physicians, physical therapists, athletic trainers, coaches, and players.
2. Special training on proper techniques for weight lifters and racquet sports. Emphasis on proper mechanics—especially in young baseball players, swimmers, and racquet sports participants.
3. Careful monitoring of the very young (10 to 15 years) athlete. Limits on games, practices and innings pitched.
4. Immediate and aggressive conservative treatment of all *sore shoulders*—which includes strengthening exercises designed to improve the dynamic stabilization and control of the shoulder.

These measures should be enforced to prevent the irreversible changes associated with athletically accelerated aging and the resultant increased risk of traumatic avulsive tears of the rotator cuff.

# REFERENCES

1. Andrews JR, Carson WG Jr: Arthroscopy of the shoulder in the management of partial tears of the rotator cuff: a preliminary report. Presented at Sports Medicine Conference, Cleveland, 1986
2. Jobe FW, Jobe CM: Painful athletic injuries of the shoulder. Clin Orthop 173:117, 1983
3. Jobe FW, Bradley JP: The diagnosis and nonoperative treatment of shoulder injuries in athletes. Clin Sports Med 8:419, 1989
4. Bateman JE: Cuff tears in athletes. Orthop Clin North Am 4:721, 1973
5. Hawkins RJ, Kennedy JC: Impingement syndrome in athletes. Am J Sports Med 8:151, 1980
6. Tibone JE, Elrod B, Jobe FW et al: Surgical treatment of tears of the rotator cuff in athletes. J Bone Joint Surg 68A:887, 1986
7. Codman EA, Akerson TB: The pathology associated with rupture of the supraspinatus tendon. Ann Surg 93:354, 1911
8. Codman EA: The Shoulder. Thomas Todd, Boston, 1934
9. Rockwood CA Jr, Matsen FA III: The Shoulder. Vol. 2. WB Saunders, Philadelphia, 1990
10. Uhthoff HK, Loehr J, Sarkar K: The pathogenesis of rotator cuff tears. In Proceedings of the Third International Conference on Surgery of the Shoulder, Fukuora, Japan, October 27, 1986
11. Codman EA: Rupture of the supraspinatus tendon (1911 Classic article). Clin Orthop 254:3, 1990
12. Codman EA: Rupture of the supraspinatus—1834–1934. J Bone Joint Surg 19:643, 1937
13. DePalma AF, Gallery G, Bennett CA: Variational anatomy and degenerative lesions of the shoulder joint. Instr Course Lect 6:255, 1949
14. Neer CS II: Anterior acromioplasty for the chronic impingement syndrome in the shoulder. J Bone Joint Surg 54A:41, 1972
15. Neer CS II: Impingement lesions. Clin Orthop 173:70, 1983
16. Neviaser JS: Ruptures of the rotator cuff. Clin Orthop 3:92, 1954
17. McLaughlin HL: Rupture of the rotator cuff. J Bone Joint Surg 44A:979, 1962
18. Codman EA: Complete rupture of the supraspinatus tendon. Operative treatment with report of two successful cases. Boston Med Surg J 164:708, 1911
19. Codman EA: Rupture of the supraspinatus. Am J Surg 42:603, 1938
20. Meyer AW: The minute anatomy of attrition lesions. J Bone Joint Surg 13A:341, 1931
21. DePalma AF: Surgery of the Shoulder. JB Lippincott, Philadelphia, 1950
22. DePalma AF: Surgical approaches to the region of the shoulder joint. Clin Orthop 20:163, 1961
23. DePalma AF: Surgery of the Shoulder. 2nd Ed. JB Lippincott, Philadelphia, 1973
24. Neviaser JS: Ruptures of the rotator cuff of the shoulder. New concepts in the diagnosis and operative treatment of chronic ruptures. Arch Surg 102:483, 1971
25. Neviaser RJ: Tears of the rotator cuff. Orthop Clin North Am 11:295, 1980
26. Hawkins RJ: Surgical management of rotator cuff tears. p. 161. In Bateman JF (ed): Surgery of the Shoulder. EC Decker, Philadelphia, 1984
27. Hawkins RJ, Misamore GW, Hobeika PE: Surgery of full thickness rotator cuff tears. J Bone Joint Surg 67A:1349, 1985
28. Scarpinato DF, Brauhall JP, Andrews JR: Arthroscopic management of the throwing athletes shoulder: indications, techniques and results. Clin Sports Med 10:913, 1991
29. Moseley HF, Goldie I: The arterial pattern of the rotator cuff of the shoulder. J Bone Joint Surg 45B:780, 1963
30. Rathbun JB, Macnab I: The microvascular pattern of the rotator cuff. J Bone Joint Surg 52B:540, 1970
31. Reeves B: Arthrography of the shoulder. J Bone Joint Surg 48B:424, 1966
32. Moseley HF: Ruptures to the Rotator Cuff. Charles C Thomas, Springfield, IL, 1952.
33. Bateman JE: Shoulder and Neck. WB Saunders, Philadelphia, 1972
34. Cofield RH: Current concepts review rotator cuff disease of the shoulder. J Bone Joint Surg 67:974, 1985
35. Pettersson G: Rupture of the tendon aponeurosis of the shoulder joint in anterior inferior dislocation. Acta Chir Scand (Suppl) 77:1, 1942
36. McMasters PE: Tendon and muscle ruptures: clinical and experimental studies on the causes and location of subcutaneous ruptures. J Bone Joint Surg 15A:705, 1933
37. Meyer AW: Further evidence of attrition in the human body. Am J Anat 34:241, 1924
38. Nixon JE, DiStefano V: Ruptures of the rotator cuff. Symposium on surgery of the shoulder. Orthop Clin North Am 6:423, 1795
39. Lindblom K: On pathogenesis of ruptures of the tendon aponeurosis of the shoulder joint. Acta Radiol 20:563, 1939

40. Cotton RE, Rideout DF: Tears of the humeral rotator cuff. A radiological and pathological necropsy survey. J Bone Joint Surg 46B:314, 1964

41. Andrews JR, Gillogly MD: Physical Examination of the Shoulder in Throwing Athletes. Injuries To the Throwing Arm. WB Saunders, Philadelphia, 1985

42. Andrews JR, Gidamah RH: Shoulder arthroscopy in the throwing athlete. Perspective and progress. Arthroscopy 6:565, 1987

## SUGGESTED READINGS

Bassett RW, Cofield RH: Acute tears of the rotator cuff. The timing of surgical repair. Clin Orthop 175:98, 1983

Bateman JE: The diagnosis and treatment of ruptures of the rotator cuff. Surg Clin North Am 43:1523, 1963

Bateman JE: Neurological painful conditions affecting the shoulder. Clin Orthop 174:44, 1983

Cofield RH: Tears of rotator cuff. Instr Course Lect 30:258, 1981

DeSmet AA, Ting YM: Diagnosis of rotator cuff tear on routine radiographs. J Assoc Can Radiol 28:54, 1977

Hoppenfeld S: Physical Examination of the Spine and Extremities. Appleton-Century-Crofts, East Norwalk, CT, 1976

Inman VT, Saunders JB de CM, Abbott LC: Observations on the function of the shoulder joint. J Bone Joint Surg 26A:1, 1944

Lindblom K: Arthrography and roentgenography in rupture of the tendons of the shoulder joint. Acta Radiol 20:548, 1939

McLaughlin HL: Lesions of the musculotendinous cuff of the shoulder. I. The exposure and treatment of tears with retraction. J Bone Joint Surg 26:31, 1944

McLaughlin HL: Repair of major cuff ruptures. Surg Clin North Am 43:1535, 1939

Moseley HF: Shoulder Lesions. 3rd Ed. Churchill Livingstone, Edinburgh, 1969

Poppen NK, Walker PS: Normal and abnormal motion of the shoulder. J Bone Joint Surg 58A:195, 1976

Rothman RH, Parke WW: The vascular anatomy of the rotator cuff. Clin Orthop 41:176, 1965

# 14
# Calcifying Tendonitis

*LAWRENCE J. LEMAK*

A pathology occasionally seen in shoulders is calcifying tendonitis, most often identified as a reactive process of self-healing. Calcium deposits appear in the shoulder more often than in any other joint, but why the shoulder and why do these deposits have clinical relevance?

To understand calcification of the rotator cuff completely, we must have knowledge of the anatomy of the rotator cuff, the pathomechanics of rotator cuff motion, and the much discussed area of decreased blood supply to the rotator cuff and the Codman's critical zone. Also, we review the mechanisms of cellular calcium handling to understand the mechanisms of rotator cuff calcification.

The gross anatomy consists of the four muscles of the rotator cuff, their innervation, and their blood supply. The rotator cuff tendon is generally referred to as that of the subscapularis muscle and tendon, the supraspinatus muscle and tendon, the infraspinatus muscle and tendon, and the teres minor muscle and tendon. Innervation of the subscapularis is by the upper and lower subscapular nerves. The supraspinatus innervation is by the subscapular nerve after it passes through the subscapular notch. The infraspinatus is innervated by the suprascapular nerve. The teres minor is innervated by a branch of the axillary nerve.

Much has been written about the vascularity of the rotator cuff tendon, and it has been studied in depth by several investigators. Codman's critical zone, the area of the supraspinatus prone to rupture and calcification, was believed by many to be an avascular area. Some take exception to this. Moseley and Goldie[1] believed that this area had a rich vascular pattern and that the tendon of the supraspinatus was not much less vascularized than other parts of the cuff. The study by Rathbun and Macnab[2] offered a different thesis. They

showed that the filling of the cuff vessels was dependent on the position of the arm at the time of injection. They noted that the zone of poor filling was near the tuberosity attachment of the supraspinatus when the arm was adducted, and they believed that when the arm was in abduction, there was almost full filling of the vessels except for the superior portion of the supraspinatus. This was not seen in the other tendons of the rotator cuff. The authors suggested that tendon failure might be caused by constant pressure of the head of the humerus, which tends to wring out the blood supply to these tendons when the arm is held in a resting position of adduction and neutral rotation. Other authors[3] thought that the critical zone was an area that corresponded to the area of anastamosis between the osseous vessel as the anterior branch of the anterior humeral circumflex, the posterior humeral circumflex, and the muscular, suprascapular, and subscapular vessels.

As we review the literature, we find that the location of calcification of the rotator cuff tendon varies from study to study but is usually in the area Codman described as the critical portion, which was later renamed by Moseley and Goldie as the critical zone. Rothman and Parkes[4] reported that the critical zone was markedly undervascularized.

In most studies, calcification of the rotator cuff tendon was much more prevalent in the supraspinatus tendon. Plenk[5] showed that 82 percent of the calcification appeared in the supraspinatus, and Bosworth[6] found greater than 90 percent in the supraspinatus and the infraspinatus. DePalma and Kruper[7] reported 74 percent in the supraspinatus alone. Uhthoff and Sarkar[8] stated that there is no relationship between calcifying tendinitis and trauma. They found it interesting that most calcification is around the bursal side of the tendon and will rupture into the subacromial bursa (Fig. 14-1), whereas in a few cases, the calcific deposit ruptures into the glenohumeral side. Patte and Goutallier,[9] reported two cases of glenohumeral rupture.

The pathogenesis in the cellular function of calcification is not well understood, but the report by Messler et al casts some light on calcium metabolism at the cellular level (personal communication). Messler stated that the calcifying configurations in the rotator cuff tendons are not calcifying necrosis or calcium soaps in the classic sense. Even though the specific composition of the calcific deposits is still unknown, we know that the main mineral ingredient of the calcific deposits is hydroxyapatite.

Histologic observations of calcifying deposits showed a metaplastic transformation from tenocytes to chondrocytes as well as the increase of mucopolysaccharides and the disintegration of collagen in the surrounding matrix. The histomorphologic aspect seems to be similar to that of enchondral ossification. This calcifying tendonitis is the result of an active cell calcifying process.

The combination of the anatomic aspects, decreased blood supply, and microtrauma of the rotator cuff leads to a repetitive hypoxia of the cells and their surrounding tissue. As a result, on the cellular level the fibrocytes are transformed to chondrocytes, and the matrix of the tendon tissue shows a disintegration of collagen and an accumulation of mucopolysaccharides. The chondrocytes proceed in a way similar to enchondral ossification.

Because of the collapsing calcium gradient, hydroxyapatite is accumulated in the suborganelles of the chondrocyte in the economical bioenergetic form of hydroxyapatite. After the degeneration of the chondrocyte microglobules or matrix, vesicles are set free into the intercellular space, and the formation of hydroxyapatite mineral deposits is initiated.

Most authors have found that in the past few years the incidence of calcifying tendonitis has decreased in the population we have observed. This is believed to be directly proportional to patients in our population seeking earlier treatment and receiving good aggressive rehabilitation with active rest. Colleagues with similar practices are also finding a decreased incidence of calcifying tendonitis.

Uhthoff and Sarkar[8] revealed that calcific tendonitis can be self-healing and that different aspects of its pathology are not characteristic of degenerative disease. These authors break down the calcific tendonitis into three stages: precalcific, calcific, and postcalcific.

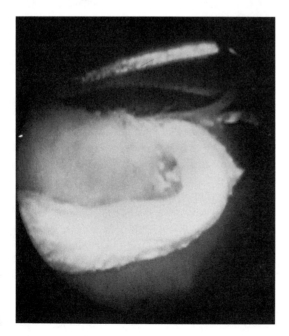

A

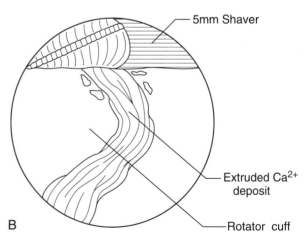

B

**Fig. 14-1. (A)** Arthroscopic view of supraspinatus muscle exhibiting calcific deposit extruding into subacromial space. **(B)** Illustration of arthroscopic view.

Some also believe that there may be genetic susceptibility to this condition.

Calcific tendonitis is a late occurring stage of tendonitis of the rotator cuff. To understand calcific tendonitis, one must understand the basic pathogenesis of rotator cuff tendonitis in the shoulder, specifically in the athletic shoulder. Athletic techniques are often a main factor in tendonitis of the rotator cuff, and subsequently we can see the late stage, which is calcific tendonitis, even in the younger age groups. We again have to refer to Codman's initial work and search the literature, finding the contributions by Moseley through the work of Neer, Jobe, and Nirschl on tendonitis of the shoulder. More extensive data are being reported from laboratories across the country with sophisticated throwing analysis equipment, both in Jobe's and his associates' laboratory and in our own laboratory at American Sports Medicine Institute in Birmingham, Alabama. The mechanics of throwing can be analyzed to show that abnormal mechanics of throwing and training can be associated with rotator cuff tendonitis. Now, in-depth studies of overhead sports can be analyzed along with their motions to identify causes of rotator cuff tendonitis secondary to poor mechanics. Many centers are showing that, through rehabilitative exercise of the rotator cuff, healing of the rotator cuff is very successful. This would include a combination of active rest and exercise for the acute tendonitis as well as the later stages of calcific tendonitis. This treatment can be shown to give symptomatic relief by developing a healthy rotator cuff tendon, probably because this treatment enhances the blood supply and the subsequent healing process.

In the athlete's shoulder, internal rotation (at 90 degrees abduction) puts a tremendous pressure on the rotator cuff. One of two mechanisms of injury can come into play: (1) direct pressure leading to tearing, either by traction or compression, or (2) the mechanism of blocking the blood supply to areas of the cuff leading to necrosis. Sarkar and Uhthoff believed that a brief calcific stage can be caused by either hypoxia (which was also suggested by Codman) or pressure, which can occur with athletic activity. Messler (personal communication) further elaborated on this at the cellular level of damage to the rotator cuff. Athletes can be very susceptible to either one of these two mechanisms. This suggests that an etiology of calcific tendonitis in the athlete may be due to pressure with secondary hypoxia to the tendon. When studying clinical presentations, we must remember that the rotator cuff can be subjected to tensile overload, compression, and shear stresses in many activities because of the repetitive overhead motions and, thus, repetitive microtrauma. Also, we must not forget the predisposition to irritation of the rotator cuff secondary to compressive mechanical forces, such as a hooked-type acromion or acromioclavicular spur.

When we review the clinical presentations, we must remember the natural history of rotator cuff tendonitis. In later stages, it can turn into calcific tendonitis. A thorough history is important, because rotator cuff tendonitis can be secondary to tension overload. This can be treated with good clinical results by rehabilitative exercises designed to restore the tendon to proper health and function.

When the patient or athlete presents with calcifying tendonitis, the symptoms may range from simple discomfort to severe pain. The patients with severe pain present with such acute and severe pain that it constitutes an emergency. In these cases, the calcium deposit in the tendon is under tremendous pressure. Other patients may present simply with other problems in the shoulder, and the calcific deposits are seen as an incidental radiographic finding. Authors such as Lippmann[11] and others suggested that different forms of calcium found in the shoulder can be associated with different presentations. Calcium can be present in the shoulder as a soft, toothpaste-like material under pressure but also can be present as a hard, chalky, uninflamed area. The clinical presentation can also be one part of a symptom complex that is associated with tendonitis. We also see calcification in association with impingement syndrome of the shoulder and with complete rupture of the rotator cuff. During the acute phase, symptoms persist for up to 2 weeks. The subacute and chronic phase symptoms can last 3 to 8 weeks, and very chronic phase symptoms have been confirmed for 3 months or longer. Also consider that during the subacute and chronic phases, the calcific tendonitis may lead to a secondary impingement because of the localized hyperemia of the supraspinatus tendon. Therefore, the patient will present with pain similar to a classic impingement syndrome. Often it is difficult to separate the two conditions to decide exactly which pathology came first. For instance, as we previously described, the etiology that impingement pressures on the rotator cuff may lead to secondary calcification after a period of time. Patients in the acute phase will often not allow their shoulder to be moved. They also will be very discretely tender over the calcific area. A thorough physical examination sometimes cannot even be conducted until the more subacute or chronic phases. Secondary problems other than the calcific tendonitis can be delineated much easier with a thorough physical examination. Frozen shoulders may also be part of the clinical presentation with calcific tendonitis.

The physical examination for calcifying tendonitis consists of the routine physical examination of the shoulder. As mentioned, in some of the very acute phases a thorough physical examination cannot be performed until the calcifying tendonitis is in the subacute phase. The examination consists of range of motion, impingement testing, and cross-arm testing for acromioclavicular joint stability. Tests for instability, such as Jobe's maneuver, are also important, because the calcifying tendonitis can be a secondary problem with the underlying pathology being instability or impingement, or both. Strength testing of all the shoulder girdle muscles is critical to determine if the rotator cuff is intact. Careful delineation of all historical data must be included in the workup of the patient, along with the physical examination.

The radiologic evaluation is imperative for diagnosis of calcific deposits in the tendon of the rotator cuff. Initial radiographs should include a routine shoulder series (Fig. 14-2). In our institution, we use what we call the thrower's series. This includes an internal rotation anteroposterior, an external rotation anteroposterior, a Stryker, and a Westpoint view. In the radiographs, deposits of calcium in the supraspinatus tendon can easily be seen on neutral rotation; deposits in the infraspinatus and teres minor are best seen in internal rotation; and calcification of the subscapular tendon will be seen in external rotation. Studies including magnetic resonance imaging can be helpful in assessing the extent and exact location of calcification. Computed tomographic studies will not be useful; however, when combined with the arthrogram, they can further help to determine if there is a rupture or tear of the rotator cuff. Although the size and location of the calcific deposit will not necessarily lead directly to the prognosis of calcifying tendonitis, it can be helpful.

DePalma and Kruper[7] described two radiologic types of calcific tendonitis. Type I was fluffy and appeared with the periphery poorly defined. They believed this was consistent with the acute phase. Type II was less discrete and homogeneous with more uniform density, and they believed this was the subacute and chronic stages. Not all authors agree that classification is so easy to determine from radiographs; however, it is a good starting point for evaluation.

In reviewing the differential diagnosis and the associated pathology in the athlete, it would be unusual not to have associated pathology in the patient with calcifying tendonitis. Usually it is secondary to a long-standing tendonitis, associated impingement syndrome, or rupture of the rotator cuff. When calcifica-

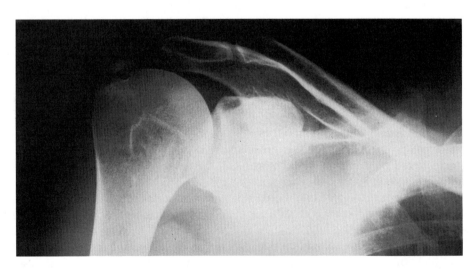

**Fig. 14-2.** Radiographic anterior to posterior view of right shoulder with calcific tendonitis.

tion occurs in a rupture of the rotator cuff, it is usually a long-standing rupture. This is seen especially in the older patient-athlete. An example is an older golfer with long-standing rotator cuff problems who has not been treated by a physician and therapist. Other problems inlcude calcifications secondary to impingement syndrome, and impingement that sometimes can be associated with the subluxing or unstable shoulder. The diagnosis of frozen shoulder (adhesive capsulitis) is unlikely to be seen in the highly competitve athlete, but in the recreational athlete it is not an uncommon presentation for calcific tendonitis. Also remember that we may be seeing a chronic calcifying tendonitis that is absolutely asymptomatic, only a radiographic finding, and may not be secondary to underlying pathology presenting in the shoulder. Therefore, a careful history and physical examination establishing the differential diagnosis is always critical.

## TREATMENT

The goals of treatment are to restore health and function to the rotator cuff with the calcifying tendonitis and to prevent further complications of the calcium deposits in the rotator cuff. One complication could be rupture of the tendon secondary to structural weakness in the calcified area. Another complication seen is secondary inflammatory reaction in the bursa, with bursitis after rupture of the calcific deposit into the bursa, and synovitis of the shoulder precipitated by a secondary rupture of the bursa into the glenohumeral joint. Rupture into the glenohumeral joint is a fairly unusual presentation. However, Patte and Goutallier[9] described a rupture of a deposit into the glenohumeral joint. Most of these patients will respond to good conservative measures including physiotherapy and a comprehensive rehabilitation program to restore function and motion to the shoulder and to the rotator cuff tendons.

The goals for treatment also include correcting any underlying pathology and treatment of the calcifying tendonitis itself, whether it is an isolated problem or a secondary problem. In the author's experience, calcifying tendonitis can be treated in most athletes by conservative measures with very satisfactory results. Treatment includes physical therapy and comprehensive rehabilitation including range of motion and strengthening exercises. In acute cases, however, more

aggressive measures may be indicated. Ultrasound can be used to help break up the calcium. Although there is no scientific randomized study to prove the efficacy of this treatment, most patients have experienced pain relief from the use of ultrasound. In some acute cases, relief of pain secondary to the calcific tendonitis has to be the overriding concern. Some authors have claimed success with steroid injections into the deposit. Others have achieved excellent results in patients with injections of Xylocaine alone. Some authors prefer to inject corticosteroids; however, caution in the use of corticosteroids must continue to be a concern among treating physicians. There is no hard scientific evidence for the successful use of injections in calcifying tendonitis. Moreover, we must remember that any injection of any nature must be used judiciously because complications from injection, such as infection and rupture of tendons, must always be kept in mind. Judicious use of a short-term course of nonsteroidal anti-inflammatory drugs can also help in the acute and subacute phases of this condition, when the generalized inflammatory response can be decreased by use of this class of drug.

Most authors have thought that surgical treatment may be necessary, but only in a few very specific cases. Most of the present literature describes an open surgical technique using a deltoid-splitting approach to the calcification for excision. If a surgical intervention is indicated, this can be readily accomplished by arthroscopic technique in the hands of a competent arthroscopic surgeon, thereby minimizing the morbidity of open deltoid-splitting surgery. Before a surgical approach is undertaken to remove calcium, the surgeon must anticipate any underlying pathology that should be addressed at the same time, such as an associated impingement syndrome and intra-articular problems that can be corrected using arthroscopic techniques. If arthroscopy is performed, the calcium can sometimes be readily assessed and identified simply by observing the subacromial bursa. However, if the presentation of calcification is unusual or is in the infraspinatus or teres minor tendon, a simple approach is to use c-arm fluoroscopy in the operating room to identify the calcification, using a needle for localization. Then the needle placement is observed with the arthroscope once the needle has been identified to be in the calcifying portion of the tendon. In rare cases, the calcific bursa can present with decompression in the glenohumeral side of the joint. With debridement of the calcific portion of the tendon, the necrotic portion of the tendon should be removed, and this will allow the tendon to heal normally. Because most of these are partial tears of the rotator cuff, once the calcification has been debrided, the partial tears of the rotator cuff can readily heal with proper rehabilitation and strengthening. In the subacromial bursa, once the calcification has been identified, it can be readily removed. The calcium usually comes out in a toothpaste-like consistency, but occasionally chalk-like material is also found. After the calcium is arhtroscopically removed, the necrotic rotator cuff tendon should be debrided back to the good tendon so that this partial tear can heal. After the calcification has been identified in the subacromial bursa and removed, an active immediate range of motion and physiotherapy program should be started.

Physical therapy and rehabilitation are described in detail in later chapters.

## SUMMARY

To understand and treat successfully the athlete with calcific tendonitis and to determine its cause, there must be a thorough understanding of the anatomy, pathology, and mechanics of associated disorders. Only then can a comprehensive rehabilitation and treatment program begin.

## REFERENCES

1. Moseley HF, Goldie I: The internal pattern of the rotator cuff of the shoulder. J Bone Joint Surg 45B:780, 1963
2. Rathbun JB, MacNab I: The microvascular pattern of the rotator cuff. J Bone Joint Surg 52B:540, 1970
3. Nixon J, DiStefano V: Ruptures of the rotator cuff. Orthop Clin North Am 6:423, 1975
4. Rothman RH, Parkes WW: The vascular anatomy of the rotator cuff. Clin Orthop 41:176, 1965
5. Plenk HP: Calcifying tendonitis of the shoulder. Radiology 59:384, 1952
6. Bosworth BM: Calcium deposits in the shoulder and subacromial bursitis. JAMA 116:2477, 1941
7. DePalma AF, Kruper JS: Long term study of shoulder joints afflicted with and treated for calcific tendonitis. Clin Orthop 20:61, 1961
8. Uhthoff HK, Sarkar K, Maynard JA: Calcifying tendonitis—a new concept of pathogenesis. Clin Orthop 188:164, 1976
9. Patte D, Goutallier D: Calcifications. Rev Chir Orthop 74:277, 1988
10. Messler HH, Kock W, Münzenberg KJ: Analogous effects of organic calcium antagonists and magnesium on the epiphyseal growth plate. Clin Orthop 258:135, 1990
11. Lippmann RK: Observations concerning the calcific cuff deposits. Clin Orthop 20:49, 1961

# 15

# Open Repair of the Rotator Cuff

*SANFORD S. KUNKEL*
*RICHARD J. HAWKINS*

Management of a rotator cuff tear in an athlete presents a unique and challenging problem. The etiology, pathophysiology, and treatment may depend on the athlete's level of competition.

The presence of a rotator cuff tear may be determined clinically or by diagnostic studies such as arthrogram, ultrasound, or magnetic resonance imaging. Often an arthroscopic evaluation allows us to evaluate the extent of the rotator cuff tear and other associated pathology. At times, small rotator cuff tears may be managed with a mini-repair, which is described in Ch. 16. The traditional technique for an open rotator cuff repair is described in this chapter.

In the athlete, the primary goal for operating is most often to relieve pain, the secondary goal being to improve function. In the competitive overhead athlete, the primary complaint may be loss of endurance or fatigue. The goal is then to return the athlete to previous level of competition. In most cases, impingement plays an important role, the vascularity compromises healing, and there may be associated supraspinatus outlet stenosis. A rotator cuff tear is usually the result of overuse, eccentric overload, and fiber failure, resulting in proximal migration of the humeral head and secondary impingement. With repetitive overhead athletes, the rotator cuff pathology may be secondary to anterior glenohumeral instability with a secondary rotator cuff tendinitis or cuff tear. The impingement sign described by Neer and Welsh[1] and Hawkins and Abrams[2] and the relocation test describe by Jobe et al[3] can help us to differentiate the primary etiology of cuff pathology. If the primary pathology is anterior instability, an anterior capsulolabral reconstruction may be indicated.[3] If only pure impingement is present, decompression and rotator cuff repair may be indi-

cated. Decompression is performed by an anterior acromioplasty for the following reasons: (1) to remove the offending structure; (2) to protect the rotator cuff repair; and (3) to prevent disease progression.

## OPERATIVE PROCEDURE

If diagnostic arthroscopy is performed before rotator cuff surgery, it may be in the sitting or the lateral recumbent position. Once the arthroscopy is completed, the patient is positioned in the beach chair position (Fig. 15-1). The patient's head is rotated to the contralateral side, and a pillow is placed behind the knees with a strap across the thighs for stability. The bladder of a blood pressure cuff or a sand bag may be used to elevate the ipsilateral scapula, bringing the shoulder into an advantageous position for the surgical approach. A sterile drape is placed across the base of the neck to prevent hair and saliva from contaminating the wound. Intravenous antibiotics are administered to the patient before the skin incision is made. The procedure may be carried out with general anesthesia, interscalene block, or general anesthetic supplemented with an interscalene block for postoperative pain. The shoulder, axilla, and hemithorax are prepared, and the upper extremity is draped free. A sterile stockinette allows for free manipulation of the arm. A large sterile drape is applied anteriorly and then wrapped completely and circumferentially to seal off the axilla and hold the drapes in the appropriate positions.

Bony landmarks are outlined, and the skin incision bisects the anterior acromion approximately midway between the acromioclavicular joint and the lateral

141

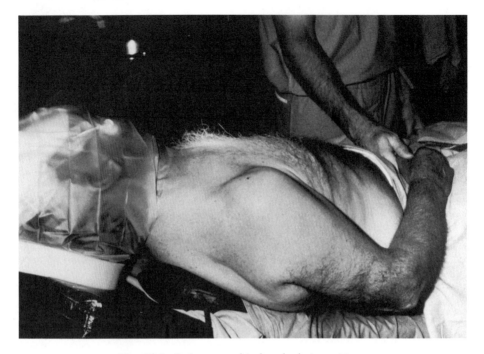

**Fig. 15-1.** Patient seated in beach chair position.

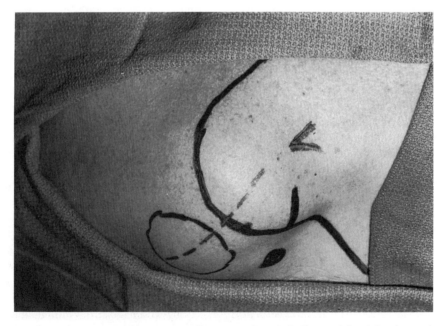

**Fig. 15-2.** Skin incision for rotator cuff repair in line with fibers of the deltoid muscle.

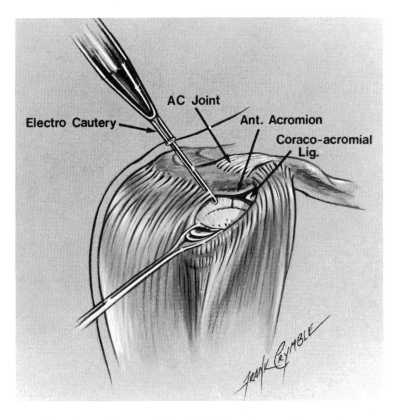

**Fig. 15-3.** Reflection of the deltoid from the anterior acromion.

border of the acromion. It covers a distance of approximately 4 cm with two-thirds below and one-third above the anterior acromion (Fig. 15-2). The skin incision is made in the direction of the deltoid fibers to allow for appropriate release of the deltoid muscle as required. Self-retaining retractors allow for exposure and secure hemostasis. After sharp dissection through the subcutaneous layer, the white aponeurotic fibers overlying the acromion can be visualized along with the red fleshy fibers of the deltoid muscle. The deltoid muscle may be detached from the anterior acromion with electrocautery extending from the acromioclavicular joint to the lateral border of the acromion, a distance of approximately 2.5 cm (Fig. 15-3). In the athlete, it may be advantageous to split the deltoid longitudinally with less chance of retraction, improved reattachment, and perhaps better postoperative function (Fig. 15-4).

## ANTERIOR ACROMIOPLASTY

The detached deltoid muscle is retracted from the anterior acromion, and an anterior acromioplasty is performed. A 1-in.-wide osteotome or an oscillating saw is used for the formal acromioplasty as described by Neer.[4] The acromioplasty begins at the anterior superior aspect of the acromion and extends to the apex of the undersurface of the acromion, a distance of approximately 1.5 cm. The direction is usually perpendicular to the floor, with the patient in the beach chair position (Fig. 15-5). Care must be taken to remove any anterior beaking of the acromion. The acromial fragment is then removed with the accompanying coracoacromial ligament, which is attached to the undersurface of the anteromedial corner of the acromial fragment. The acromial branch of the thoracoacromial

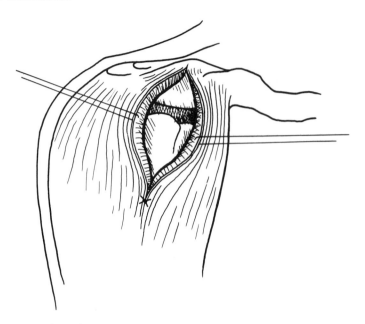

**Fig. 15-4.** Deltoid fascia split and retracted from underlying acromion.

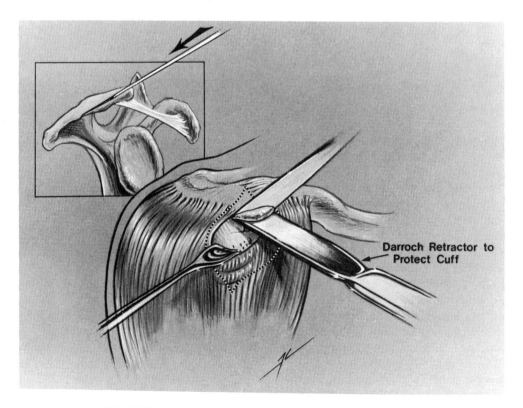

Darroch Retractor to Protect Cuff

**Fig. 15-5.** Acromioplasty removing anterior inferior acromion.

artery often runs with the ligament and may need to be cauterized.

## RESECTION OF SCAR TISSUE

After the acromioplasty, the surgeon releases the scar tissue by blunt dissection. The bursa is identified and resected along with any other scar tissue for better definition of the rotator cuff defect. Recent studies suggest the undersurface of the bursa may contain regenerative cells; therefore, only enough bursa should be excised to visualize the rotator cuff tear.[5] With rotation of the arm, the rotator cuff tear is identified. If the tear is small, the deltoid muscle may not need to be split to facilitate more exposure. With a moderate or large tear, the deltoid muscle should be split at the junction of the anterior and lateral thirds, extending a distance of approximately 5 cm (Fig. 15-6). This allows the deltoid muscle to be opened like a book for a greater exposure, particularly anteriorly in the area of the subscapularis and over the greater tuberosity for preparation of a trough. A suture is placed in the apex of the

deltoid split to prevent the split from extending. A second suture should be placed laterally in the deltoid so that the deltoid does not retract laterally under the skin making subsequent closure difficult.

The acromioclavicular joint is then examined. Any prominent osteophytes on the undersurface are removed with an osteotome or rongeur. In chronic rotator cuff tears, often seen in the recreational athlete, a distal clavicle resection may rarely be indicated, based on the patient's localization of pain and response to preoperative local injections. The acromioclavicular joint generally does not need to be resected for increased exposure.

The extent of the rotator cuff tear is ascertained at this time, and the torn edges of the rotator cuff are identified. In a large or chronic tear, stay sutures are placed in the edge of the rotator cuff tendons to facilitate subsequent repair and reconstruction (Fig. 15-7). Often athletes will present with partial rotator cuff tears that may be repaired in a side-to-side fashion after debridement of degenerative tissue. It is unusual to be able to repair a chronic or large rotator cuff tear in a side-to-side or end-to-end fashion because the tear

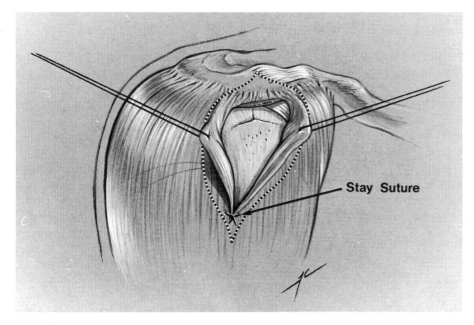

**Fig. 15-6.** Deltoid muscle split in line with its fibers for repair of moderate and large tears.

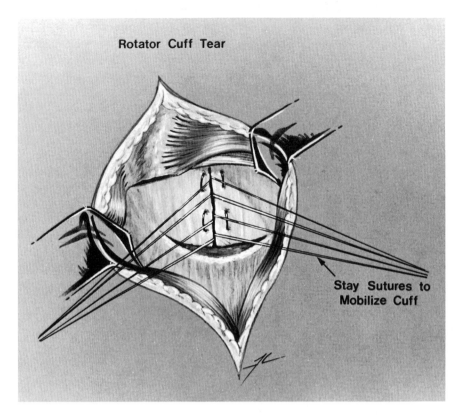

**Fig. 15-7.** Stay sutures placed in free margin of rotator cuff for mobilization.

commences as an avulsion from the greater tuberosity and thus there is not enough tissue to be repaired on the humeral side. Most full-thickness tears are repaired to a trough in bone from where they began. We divide cuff tears into small (less than 1 cm), moderate (1 to 3 cm), large (3 to 5 cm), and massive (greater than 5 cm). Massive tears may be impossible to repair, and the surgeon may be able to perform debridement and decompression only. In our experience,[6] better pain relief is achieved if the tear is repaired; therefore, it is important to strive for repair in all cuff tears.

## MOBILIZATION OF THE ROTATOR CUFF

The general principle we follow for repair of most rotator cuff tears consists of superior mobilization of the subscapularis from the front, superior mobilization of the infraspinatus from behind, and mobilization of the supraspinatus, when present, from under the acromioclavicular joint. All are repaired to a trough in bone at the area of the anatomic neck adjacent to the greater tuberosity.[7,8]

The use of a small elevator may help to mobilize the cuff with both extra-articular and intra-articular dissection. The subscapularis may be mobilized from its attachment on the neck of the scapula, and the supraspinatus may be mobilized with dissection to the point of the supraspinatus notch. In chronic cuff tears, the coracohumeral ligament, which runs from the coracoid process to the rotator interval, should be released. This often provides significant mobilization. The supraspinatus tendon is often retracted into its fossa under the acromioclavicular joint and may not be available for repair. Often a cuff tear will extend posteriorly into the infraspinatus tendon. The subscapularis is usually spared, maintaining its normal anatomic insertion into the lesser tuberosity. Tension is placed with stay sutures in the edge of the cuff, and a rubbery tension of the attached muscles can be appreciated, which gives one a sense of the degree mobilization that can be achieved. Occasionally, the infraspinatus needs to be taken off the posterior aspect of the intra-articular portion of the glenoid cavity along with some of the capsule for a more definitive mobilization. Care should be exercised not to dissect below the level of the teres minor tendon to avoid injury to the axillary nerve as it exits from the quadrangular space.

## PLACEMENT OF THE BONY TROUGH

At this point, the amount of mobilization can be assessed and location of the bony trough determined. Because the lateral surface of the greater tuberosity possesses no firm cuff tissue that will hold suture material, a trough in bone is used at the junction of the anatomic neck of the greater tuberosity. If the anatomic neck cannot be reached with the tendinous tissue, the trough may be placed more proximally on the articular surface. The trough is fashioned with a gentle slope toward the articular surface margin (Fig. 15-8). A power burr is used to debride the articular surface margin of the trough for subsequent healing of the cuff. A drill is then used to make several drill holes directed from the humerus into the trough from the lateral side. Care must be taken not to break the bony bridge of the tuberosity because this bone may be quite osteoporotic. If possible, the free edge of the cuff tear should be reapproximated into the trough directly. If the tear is fairly large with an extension into the supra- or infraspinatus, a shoe lace type of interrupted repair is performed using absorbable or nonabsorbable suture, depending on the surgeon's preference (Fig. 15-9).

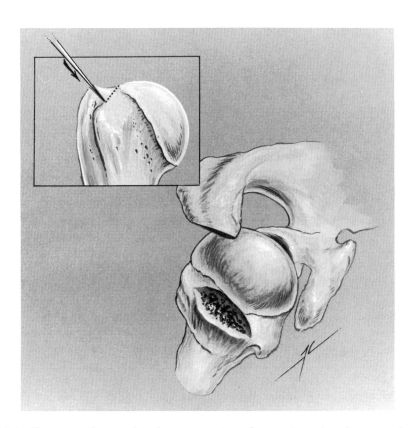

**Fig. 15-8.** Placement of a trough in bone at junction of anatomic neck and greater tuberosity.

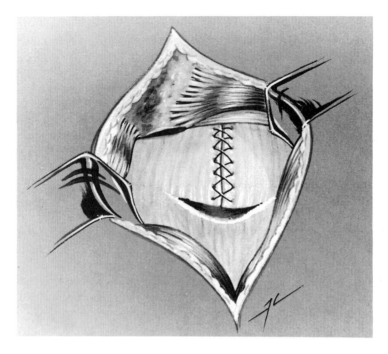

**Fig. 15-9.** Repair of rotator cuff extending into supraspinatus or infraspinatus.

The suture is directed from the tendon into the trough through a drill hole in the greater tuberosity, back through a different hole, through the trough, and again into the free edge of the tendon. This may be performed in reverse fashion, but we have found this allows for secure closure as the knot is tied down while pushing the free edge of the tendon into the trough. Often, three or four sutures are adequate (Fig. 15-10). On completion, the repair should be watertight and should be checked for secureness. The repair may be performed with the arm in the abducted position secondary to excessive tension on the cuff. The point at which the cuff comes under excessive tension should be noted for postoperative positioning and rehabilitation. Hopefully, the repair is performed without tension and can be positioned down at the side.

After the wound is thoroughly irrigated, the detached deltoid muscle is reapproximated to the remaining cuff of tissue on the anterior acromion. If a secure repair cannot be achieved, the deltoid muscle can be reapproximated to the acromion using several small drill holes through the acromion and horizontal mattress sutures (Fig. 15-11). As commonly used now, if the deltoid has been split in the direction of its fibers, it hopefully can be closed side to side without reattachment to anterior acromion. Subcutaneous layer is closed with 2-0 absorbable sutures, and the skin is reapproximated with a running subcuticular 3-0 absorbable suture. A nonadherent dressing is placed on the shoulder, and the arm is placed in a sling. If excessive tension on the repair is noted intraoperatively, an abduction brace may be considered.

## POSTOPERATIVE CARE

Most athletes have small- or medium-sized rotator cuff tears, which may be managed in a sling postoperatively. If the tear is massive in an older athlete, an abduction pillow may be necessary. We prefer not to use a brace and encourage early range of motion exercises, but this is not always possible. If the patients are placed in an abduction brace, we encourage assisted elevation and external rotation above the brace until the brace

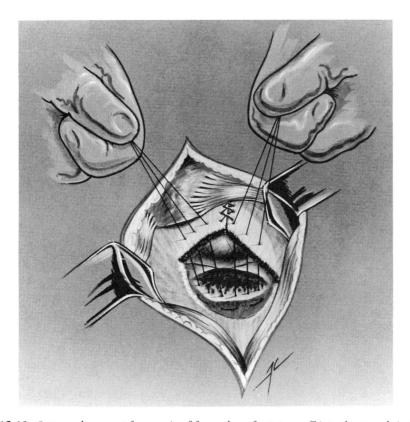

**Fig. 15-10.** Suture placement for repair of free edge of rotator cuff into the trough in bone.

is removed at 4 to 6 weeks. Active motion may be implemented after the brace is removed.

## REHABILITATION

Rehabilitation consists of assisted motion until the repair is secure. Active motion is then allowed after 6 to 8 weeks. Once active motion is instituted, terminal stretching is required, but resisted motion is delayed until appropriate active motion has been achieved, usually during the third month. It is important to remind patients that rehabilitation after rotator cuff surgery takes many months; often 6 months go by before patients can elevate their arms above the horizontal position with comfort and efficiency.[9,10] (See Appendix 15-1.)

The initial rehabilitation consists of assisted elevation and external rotation, followed by pendulum exercises, extension, and internal rotation. Active motion begins depending on the size of the tear and secureness of the repair. Prolonged rehabilitation emphasizing range of motion and strengthening exercises is continued for a minimum of 2 years. Those athletes who are involved in repetitive overhead athletics are often involved in a prolonged and intense rehabilitation program for a minimum of 1 and up to 2 years before return to the competitive arena.[11] Throwing athletes are not permitted to throw for a minimum of 12 months and are taken through a specific rehabilitation program that emphasizes mobility and strength followed by a progressive throwing program. Preoperative consultation involving time parameters is helpful for patient cooperation and understanding.

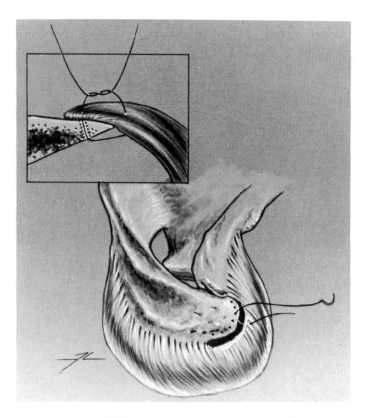

**Fig. 15-11.** Re-approximation of deltoid fascia to anterior acromion through vertical drill holes.

## SUMMARY

The technique of open rotator cuff repair[7,8] is a well-accepted technique for rotator cuff repair. This technique provides secure fixation of the ruptured ends of the rotator cuff with a watertight closure. Neer et al[12] and Hawkins et al[6] have reported good results with this technique using a rotator cuff repair secured to a trough in bone. Decompression is considered to be an important component of all rotator cuff repairs. Rotator cuff pathology caused by anterior instability needs to be evaluated preoperatively. Anterior capsulolabral reconstruction may be necessary for those with an underlying instability pattern.

The goals in rotator cuff surgery are first to relieve pain and second to improve function. Appropriate patient selection and meticulous surgical repair, coupled with an intense rehabilitation program, are the keys to success in open repair of the rotator cuff.

## REFERENCES

1. Neer CS II, Welsh RP: The shoulder in sports. Orthop Clin North Am 8:583, 1977
2. Hawkins RJ, Abrams JS: Impingement syndrome in the absence of rotator cuff tear (stages 1 and 2). Orthop Clin North Am 18:373, 1987
3. Jobe FW, Giangarra CE, Kvitne RS, Glousman RE: Anterior capsulolabral reconstruction of the shoulder in athletes in overhand sports. Am J Sports Med 19:428, 1991
4. Neer CS II: Anteror acromioplasty for the chronic impingement syndrome in the shoulder: a preliminary report. J Bone Joint Surg 54A:41, 1972

5. Uhthoff HK, Sarkar K: Classification and definition of tendinopathies. Clin Sports Med 10:707, 1991

6. Hawkins RJ, Misamore GW, Hobeika PE: Surgery for full thickness rotator-cuff tears. J Bone Joint Surg 67A:1349, 1985

7. Kunkel SS, Hawkins RJ: Rotator-cuff repair utilizing a trough in bone. Techniques Orthop 3:51, 1989

8. McLaughlin HL, Asherman EG: Lesions in the musculotendinous cuff of the shoulder: IV. Some observation based on the results of surgical repair. J Bone Joint Surg 33A:76, 1951

9. Hawkins RJ: The rotator cuff and biceps tendon. p. 1393. In Evarts CM (ed): Surgery of the Musculoskeletal System. 2nd Ed. Churchill Livingstone, New York, 1990

10. Hawkins RJ: Surgical management of rotator cuff tears. p. 161. In Bateman JE, Welsh RP (eds): Surgery of the Shoulder. BC Dekker, Philadelphia, 1984

11. Hawkins RJ, Kunkel SS: Rotator cuff tears. p. 395. In Torg JS, Welsh RP, Shepard RJ (eds): Current Therapy in Sports Medicine. 2nd Ed. BC Decker, Toronto, 1990

12. Neer CS II, Flatow EL, Lech O: Tears of the rotator cuff: long term results of anterior acromioplasty and repair. Paper read at the 55th Annual Meeting of the American Academy of Orthopaedic Surgeons, Atlanta, GA, February 5, 1988

# Appendix 15-1

# Shoulder Conditioning/Therapy Checklist

## POSTOPERATIVE PROGRAM: ROTATOR CUFF REPAIR

| ICE PHASE I, II, III | Days per week _____ Times per day _____ | 15–20 minutes "on" 60 minutes "off" |
|---|---|---|

### PHASE I

### (0–6 Weeks or 8 Weeks, Depending on Size of Tear)

### Small—6 weeks

### Large—8 weeks

Days per Week _____

Times per Day _____

| PASSIVE MOTION | Sets | Reps |
|---|---|---|
| Pendulum Exercises | 1–2 | 20–30 |
| External Rotation | 1–2 | 10–15 |
| Internal Rotation | 1–2 | 10–15 |
| Overhead Elbow Lift | 1–2 | 5–10 |

### PHASE II

### (Week 6 or 8, Depending on Size of Tear)

Days per Week _____

Times per Day _____

| ACTIVE MOTION (WITH TERMINAL STRETCH) | Sets | Reps |
|---|---|---|
| Pendulum Exercises | 1–2 | 20–30 |
| External Rotation | 1–2 | 10–15 |
| Internal Rotation | 1–2 | 10–15 |
| Overhead Elbow Lift | 1–2 | 5–10 |

### PHASE III

### (Week 10 or 12, Depending on Size of Tear)

Days per Week _____

Times per Day _____

| ACTIVE MOTION (WITH TERMINAL STRETCH) | Sets | Reps |
|---|---|---|
| Pendulum Exercises | 1–2 | 20–30 |
| External Rotation | 1–2 | 10–15 |
| Internal Rotation | 1–2 | 10–15 |
| Overhead Elbow Lift | 1–2 | 5–10 |

| SPORT CORD STRENGTHENING | Sets | Reps |
|---|---|---|
| External Rotation | 1–2 | 10–15 |
| Internal Rotation | 1–2 | 10–15 |
| Forward Punch | 1–2 | 10–15 |
| Overhead Punch Press | 1–2 | 10–15 |

### Comments

1. Return to supine position for phase II active motion program (especially for massive defects).

# 16

# Mini-Open Repair of the Rotator Cuff

*LAURA A. TIMMERMAN*
*JAMES R. ANDREWS*
*KEVIN E. WILK*

The traditional open acromioplasty and rotator cuff repair requires at least a partial takedown of the deltoid insertion on the acromion to complete the acromioplasty and to gain exposure to the rotator cuff. With the development of shoulder arthroscopy, the subacromial decompression can be completed arthroscopically without significant disruption of the deltoid insertion or the trapezo-deltoid fascia. This is advantageous, as an early rehabilitation program to regain shoulder motion and strength is possible because the deltoid insertion is intact and only minimal arthroscopic portal incisions were made. Also, an arthroscopic examination of the glenohumeral joint allows evaluation of other pathologic conditions, including complete inspection of the rotator cuff. If a rotator cuff tear is present, its extent can be determined from both the undersurface and subacromial areas, and the decision regarding the indications for open repair can be made with accurate information.

## INDICATIONS

Before performing open repair of a rotator cuff tear, one must carefully consider the patient's subjective complaints. If the primary symptom is pain, an adequate subacromial decompression will often offer relief, especially for the older patient with a chronic rotator cuff tear. If the primary complaint is that of weakness, repair of the rotator cuff may be indicated.

A patient will often complain of pain and weakness, and the clinical examination is important in sorting out the primary symptom; weakness to motor strength testing may be secondary to pain and not to an actual deficit in the muscle/tendon unit. If an injection in the subacromial space relieves the pain and normal strength is present, a decompression may be all that is necessary; conversely, if weakness is still present after the pain is blocked by an injection, repair of a rotator cuff tear should be considered.

Other important factors involved in the decision to openly repair a rotator cuff tear include whether the tear is full or partial thickness; the size of the tear, usually greater than 1 cm in length but not too extensive to allow reapproximation of tendon into bone; the mobility of the tissue involved in the tear; and the age, occupation, and activity level of the patient.

## SURGICAL TECHNIQUE

After general endotracheal anesthesia is administered, the patient is positioned in the lateral decubitus position with the torso supported by a vacuum bean bag. The involved extremity is suspended overhead with a prefabricated wrist gauntlet at approximately 70 degrees abduction and 15 to 20 degrees of forward flexion. Approximately 10 to 15 lb of traction is used for distraction to provide adequate visualization of the glenohumeral joint. The surgeon stands posterior to the patient, with the first assistant positioned toward the patient's feet and the second assistant or surgical nurse opposite the surgeon on the other side of the patient.

After the shoulder is prepared and draped, the bony landmarks are outlined using a marking pen. It is important to place an 18-gauge spinal needle in the acromioclavicular joint to allow for identification of the acromioclavicular joint during the subacromial space arthroscopy. Routine diagnostic and operative arthroscopy of the glenohumeral joint is then performed, with careful evaluation of other evidence of pathology. This is especially important in the young athletic patient, in whom a partial, tensile-type rotator cuff tear may be secondary to anterior instability and not a primary process. The rotator cuff tear can be debrided to bleeding tissue on the undersurface with use of a motorized debrider.

The subacromial space is then entered, where resection of the scarred or redundant bursal tissue is usually necessary before the rotator cuff can be visualized. With very large tears, the glenohumeral joint and subacromial space become one area and the diagnosis is obvious. The rotator cuff is then inspected, and the decision of whether to proceed with an open repair is made. If an open repair is indicated, the arthroscopic

subacromial decompression should be completed without delay to prevent excessive extravasation of fluid into the soft tissues. We prefer to perform the subacromial decompression arthroscopically because less soft tissue dissection is necessary and the extent of the decompression can easily be directly visualized.

After the subacromial decompression is completed, the arthroscopic equipment is removed from the subacromial space. The arm is left suspended in the overhead position, with slightly less abduction to approximately 30 to 40 degrees. A sterile betadine impregnated adhesive plastic wrap is then placed over the shoulder to cover the exposed skin completely. The patient is given an additional dose of intravenous prophylactic antibiotics; we have not found that separate preparation and drape are necessary for the open repair, although this depends on the surgeon's preference.

A transverse saber-type incision is made through the skin in Langer's lines approximately 4 to 6 cm long. The incision begins at the anterolateral corner of the acromion and is continued posteriorly to the posterolateral corner (Fig. 16-1). Previously, we used a straight longitudinal incision based off the acromion in the line of the deltoid fibers, but we found that this incision was not as aesthetically pleasing. Also, with the incision in the same plane as the split in the deltoid fibers, on

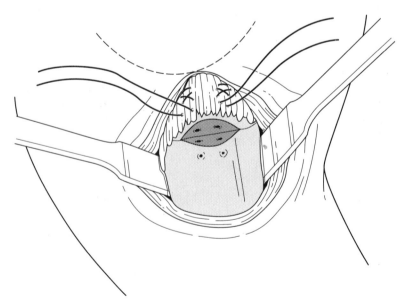

**Fig. 16-1.** A longitudinal incision 4 to 5 cm long is made from the base of the acrmion through the fibers to expose the torn rotator cuff.

occasion painful scar adhesions formed in this area. The skin is then retracted in the anterior and posterior plane to reveal the underlying deltoid, which is split in line with its fibers off the anterolateral corner of the acromion. If a posterior cuff tear is present, the location of the incision and the deltoid split can be modified; a helpful aid is to leave the arthroscopic cannula in the tear defect at the completion of the acromioplasty to allow for identification of the tear location externally. Care is taken not to split the deltoid farther than 5 cm distally to avoid damage to the axillary nerve. A self-retaining retractor is then placed to retract the deltoid in the anterior and posterior direction, with an assistant holding an additional retractor distally to expose the humerus. The rotator cuff tear is then identified, and any additional bursal tissue is resected. The adequacy of the subacromial decompression can be assessed.

The edge of the torn tendon is then identified and is incised with a sharp blade to allow for bleeding tissue. The area for repair into bone is selected, located just lateral to the articular surface in the region of cancellous bone. A high-speed burr is used to make a trough long enough to contain the torn tendon edge, approximately 3 to 4 mm deep. The trough is undercut slightly to allow a bony cortical roof over the top of the defect for suture ties. A double-layer suture to bone repair is then performed. Using no. 2 Tevdek sutures, Bunnell-type sutures are placed in the tendon edge to achieve an optimal hold on the tendon. Holes then are made in the trough to connect with the bony bridge superiorly, in the fashion of a Bankart repair. A minimum of three holes usually are used, or roughly one hole every 5 mm. A towel clip-type device facilitates making these holes; we have found the Concept Rotator Cuff Repair System (Linvatec Corporation, Largo, Florida) instruments to be especially helpful. The double layer of sutures allows for more contact area between the rotator cuff and the raw bed of bone.

The next step is to place bony soft tissue suture anchors into the most medial edge of the bony trough (Fig. 16-2). This will help to hold the tendon into the trough with an additional attachment to bone. Depending on the size of the trough, two to four suture anchors are placed into the bone, with the drill directed toward the more substantial subchondral bone, which affords a superior hold. These sutures from the suture anchors then are brought through the tendon, approximately 1.5 cm proximal to the tendon edge. Care is taken to avoid the other sutures already in the tendon edge. The sutures in the tendon edge are then passed from inside the trough to the exterior cortical bone,

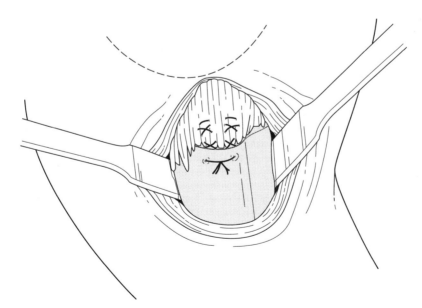

**Fig. 16-2.** Once the bony trough is made, the resected supraspinatus tendon is sutured with #2 Tevdek sutures with Bunnell-type sutures into the bone.

thereby pulling the tendon edge deep into the trough. These sutures then are tied over the bony bridges. The anchor sutures located in the base of the trough are then tied over the top of the tendon for additional stability. The arm has been left in the overhead abducted position for the surgical repair; when necessary the arm can be brought back to approximately 70 degrees of abduction for ease of tying the sutures. The stability of the repair can then be directly assessed by removing the arm from traction. If the repair is stable with minimal abduction of the arm, a shoulder immobilizer is all that is needed postoperatively, and early aggressive rehabilitation is possible. With cases of a very large tear or one that was difficult to mobilize, the arm may need to be maintained in abduction for 4 to 6 weeks during the early healing period.

Any further defects in the rotator cuff, including longitudinal tears, are then closed with absorbable suture, with care taken to avoid tying down the biceps tendon. The deltoid defect is then closed with absorbable suture. A small Hemovac drain is placed in the subacromial space before closure. The skin is then closed with subcutaneous sutures, and Steri-Strips are applied. The arm is then placed in a shoulder immobilizer for the initial postoperative period, with a sling for use during the day, or into an abduction-type splint, depending on the nature of the rotator cuff tear.

The patient is given a minimum of 24 hours of prophylactic antibiotics postoperatively, and the drain is pulled the next morning.

# REHABILITATION

The rehabilitation program after the mini-open (deltoid splitting) rotator cuff repair depends on several factors (Table 16-1). Generally, the older the patient, the more extensive the rehabilitation is required to return to a desirable activity level. This is often true because of degenerative osseous changes, rotator cuff degeneration, and an overall decrease in shoulder strength.

The onset of the injury is another important factor to consider. When an acute repair is performed, the residual rotator cuff tissue is viable and a satisfactory tissue-to-bone fixation is accomplished with little difficulty. When a large degenerative chronic tear is present, the repair process is often difficult, and thus, the

**Table 16-1. Factors Influencing Rehabilitation After Rotator Cuff Repair**

| |
| --- |
| Age of patient |
| Onset of injury |
| Size of tear |
|     Small   (<1 cm) |
|     Medium (1–3 cm) |
|     Large   (3–5 cm) |
|     Massive (>5 cm) |
| Work requirements |
| Desired activity level |
| Rehabilitation potential |
|     Patient motivational level |

rehabilitation process is much slower than the acute tear. Basset and Cofield[1] reported that an early repair led to a better functional outcome than a chronic repair.

The third factor is the size of the rotator cuff tear. The repair of a small- to medium-sized tear allows the patient to rehabilitate in an accelerated fashion (see Appendix 16-1) called the type 1 rehabilitation program. When a repair is performed on a large-sized tear, the rehabilitation is much slower than the type 1 program; this rehabilitation program is referred to as the type 2 program (see Appendix 16-2). The type 3 rehabilitation program (see Appendix 16-3) represents the program prescribed for an individual with a large to massive tear when a tenuous repair was performed. In this type of patient, it is difficult for the physician to resect the torn muscle back to healthy tissue. Consequently, the repair is often dependent on the remaining tissue quality (bone and muscle) and the amount of resection required.

The fourth and fifth factors affecting the rehabilitation process is the desired activity level after surgery and the requirements of work on the shoulder joint. Often, rotator cuff repairs are performed on the recreational athlete, such as the golfer or tennis player. Bigliani et al[2] reported on 23 tennis players who underwent a rotator cuff repair. The size of tears included eight small, five moderate, two large, and eight massive tears. After surgery and extensive rehabilitation, 83 percent achieved a good result (pain-free, able to play tennis), 13 percent a satisfactory result (able to play at less competitive level), and 4 percent (one patient) had an unsatisfactory result. Bigliani et al reported a correlation between size of the tear and outcome of surgery. The last variable considered is the patient's rehabilitation potential. This variable addresses the patient's motivational level to comply to the rehabilitation program. We believe a possible contraindication to rotator cuff repair surgery is a patient who presents with a behavior that is independent, unable to follow instructions, and will not comply to the rehabilitation program. The rehabilitation after a repair of the rotator cuff is lengthy and somewhat strict, and adherence to the program is vital to the ultimate surgical success.

The rehabilitation program after rotator cuff using a deltoid splitting is much faster than that of a rotator cuff repair when the deltoid is detached from the acromion. The role of the rotator cuff muscles is to provide stability to the humeral head during arm movement. The rotator cuff muscles control and steer the humeral head. Additionally, they maintain point surface compression during arm movements.[3,4] Based on this concept, we believe a patient should not perform isotonic dumbbell exercises for the glenohumeral muscles until the patient can perform active assisted shoulder flexion with a bar without scapula elevation (scapulae hiking). If substitution of the scapulothoracic muscles occur, the patient should be placed on a humeral head stabilizing exercise program. In addition, flexibility of the capsule is important to ensure proper glenohumeral joint kinematics.[5] A gradual progressive return to sport or strenuous work activities is also recommended in an attempt to prevent fatigue microtrauma or overload failure.

## SUMMARY

The mini-open rotator cuff repair, in conjunction with an arthroscopic inspection of the shoulder joint and an arthroscopic subacromial decompression, offers the advantages of improved visualization of the pathology and lesser surgical dissection. This allows for an earlier aggressive rehabilitation program, with more rapid return to activities. We have found this technique to be successful in the treatment of repairable rotator cuff tears.

## REFERENCES

1. Bassett RW, Cofield RH: Acute tears of the rotator cuff: the timing of surgical repair. Clin Orthop 175:12, 1983
2. Bigliani LU, Kimmel J, McCann PD, Wolf I: Repair of rotator cuff tears in tennis players. Am J Sports Med 20:112, 1992
3. Matsen FA, Arntz CT: Subacromial impingement. p. 623. In Rockwood CA, Matsen FA (eds): The Shoulder. WB Saunders, Philadelphia, 1990
4. Neer CS: Impingement lesions. Clin Orthop 173:70, 1983
5. Wilk KE, Andrews JR: Rehabilitation following arthroscopic shoulder subacromial decompression. Orthopedics 16:349, 1993

# Appendix 16-1

# Type 1 Rehabilitation Program for Rotator Cuff Repair (Deltoid Splitting)

I. *Phase 1—Protective Phase* (Weeks 0–6)
   Goals: Gradual return to full range of motion
   Increase shoulder strength
   Decrease pain
   A. Weeks 0–3
   1. Sling for comfort (1–2 weeks)
   2. Pendulum exercises
   3. Active assisted range of motion exercises* (L-bar exercises)
   4. Rope and pulley for flexion (only)
   5. Elbow range of motion, hand gripping
   6. Isometrics (submaximal, subpainful isometrics)
      a. Abductors
      b. External rotators
      c. Internal rotators
      d. Elbow flexors
      e. Shoulder flexors
   7. Pain control modalities (ice, high-voltage galvanic stimulation)
   * Range of motion exercises are used in a nonpainful range, with a gentle and gradual increase of motion to tolerance
   B. Weeks 3–6
   1. Progress all exercises (continue all above exercises)
   2. Active assisted range of motion L-bar exercises
      External rotation/internal rotation (shoulder at 45° abduction)

   3. Surgical tubing external rotation/internal rotation (arm at side)
   4. Initiate humeral head stabilizing exercises

II. *Phase 2—Intermediate Phase* (Weeks 7–12)
   Goals: Full nonpainful range of motion
   Improvement of strength and power
   Increase of functional activities
   Decrease of residual pain
   A. Weeks 7–10
   1. Active assisted range of motion exercises* (L-bar)
      a. Flexion to 170°–180°
      b. External rotation/internal rotation performed at 90° abduction of shoulder
         External rotation to 75°–90°
         Internal rotation to 75°–85°
      c. External rotation exercises performed with 0° abduction
         External rotation to 30°–40°
   * Full range of motion is goal of weeks 8 to 10
   2. Strengthening exercises for shoulder
      a. Exercise tubing external rotation/internal rotation arm at side
      b. Isotonics dumbbell exercises for
         Deltoid
         Supraspinatus
         Elbow flexors

Scapula muscles
3. Upper body ergometer
B. Weeks 10–12
1. Continue all above exercises
2. Initiate isokinetic strengthening (scapulae plane)
3. Initiate sidelying external rotation/internal rotation exercises (dumbbell)
4. Initiate neuromuscular scapulae control exercises

III. *Phase 3—Advanced Strengthening Phase* (Weeks 13–21)
Goals: Maintain full nonpainful range of motion
Improve shoulder complex strength
Improve neuromuscular control
Gradual return to function activities
A. Weeks 13–18
1. Active stretching program for the shoulder
Active assisted range of motion L-bar flexion, external rotation, internal rotation
2. Capsular stretches
3. Aggressive strengthening program (isotonic program)

a. Shoulder flexion
b. Shoulder abduction
c. Supraspinatus
d. External rotation/internal rotation
e. Elbow flexors/extensors
f. Scapulae muscles
4. Isokinetic test (modified neutral position) [week 14]
External rotation/internal rotation at 180° and 300°/s
5. General conditioning program
B. Weeks 18–21
1. Continue all exercises listed above
2. Initiate interval sport program

IV. *Phase 4—Return to Activity Phase* (Weeks 21–26)
Goals: Gradual return to recreational sport activities
A. Weeks 21–26
1. Isokinetic test (modified neutral position)
2. Continue to comply to interval sport program
3. Continue basic 10 program for strengthening and flexibility

# Appendix 16-2

# Type 2 Rehabilitation Program for Rotator Cuff Repair (Deltoid Splitting)

I. *Phase 1—Protection Phase* (Weeks 0–6)
   Goals:  Gradual increase in range of motion
   Increase shoulder strength
   Decrease pain and inflammation
   A. Weeks 0–3
      1. Brace or sling (physician determines)
      2. Pendulum exercises
      3. Active assisted range of motion exercises (L-bar exercises)
         a. Flexion to 125°
         b. External rotation/internal rotation (shoulder at 40° abduction) to 30°
      4. Passive range of motion to tolerance
      5. Rope and pulley flexion
      6. Elbow range of motion and hand gripping exercises
      7. Submaximal isometrics
         a. Flexors
         b. Abductors
         c. External rotation/internal rotation
         d. Elbow flexors
      8. Ice and pain modalities
   B. Weeks 3–6
      1. Discontinue brace or sling
      2. Continue all exercises listed above
      3. Active assisted range of motion exercises
         a. Flexion to 145°
         b. External rotation/internal rotation (performed at 65° abduction) range to tolerance

II. *Phase 2—Intermediate Phase* (Weeks 7–14)
    Goals:  Full nonpainful range of motion (week 10)
    Gradual increase in strength
    Decrease pain
    A. Weeks 7–10
       1. Active assisted range of motion L-bar exercises
          a. Flexion to 160°
          b. External rotation/internal rotation (performed at 90° shoulder abduction) to tolerance (>45°)
       2. Strengthening exercises
          a. Exercises tubing external rotation/internal rotation (arm at side)
          b. Initiate humeral head stabilizing exercise
          c. Initiate dumbbell strengthening exercises*
          Deltoid
          Supraspinatus
          Elbow flexion/extension
          Scapulae muscles
       * Patient must be able to elevate arm without shoulder and scapular hiking before initiating isotonics; if unable, maintain on humeral head stabilizing exercises
    B. Weeks 10–14 (full range of motion desired by weeks 10–12)
       1. Continue all exercises listed above

2. Initiate isokinetic strengthening (scapulae plane)
3. Initiate sidelying external rotation/internal rotation strengthening exercises
4. Initiate neuromuscular control exercises for scapular

III. *Phase 3—Advanced Strengthening Phase* (Weeks 15–26)
   Goals:   Maintain full nonpainful range of motion
            Improve stength of shoulder
            Improve neuromuscular control
            Gradual return to functional activities
   A. Weeks 15–20
      1. Continue active assisted range of motion exercises with L-bar
         Flexion, external rotation/internal rotation
      2. Self capsular stretches
      3. Aggressive strengthening program
         a. Shoulder flexion

b. Shoulder abduction (to 90°)
c. Supraspinatus
d. External rotation/internal rotation
e. Elbow flexors/extensors
f. Scapula strengthening
4. Conditioning program
B. Weeks 21–26
   1. Continue all exercises listed above
   2. Isokinetic test (modified neutral position) for external rotation/internal rotation at 180° and 300°/s
   3. Initiate interval sport program

IV. *Phase 4—Return to Activity Phase* (Weeks 24–28)
   Goals:   Gradual return to recreational sport activities
   A. Weeks 24–28
      1. Continue all strengthening exercises
      2. Continue all flexibility exercises
      3. Continue progression on interval programs

# Appendix 16-3

# Type 3 Rehabilitation Program for Rotator Cuff Repair (Deltoid Splitting)

I. *Phase 1—Protection Phase* (Weeks 0–8)
   A. Weeks 0–4
      1. Brace or sling (determined by physician)
      2. Pendulum exercises
      3. Passive range of motion to tolerance
         a. Flexion
         b. External rotation/internal rotation (shoulder at 45° abduction)
      4. Elbow range of motion
      5. Hand gripping exercises
      6. Continuous passive motion
      7. Submaximal isometrics
         a. Abductors
         b. External rotation/internal rotation
         c. Elbow flexors
      8. Ice and pain modalities
      9. Gentle active assisted range of motion with L-bar at week 2
   B. Weeks 4–8
      1. Discontinue brace or sling
      2. Active assisted range of motion with L-bar
         a. Flexion to 100°
         b. External rotation/internal rotation (shoulder 45° abduction) 40°
      3. Continue pain modalities

II. *Phase 2—Intermediate Phase* (Weeks 8–14)
   Goals: Establish full range of motion (week 12)
          Gradually increase strength
          Decrease pain
   A. Weeks 8–10
      1. Active assisted range of motion L-bar exercises
         a. Flexion to tolerance
         b. External rotation/internal rotation (shoulder 90° abduction) to tolerance
      2. Initiate isotonic strengthening*
         a. Deltoid to 90°
         b. External rotation/internal rotation sidelying
         c. Supraspinatus
         d. Biceps/triceps
         e. Scapula muscles
      * If patient is unable to elevate arm without shoulder hiking (scapulothoracic substitution), maintain on humeral head stabilizing exercises
   B. Weeks 10–14
      1. Full range of motion desired by weeks 12–14
      2. Continue all exercises listed above
      3. Initiate neuromuscular control exercises

III. *Phase 3—Advanced Strengthening Phase* (Weeks 15–26)
   Goals: Maintain full nonpainful range of motion
          Improve strength of shoulder
          Improve neuromuscular control
          Gradual return to functional activities
   A. Weeks 15–20

1. Continue active assisted range of motion exercises with L-bar—Flexion, external rotation/internal rotation
2. Self capsular stretches
3. Aggressive strengthening program
   a. Shoulder flexion
   b. Shoulder abduction (to 90°)
   c. Supraspinatus
   d. External rotation/internal rotation
   e. Elbow flexors/extensors
   f. Scapula strengthening
4. Conditioning program

B. Weeks 21–26

1. Continue all exercises listed above
2. Isokinetic test (modified neutral position) for external rotation/internal rotation at 180° and 300°/s
3. Initiate interval sport program

IV. *Phase 4—Return to Activity Phase* (Weeks 24–28)
   Goals: Gradual return to recreational sport activities
   A. Weeks 24–28
   1. Continue all strengthening exercises
   2. Continue all flexibility exercises
   3. Continue progression on interval programs

# 17

# Arthroscopic Debridement of Rotator Cuff Injuries

*PETER E. LOEB*
*JAMES R. ANDREWS*
*KEVIN E. WILK*

This chapter discusses the role of arthroscopy in the debridement of rotator cuff lesions in the athletic shoulder. We review the pertinent history and physical examination associated with lesions to the rotator cuff in the athlete. The goals of the procedure, surgical indications and contraindications to arthroscopic management of rotator cuff problems, the operative technique, and postoperative rehabilitation are also discussed.

## ARTHROSCOPY

Within the past decade, the indications and capabilities of arthroscopy have expanded. As technical ability has improved, paralleling development of better instrumentation, orthopaedists have expanded the use of arthroscopy.

Arthroscopy about the shoulder has multiple indications and uses. These range from diagnostic surgery to debridement and stabilization procedures.[1,2] Direct visualization of the rotator cuff has allowed precise diagnosis of partial-thickness rotator cuff tears as described by Andrews et al.[3] Partial tearing of the rotator cuff or tensile tearing is felt to be an undersurface tensile failure of the cuff at its insertion. The tendon fails through several millimeters of its undersurface thickness in an "onion stir" peeling fashion.[3] Although magnetic resonance imaging and arthrography have become valuable tools by which to diagnose rotator cuff lesions,[2,4–6] arthroscopy allows direct visualization of the lesion from both intra-articular and subacromial space.[2,3,5,7–9] Direct examination and probing using the arthroscope give valuable information regarding the integrity of the rotator cuff. The throwing athlete is the best model to study the pathophysiology of this type of rotator cuff injury.

## HISTORY AND PHYSICAL EXAMINATION

The throwing athlete will often be referred to the orthopaedist or trainer because of "pain or weakness" while throwing. Although these rotator cuff problems often involve baseball players (i.e., pitchers), they may involve any athlete involved in throwing sports. The player may not be able to describe a certain position associated with the change in throwing function but may mention a feeling of weakness and "catching" within their shoulders. Positional complaints during throwing may indicate instability or rotator cuff impingement.[10] Although many throwers show some form of "looseness about the shoulder," it is important to differentiate carefully a history of instability versus weakness or pain.

On physical examination, the most common finding by Andrews et al.[3] was a catching in the shoulder and pain in the straightforward flexion plane between 160 and 180°. With the arm completely forward flexed and abducted, internally and externally rotating the humerus, a painful catching may be reproduced. This was elicited in more than 80 percent of Andrews' patients with partial-thickness tears.[3] Although full-thickness tears do occur in athletes, they are rare. Full-thickness tears present with profound weakness and are associated with an acute onset of symptoms. Partial thickness tears often result from repetitive microtrauma with an insidious onset of decreasing throwing function. Some throwers may recall an actual injury or type of throw in which they developed a partial rotator cuff tear. Examination of muscle strength with partial tears may show mild to moderate weakness, but often no clinical weakness is found. Isokinetic testing may be used to study specific muscle groups. This information is useful in following injuries as well as rehabilitation. Muscle testing will also guide us as to when an athlete may return to his or her throwing sport.

## GOALS OF ARTHROSCOPIC DEBRIDEMENT

The goals of surgery are to define carefully the pathology present and to intervene in the appropriate manner to aid in healing of the tissues. Full-thickness tears in

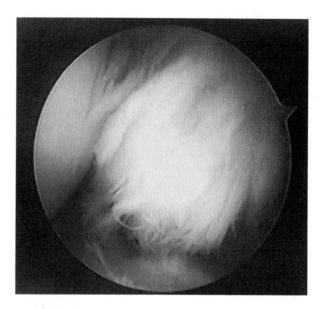

**Fig. 17-2.** Large amount of partial-thickness rotator cuff tear.

young athletes should be repaired by an open incision. Arthroscopy of the shoulder is very effective for performing bursectomy and debriding partial-thickness tears of the rotator cuff.[1,3,7–9,11] Debridement of partial-thickness tears (tensile tearing) of the rotator cuff removes the abnormal tissue and allows a healing response to this area of the cuff.[3,11–14] Inflammation and increased vascular response after debridement allows a healing response.[15]

Although the area of the supraspinatus insertion is often involved (Figs. 17-1 and 17-2), the posterior rotator cuff may also be involved.[3] Once debrided, it is expected that the athlete will proceed to heal the area and return to active throwing in the ensuing months, after effective, progressive rehabilitation.

## SURGICAL INDICATIONS AND CONTRAINDICATIONS

Surgery is indicated in the athlete with symptoms after a full, conservative rehabilitation program. Athletes who present with shoulder symptoms should be thoroughly examined and, if a rotator cuff problem is suspected, should be placed on a planned rotator cuff rehabilitation program. If after an adequate trial of rest and

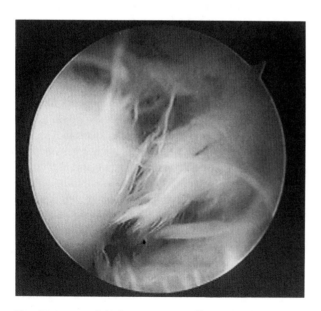

**Fig. 17-1.** Partial-thickness rotator cuff tear; view from posterior portal.

rehabilitation the patient continues with symptoms, he or she may be a candidate for examination under anesthesia and diagnostic and possibly operative arthroscopy.

Contraindications include patients who have not attempted rehabilitation or those whose problems are a result of an instability pattern. Orthopaedists must understand that any arthroscopic intervention will affect the patient's return to athletics for several weeks to months, even without operative arthroscopy.

## TECHNIQUE

The athlete under anesthesia is examined carefully, noting range of motion and instability patterns. The uninvolved shoulder should also be examined. Care must be taken to compare these examination findings with those of the patient's office examination.

After examination, the patient is placed on a bean bag in the lateral decubitus position with an axillary pad.[2] The arm is then suspended by an arm holder in 15 to 20 degrees of forward flexion and approximately 70 degrees of abduction. The arm is suspended by 10 to 15 lb of traction. The coronal position of the thorax is with approximately 15 degrees of angulation posteriorly when in the lateral decubitus position.[16] An 18-gauge spinal needle is used posteriorly to insufflate the joint with 60 ml saline.

The posterior portal is made as described by Andrews and Carson.[16] Diagnostic arthroscopy is then performed, examining the entire joint. An anterior portal is used, and the arthroscope is placed anteriorly to observe the posterior rotator cuff.

Motorized shavers can be placed within the portals to allow debridement of the partial tearing of the rotator cuff under direct visualization. The posterior portal is used to enter the subacromial space. A lateral portal may be used for bursectomy and debridement of the subacromial cuff disease when indicated.

With intra-articular rotator cuff disease, shavers are used to debride to a bleeding surface (Fig. 17-3). This usually involves only removing several millimeters of the superficial degenerated avascular undercuff surface.

When in the subacromial space, evaluation of impingement may be made. The space between the acro-

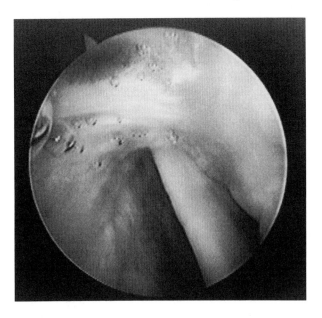

**Fig. 17-3.** View of supraspinatus insertion after debridement of partial-thickness tear; view from posterior portal.

mion and the humeral head and the rotator cuff is examined critically. Abrasion of the subacromial surface of the rotator cuff may indicate impingement. If found, debridement of the bursa and the roughened area may relieve the patient's symptoms. If a hooked type II or beaked type III[17] acromion is found, a decompression (acromioplasty) of the anterior lateral edge of the acromion may be performed.[7,8,11,18]

The impingement complex described by Neer[10] (stage II or stage III) occurs less often in young athletes. One must carefully evaluate patients and their complaints before performing a decompression on a throwing shoulder. Decompression of a multidirectionally unstable shoulder may lead to greater instability and a very poor result.[15,19]

Full-thickness tears in athletes occur rarely. These are managed by open repair or by arthroscopically aided "mini"-open repair, which results in less operative morbidity.[20] In the older population with full-thickness tears, arthroscopic debridement has been beneficial (84 percent rated good or excellent). Levy et al.[7] reported on patients with an average age of 51 years and stated that 88 percent of patients were satisfied with their results.

# REHABILITATION AFTER ARTHROSCOPIC DECOMPRESSION

The rehabilitation program after arthroscopic decompression can be divided into five specific phases. The specific phases of this rehabilitation can be found in Appendix 17-1. The rehabilitative process after arthroscopic decompression is associated with minimal tissue morbidity because the deltoid insertion is not violated.[21,22] It permits early rehabilitation, which will allow an earlier return to functional activities. We briefly discuss the rehabilitation process after arthroscopic decompression and/or debridement.

The first phase of rehabilitation process is the immediate motion phase, which usually comprises the first 7 to 14 days after surgery. The patient generally exhibits postsurgical pain, inflammation, a loss of motion, and muscular weakness. The goals of this phase are to (1) prevent the deleterious effects of immobilization, (2) regain full nonpainful range of motion, (3) retard muscular atrophy, and (4) reduce the postsurgical pain and inflammation.

Immediately postsurgery, the patient is placed on motion exercises, which include pendulum exercises to promote early motion and minimize shoulder pain. Also, active assisted motion exercises are initiated with an L-shaped bar (Breg Corporation, Vista, CA)

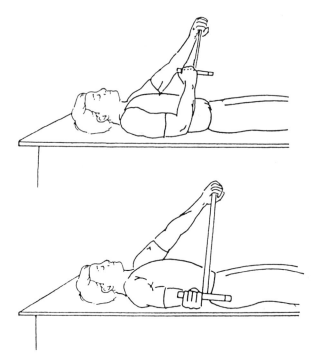

**Fig. 17-5.** Active assisted external rotation performed with the arm at 0 to 20 degrees of abduction.

(Fig. 17-4). The exercises we routinely prescribe are external shoulder rotation. The internal/external rotation motions are initiated with the shoulder at 0 to 20 degrees of shoulder abduction (Fig. 17-5), and then as the patients progress, they are performed at 45 de-

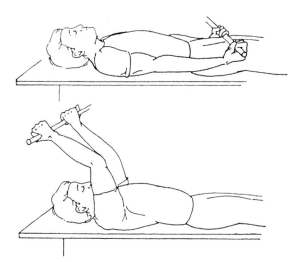

**Fig. 17-4.** Active assisted shoulder flexion using an L-shaped bar.

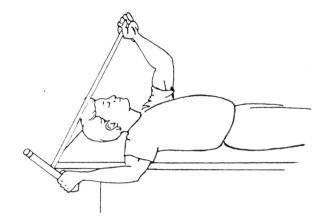

**Fig. 17-6.** Active assisted external rotation being performed at 90 degrees of shoulder abduction.

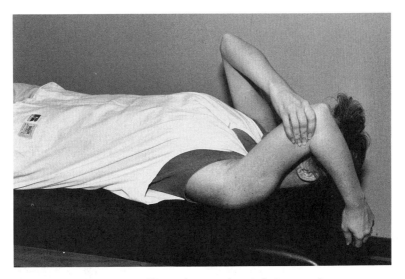

**Fig. 17-7.** Self capsular stretches, inferior stretch.

grees and finally at 90 degrees of abduction (Fig. 17-6). The patients' signs and symptoms must be carefully monitored during this progression. Self-performed capsular stretches are also used for the anterior, inferior, and posterior capsule using the opposite arm to create an overpressure[23] (Figs. 17-7 to 17-9).

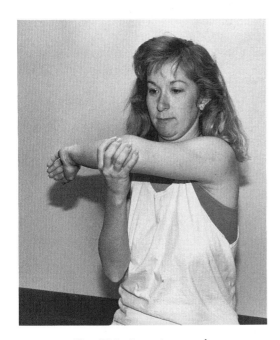

**Fig. 17-8.** Posterior stretch.

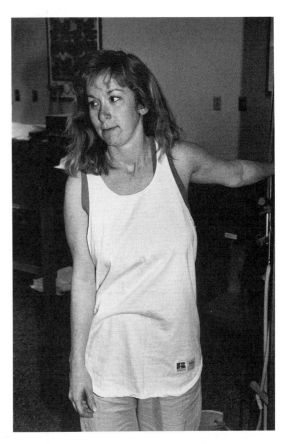

**Fig. 17-9.** Anterior stretch.

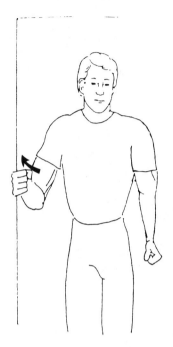

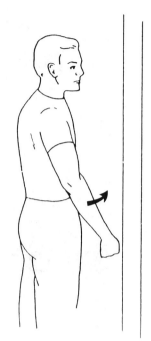

**Fig. 17-10.** Isometric muscular contraction for the shoulder abductors.

**Fig. 17-12.** Isometric muscular contraction for the shoulder flexors.

Immediate strengthening exercises are used during this phase. These exercises are isometrics for the shoulder external rotators, internal rotators, flexors abductors, and biceps brachii. Then exercises are performed submaximally, in a pain-free position with moderate force generated. Also, modalities such as ice, high-voltage galvanic stimulation, ultrasound, and nonsteroidal anti-inflammatory drugs are used for the postsurgical inflammation and pain.

During this phase, we believe it to be vital for the

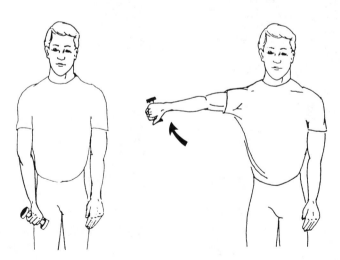

**Fig. 17-11.** Supraspinatus strengthening with a dumbbell weight (scaption plane).

patient to initiate immediate motion and strengthening exercises to prevent the deleterious effects of relative immobilization.[24,25] Also, we believe it critical to re-initiate humeral head control through the rotator cuff as quickly as possible. This is imperative to prevent excessive, uncontrollable humeral head migration. The primary function of the rotator cuff is to dynamically stabilize and steer the humeral head during shoulder movements.[26] Thus, early isometric exercises for the rotator cuff are intended to re-establish voluntary humeral head control.

When the patient exhibits minimal pain and tenderness, nearly complete shoulder motion, and strength that has returned to at least the "good" (4/5) grade, phase 2 of the program may be initiated. The goals of this second phase are to (1) normalize full nonpainful motion and re-establish normal arthrokinematics of shoulder complex; (2) regain and improve muscular strength; (3) improve the patients' neuromuscular control of the shoulder complex; and (4) eliminate residual pain and inflammation.

In this phase, strengthening exercises are progressed from isometric muscular contractions to isotonic dumbbell exercises. The exercises we routinely emphasize are shoulder abduction to 90 degrees, supraspinatus (scaption), shoulder flexion to 90 degrees, internal/external rotation, and elbow flexion (Figs. 17-10 to 17-15). Also, scapular strengthening is emphasized, especially scapula retraction and depression to reposition the scapula on the thoracic wall.

Additional strengthening exercises in the later portion of this phase include submaximal isokinetics in the plane of the scapulae or modified neutral,[27] proprioceptive neuromuscular facilitation exercises such as $D_2$ flexion with rhythmic stabilization,[28] and cardiovascular endurance exercises such as rowing or the upper body ergometer.

Also in this phase, aggressive stretching is performed to eliminate capsular restrictions, especially of the posterior capsule. The impingement patient commonly

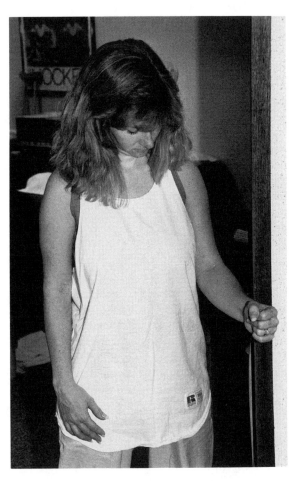

**Fig. 17-13.** External rotators.

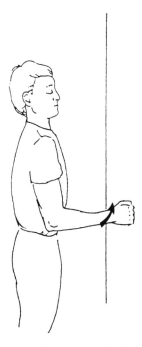

**Fig. 17-14.** Isometrics for the shoulder's internal rotators.

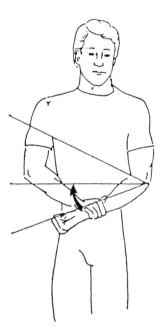

**Fig. 17-15.** Elbow flexors being exercised at multiple angles during isometrics.

exhibits posterior capsular tightness, which restricts glenohumeral internal rotation and elevation.[29] Posterior capsular tightness will cause the humeral head to migrate anteriorly during shoulder elevation, which may contribute to the impingement of the supraspinatus on the coracoacromial arch. We commonly refer to this as the humeral head "rolling up." Thus, one of the primary goals is the re-establishment of full internal rotation (85°) of the shoulder at 90 degrees of abduction.

Phase 3 (dynamic strengthening) is begun when the patient exhibits four specific criteria. These criteria include (1) full nonpainful range of motion, (2) no pain or tenderness, (3) strength 70 percent of contralateral side, and (4) a satisfactory clinical examination. The goals of this phase are to improve strength, power, and endurance, improve the neuromuscular control of the shoulder, and prepare the individual for a gradual return to functional activities.

In this phase, capsular stretches are used to maintain range of motion of the shoulder, and a strengthening program is progressed from dumbbells to exercise tubing, which provides constant loading (concentric/eccentric) of the shoulder musculature. Appendix 17-1 illustrates the basic glenohumeral and scapulothoracic strengthening exercises used in this phase. These exercises have been chosen because of reported electromyogram activity during these movements.[30,31]

During this phase, isokinetics, manual resistance, eccentrics, and neuromuscular control exercises are progressed. For the competitive athlete who requires enhanced strength, especially the throwing athlete, a plyometric program to improve the athlete's strength, power, and coordination may be used.[32]

The last phase of the rehabilitation program is the return to activity phase (usually 12 to 20 weeks postsurgery). The patient must exhibit the following criteria to progress into this phase: (1) full nonpainful range of motion, (2) no pain or tenderness, (3) muscular strength that fulfills our pre-established criteria, and (4) a satisfactory clinical examination.

The goals of this phase are a progressive return to unrestricted activities and a maintenance program to ensure normal shoulder motion and strength. During this phase, the exercises are progressed to include functional patterns commonly performed by the patient. Also, for the competitive or recreational athlete, the patient is placed on an interval program for throwing, tennis, golf and/or racquet ball (see Ch. 52). Once the patient returns to unrestricted activities, we encourage the continuation of an exercise program for 1 year from the date of surgery.

## CONCLUSION

Arthroscopic debridement of partial tears in the rotator cuff is an important tool in the management of the throwing shoulder. It is important to diagnose rotator cuff disease correctly and to begin an effective rehabilitation program. Tensile tearing of the rotator cuff can be well managed with arthroscopic debridement and is followed by intensive physical therapy. The goal of this management is to return the athletic throwing shoulder to sport as soon and as safely as possible.

The successful outcome after arthroscopic shoulder decompression is dependent on several factors including (1) an accurate differential diagnosis, (2) the appropriate surgical technique, (3) the identification of all involved tissues, (4) identifying capsular laxity or tightness, (5) the appropriate rehabilitation program that is progressive and sequential, and (6) a team approach with the patient, physician, and therapist all working together with the common goal of a full return to unrestricted activities.

# REFERENCES

1. Ellman H: Shoulder arthroscopy: current indications and techniques. Orthopedics 11:45, 1988
2. Ogilvie-Harris DJ, D'Angelo G: Arthroscopic surgery of the shoulder. Sports Med 9:120, 1990
3. Andrews JR, Broussard TS, Carson WG: Arthroscopy of the shoulder in the management of partial tears of the rotator cuff: a preliminary report. Arthroscopy 1:117, 1985
4. Evancho AM, Stiles RG, Fajman WA et al: MR imaging diagnosis of rotator cuff tears. AJR 151:751, 1988
5. Kneisl JS, Sweeney HJ, Paige ML: Correlation of pathology observed in double contrast arthrotomography and arthroscopy of the shoulder. Arthroscopy 4:21, 1988
6. Morrison DS, Ofstein R: The use of magnetic resonance imaging in the diagnosis of rotator cuff tears. Orthopedics 13:633, 1990
7. Levy HF, Gardner RD, Lemak LJ: Arthroscopic subacromial decompression in the treatment of full-thickness rotator cuff tears. Arthroscopy 7:8, 1991
8. Gartsman GM: Arthroscopic acromioplasty for lesions of the rotator cuff. J Bone Joint Surg 72A:169, 1990
9. Snyder SJ, Pachelli AF, Del Pizzo W et al: Partial thickness rotator cuff tears: results of arthroscopic treatment. Arthroscopy 7:1, 1991
10. Neer CS: Anterior acromioplasty for the chronic impingement syndrome in the shoulder. J Bone Joint Surg 54A:45, 1972
11. Esch JC, Ozerkis LR, Helgager JA et al: Arthroscopic subacromial decompression: results according to the degree of rotator cuff tear. Arthroscopy 4:241, 1988
12. Cofield RH: Tears of rotator cuff. Instr Course Lect 30:258, 1981
13. Hurley JA, Anderson TE: Shoulder arthroscopy: its role in evaluating shoulder disorders in the athlete. Am J Sports Med 18:480, 1990
14. Souryal TO, Baker CL: Anatomy of the supraclavicular fossa portal in shoulder arthroscopy. Arthroscopy 6:297, 1990
15. Jobe FW, Ling B: The Shoulder: Surgical and Nonsurgical Management. Lea & Febiger, Philadelphia, 1988
16. Andrews Jr, Carson WG: Shoulder joint arthroscopy. Orthopedics 6:1157, 1983
17. Bigliani LU, Morrison DS, April EW: The morphology of the acromion and its relationship to rotator cuff tears. Orthop Trans 10:216, 1986
18. Ellman H: Diagnosis and treatment of incomplete rotator cuff tears. Clin Orthop 254:64, 1990
19. Rathbun JB, Macnab I: The microvascular pattern of the rotator cuff. J Bone Joint Surg 52B:540, 1970
20. Levy HJ, Uribe JW, Delany LG: Arthroscopic assisted rotator cuff repair: preliminary results. Arthroscopy 6:55, 1990
21. Paulos LE, Franklin JL: Arthroscopic shoulder decompression development and application; a five year experience. Am J Sports Med 18:235, 1990
22. Johnson LL: Shoulder arthroscopy. In Johnson LL (ed): Arthroscopic Surgery Principles and Practices. CV Mosby, St Louis, 1986
23. Wilk KE, Arrigo CA, Courson R et al: Preventive and Rehabilitative Exercises for the Shoulder and Elbow. American Sports Medicine Institute, Birmingham, AL, 1991
24. Akeson WH, Woo SLY, Amiel D: The connective tissue response to immobility: biomechanical changes in periarticular connective tissue of the immobilized rabbit knee. Clin Orthop 93:356, 1973
25. Dehne E, Tory E: Treatment of joint injuries by immediate mobilization; based upon the spinal adaption concept. Clin Orthop 77:218, 1971
26. Matsen FA, Arntz CT: Subacromial impingement. p. 623. In Rockwood CA, Matsen FA (eds): The Shoulder. WB Saunders, Philadelphia, 1990
27. Wilk KE, Arrigo CA: Isokinetic testing and exercises for microtraumatic shoulder injuries. In Davies GJ (ed): The Compendium of Isokinetics. 4th Ed. S & S Publishing, Onalaska, WI, 1992
28. Knott M, Voss DE: Proprioceptive neuromuscular facilitation. Harper & Row, New York, 1956
29. Wilk KE, Andrews JR: Conservative treatment of the stage II and stage III shoulder impingement patients. J Orthop Sports Phys Ther (submitted for publication)
30. Mosely JB, Jobe FW, Pink M et al: EMG analysis of the scapular muscles during a shoulder rehabilitation program. Am J Sports Med 20:220, 1992
31. Townsend H, Jobe FW, Pink M, Perry J: EMG analysis of the glenohumeral muscles during a baseball rehabilitation program. Am J Sports Med 19:264, 1991
32. Wilk KE, Voight M, Keirns MA et al: Plyometrics for the upper extremity, the theory and clinical application. J Orthop Phys Ther (accepted for publication)

# Appendix 17-1

# Postsurgical Rehabilitation After Arthroscopic Decompression/Debridement

This rehabilitation program's goal is to return the patient/athlete to his or her activity/sport as quickly and safely as possible. The program is based on muscle physiology, biomechanics, anatomy, and healing response.

I. *Phase 1—Motion Phase*
 Goals: Re-establish nonpainful range of motion
  Retard muscular atrophy
  Decrease pain and inflammation
 A. Range of Motion
  1. Pendulum exercises
  2. Rope and pulley (flexion/extension only)
  3. T-bar exercises
   a. Flexion/extension
   b. Abduction/adduction
   c. External rotation/internal rotation (begin at 0°, progress to 45°, then 90° of abduction
  4. Self stretches (capsular stretches)
 B. Strengthening Exercises
  1. Isometrics
  2. May begin tubing for external rotation/internal rotation at 0° late phase
 C. Decrease Pain and Inflammation
  1. Ice, nonsteroidal anti-inflammatory drug, modalities

II. *Phase 2—Intermediate Phase*
 Goals: Regain and improve muscular strength
  Normalize arthrokinematics
  Improve neuromuscular control of shoulder complex
 A. Criteria to Progress to Phase 2
  1. Full range of motion
  2. Minimal pain and tenderness

  3. "Good" manual muscle test of internal rotation, external rotation, flex
 B. Initiate Isotonic Program with Dumbbells
  1. Shoulder musculature
   External/internal rotator strengthening
    shoulder abduction/flexion to 90°
   Supraspinatus strengthening
   Biceps/triceps
  2. Scapulothoracic musculature
   Retractors/protractors
   Elevators/depressors
 C. Normalize Arthrokinematics of Shoulder Complex
  1. Joint mobilization (GH, AC, SC, ST joints)
  2. Control T-bar range of motion
 D. Initiate Neuromuscular Control Exercises
 E. Initiate Trunk Exercises
 F. Initiate Upper Extremity (UBE) Endurance Exercises
 G. Continue Use of Modalities, Ice as Needed

III. *Phase 3—Dynamic Strengthening Phase*
 (Advanced Strengthening Phase)
 Goals: Improve strength/power/endurance
  Improve neuromuscular control
  Prepare athlete to begin to throw, etc.
 A. Criteria to Enter Phase 3
  1. Full nonpainful range of motion
  2. No pain or tenderness
  3. Strength 70 percent compared with contralateral side
 B. Emphasis of Phase 3
  1. High-speed, high-energy strengthening exercises
  2. Eccentric exercises
  3. Diagonal patterns

C. Exercises
1. Continue dumbbell strengthening (supraspinatus, deltoid)
2. Initiate tubing exercises in the 90°/90° position for internal rotation/external rotation (slow/fast sets)
3. Tubing exercises for scapulothoracic musculature
4. Tubing exercises for biceps
5. Initiate plyometrics for rotator cuff muscles
6. Initiate diagonal patterns (proprioceptive neuromuscular facilitation) PNF $D_2$ flexion/extension patterns
7. Initiate isokinetics external/internal rotation in scapular plane
8. Continue endurance exercises; neuromuscular control exercises

IV. *Phase 4—Return to Activity Phase*
   Goals: Progressively increase activities to prepare patient for full functional return
   A. Criteria to Progress to Phase 3
      1. Full range of motion
      2. No pain or tenderness
      3. Isokinetic test that fulfills criteria to throw
      4. Satisfactory clinical examination
   B. Initiate Interval Program
   C. Continue All Exercises as in Phase 3
      1. Throw and train on same day
      2. Lower extremity and range of motion on opposite days
   D. Progress interval program
V. *Follow-Up Visits* (6 months, 1 and 2 years)
   A. Isokinetic Tests
   B. Clinical Examination

# 18

# Anterior Instability of the Shoulder

STEPHEN J. O'BRIEN
MICHAEL J. PAGNANI
ROBERT A. PANARIELLO
HUGH M. O'FLYNN
STEPHEN FEALY

## ANATOMY OF THE STABLE AND UNSTABLE SHOULDER

The cornerstone to evaluating and treating anterior instability of the glenohumeral joint is a thorough understanding of both normal and abnormal anatomy. We certainly have made strides in the last ten years in this area, aided significantly by the availability of the arthroscope and by recent anatomic and biomechanical studies.[1–8] This has had a direct effect on surgical treatment, leading to a shift in surgical techniques that primarily address restoring normal anatomy, rather than previous "non-anatomical" techniques.

Two basic factors to consider when attempting to distinguish the primary direction of clinical instability in a particular patient are (1) distinguishing normal laxity from instability and (2) establishing positions and circumstances in which clinical instability occurs. Armed with the proper anatomic background, we should be able to address both of these concerns.

The human glenohumeral anterior shoulder joint is formed by the humeral head and the glenoid surfaces of the scapula (Fig. 18-1). This unique glenometrical relationship allows for remarkable ranges of motion, which were so important for adapting phylogenetically erect arthrograde postures, but at the expense of the intrinsic stability.

Both static and dynamic constraints directly affect glenohumeral stability. Static mechanics include bony joint conformity, negative intra-articular pressure, the glenoid labrum, and capsuloligamentous restraints. Dynamic mechanisms include the rotator cuff muscles, the long head of the biceps tendon, and the surrounding shoulder musculature traversing the glenohumeral joint, which affects proximal humeral motion.[9] These muscles and tendons create both joint compressive loads and other forces, limiting excessive translation of the humeral head on the glenoid. Attention to all of these details must be part of the diagnosis, corrective treatment, and rehabilitation of the athlete with problems related to shoulder instability.

Problems regarding stability of the shoulder in the athlete would best be understood by thinking of two basic categories, *symptomatic laxity* and *overt instability*. Athletes with symptomatic laxity often have problems with repetitive edge loading or traction on the glenoid labrum, depending on the sport and positions in which the load is applied. For example, a football lineman may develop posterior pain and labral injuries from blocking with the arms held forward flexed with elbows locked in extensor, while a thrower may injure the posterior labrum of the superior labral-biceps complex from traction in the follow-through phase of throwing. Symptomatic laxity may also involve

177

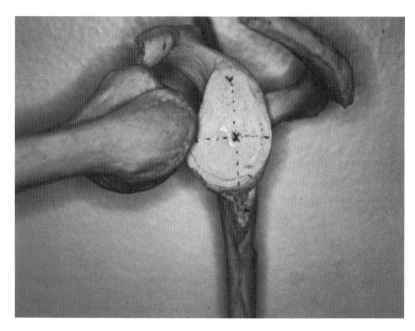

**Fig. 18-1.** Sagittal view of the glenohumeral joint.

rotator cuff tendonitis (impingement instability) as the lax shoulder puts excessive eccentric load on the rotator cuff, or dead arm symptoms from traction on the brachial plexus in the lax shoulder as it subluxes inferiorly or anteroinferiorly.

*Instability,* on the other hand, refers to problems in which the athlete cannot contain the humeral head and clearly dislocates. This puts athletes in a fully compromised position in which they are incapacitated until the shoulder is reduced. The athlete has no interval pain but is at risk for more serious nerve, bone, or joint injuries, which will require surgical correction. In this chapter, we focus on the *instability* group, particularly those athletes who dislocate anteriorly and those who have multidirectional laxity but who are primarily unstable anteriorly or anteroinferiorly.

The most common etiology for anterior shoulder instability is failure of the capsuloligamentous structures. The contribution of the shoulder capsule to stability depends on the collagen integrity, attachment sites on the glenoid and humeral head, and the position of the arm. Certain areas of the capsule are thicker than others, are ligamentous-like, and are called the glenohumeral ligaments (Fig. 18-2).

The superior glenohumeral ligament is a fairly constant structure with the shoulder capsule arising just anterior to the long head of the biceps tendon origin. It inserts into the forearm capitis, lying just superior to the lesser tuberosity (Fig. 18-3). Its size and integrity are quite variable and are usually not visualized well arthroscopically with the joint distended with saline (Fig. 18-4). Its contribution as a primary restraint to glenohumeral stability is greatest with the arm suspended at the side (i.e., at 0 degrees abduction).[8] As the shoulder is abducted to 45 degrees, it plays a secondary role when the arm is internally or externally rotated, creating a "wind up" effect around the humeral head. In 90 degrees of abduction it plays no role in glenohumeral stability.[4]

The middle glenohumeral ligament is quite variable in size and shape and may be present as a thin wisp of tissue or as tissue as thick as the biceps tendon (Figs. 18-1, 18-3). It is absent in approximately 20 percent of shoulders. When present, it arises either from the

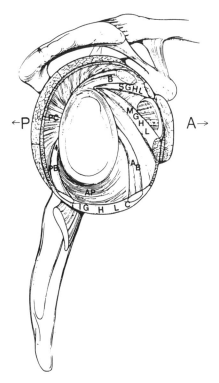

**Fig. 18-2.** Anatomic depiction of the glenohumeral ligaments and the inferior glenohumeral ligament complex (*IGHLC*). (*P,* posterior; A, anterior; *SGHL,* superior glenohumeral ligament; MGHL, middle glenohumeral ligament) (From Rockwood and Matsen,[21] with permission.)

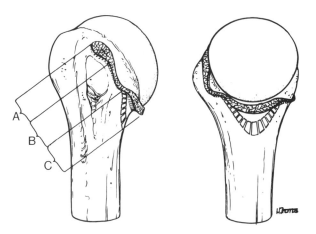

**Fig. 18-3.** The attachment sites of the glenohumeral ligaments. *Left,* the superior glenohumeral ligament inserts into the fovea capitis line just superior to the lesser tuberosity (*A*). The middle glenohumeral ligament inserts into the humerus just medial to the lesser tuberosity (*B*). The inferior glenohumeral ligament complex has two common attachment mechanisms (*C*). It may attach in a collar-like fashion, or it may have a **V**-shaped attachment to the articular edge, *right.* (From Rockwood and Matsen,[21] with permission.)

labrum immediately below the superior glenohumeral ligament or from the adjacent glenoid neck. As it traverses the joint anteriorly, it crosses the tendon of the subscapularis and inserts into the humerus just medial to the lesser tuberosity. The middle glenohumeral ligament plays a secondary role in 0, 45, and 90 degrees of abduction, although this role may be substantial when the ligament is quite thick.

The inferior glenohumeral ligament complex (IGHLC) is a hammock-like structure that cradles and supports the humeral head (Figs. 18-2, 18-5, 18-6). It consists of three parts: anterior band, axillary pouch, and posterior band.[3] The IGHLC takes its origin from either the glenoid labrum or glenoid neck and inserts into the anatomic neck of the humerus. The anterior band originates at the comma-like portion of the ante-

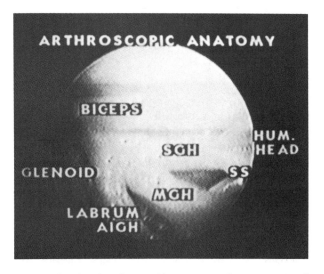

**Fig. 18-4.** The glenohumeral ligaments are best appreciated with arthroscopic visualization without distension with air or saline. In this view, the various glenohumeral ligaments are seen as they appear from a posterior portal view. (From Rockwood and Matsen,[21] with permission.)

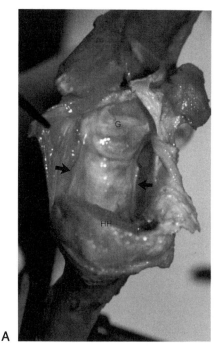

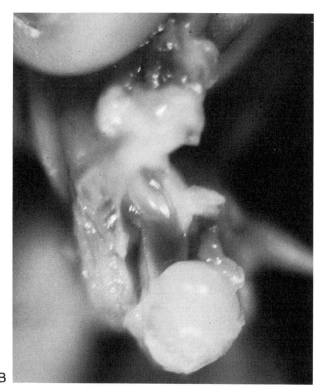

A    B

**Fig. 18-5.** (**A**) The anterior and posterior ends of the inferior glenohumeral ligament complex (*arrows*) are clearly defined in this picture of an abducted shoulder specimen with the humeral head (HH) partially resected. (From Rockwood and Matsen,[21] with permission.) (**B**) The inferior glenohumeral ligament complex is the only capsular ligamentous structure that can be seen in the fetal shoulder. The anterior and posterior bands are seen as thick bands macroscopically.

rior glenoid, often referred to as the transepiphyseal line, while the posterior band commonly attaches slightly more inferior, below this transepiphyseal line posteriorly[10] (Fig. 18-7). On the humeral head side, the IGHLC attaches in a 90-degree arc below the articular margin of the humeral head. This is either in a collar-like or **V** shaped attachment (Fig. 18-8).

The concept of the IGHLC functioning as a hammock-like sling to support the humeral head gives a unifying mechanism for understanding anterior and posterior instability in the abducted shoulder, where most clinical instability occurs (Fig. 18-9). Biomechanical studies confirm the IGHLC to be the prime stabilizer with regard to the anterioposterior translation in the abducted shoulder, with the anterior band the prime

stabilizer in abduction and extension, and the posterior band the prime stabilizer in abduction and forward flexion.[4] In the 90-degree abducted position, there is reciprocal tightening of the IGHLC. With 90 degrees abduction and internal rotation, the posterior band and the axillary pouch fan out like a sail to support the humeral head posteriorly. The tension in the anterior band depends on the degree of horizontal flexion or extension, as well as the degree of rotation and elevation. With the arm abducted and forward flexed, the anterior band is relaxed, but with increasing horizontal extension the anterior band progressively tightens to become card-like. With 90 degrees of abduction and external rotation, the converse is true. The anterior band and axillary pouch fan out to cradle the humeral

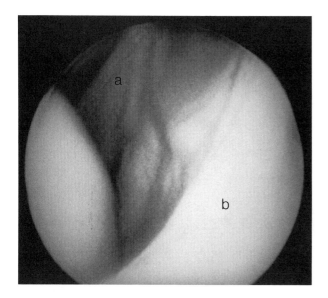

**Fig. 18-6.** An arthroscopic view anteriorly of the inferior glenohumeral ligament complex showing the anterior and posterior bands (*a,* anterior band; *b,* posterior band) and the intervening axillary pouch. (From Rockwood and Matsen,[21] with permission.)

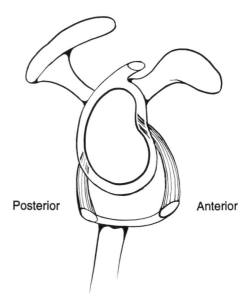

**Fig. 18-7.** View of the attachment sites for the anterior and posterior bands of the inferior glenohumeral ligament complex on the glenoid. Note that the anterior band attaches higher up on the comma-like glenoid than the posterior band.

head, and the posterior band tension changes from being tight and card-like in forward flexion to being fully relaxed in extension.

Surgically, to restore stability to the glenohumeral joint, the competence of the IGHLC must be restored. This means restoring an anterior anchor point on the glenoid and humerus (anterior band), a posterior anchor point (posterior band), and a competent axillary pouch in between. *All three* components must be present to restore full anatomic stability.

To understand the role the shoulder capsule plays in shoulder stability, it is often helpful to think of the shoulder capsule between the glenoid and humeral head as a circle (Fig. 18-10). For dislocation to occur in one direction, there must be damage to both sides of the capsule. Therefore, in cases of anterior instability to the shoulder, it is not surprising to see some increase in posterior laxity. Conversely, posterior dislocation cannot occur without anterior damage. Remember that the IGHLC is *one* structure, an inferior structure that spans both anteriorly *and* posteriorly.

Two areas of the capsule that we have not addressed yet are the posterior superior capsule above the posterior band of the IGHLC, and the rotator interval, which is the area between the subscapularis tendon and the supraspinatus. The posterior superior capsule plays a secondary role to the posterior band with regard to both anterior-posterior and superior-inferior stability.[4,8] This tissue also lacks the structural integrity of the IGHLC. Similarly, the tissue in the rotator interval lacks structural integrity. The coracohumeral ligament represents the capsule fold at the apex of the rotator interval. Warner et al[8] showed that this was a significant restraint to inferior translation in only one of 11 shoulders tested. However, in multidirectional instability, closing the rotator interval may make a significant difference because it effectively tightens the superior glenohumeral ligament region and also removes any redundancy in the midcapsular portion of the IGHLC. This effectively eliminates the sulcus sign. The senior author recently had a patient who had significant inferior instability with the arm at the side but had full

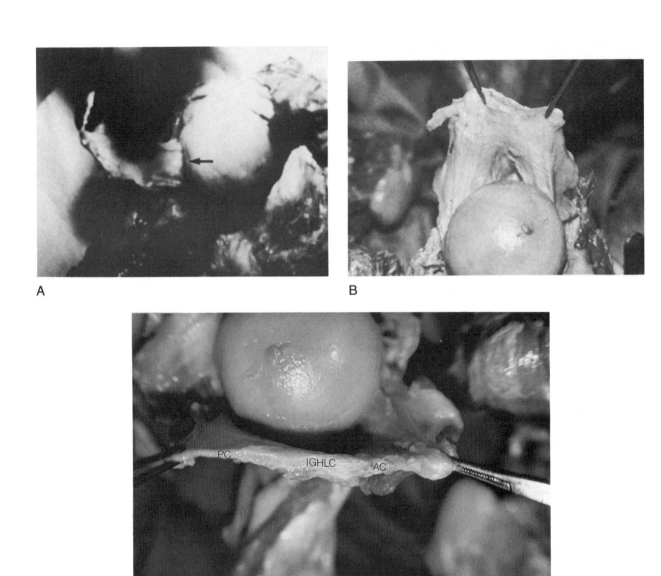

**Fig. 18-8.** (**A**) An example of a collar-like attachment of the inferior glenohumeral ligament complex just inferior to the articular edge and closer to the articular edge than the remainder of the capsule. Matsen, (**B**) A **V**-shaped attachment of the inferior glenohumeral ligament complex of the humerus, with the axillary pouch attaching to the humerus at the apex of the **V** farther from the articular edge. (**C**) The inferior glenohumeral ligament complex (*IGHLC*) is thicker than both the anterior capsule (*AC*) and the posterior capsule (*PC*). (From Rockwood and Matsen,[21] with permission.)

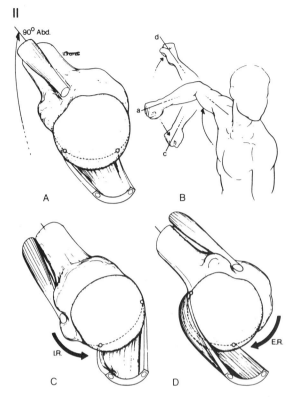

**Fig. 18-9. (A)** The inferior glenohumeral ligament complex is tightened during abduction. **(B)** During abduction and internal or external rotation different parts of the band are tightened. **(C)** With internal rotation the posterior band fans out to support the head, and the anterior band becomes cord-like or relaxed, depending on the degree of horizontal flexion or extension. **(D)** Upon abduction and external rotation, the anterior band fans out to support the head and the posterior band becomes cord-like or relaxed, depending on the degree of horizontal flexion or extension. (From Rockwood and Matsen,[21] with permission.)

stability when abducted to 90 degrees. This patient did quite well with closure of the rotator interval alone.

In trying to decide whether a particular case of anterior instability should be treated arthroscopically or open, it is important to recall the patient's history and demands on his shoulder. Do a thorough examination under anesthesia in varying degrees of abduction, flexion-extension, and internal-external rotation. Also

look for certain arthroscopic findings, especially whether the instability is from a detachment of the anterior band alone, from plastic deformation of the capsule, or both. Another sign of instability is a positive "drive-thru" sign, in which the arthroscope passes easily between the glenoid and humeral head. Elimination of this sign is an important endpoint for a technically successful arthroscopic stabilization.

Generally, a patient with low demand (non-contact sport), unidirectional instability, no excessive ligamentous laxity, and a lesion of the anterior band alone without excessive laxity of the axillary pouch is the ideal candidate for arthroscopic stabilization. Unfortunately, this does not represent the way in which the majority of patients present to the treating physician.

# SURGICAL TECHNIQUES TO CORRECT ANTERIOR INSTABILITY

Many operative procedures have been described to correct anterior shoulder instability. We will divide these into what we consider anatomic vs. non-anatomic techniques. Anatomic reconstructions seek to address primarily the pathologic anatomy, whereas non-anatomic reconstructions seek to create functional restraints that would limit excessive translation.

## Anatomic Reconstructions: Open

Anatomic anterior stabilizations include restoring competency to the IGHLC in patients with pure anterior instability, and to the IGHLC *plus* the superior glenohumeral ligament-rotator interval region in patients with multidirectional instability whose primary direction of instability is anterior. Restoring competency to the IGHLC involves a competent anterior band, competent posterior band, and competent axillary pouch. All three elements need to be addressed.

The concept of repairing the capsular-periosteal separation at the anterior glenoid neck was first proposed by Perthes, and later expounded upon by Bankart.[11–14] This technique attacks the pathology at its most com-

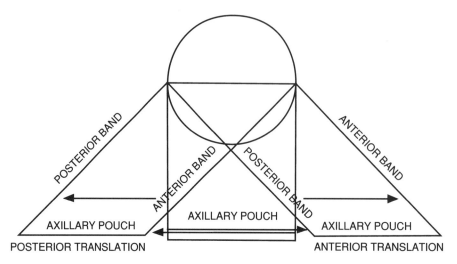

**Fig. 18-10.** The circle concept as a means to understand the role that the shoulder capsule plays in shoulder stability. Damage to both sides of the capsule, anterior and posterior, is required to produce dislocation in one direction.

mon site and is directed at reconstitution of the primary static stabilizer of the shoulder, the IGHLC. In this technique, the capsule is entered vertically at the junction of the capsule and the glenoid attachment medially. The anterior glenoid neck is then stripped of its periosteal soft tissue attachments and abraded to a roughhead bleeding surface. Three holes are then drilled in the glenoid margin and sutures are passed to advance the capsule medially and superiorly to address any redundancy. This glenoid periosteal soft tissue is then sutured back over the advanced reattached medial capsule. In a long-term review of 50 patients treated by Bankart and his colleagues between 1925 and 1954, recurrent instability occurred in only two patients.[15] Rowe et al[16] noted a 3.5 percent recurrence rate in 145 patients with the Bankart procedure with 69 percent of the patients regaining full range of motion. DuToit popularized a similar procedure (Fig. 18-11) in which the detached capsule secured back to the glenoid using staples.[17,18] However, the use of staples for surgical repairs may be associated with major complications.[19]

Although the Bankart procedure has been the gold standard for anatomic repairs, it does not address situations in which excessive laxity is present in addition to a Bankart lesion, or the many cases of multidirectional

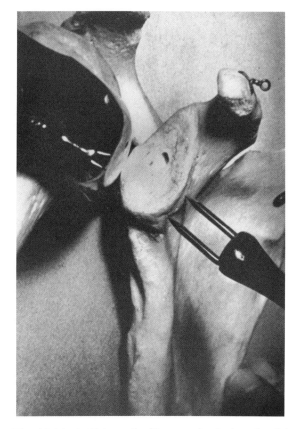

**Fig. 18-11.** DuToit staple. (See text for further details.)

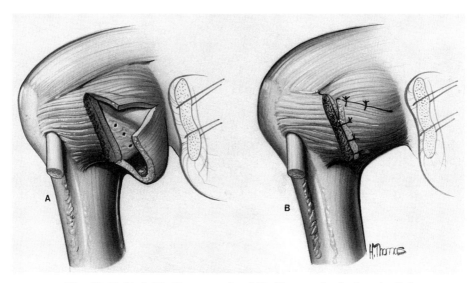

**Fig. 18-12 (A & B).** Neer capsular shift. (See text for further details.)

instability in which no Bankart lesion is present. Addressing these situations, and in some part because of the ease of exposure, lateral capsular procedures were developed. Neer and Foster[20] developed an inferior capsular shift procedure for multidirectional instability where laxity is addressed on the lateral margin of the capsule at the humeral neck, and the tissue is advanced laterally and superiorly (Fig. 18-12). Matsen and Thomas also popularized a lateral approach in which the subscapularis is taken down as one unit (Fig. 18-13). With these techniques, a Bankart lesion must be repaired as a separate step. Altchek et al[22] described a T-plasty modification of the Bankart procedure for multidirectional instability in which two capsular incisions are used: a transverse one in the mid portion of the capsule and a vertical one at the glenoid margin. The vertical incision is made first to inspect the joint for a Bankart lesion with repair as needed. The T portion allows for an inferior flap to be advanced superiorly, and a superior flap inferiorly (Fig. 18-14). Finally, Rockwood and Matsen[21] described a midcapsular repair in which the capsule is divided vertically midway between its usual attachment on the glenoid rim and the humeral head (Fig. 18-15). A Bankart type of repair is performed medially if necessary, and the capsule is "double-breasted" by taking the medial capsule later-ally and superiorly, and the lateral capsule medially and superiorly.

## Authors' Preferred Method of Treatment

### Rotator Interval Approach

The subscapularis is divided in its tendinous portion to fully expose the anterior capsule. The lower-most muscular fibers of the subscapularis are left intact, however, below the tendinous portion. This allows for full visualization of the thin rotator interval and region of the superior glenohumeral ligament. Often there is a natural opening in this rotator interval, which varies in size and shape and which corresponds to the subscapularis bursa opening. The senior author takes advantage of this open and/or thin area to enter the glenohumeral joint. This is an area that he will close anyway and it allows him to visualize the joint to decide if he will approach the joint laterally or medially. For this reason he does not use the Jobe subscapularis split.[23] It is difficult with that technique to adequately visualize and tension a large rotator interval in his hands.

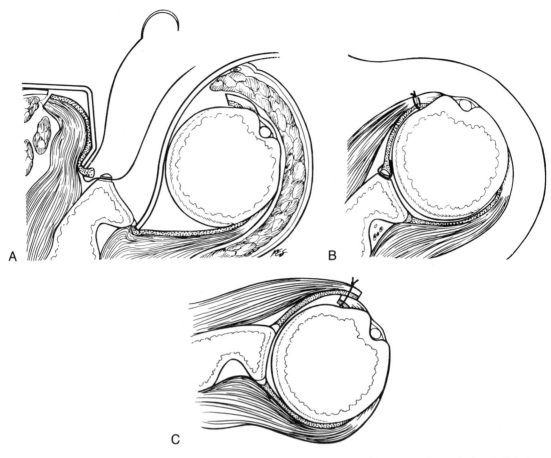

**Fig. 18-13.** (**A**) Transverse plane section passage of a No. 2 nonabsorbable suture through the drill hole and into the capsule. Note the use of a deep right-angle retractor on the subscapularis and superficial capsule to afford the necessary exposure for proper placement of the suture. (**B**) Transverse plane section showing the completed repair of a Bankart lesion and the anatomical repair of an incision through the subscapularis and the capsule. (**C**) Transverse plane secton showing reefing of the subscapularis tendon and capsule in a situation where no Bankart lesion is found with isolated anterior instability. Note the intact anterior glenoid rim and the strong repair of the subscapularis tendon. (Modified from Matsen and Thomas,[51] with permission.)

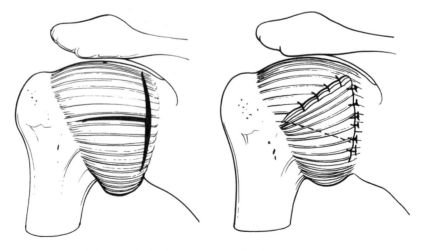

**Fig. 18-14.** T-plasty. (See text for further details.)

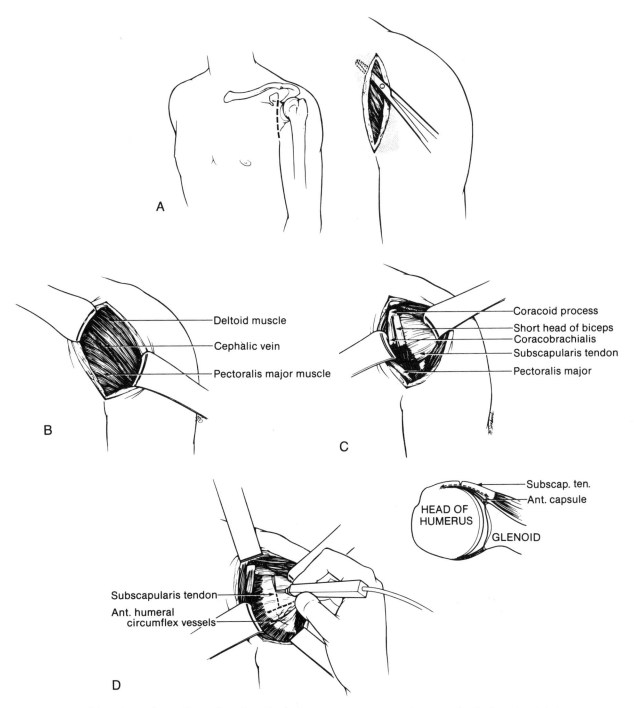

**Fig. 18-15 (A–S).** Rockwood's preferred method of operative treatment. (See text for further details.) (*Figure continues.*)

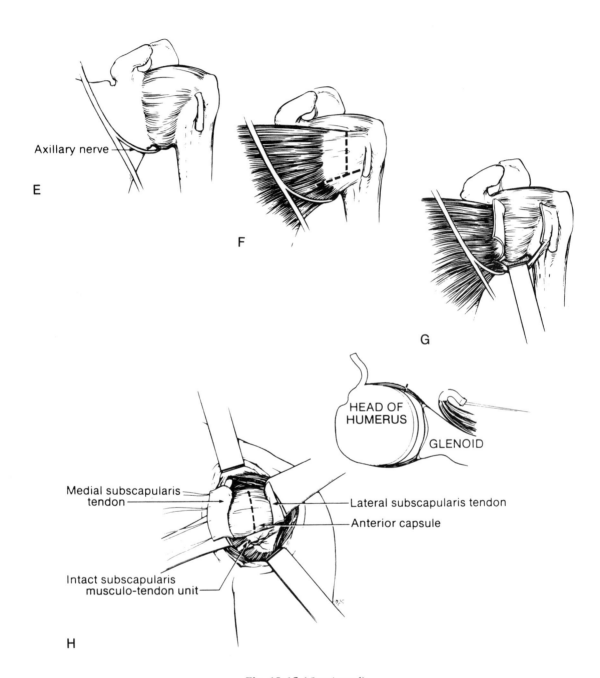

Fig. 18-15 (*Continued*).

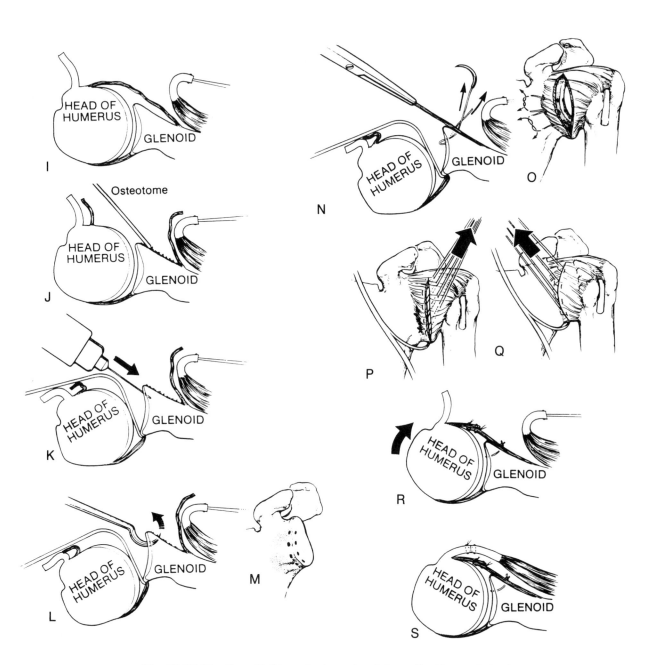

**Fig. 18-15** (*Continued*). (From Rockwood and Green,[52] with permission.)

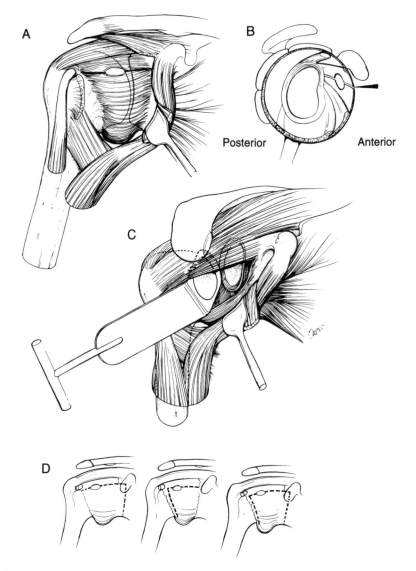

**Fig. 18-16.** Author's (SJO) preferred method of operative treatment. (See text for further details.)

A transverse incision is made in the thin rotator interval using any natural opening and is carried medially to the capsulolabral edge. A Facuda retractor is then placed inside the glenohumeral joint to visualize the anterior labrum and capsule inferiorly without making a linear incision (Fig. 18-16). If there is no Bankart lesion, then either a lateral capsular shift or a pants-over-vest closure of the rotator interval will be performed, depending on the degree of laxity encountered. This will advance the anterior band in the mid-capsule axillary pouch superiorly, eliminating anterior and inferior laxity.

If a Bankart lesion is encountered, then this area is exposed, not by a vertical incision medially, but rather by a stripping of the whole capsulo-labral-periosteal envelope. This envelope is peeled off the

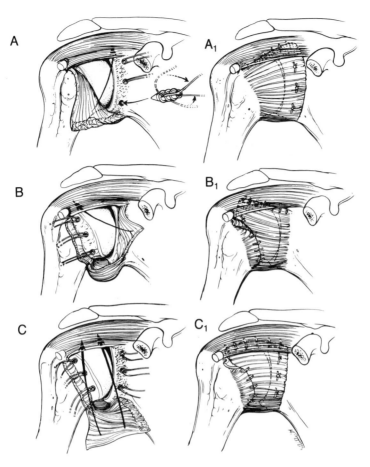

**Fig. 18-17.** (**A**) Medial capsular advancement on glenoid neck with rotator interval imbrication; (**B**) Lateral advancement; (**C**) H-plasty. (See text for further details.)

anterior glenoid rim and neck as one unit. With tension generated with the Facuda retractor, a scalpel tears this tissue carefully off the glenoid neck down to the 6 o'clock position, which represents the middle of the axillary pouch of the IGHLC. This technique avoids inadvertently risking limiting external rotation by making a vertical incision too far laterally in the capsule, especially in the lower portion of this incision where it often can be quite difficult to stay medially at the capsular-labral edge.

The anterior glenoid neck is then abraded with a power burr, and three suture anchors are used at the edge of the glenoid rim.[24] Next, the medial capsular complex is advanced superiorly and secured. The remaining laxity is then eliminated by a pants-over-vest

closure of the rotator interval, or in extreme circumstances, by a vertical lateral incision, which creates a type of H plasty in which the capsular advancement simulates the bottom half of the letter H (Fig. 18-17). This inferior tissue is then advanced superiorly and laterally, followed by the pants-over-vest rotator interval closure. The arm is then put through a range of motion to ensure proper tensioning, and the subscapularis tendon is repaired without advancement.

## Non-anatomic Reconstructions: Open

Over the years, many non-anatomic operative procedures have been described for treatment of anterior instability. In these procedures, stability is achieved

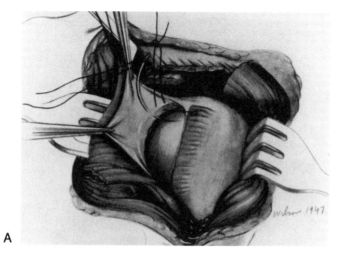

A

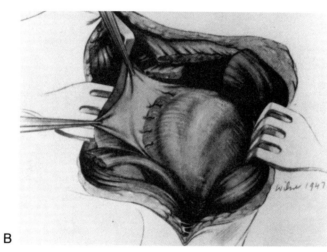

B

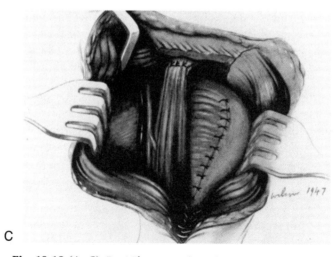

C

**Fig. 18-18** (**A–C**). Putti-Platt procedure. (See text for further details.)

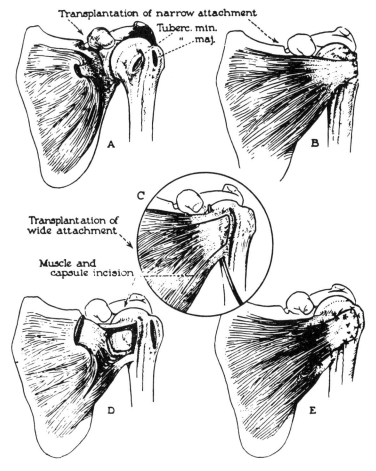

Transplantation of narrow attachment
Tuberc. min.
" ...maj.

A

B

C

Transplantation of
wide attachment

Muscle and
capsule incision

D

E

**Fig. 18-19 (A–E).** Magnuson-Stack procedure. (See text for further details.)

either by restricting range of motion, creating a bony buttress to excessive translation, creating new suspensory ligaments, or by osteotomy of the proximal humerus. Although most of these procedures are no longer used routinely by most shoulder surgeons, a few have survived the test of time and are, therefore, noteworthy.

### Subscapularis Muscle Procedures

In 1956, Carr stated, "I wish to emphasize that completely normal scapulohumeral motion should not be the requirement for an excellent result . . . restriction of movement is the price paid willingly for stability and full confidence in the shoulder."[25] DePalma believed that the limitation of external rotation was the

key to preventing recurrent anterior instability of the shoulder and that the surgeon should adopt the simplest procedure that accomplished this limitation.[26] It was in this spirit that the Putti-Platt and Magnuson-Stack procedures became popular.

In the Putti-Platt procedure, the subscapularis tendon and capsule are divided 2.5 cm medial to the bony insertion (Fig. 18-18). The lateral edge of the tendon and capsule are then sutured to the tissue and labrum at the glenoid rim or undersurface of the capsule and subscapularis medially. The medial edge of the incised tissue is then pulled laterally and sutured to the cuff at the greater tuberosity.

The Magnuson-Stack procedure involves transfer of the subscapularis tendon and lateral capsule down-

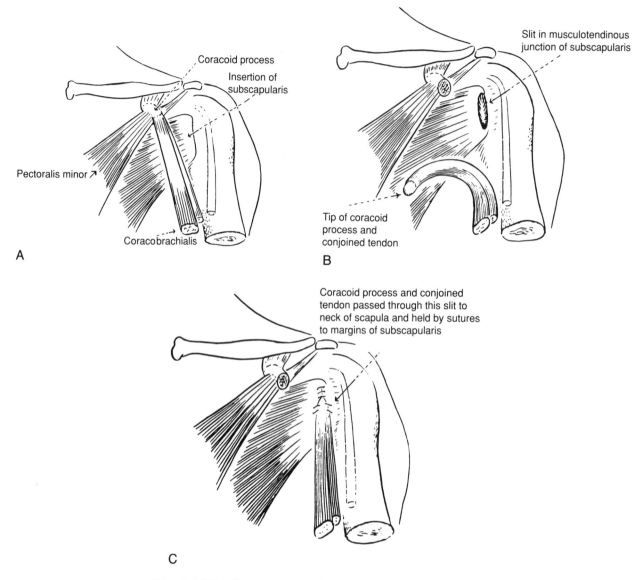

**Fig. 18-20 (A–C).** Bristow procedure. (See text for further details.)

ward and outward to a position lateral to the bicipital groove, and just below the greater tuberosity (Fig. 18-19). This is attached to the shaft of the humerus into a bone through use of sutures, a staple, or a boat nail. This was designed to be a static and dynamic muscle sling anteroinferiorly to stabilize the glenohumeral joint.[27]

Although both of these procedures may be effective in unidirectional anterior instability, the often severe limitations to motion and function may accelerate wear in the joint, making these procedures unacceptable, especially for an athlete who requires full or near-full range of motion.

## Bone Block Procedures

Two bone block procedures have been popular: the Bristow procedure, a type of coracoid transfer procedure, and the Eden-Hybbinette procedure in which the bone block is obtained from a distant site, the iliac crest.[28–30]

The Bristow procedure was first described in 1958 by Helfet, who credited Bristow with a bone-block coracoid transfer operation in which the tip of the coracoid with the conjoined tendon attached is trans-ferred to the inferior aspect of the glenoid rim (Fig. 18-20).[29] The procedure was designed to reinforce the defective anterior portion of the joint and create a bone block to restrict translation. It was also felt to have a tendonizing effect on the subscapularis, preventing the subscapularis from moving upward as the arm is ab-

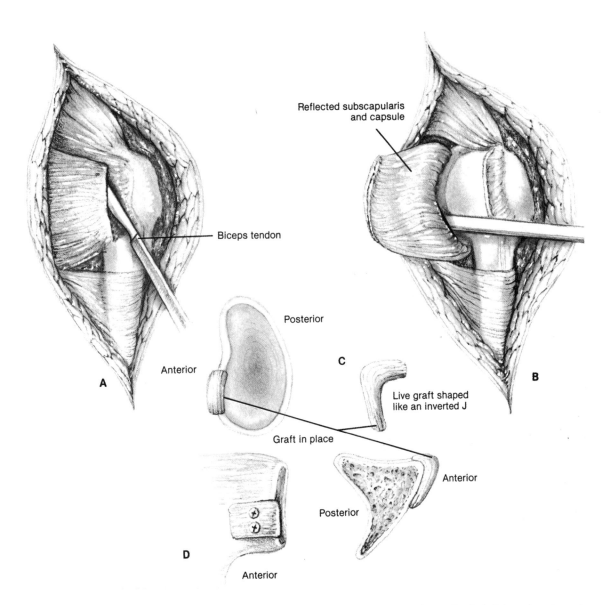

**Fig. 18-21.** Eden-Hybbinette operation. (**A**) The subscapularis tendon and capsule are divided. (**B**) A subperiosteal pocket is developed in the anteroinferior aspect of the neck of the scapula; the osteotome is under the labrum. (**C**) The iliac graft is shaped like an inverted **J** and inserted into the pocket and fixed with one or two screws. (**D**) The graft is anchored to the glenoid neck with two screws. (From DePalma,[26] with permission.)

ducted. Many modifications of the procedure have been described; in the most popular, by May,[31] the subscapularis is divided vertically in the tendinous portion and then horizontally into superior and inferior halves that are then reattached around the transferred coracoid, half above and half below the fixed coracoid tip on the glenoid.

The Eden-Hybinette operation creates an anterior buttress with a J-shaped iliac crest graft on the anterioinferior portion of the glenoid, which is transfixed with one or two screws (Fig. 18-21). This may be efficient in cases of glenoid deficiency. The goal of the procedure is to increase the buttress effect of the anterior glenoid.

Bone-block procedures, when done in isolation, also fail to address anteroinferior capsulolabral insufficiency. The concept of an anterior bony buttress may be invalid, particularly in patients who are subluxing. Hardware problems are common and injuries to the musculoskeletal nerve have been reported with the Bristow procedure from traction with the coracoid transfer.[19,32,33] In addition, a revision stabilization procedure is difficult following a failed Bristow procedure due to extensive scarring of the anterior capsular and subscapularis tendon.[34]

## Suspensory Procedures

Suspensory procedures propose to create a suspensory ligament for holding the humeral head suspended

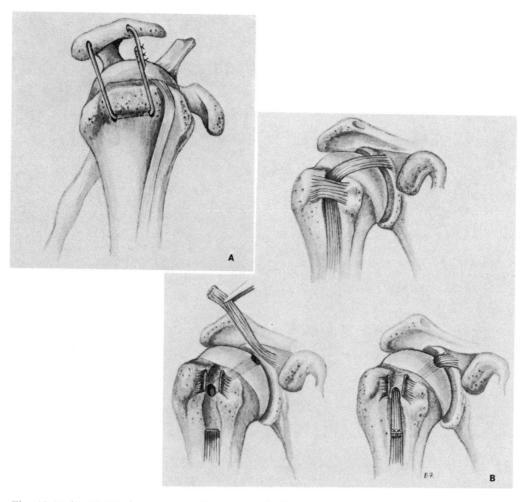

**Fig. 18-22 (A–B).** Nicola procedure. (See text for further details; from DePalma,[26] with permission.)

from the glenoid fossa. The Nicola and the Gallie procedures are the best known of these.[35,36]

In the Nicola procedure the long head of the biceps tendon is used as a suspensory ligament (Fig. 18-22).[36] The biceps tendon is divided at the distal end of the bicipital groove and then passed through a drill hole in the humeral head and reattached to its distal stump.

In the Gallie procedure (Fig. 18-23), a slug of fascia lata is used to suspend the humeral head by passing the fascia lata through a drill hole in the inferior half of the glenoid, then up through the humeral head, and then further up through a drill hole in the acromion.[35]

The Nicola procedure has had high recurrence rates (between 30 and 50 percent) and is no longer used, although the Gallie procedure and modifications of it, using the semitendinous and gracilis muscles, have been used as salvage procedures in cases of current instability as an alternative to shoulder fusion.[37,38]

### Osteotomy of the Proximal Humerus

Weber reported in 1969, and again in 1984, on rotational osteotomy in patients who have concurrent anterior instability and large defects in the posterolateral humeral head (Hill Sach's deformity.[39,40] This increases the retroversion of the humeral head, limiting the amount of exposed humeral head over the anterior glenoid and avoiding contact of the large head defect

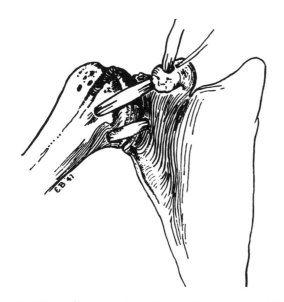

**Fig. 18-23.** Gallie procedure. (See text for further details.)

on the glenoid rim (Fig. 18-24). This procedure was combined with a shortening of the subscapularis muscle and anterior capsular reefing. Although the reported redislocation rate is low (5.7 percent), it is hard to determine how much of an effect the osteotomy itself had because of the concomitant capsular reefing. Also, most patients required reoperation for plate removal.

### Arthroscopic Stabilization Procedures

Arthroscopic stabilization techniques have generated a great deal of interest in the orthopaedic community since the introduction of arthroscopic staple capsulorraphy by Johnson in the early 1980s.[41] Arthroscopic techniques offer the advantage of less perioperative pain and morbidity. The reported risk of recurrence after arthroscopic stabilization, however, is higher (between 15 and 20 percent) than that after an open procedure.[42-45] Recently, Morgan and Bidenstab[43] reported a recurrence rate of only 5 percent after 1- to 7-year follow-up of 175 patients who had undergone an anterior stabilization using a transglenoid suture technique.

Currently, the indications for an arthroscopic stabilization is fairly narrow. The ideal candidate is a patient with recurrent anterior subluxation or dislocation who has demonstrated detachment of a stout, well defined IGHLC-labral complex on arthroscopic examination, without significant sulcus sign on preoperative examination. Patients with a positive sulcus sign or an attenuated, patulous anterior and inferior capsule are less likely to have a favorable result.[46] In properly selected candidates, however, there is a strong possibility that arthroscopic techniques will improve the results of the operative treatment of instability in throwers. In the series by Rowe et al,[16] only 69 percent of those patients treated by open Bankart procedure regained full motion, and less than one-third of the throwing athletes were able to return to their premorbid level of pitching. On the other hand, Morgan[47] reported recovery of full range of motion in 87 percent of the first 55 patients that he treated arthroscopically, and Warner et al[46] recently reported that 75 percent of overhead athletes stabilized arthroscopically with a biodegradable tac were able to return to their preinjury level of function.

Currently most of the experience with arthroscopic techniques is with two procedures. The first type of

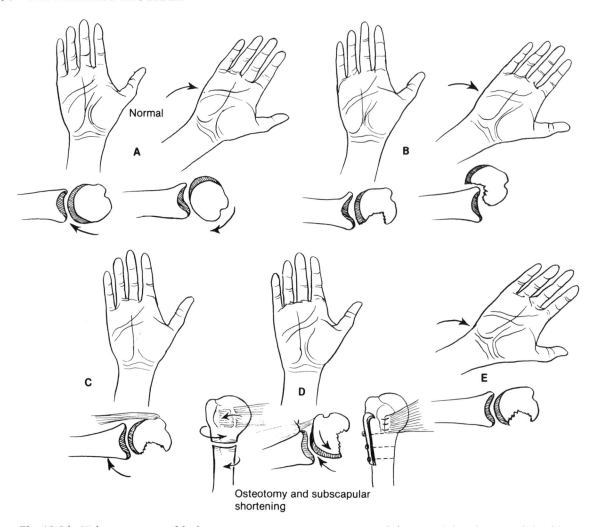

**Fig. 18-24.** Weber osteotomy of the humerus to prevent recurrent anterior dislocation. (**A**) In the normal shoulder, during external rotation, the posterior articular surface of the humeral head is in contact with the glenoid fossa. (**B**) In the presence of a large defect in the posterolateral aspect of the humeral head, the articulating surface area is decreased so that on external rotation the anterior glenoid rim drops into the defect. (**C–E**) By increasing the retroversion of the humeral head by an osteotomy and shortening the subscapularis tendon, on external rotation the defect does not engage the glenoid rim. (Modified from Weber,[39] with permission.)

stabilization employs sutures that are passed through drill holes in the glenoid neck and tied posteriorly. The second type of stabilization involves the use of a biodegradable tac. The use of metal hardware around the shoulder is not recommended for routine use because of problems with implant loosening over time and the potential for articular injury.[19]

The arthroscopic suture technique involves an ana-tomic repair of the anterior band of the IGHLC, taking whatever laxity out of the axillary pouch that can be achieved by advancing the anterior band superiorly (Fig. 18-25).[43,47]

Morgan and Caspari[48] have reported good results with this technique in carefully selected patients. Mor-gan reported a recurrence rate of only 5 percent in 175 patients with one- to seven-year follow-up. Of-

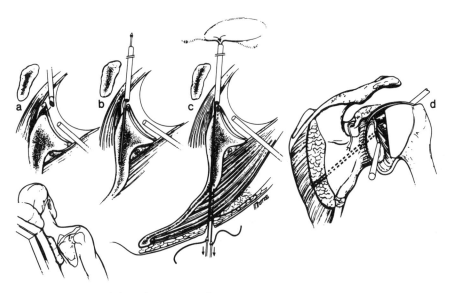

**Fig. 18-25 (A–D).** Suture technique. (See text for further details.)

falmeier and Caspari similarly reported a 4 percent recurrence rate in over 200 patients (unpublished data). Potential complications of the suture technique include injury to the suprascapular nerve posteriorly and the potential for a sinus and subsequent cyst posteriorly (S. J. O'Brien, personal communication). Trans-

glenoid drilling can also be technically quite difficult, especially when multiple drill holes are used and sutures from separate holes need to be tried posteriorly.

The use of a cannulated biodegradable tac (Acufex Inc., Norwood, MA) made from polyglyconate has been designed and popularized by Warren (Fig. 18-26).[49,50]

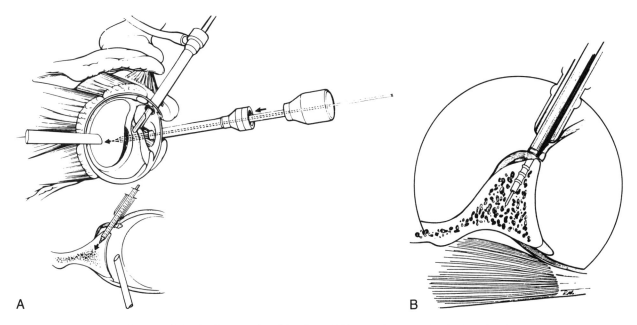

**Fig. 18-26 (A & B).** Cannulated biodegradable tax. (See text for further details.)

The early results are currently being reviewed but appear to be similar to the transglenoid suture technique (M. J. Pagnani, personal communication). It also avoids potential problems posteriorly from transglenoid drilling. The surgical technique involves a Bankart-type advancement similar to the suture technique. The strength of the tac diminishes over a four-week period. Robs on the shaft of the tac increase its pullant strength to approximately 100 Newton. The tac also has a broad flat head, allowing it to capture soft tissue. In some patients a combination of the suture and tac techniques may be needed for optimum tensioning of the tissue. In this situation, sutures are used superiorly to tension the tissues, and then a tac is placed at the four o'clock position to close the defect.

## REHABILITATION FOLLOWING ANTERIOR STABILIZATION PROCEDURE

Successful rehabilitation following anterior stabilization procedures requires a physical therapist with knowledge and experience in this area. The "feel" that is needed to progress a patient is a result of proper supervised training in this area and substantial patient experience.

Most patients require sling immobilization for three to four weeks, depending on the surgeon's confidence in the repairs. The patient then starts a program of progressive passive, active assisted, and active range of motion. Appendix 18-1 outlines the timetable for progression of therapy. It must be emphasized that normal scapulohumeral rhythm requires a complete parascapular muscle strengthening program, and that functional rehabilitation includes total body conditioning during the rehabilitation process, especially in throwing athletes.

## ACKNOWLEDGMENT

The authors would like to thank Stephen Fries, P.A., for his technical assistance.

## REFERENCES

1. Harryman DT, Sidles JA, Clark JM, McQuade KJ: Translation of the humeral head on the glenoid with passive glenohumeral motion. J Bone Joint Surg 72A:1334, 1990
2. Harryman DT, Sidles JA, Harris SL, Matsen FA: Role of the rotator interval capsule in passive motion and stability of the shoulder. J Bone Joint Surg 72A:53, 1990
3. O'Brien SJ, Neves MC, Arnoczky SP, et al: The anatomy and histology of the inferior glenohumeral ligament complex. Am J Sports Med 18:449, 1990
4. O'Brien SJ, Schartz R, Warren RF, Torzilli PT: Capsular restraints to anterior-posterior motion of the abducted shoulder: a biomechanical study. (submitted)
5. Oveson J, Nielson S: Experimental distal subluxation in the glenohumeral joint. Arch Orthop Trauma Surg 104:78, 1985
6. Oveson J, Nielson S: Anterior and posterior instability: a cadaver study. Acta Orthop Scand 57:324, 1986
7. Oveson J, Nielson S: Posterior instability of the shoulder: a cadaver study. Acta Orthop Scand 57:436, 1986
8. Warner JJP, Warren RF: Arthroscopic Bankart repair using a cannulated, absorbable fixation device. Operative Tech Orthop 1:192, 1991
9. Pagnani MJ: The effects of the long head of the biceps brachii on glenohumeral translation. Paper presented at The Fellows Research Program, The Hospital for Special Surgery, New York, NY, June, 1993
10. DePalma AF, Callery G, Bennett GA: Variational anatomy and degenerative lesions of the shoulder joint In AAOS Instr Course Lect 7:255, 1949
11. Bankart ASB: Recurrent or habitual dislocation of the shoulder joint. Br Med J 2:1132, 1923
12. Bankart ASB: The pathology and treatment of recurrent dislocation of the shoulder joint. Br J Surg 26:23, 1938
13. Bankart ASB: Discussion on recurrent dislocation of the shoulder. J Bone Joint Surg 30B:46–47, 1948
14. Perthes G: Uber operationen der habituellen Schulterluxation. Deutsche Ztschr f Chir 85:199, 1906
15. Dickson JW, Duvas MB: Bankart's operation for recurrent dislocation of the shoulder. J Bone Joint Surg 39B:114, 1957
16. Rowe CR, Patel D, Southmayd WW: The Bankart procedure: a long term end-result study. J Bone Joint Surg 60A:1, 1978
17. DuToit GT, Roux D: Recurrent dislocation of the shoulder. A 24-year study of the Johannesburg stapling operation. J Bone Joint Surg 38A:1, 1956
18. Sisk TD, Boyd HB: Management of recurrent anterior dislocation of the shoulder. DeToit type or staple capsulorraphy. Clin Orthop 103:150, 1974

19. Zuckerman JD, Matsen FA: Complications about the glenohumeral joint related to the use of screws and staples. J Bone Joint Surg 66A:175, 1984

20. Neer CS, Foster CR: Inferior capsular shift for involuntary inferior and multidirectional instability of the shoulder. A preliminary report. J Bone Joint Surg 62A:897, 1980

21. Rockwood CA, Jr., Matsen FA: The Shoulder. WB Saunders, Philadelphia, 1990

22. Altchek DW, Warren RF, Skyhar MJ, Ortiz G: T-plasty modification of the Bankart procedure for multidirectional instability of the anterior and inferior types. J Bone Joint Surg 73A:105, 1991

23. Jobe FW, Giangarra CE, Kvitne RS, Glousman RE: Anterior capsulolabral reconstruction of the shoulder in athletes in overhead sports. Am J Sports Med 19:428, 1991

24. Richmond JC, Donaldson WR, Fu FH, Harner CD: Modification of the Bankart reconstruction with a suture anchor. Report of a new technique. Am J Sports Med 19:343, 1991

25. Carr CR: In discussion of prognosis in dislocations of the shoulder. J Bone Joint Surg 38A:977, 1956

26. DePalma AF: Surgery of the Shoulder. JB Lippincott, Philadelphia, 1950

27. Regan WD, Webster-Bogaert S, Hawkins RJ, Fowler PJ: Comparative functional analysis of the Bristow, Magnuson-Stack, and Putti-Platt procedures for recurrent dislocation of the shoulder. Am J Sports Med 17:42, 1989

28. Eden R: Zur operativen Behandlung der habituellen Schulterluxation unter mitteilung, eines neuen Verfahrens bei abriss am inneren Pfannenrande. Deutsche Z Chir 144:269, 1918

29. Helfet AJ: Coracoid transplantation for recurring dislocation of the shoulder. J Bone Joint Surg 40B:198, 1948

30. Hybbinette S: De la transplantation d'un fragment osseux pour remedier aux luxations recidivantes de l'epaule; constatations et resultats operatiores. Acta Chir Scand 71:411, 1932

31. May VR: A modified Bristow operation for anterior recurrent dislocation of the shoulder. J Bone Joint Surg 52A:1010, 1970

32. Bach BR, O'Brien SJ, Warren RF, Leighton M: Unusual neurological complications of the Bristow procedure: a case report. J Bone Joint Surg 70A:3, 1988

33. Schauder KS, Tullos HS: Role of the coracoid bone block in the Bristow procedure. Am J Sports Med 20:31, 1992

34. Young DC, Rockwood CA: Complications of a failed Bristow procedure and their management. J Bone Joint Surg 73A:969, 1991

35. Gallie WE, Le Mesurier AB: An operation for the relief of recurring dislocation of the shoulder. Trans Am Surg Assoc 45:392, 1927

36. Nicola T: Recurrent dislocation of the shoulder: its treatment by transplantation of the long head of the biceps. Am J Surg 6:815, 1929

37. Carpenter GI, Millard PH: Shoulder subluxation in elderly inpatients. J Am Geriatr Soc 30:441, 1982

38. Jones FW: Attainment of upright position of man. Nature 146:26, 1940

39. Weber BG: Operative treatment of recurrent dislocation of the shoulder. Injury 1:107, 1969

40. Weber BG, Simpson LA, Hardegger F: Rotational humeral osteotomy for anterior dislocation of the shoulder associated with a large Hill-Sachs lesion. J Bone Joint Surg 66A:1443, 1984

41. Johnson LL: Symposium on Arthroscopy. Arthroscopic Association of North America Annual Meeting, San Francisco, CA, March, 1986

42. Hawkins RB: Arthroscopic stapling repair for shoulder instability: a retrospective study of 50 cases. Arthroscopy 5:122, 1989

43. Morgan CD, Bodenstab AB: Arthroscopic Bankart suture repair: technique and early results. Arthroscopy 3:111, 1987

44. Wiley AM: Arthroscopy for shoulder instability and a technique for arthroscopic repair. Arthroscopy 4:25, 1988

45. Yahiro MA, Matthews LA: Arthroscopic stabilization procedures for recurrent anterior shoulder instability. Orthop Rev 11:1161, 1989

46. Warner JJP, Xiang-Hua D, Warren RF, Torzilli PA: Static capsuloligamentous restraints to superior-inferior translation of the glenohumeral joint. Am J Sports Med 20:675, 1992

47. Morgan CD: Arthroscopic transglenoid Bankart suture repair. Operative Tech Orthop 1:171, 1991

48. Caspari R, Savoie F: Arthroscopic reconstruction of the shoulder: the Bankart repair. p. 507. In McGinty J et al (eds): Operative Arthroscopy Raven Press, 1991

49. Warner JJP, Pagnani MJ, Warren RF, Kavanaugh J, Montgomery W: Arthroscopic Bankart repair with an absorbable, cannulated fixation device Orthop Trans 15:761, 1991

50. Warren RF: Surgical technique for Suretac. Acufex Microsurgical, Inc., Mansfield, MA, 1991

51. Matsen FA, Thomas SC: Glenohumeral instability. In Evarts CM (ed): Surgery of the Musculoskeletal System. 2nd Ed. Churchill Livingstone, New York, 1989

52. Rockwood CA, Green DP (eds): Fractures. 2nd Ed. JB Lippincott, Philadelphia, 1984

# Appendix 18-1

# Anterior Stabilization Rehabilitation

### Phase 1 (0–6 Weeks)

*Weeks 1–3*
 Sling for 4 weeks
 Pendulum exercises (Day 1)
 Submaximal isometrics in the neutral position
  (Week 1–3)
  Include scapular stabilizing musculature
 Protect anterior capsule from stretch
  Passive range of motion external rotation to 30°
   (Week 3)

*Weeks 4–6*
 Modalities as needed
 Active assistive upper body ergometer
  Range of motion
  Warmup
 Active assistive range of motion exercises for forward
   flexion
  Pulleys
  Wand exercises
 Passive range of motion
  Forward flexion to 140° (Week 4–5)
  Forward flexion to 180° (Week 6)
  External rotation to 45°–50° (Week 6)
  Passive range of motion isokinetics Continuous
   passive motion mode (Week 4)
 Joint mobilization
  Glenohumeral joint (posterior glides)
  Sternoclavicular joint
 Theraband exercises (Week 4–6)
  Internal rotation
  External rotation to 20°
  Scapular stabilizers

### Phase 2 (6–10 Weeks)

Continue with present treatment program
Active range of motion for full range of motion
 Forward flexion
 Internal rotation
 Horizontal adduction
Passive range of motion external rotation to 65°–70°
 (Week 10)
Theraband (light dumb-bells)
 Full internal rotation
 External rotation to 45°
 Scapular stabilizers
Isokinetics
 Continuous passive motion mode
  "Light" eccentrics (limited arc) (Week 8)
   Active assisted range of motion progressive
    resistance exercises (limited arc) (Week 8)

### Phase 3 (Weeks 10–16)

Full external rotation (12 Weeks)
 Pitcher external rotation to 110°–120° (Week 16)
Restore scapulohumeral rhythm
Isokinetics
 Sub-maximal (60°–90°/sec) (10 Weeks)
 Limited arc
 Neutral position
Isotonics/progressive resistance exercises
 Pain free/limited arcs
 Light weight/high reps
 Deltoid
 Rotator cuff

Scapular stabilizers
Kinesthetic training
Advance eccentric training (12 Weeks)

### Phase 4 (16–24 Weeks)

Advance isokinetics
Advance progressive resistance exercises
Increase weights
Decrease reps
Start overhead and abduction progressive resistance exercises
Start power activities
Free weight/medicine balls
Isokinetic testing (20 Weeks)

Ratio of internal rotation : external rotation
3 : 2
3 : 3
All others 80%–85% strength
Endurance program
Sport specific activities
Upper body ergometer
Intergrate strength/power program
Whole upper quarter
Lower extremities
Begin supervised throwing/racquet program

### Phase 5 (24–28 Weeks)

Eliminate strength/power deficits
Return to full activity

# 19

# Posterior Instability of the Shoulder

*DOROTHY F. SCARPINATO*
*JAMES R. ANDREWS*

Shoulder instability was a recognized entity as early as 3000 BC, as the murals in Egyptian tombs depicted glenohumeral dislocations.[1] In the fifth century BC, Hippocrates described dislocations resulting from injury and classified these as "traumatic"; he classified voluntary dislocations as "atraumatic." Another category has been added to the classification scheme, which has been called "acquired." In this group, repetitive activities have led to loosening of the shoulder, such as throwing, swimming, weight lifting, and gymnastics. Most of these instabilities are anterior, but in the athlete, posterior instability is increasingly being recognized as a separate and real entity.

The incidence of posterior instability varies in the literature and has been reported in 2 to 4 percent of patients presenting with an unstable shoulder.[2,3] The literature on posterior dislocation and subluxation is not very extensive; therefore, the exact incidence is difficult to determine.

In this chapter, the etiology, mechanism of injury, diagnosis, and treatment modalities of posterior instability in the athlete are discussed.

## ANATOMY AND BIOMECHANICS
### Glenohumeral Joint

The glenohumeral joint is composed of the articular surfaces of the glenoid cavity and the head of the humerus.[4] Alone, these two bony structures have very little inherent stability. The joint is surrounded by a thin articular capsule, within which are thickened bands anteriorly known as the glenohumeral ligaments. The posterior capsule is quite thin and does not possess any distinct capsular bands of reinforcement. The capsule attaches to the glenoid labrum, which attaches to the edge of the glenoid circumferentially. The labrum augments the glenoid cavity, which deepens the socket and cushions the bony impact as the joint moves through a range of motion.[5] The glenoid is approximately one-quarter to one-half the diameter of the humeral head; with the addition of the labrum, the diameter of the glenoid surface increases to 75 percent of the humeral head.[6]

### Rotator Cuff

The rotator cuff surrounds the capsule superiorly, anteriorly, and posteriorly and is closely apposed to it. It comprises the supraspinatus, subscapularis, infraspinatus, and teres minor, which with their tendinous attachments aid in stabilizing the joint by holding the head of the humerus in the glenoid cavity. The infraspinatus and teres minor provide passive restraints posteriorly.

Warren et al[3,7] dissected the structures responsible for static posterior shoulder stability. Incising the infraspinatus and teres minor did not cause significant posterior instability. They also selectively cut the posterior capsule from the 9-o'clock to the 12-o'clock position and found no increase in posterior instability. When the capsule was cut to the 6-o'clock position, the shoulder started to sublux posteriorly. It was not until the capsule was incised from 1 to 3 o'clock, including the superior glenohumeral ligament, that the shoulder dislocated posteriorly. They also found posterior subluxation occurred when the entire inferior capsule was cut from the anterior border of the inferior glenohumeral ligament to the superior edge of the posterior porch of the inferior glenohumeral ligament.

## Athletic Movements/Throwing Motion

As the shoulder exceeds the limits of its physiologic range of motion, it begins to strain the capsule and ligaments; with further motion, it can ride out of the glenoid and over the labrum. A subluxation may be so transient that the athlete does not recognize the event. The degree of flexibility and normal joint motion varies; those who have an increased degree of motion may have generalized ligamentous laxity.[8] In these individuals, the humeral head can lose contact with the glenoid at extremes of motion. Physiologic subluxation is necessary to perform certain athletic events, such as gymnastics. Thus, the division between shoulder stability and subluxation can be difficult to define.[8]

During pitching, throwing, and use of the racquet in tennis, the arm undergoes three phases of action: cocking, acceleration, and follow-through. During follow-through, the arm continues forward into internal rotation and horizontal adduction after the ball has left the hand.[6] The posterior musculature creates a decelerating torque that has been calculated to equal approximately one times the body weight of the thrower. The follow-through phase of throwing appears to stress the posterior and inferior capsule.[7] This is a result of the internal rotation that occurs during this phase of throwing. Swimming will similarly stress the posterior structures in the pull-through phase of the freestyle stroke. Tennis players stress the posterior structures during the follow through phase of a tennis serve or a backhand stroke.

## Pathomechanics

The functional anatomy of the throwing athlete's shoulder undergoes changes that set it apart from the nonthrowing shoulder.[9] There is an increased hypertrophy of the shoulder girdle and an increase in external rotation with a relative loss of internal rotation when compared with the contralateral shoulder. This characteristic of the throwing shoulder may contribute to subtle

instability. The competitive throwing athlete probably performs at a level of stress just below the maximum threshold of the tissues. When there is an imbalance or an excess in the tolerance of the supportive structures, injury may occur. By having an understanding of basic throwing, swimming, or racquet sport mechanics, the physician, therapist, and trainer can diagnose, treat, and rehabilitate the injured shoulder, as well as aid in prevention of recurrence.

# DIAGNOSIS
## History and Mechanism of Injury

The initial step in the examination is the patient's history. In a traumatic dislocation, details of the mechanism of injury, position of the arm, and method of reduction are important in helping identify the direction of instability. The mechanism of injury of posterior dislocation is usually an indirect force applied to the shoulder in flexion, adduction, and internal rotation, such as a fall on the oustretched hand. Less common, a direct blow to the anterior shoulder can cause a posterior dislocation.

In the athlete, recurrent posterior subluxation is more commonly seen than acute posterior dislocation. The etiology may be traumatic or atraumatic, and ligamentous laxity may play a role.[3] Most patients with posterior subluxation present initially with a complaint of pain, with instability as a secondary complaint.[3]

Recurrent posterior subluxation is often associated with high forces generated in the follow-through phase of different sports activities. Again, the humerus is in adduction, flexion, and internal rotation. This may be seen in pitchers, swimmers, and tennis players. The pain with posterior instability may be posterior, anterior, or both. Recurrent posterior subluxation can cause reverse Bankart lesions presenting as posterior pain. Pain may also be secondary to traction applied to the anterior capsule.[3]

The patient with posterior instability often describes a sensation of crepitation or clicking in the shoulder in the appropriate position. They may describe the shoulder "coming out" with certain maneuvers, such as when the arm is elevated forward in internal rotation.

The athlete should be asked, if possible, to demonstrate at what phase in the throwing motion, swimming stroke, or racquet swing symptoms occur.

Patients who present with pain that is related to

overuse in overhead sports may have an overworked rotator cuff that is trying to maintain shoulder stability. Therefore, a patient with rotator cuff tendonitis may have underlying instability that should not be overlooked.

## Physical Examination

The physical examination of the athlete's shoulder should be carried out systematically and compared with the uninjured shoulder. Initial examination begins with inspection and palpation of the shoulder contours with the patient sitting and the examiner standing behind the patient looking for asymmetry, atrophy, hypertrophy, and swelling. Palpation of the shoulder may elicit tenderness along the posterior capsule. The posterior musculature can be accentuated by having patients place their hands on their hips and tighten their muscles.[9]

Range of motion is assessed next, again with comparison with the contralateral shoulder. Patients with recurrent posterior subluxation usually have loss of internal rotation, particularly with the arm at 90 degress abduction.[7]

With the patient sitting still, translation of the humeral head can be assessed. With the patient relaxed, the examiner places one hand on the clavicle and scapula to fix the shoulder girdle[5] (Fig. 19-1). The other hand grasps the humeral head and displaces it anteriorly and posteriorly. The amount of translation is assessed and graded, comparing it with the opposite shoulder. Any clicking or pain is observed. Approximately 25 percent of translation is considered normal.

The sulcus sign can also be performed in this sitting position to assess multidirectional instability. The examiner applies a longitudinal force in line with the humerus in an inferior direction.[5]

Rotator cuff strength can be assessed with the patient sitting. The supraspinatus test is performed with both arms abducted 90 degrees, forward flexed 15 degrees, and thumbs pointing to the floor. The internal and external rotators are tested with the arms at the patient's side and elbows flexed. Comparison is made with the opposite shoulder. Patients with posterior instability may show external rotator weakness (Fig. 19-2).

With the patient supine, the posterior draw test can be demonstrated.[10] The examiner grasps the patient's forearm with the shoulder in 90 degrees of abduction and 20 to 30 degrees forward flexion. The examiner's other hand cups the scapula posteriorly, with the thumb on the anterior humeral head. The upper arm

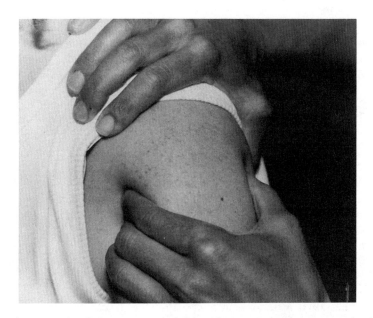

**Fig. 19-1.** Translation testing for posterior instability with patient sitting (posterior load and shift test).

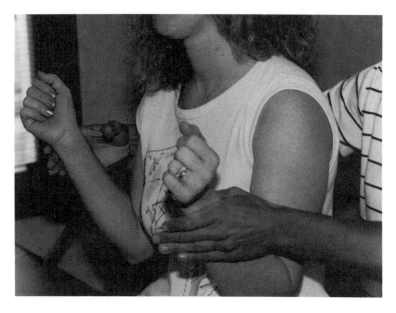

**Fig. 19-2.** External rotator muscle strength testing.

is then flexed 60 to 80 degrees and internally rotated while the thumb subluxes the humeral head posteriorly (Fig. 19-3). The amount of translation or instability can be graded as a percentage of the humeral head diameter coming out of the glenoid.

Another test with the patient supine is performed in adduction and 90 degrees forward flexion, again pushing the humeral head posteriorly. Frequently, throwing athletes show posterior laxity.[9]

Rarely, a patient may present with an unreduced posterior dislocation. The arm usually is held internally rotated and adducted, with loss of external rotation

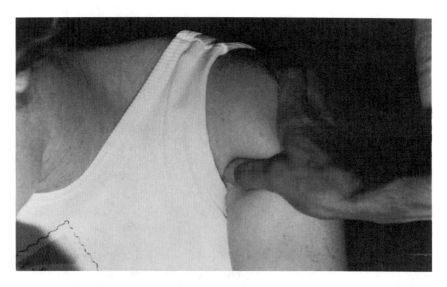

**Fig. 19-3.** Posterior draw test performed with patient supine.

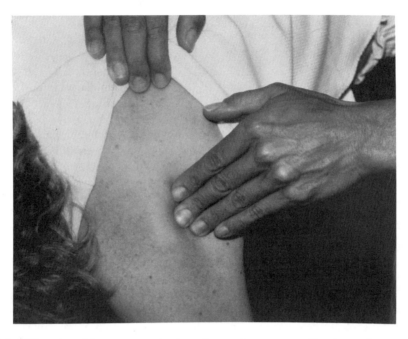

**Fig. 19-4.** With patient lying prone, palpation of posterior rotator cuff and capsule is performed.

and abduction. The coracoid is usually prominent. The importance in the recognition of a posterior dislocation cannot be overemphasized.

The final position in the examination of the athlete's shoulder is prone. The arm should be allowed to relax and drop over the side of the examining table with the elbow extended (Fig. 19-4). In this position, the posterior deltoid falls out of the way of the posterior cuff so that palpation of the rotator cuff and capsule is possible.

# RADIOGRAPHIC EVALUATION

## Roentgenograms

Further diagnostic studies are usually required in the athlete's shoulder examination to help confirm and support the physical findings so that a conclusive diagnosis can be made and appropriate treatment instituted. This usually begins with radiographs, which should include anteroposterior views in internal and external rotation, an axillary lateral, and the West Point view.[8,9] A Stryker Notch view may also be helpful.[3] The anteroposterior view in external rotation may be helpful to identify a reverse Hill-Sachs lesion of the

humeral head. On the axillary view, calcification along the posterior aspect of the capsule and glenoid labrum may hint that posterior instability is present.[3] Also, on this view bony erosion of the posterior glenoid view may be appreciated. Obviously, an unreduced posterior dislocation is readily evident on the axillary lateral projection.

## Computed Tomography Scan/Computed Tomography–Arthrogram

A Computed Tomography scan of the shoulder helps to assess the amount of version of the glenoid and humeral head.[3] Marked glenoid retroversion may suggest posterior instability. Computed Tomography-arthrography helps to assess the glenoid labrum, especially a reverse Bankart lesion.

## Magnetic Resonance Imaging

Magnetic Resonance Imaging of the shoulder is evolving as a reliable diagnostic tool, especially in the assessment of rotator cuff pathology. However, its usefulness in the workup of posterior instability is not clearly defined at this point.

## EXAMINATION UNDER ANESTHESIA

The athlete with shoulder pain and suspected posterior instability may have a negative or inconclusive physical examination, which may be secondary to muscle guarding or apprehension. Then, examination under anesthesia, which affords total muscle relaxation, may be used to assess the amount of laxity.

The examination under anesthesia should be performed systematically as stressed before, and comparison made with the opposite shoulder. Range of motion (ROM) is noted bilaterally, followed by translation tests and the posterior drawer test. For the translation test, the scapula is stabilized as previously described, the humeral head is "pushed" anteriorly and posteriorly, and the amount of excursion is noted. The posterior drawer test is performed as previously described (Fig. 19-5). After the drawer test, the arm is lowered and externally rotated to reduce the humeral head.[1] At times it may be difficult to tell whether the shoulder is subluxed posteriorly and the examiner is reducing it or if he or she is pushing the head out anteriorly

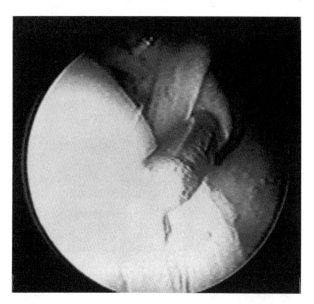

**Fig. 19-5.** Arthroscopic evaluation and debridement of the posterior undersurface (articular) of the rotator cuff.

from a reduced position.[7] The starting position with the humeral head seated in the glenoid should be strived for, so that an accurate diagnosis is made.

The examiner should be cautious in the interpretation of the examination under anesthesia. When the patient is asleep, there is frequently more shoulder excursion than is usually noted on physical examination with the patient awake.[7] With experience, this interpretation is not as difficult, especially if it is compared with the opposite shoulder.

### Diagnostic Arthroscopy

After the examination under anesthesia, the patient is turned into the lateral decubitus position with the affected arm held abducted 70 degrees and forward flexed 20 degrees in the suspension system. Diagnostic arthroscopy is performed using standard posterior and anterior portals as previously described by Andrews et al.[11] The glenohumeral joint is thoroughly inspected. Attention to labral lesions and detachments, humeral head defects, and degeneration of the glenoid rim gives clues to the diagnosis.[7] In the athlete with posterior instability, a detached posterior labrum may be evident and/or a reverse Hill-Sachs lesion may be present. The posterior glenoid may appear rounded or degenerated secondary to recurrent subluxations. A posterior "pouch" may form in which the posterior-inferior capsule is distended to hold the humeral head when it is subluxed or dislocated.[1]

Arthroscopy is also used to visualize the instability dynamically. With the arthroscope in the glenohumeral joint, the humeral head is "pushed" anteriorly, posteriorly, and inferiorly with manual pressure or a probe and the amount of translation or subluxation is assessed in each direction. This has been very helpful in the patient with multidirectional instability to determine the main direction of laxity and therefore the subsequent appropriate surgical reconstruction.

## TREATMENT OF POSTERIOR INSTABILITY
### Conservative Management

After the diagnostician has determined the presence of posterior instability, a treatment plan must be initiated. Conservative treatment, initially, is the preferred approach.[12] Rehabilitation of the rotator cuff is the focus of nonoperative treatment. The goals of conservative treatment mainly are to avoid episodes of instability and to restore normal shoulder motion and strength.[3]

An acute posterior dislocation may be managed initially with sling immobilization and anti-inflammatory medication for a brief period followed by an aggressive rehabilitation program.

Frequently, posterior instability may have with it associated tendinitis and/or subacromial impingement.[7] Tendinitis is usually secondary to abnormal joint motion. In posterior instability, internal rotation may be restricted, which places abnormal stresses on the shoulder as it tries to compensate. This will result in inflammation of the rotator cuff. Inflammation may also develop in the rotator cuff and capsule secondary to impingement. In those patients with concomitant refractory subacromial impingement, a steroid injection into the subacromial bursa may be beneficial to allow the athlete to participate in the rehabilitation program.

The nonoperative rehabilitation program for posterior subluxation is designed to return the athlete to his or her sport as quickly and as safely as possible (K. Wilk, personal communication). The program consists of four phases and is outlined as follows:

*Phase 1—acute phase:* Goals are to decrease pain and inflammation and re-establish nonpainful ROM. This is accomplished through ice, heat, anti-inflammatory medication, and ROM exercises. Strengthening exercises during this phase consist of isometrics with emphasis on flexion, internal/external rotation, abduction, and extension. During this phase, any motion that stresses the posterior capsule, such as excessive internal rotation, abduction, and horizontal adduction, is minimized.

*Phase 2—intermediate phase:* Goals are to regain and improve muscular strength and to improve neuromuscular control of the shoulder. Isotonic strengthening is initiated for the shoulder flexors, abductors, internal/external rotation, and extensors. Eccentric strengthening using surgical tubing is initiated for external rotation from 0 degrees to full external rotation and internal rotation from external rotation to 0 degrees (Fig. 19-6).

*Phase 3—advanced strengthening phase:* Goals are to improve strength, power, and endurance and prepare the athlete for activity. Isotonic and eccentric

strengthening are continued. Isokinetic exercises in all planes of motion are initiated. Plyometrics using surgical tubing, plyoball, and wall push-ups are begun (see Ch. 33).

*Phase 4—return to activity:* Goals are to increase activity level progressively to return the athlete to full function in his or her sport. In the case of a thrower, an interval throwing program is initiated. This consists of warm-up throwing, starting at 45 ft, progressing to 180 ft, throwing off the mound, to finally pitching a simulated game.

Obviously, all athletes are different and therefore their rehabilitation programs should be individualized depending on their needs, symptoms, and progress.

Many patients with posterior instability will respond to an aggressive rehabilitation program, especially those with generalized ligamentous laxity and instability secondary to repetitive microtrauma.[3]

## Operative Treatment

Operative treatment should be considered in the athlete who has failed an adequate trial of conservative therapy, usually 3 to 6 months.

An examination under anesthesia is performed first, as previously discussed, followed by arthroscopy. Arthroscopy is beneficial for two reasons. First, it helps the physician make an appropriate, accurate diagnosis. Second, it allows the physician to treat labral tears by resection or repair (Fig. 19-7). This may be beneficial in the care of throwers, as arthroscopic debridement of labral tears may decrease pain sufficiently to allow them to resume throwing even though it may not affect their instability.[3,12] Arthroscopic stabilization of a detached posterior labrum may be performed as described by Caspari[13] using the suture punch technique. This may be indicated in the thrower or the recurrent subluxator with a reverse Bankart lesion.

In the athlete with recurrent posterior dislocations, subluxations, or multidirectional instability with the primary component posterior, a posterior capsular shift is usually performed, as described by Bigliani.[14] Through a posterior approach, the deltoid is detached from the posterior acromion. The infraspinatus is dissected from the capsule and cut diagonally from medial to its lateral insertion on the greater tuberosity. A T-

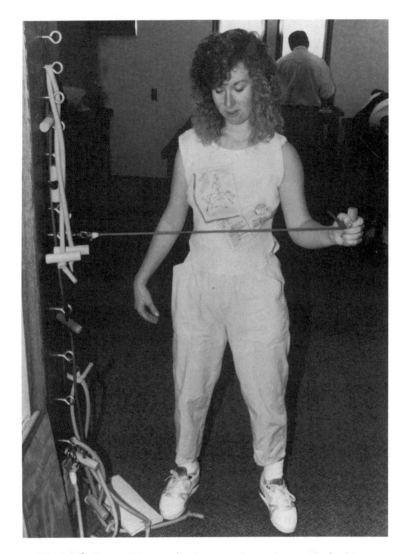

**Fig. 19-6.** Eccentric strengthening exercises using surgical tubing.

incision is made in the capsule approximately 5 mm from its insertion on the humerus. The posterior labrum is inspected. If it is detached, it is repaired to the glenoid using anchor sutures placed in the glenoid rim and passed through the labrum to tack it down.

Next, the capsular shift is performed. Currently, anchor sutures are being used for the repair. The bone is roughened on the humerus with a burr, three drill holes are made, and the anchors with sutures are placed in the holes. The sutures are passed through the capsule with the superior part of the capsule shifted inferiorly first. The arm should be held in 10 to 15 degrees of abduction and slight external rotation dur-

ing the capsular shift. The infraspinatus and deltoid are then repaired. A drain is placed, the wound is closed, and a compressive dressing is applied.

Postoperatively, the patient is placed in an abduction pillow for 4 weeks. No horizontal adduction or internal rotation is allowed for 4 weeks. On postoperative day 1 to 2, active assisted ROM to the elbow, hand, and neck is performed. On postoperative day 3 to 7, active assisted abduction and external rotation are started. Isometric shoulder exercises for adduction, abduction, flexion, and extension are used (K. Wilk, personal communication).

During weeks 2 to 4 postoperatively, active assisted

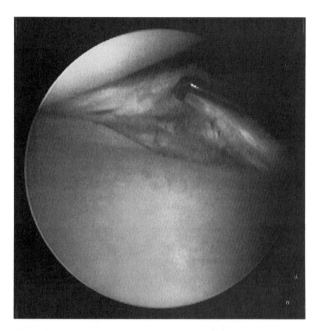

**Fig. 19-7.** Arthroscopy demonstrating posterior labral tear.

ROM exercises are progressed to 90 degrees abduction and external rotation to 90 degrees. After week 4, the splint is removed.

During weeks 4 to 8, overhead flexion and abduction exercises with pulleys and T-bar are started, as well as active internal rotation with the arm at the side. Progressive resistive exercises (PRE's) are begun for abduction, external rotation, and flexion.

During weeks 8 to 12 postoperatively, T-bar internal rotation exercises in 90/90 degree position are begun. Eccentric internal rotation, external rotation, flexion, abduction, and adduction are performed with tubing.

Horizontal adduction stretching is begun at weeks 12 to 16. A supervised free weights program is started.

After the 20th to 26th week, functional activities are begun, such as an interval sports program. Often the program is delayed because of inadequate ligamentous tissue posteriorly.

## RESULTS

Many procedures for posterior instability of the shoulder have been described. Most of these are not applicable to the athlete, as ROM may be limited postopera-

tively. Norwood and Terry[15] reviewed the results of 19 athletes with chronic recurrent posterior subluxation or anterior/posterior instability to document postoperative stability and the level of athletic participation after opening wedge posterior scapular osteotomy. At an average follow-up of 39.9 months after surgery, nine experienced instability: four anteriorly, three posteriorly, and two anteriorly/posteriorly; however, most returned to their sporting activities. Interestingly, 12 of the 19 shoulders involved the nondominant arm. They pointed out that instability caused by throwing or swinging has a less predictable result with this procedure. They also mentioned that they did not document preoperative ROM; therefore, they could not comment on the possible ROM restrictions after reconstruction.

Tibone et al[16] reported on their results of posterior shoulder staple capsulorrhaphy in 10 athletes, nine involved the dominant extremity. Eight patients had pain relief, and ROM was maintained postoperatively. However, no patient returned to former throwing status. Four patients had anterior instability postoperatively, and three patients had recurrence of posterior instability.

Neer[1] described a posterior capsular repair for posterior instability. He reported no recurrences in 23 patients treated with this procedure, with all returning to regular activities. He did not state, however, what activities that entailed.

The literature is replete on the long-term results of surgical repair for recurrent posterior instability of the shoulder, especially in the athlete. One explanation for this is that posterior instability is a relatively uncommon entity, even in the athlete.

## SUMMARY

The athlete with posterior instability of the shoulder may present in different ways, with the patient complaining of pain or a sense of instability. In throwing sports, tendinitis secondary to instability as a result of traction or compression of the rotator cuff may occur.[7] The physician must take a careful history and perform a thorough physical examination, noting ligamentous laxity, subtle loss of motion and strength, apprehension, and increased posterior translation. Standard x-ray films may be helpful, looking for humeral head defects or posterior glenoid lesions. Examination under anesthesia and diagnostic arthroscopy play a significant role in the evaluation of these patients.

Conservative management is usually the desired treatment initially.[12] Rehabilitation, with emphasis on strengthening of the rotator cuff, can help stabilize the shoulder and reduce symptoms enough to return the patient to activity.

If conservative treatment fails, arthroscopy may be beneficial in throwers and tennis players with posterior subluxation if they have a partial labral detachment or tear that can be addressed arthroscopically. At times, open reconstruction with posterior capsular shift is indicated in the chronic recurrent posterior subluxation. Excessive tightening of the capsule must be avoided, as it will limit athletic activity and may increase instability in the opposite direction.[7]

Postoperatively, a well-supervised rehabilitation program must be instituted to restore ROM and strength.

Success in the treatment of posterior instability lies in the correct diagnosis followed by adherence to strict criteria in the selection of conservative versus surgical management.

# REFERENCES

1. Neer CS: Dislocations. In: Shoulder Reconstruction. WB Saunders, Philadelphia, 1990
2. Boyd HB, Sisk TD: Recurrent posterior dislocation of the shoulder. J Bone Joint Surg 54A:779, 1972
3. Schwartz E, Warren RF, O'Brien SJ, Fronek J: Posterior shoulder instability. Orthop Clin North Am 18:409, 1987
4. Jenkins DB: Hollinshead's Functional Anatomy of the Limbs and Back. WB Saunders, Philadelphia, 1991
5. Hawkins RJ, Mohtadi N: Clinical evaluation of shoulder instability. Clin J Sport Med 1:59, 1991
6. Perry J: Anatomy and biomechanics of the shoulder in throwing, swimming, gymnastics and tennis. Clin Sports Med 2:247, 1983
7. Warren RF: Subluxation of the shoulder in athletes. Clin Sport Med 2:339, 1983
8. Zarins B, Rowe CR: Current concepts in the diagnosis and treatment of shoulder instability in athletes. Med Sci Sports Exerc 16:444, 1984
9. Andrews JR, Gillogly SD: Shoulder examination and diagnosis in the throwing athlete. In: AAOS Symposium on Upper Extremity Injuries in Athletes, Washington, DC, 1984
10. Gerber C, Ganz R: Clinical assessment of instability of the shoulder. J Bone Joint Surg 66B:551, 1984
11. Andrews JR, Carson WG, Ortega K: Arthroscopy of the shoulder: technique and normal anatomy. Am J Sport Med 12:1, 1984
12. Engle RP, Canner GC: Posterior shoulder instability: approach to rehabilitation. J Orthop Sports Phys Ther 10:488, 1989
13. Caspari RB: Arthroscopic reconstruction for anterior shoulder instability. In Paulos Le, Tiboze JE (eds): Operative Techniques in Shoulder Surgery. Aspen Publishers, Rockville, MD, 1991
14. Bigliani LU: Anterior and posterior capsular shift for multidirectional instability. In: Techniques in Orthopaedics. Aspen Publishers, Rockville, MD, 1989
15. Norwood LA, Terry GC: Shoulder posterior subluxation. Am J Sports Med 12:25, 1984
16. Tibone JE, Prietto C, Jobe FW et al: Staple capsulorrhaphy for recurrent posterior shoulder dislocation. Am J Sport Med 9:135, 1981
17. Gainor BJ, Piotrowski G, Puhl J et al: The throw: biomechanics and acute injury. Am J Sports Med 8:2, 1980
18. Hawkins RJ, Koppert G, Johnston G: Recurrent posterior instability (subluxation) of the shoulder. J Bone Joint Surg 66A:169, 1984
19. McGlynn FT, Caspari RB: Arthroscopic findings in the subluxating shoulder. Clin Orthop 183:173, 1984
20. Mosely HF: Athletic injuries to the shoulder region. Am J Surg 98:401, 1959

# 20

# Multidirectional Instability of the Shoulder

MARK S. McMAHON
BERTRAM ZARINS

In 1956 Carter Rowe[1] introduced the concept of atraumatic shoulder instability. In 1962 Rowe[2] was the first to point out that atraumatic instability can occur in more than one direction. Rowe[3,4] emphasized the importance of determining the type of shoulder instability present, because the type the patient has affects the outcome of surgical repair. Neer[5] called the combined type of instability multidirectional. This syndrome is now recognized as occurring more frequently than previously realized.

*Multidirectional instability* is defined as shoulder dislocation or subluxation that occurs in more than one direction. The instability can be a combination of anterior, posterior, and inferior excursion of the humeral head with relation to the glenoid fossa.[2,6] This group of patients represents both a diagnostic and therapeutic challenge to the physician and therapist.

Multidirectional instability can occur in patients who have congenital abnormalities or developmental problems such as Ehlers-Danlos syndrome or aplasia of the shoulder joint. Instability can develop after a nerve injury to the shoulder or after a stroke, resulting in a flail shoulder.[7] These syndromes should be ruled out, because their presence may significantly alter treatment. The physician should rule out the presence of a psychiatric disorder that occasionally coexists in a patient who has voluntary dislocations.[8]

The basic lesion in multidirectional instability is congenital or acquired enlargement of the glenohumeral joint volume and a very redundant capsule anteriorly, inferiorly, and/or posteroinferiorly. In the early stages of this instability, the anterior labrum is intact, but splitting and partial detachment of the labrum can develop. After the shoulder has dislocated many times, detachment of the glenoid labrum may occur, and a defect in the posterior aspect of the humeral head may develop.[9] Altchek et al[10] found some degree of anterior labral injury in 38 of 42 shoulders that had multidirectional instability.

## CLINICAL RECOGNITION

Dislocation of the shoulder in a patient who has multidirectional instability typically occurs without significant injury and is reduced by the patient.[11] Most initial dislocations occur either without trauma or with a trivial injury that would not ordinarily dislocate a normal shoulder.[11] The incidence of trauma as a causative factor in patients who have multidirectional instability is much lower than in patients who have recurrent anterior dislocations.[12]

Varying degrees of generalized joint laxity, manifested by hyperextension of the fingers and elbows, may be present in people who have multidirectional shoulder laxity. Generalized joint laxity should be assessed when examining a patient who has shoulder instability. Not only is the involved shoulder lax, but laxity may also be noted in the asymptomatic shoulder.[13] Excessive external rotation at a position of 90 degrees of shoulder abduction is commonly found in patients who have anterior or multidirectional shoulder instability.[14] One-half of patients who had multidirectional instability in the study by Altcheck et al[10] had generalized joint laxity. A patient who has generalized joint laxity, however, may also have a history of trauma to the shoulder.

The patient who has multidirectional instability is often an athlete, such as a swimmer or gymnast. The most common combination of factors associated with this disorder seems to be an individual who has a relatively lax shoulder who has stressed the capsule repetitively in work or in sports.[5] Occasionally, a patient who does not have inherent joint laxity acquires multidirectional shoulder instability as a result of repeated violent injuries, such as those sustained in wrestling or football. In a recent study of patients who have multidirectional instability, all 40 were injured during athletic activities.[10] Approximately one-half of the patients in Neer's series[9] were very active and had subjected their shoulders to repetitive injury.

Male and female patients are affected with equal frequency.[11] In Neer's series,[9] the average age of the patients who underwent surgery for this condition was 24 years, with a range of 15 to 54 years.

Pain is often caused by carrying loads at the side of the body or overhead. The patient may complain of pain when lifting light objects.[14] Inability to carry books, throw a ball, swim, or work with arms overhead are typical complaints. An extremely hypermobile shoulder may become symptomatic without unusual stress but merely from the activities of daily living.[5] The pain is often initially described as diffuse and poorly localized but can become disabling at rest and even interfere with sleep. It has been stated that this type of discomfort is a result of tendinitis.[15] These symptoms should be distinguished from the symptoms in a typical patient with multidirectional instability, who is comfortable between episodes of instability.

Inferior instability is the hallmark of multidirectional instability and is diagnosed by eliciting the sulcus sign.[11] Longitudinal traction is applied to the arm positioned at the patient's side; a positive sign is an abnormal widening of the acromiohumeral interval and a deep sulcus that can be seen just below the acromion in the mid-deltoid muscle area. The shoulder can also be tested with the arm abducted to 90 degrees and the elbow supported; the proximal humerus is pushed in an inferior direction.[14] It may not be possible to elicit this sign if the patient is tense and contracts the muscles. Apprehension signs in inferior, anterior, and posterior directions can be elicited in patients who have multidirectional instability.[11]

Many patients who have multidirectional instability describe paraesthesias or weaknesses of the upper extremity. Such neurologic symptoms or transitory numbness of the hand or arm is extremely common in patients who have inferior instability and should not be misinterpreted as being caused by an emotional problem.

Routine radiographic evaluation will usually be normal. Special radiograms for determining multidirectional instability include stress films or fluoroscopy performed while pressure is applied posteriorly, inferiorly, and anteriorly. Anteroposterior radiograms taken with the patient standing erect and with 25 lb of weight held in each hand can show inferior shoulder subluxation.[9] Occasionally, arthrograms can be used to assess the joint volume. Arthrograms combined with computerized tomography or magnetic resonance imaging are useful to show glenoid labrum tears.

Because muscle guarding, particularly in a muscular individual, can obscure multidirectional instability, every shoulder operated on for instability should be evaluated under anesthesia at the time of surgery to determine the exact nature of the instability pattern.[9,16] Arthroscopy can be a useful diagnostic adjunct, as fraying or detachment of the glenoid labrum is an indirect sign of the primary direction of the instability. The presence of some fraying or fibrillation of the labrum seen at arthroscopy, however, is not sufficient evidence to warrant surgical repair unless all the other aspects of the evaluation also point toward instability in a particular direction.[9]

Studies have shown that unrecognized multidirectional instability is one of the most frequent causes for the failure after repair of recurrent shoulder instability.[2,13] If the anterior capsule is tightened in a patient who has multidirectional instability, the result may be that the humeral head is displaced permanently into the opposite direction, leading to early degenerative arthritis as well as leaving the shoulder unstable inferiorly. The surgeon must also be careful not to perform too tight a capsular shift that can force the head out in the opposite direction.[7]

The surgeon should avoid operating on a shoulder that has multidirectional instability if another lesion coexists that is actually producing the patient's symptoms, such as acromioclavicular arthritis or cervical radiculitis. Most lax shoulders are painless, and when pain begins, one should look for possible causes of pain other than the instability.[9]

## CONSERVATIVE THERAPY

The first line of treatment in patients who have multidirectional instability is rehabilitation. Conservative treatment includes changing the way the patient uses the shoulder.[5] According to Matsen et al[15] shoulders that have loose capsules, as in pitchers, swimmers, and gymnasts, are more dependent on dynamic stabilizing mechanisms than tight shoulders. Many of these weaknesses respond to internal and external rotator cuff muscle strengthening exercises. Contractions of the rotator cuff muscles help stabilize the humeral head in the glenoid fossa and resist displacing forces.[15]

The ideal rehabilitation program should strengthen the muscles about the shoulder without producing further irritation. Rockwood et al[7] recommended to patients who have multidirectional instability a specific rehabilitation program designed to strengthen the three parts of the deltoid muscle, the rotator cuff muscles, and the scapular stabilizing muscles. Rotator cuff muscle strengthening exercises are most effectively performed by keeping the humerus close to the body and rotating the arm against resistance.[15] Over several months of exercise, the patient increases the amount of resistance—to 15 lb for women and 20 to 25 lb for men. Muscles that stabilize the scapula can be strengthened by performing push-ups and shoulder shrugs.

According to Jobe et al[17] the rehabilitation program of patients who have generalized joint laxity should emphasize isometric exercises. If isotonic exercises are performed, they should be done in a limited range only, beginning in a neutral position. When doing isotonic exercises, it is essential to avoid irritating the joint capsule and ligaments.

If a patient has significant pain and disability from multidirectional instability that fails to respond to a rehabilitation program of 6 to 12 months duration, surgery should be considered. A patient who has atraumatic instability and who has a history of significant trauma, pain, and swelling should not have surgical reconstruction unless he or she has undergone an adequate rehabilitation program.[7]

## SURGICAL THERAPY

If surgery is performed, laxity of the inferior capsule should be corrected, any enlargement of the opening between the middle and superior glenohumeral ligaments closed, and detachment of the glenoid labrum and capsule repaired. Detachment of the glenoid labrum and capsule from the glenoid rim is less likely to be present in a patient who has multidirectional laxity than in the patient who has unidirectional instability; when detachment occurs, it is likely to be a result rather than a cause of repeated dislocations.[11] Because the anterior portion of the glenoid labrum is the medial attachment of the inferior glenohumeral ligament, its reattachment to the glenoid rim is a prerequisite to the success of a capsular procedure. The standard surgical procedures performed to correct unidirectional anterior or posterior instability are not adequate to correct multidirectional instability because they do not reduce excessive redundancy of the inferior part of the capsule.[5,18]

The capsular shift procedure (Fig. 20-1) described by Neer[5] is designed to reduce the volume of the glenohumeral joint inferiorly, anteriorly, and posteriorly by equalizing capsular tightness on all three sides. The decision of whether to perform an anterior or posterior procedure can be difficult to make. The surgeon should determine which direction of instability causes most symptoms. A posterior capsular shift is performed if the direction of greatest instability is posterior.

In performing the inferior capsular shift procedure, the superficial half of the thickness of the subscapularis tendon is divided transversely 1 cm medial to the biceps tendon groove; a short stump of tendon is left attached to the lesser tuberosity to be used in the repair.[11] One-half of the subscapularis tendon is left attached to the anterior capsule to reinforce the anterior aspect of the capsule. A T-shaped incision is made in the capsule; the vertical segment of the T begins just medial to the lateral attachment of the capsule to the humerus and extended inferiorly and posteriorly. The inferior flap is then pulled upward to eliminate the inferior redundancy of the capsule and is reattached to the soft tissue on the lesser tuberosity. The upper flap is then pulled downward and sutured to the soft tissue on the humerus.[11]

Axillary nerve injury is a recognized complication

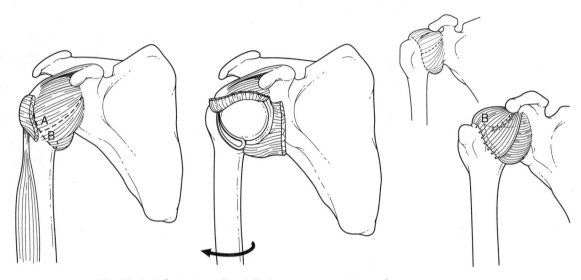

**Fig. 20-1.** Inferior capsular shift. (From Neer and Foster,[5] with permission.)

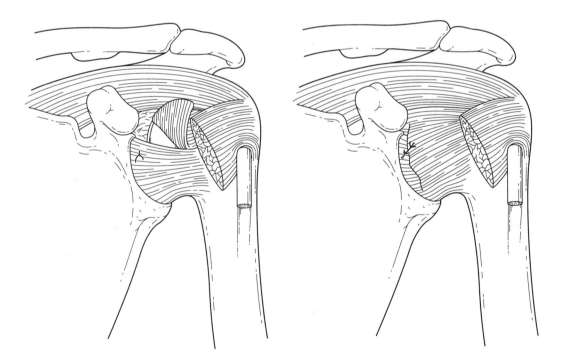

**Fig. 20-2.** T-plasty modification of Bankart procedure. (From Altchek et al,[10] with permission.)

of the capsular shift procedure for multidirectional instability of the shoulder.[19,20] The axillary nerve lies in intimate contact with the inferior capsule as it passes through the quadrilateral space.

Matsen et al[15] described a similar procedure, emphasizing that while the arm is progressively externally rotated, the anterior, inferior, and posterior aspects of the capsule are released from the neck of the humerus up to the middle of the posterior part of the humeral head. They also noted that tension of the capsular flap must reduce the inferior axillary pouch and posterior capsule redundancy until symmetric shoulder stability is restored.

Altchek et al[10] described a T-plasty in which two capsular incisions are used, a transverse one in the midportion of the capsule and a vertical one at the glenoid margin (Fig. 20-2). The inferior flap is then advanced superiorly and medially and sutured into the glenoid rim, and the superior flap is advanced distally. The remaining medial flap of capsule is sutured over the lateral flap at the glenoid rim, buttressing the repair in a manner similar to that used in the Bankart procedure.

Altchek et al[10] argued that with Neer's capsular shift procedure, a Bankart lesion must be repaired as a separate step, whereas their T-plasty makes it easier to combine shifting the capsule with performing a Bankart repair. They acknowledged that a lateral capsular incision allows easier access to the posterior portion of the capsule and may be preferable if a Bankart lesion is not present. Both Altchek et al and Neer reported that throwing athletes were unable to throw a ball with as much speed postoperatively as before surgery.

With Rockwood's procedure for treatment of multidirectional instability, the principle of the capsular shift is to divide the capsule all the way down inferiorly, midway between the attachment of the capsule to the humerus and on the glenoid rim.[15] The medial capsule is then advanced superiorly and laterally under the lateral capsule, which is then advanced superiorly and medially over the medial capsule.

## POSTOPERATIVE REHABILITATION

Postoperatively, most surgeons immobilize the patient for 6 weeks in a sling.[6,21,22] Thereafter, the patient begins passive and then active assisted range of motion exercises from 6 to 12 weeks after surgery. At 3 months, gentle strengthening exercises are begun. At 6 months, the patient may begin limited activities and then return to full throwing and overhead sports at 1 year after surgery if muscle strength and range of motion are satisfactory.

## REFERENCES

1. Rowe CR: Prognosis in dislocations of the shoulder. J Bone Joint Surg 38A:958, 1956
2. Rowe CR: Acute and recurrent dislocations of the shoulder. J Bone Joint Surg 44A:998, 1962
3. Rowe CR: Anterior dislocations of the shoulder. Surg Clin North Am 43:1609, 1963
4. Rowe CR: Complicated dislocations of the shoulder—guidelines to treatment. Am J Surg 117:549, 1969
5. Neer CS II, Foster CR: Inferior capsular shift for involuntary inferior and multidirectional instability of the shoulder: a preliminary report. J Bone Joint Surg 62A:897, 1980
6. Skyhar MJ, Warren RF, Altchek DW: Instability of the shoulder. p. 181. In Nicholas JA, Hershman EB, Posner MA (eds): The Upper Extremity in Sports Medicine. CV Mosby, St. Louis, 1990
7. Rockwood CA Jr, Thomas SC, Matsen FA III: Subluxations and dislocations about the glenohumeral joint. p. 1131. In Rockwood CA Jr, Green DP, Bucholz RW (eds): Rockwood and Green's Fractures in Adults. 3rd Ed. JB Lippincott, Philadelphia, 1991
8. Rowe CR, Pierce DS, Clark JG: Voluntary dislocation of the shoulder. A preliminary report on a clinical, electromyographic and psychiatric study of twenty-six patients. J Bone Joint Surg 55A:445, 1973
9. Neer CS II: Involuntary inferior and multidirectional instability of the shoulder: etiology, recognition, and treatment. Instr Course Lect 34:232, 1985
10. Altchek DW, Warren RF, Skyhar MJ, Ortiz G: T-plasty modification of the Bankart procedure for multidirectional instability of the anterior and inferior types. J Bone Joint Surg 73A:105, 1991
11. Neer CS II: Shoulder Reconstruction. WB Saunders, Philadelphia, 1990
12. Neer CS II, Welsh RP: The shoulder in sports. Orthop Clin North Am 8:583, 1977
13. Rockwood CA Jr, Gerber C: Analysis of failed surgical procedures for anterior shoulder instability, San Antonio, Texas. Presented to first open meeting, American Shoulder and Elbow Surgeons, Las Vegas, January 1985
14. Norris TR: Diagnostic techniques for shoulder instability. Instr Course Lect 34:239, 1985

15. Matsen FA III, Thomas SC, Rockwood CA Jr: Anterior glenohumeral instability. p. 526. In Rockwood CA Jr, Matsen FA III (eds): The Shoulder. WB Saunders, Philadelphia, 1990

16. Cofield RH, Irving JF: Evaluation and classification of shoulder instability: with special reference to examination under anaesthesia. Clin Orthop 223:32, 1987

17. Jobe FW, Moynes DR, Brewster CE: Rehabilitation of shoulder joint instabilities. Orthop Clin North Am 18:473, 1987

18. Protzman RR: Anterior instability of the shoulder. J Bone Joint Surg 62A:909, 1980

19. Bryan WJ, Schauder K, Tullos HS: The axillary nerve and its relationship to common sports medicine shoulder procedures. Am J Sports Med 14:113, 1986

20. Loomer R, Graham B: Anatomy of the axillary nerve and its relation to inferior capsular shift. Clin Orthop 243:100, 1989

21. Foster CR: Multidirectional instability of the shoulder in the athlete. Clin Sports Med 2:355, 1983

22. Mendoza FX, Nicholas JA, Sands A: Principles of shoulder rehabilitation in the athlete. p. 253. In Nicholas JA, Hershman EB, Posner MA (eds): The Upper Extremity in Sports Medicine. CV Mosby, St Louis, 1990

# 21
# Capsulolabral Reconstruction and Rehabilitation

*CLIVE E. BREWSTER*
*JUDY L. SETO*
*DIANE R. MOYNES*
*FRANK W. JOBE*

The anterior capsulolabral reconstruction is our preferred surgical procedure for treating anteriorly unstable shoulders resistent to conservative management. We have found that this technique restores stability without compromising mobility or function. The rehabilitation program is extensive and is an essential component of the overall program. Without adequate and appropriate postoperative physical therapy, the procedure will not be effective in restoring high-level performance.

This surgical procedure[1-3] restores the integrity of the joint capsule with minimal anatomic disruption. An anterior approach to the shoulder is used as the deltopectoral groove is located. An incision is made; the deltoid muscle and cephalic vein are retracted laterally, and the pectoralis muscle is retracted medially. The conjoined tendon is carefully avoided and also retracted medially. These steps allow exposure of the subscapularis muscle. The humerus is rotated externally, permitting the long head of the biceps to be placed in a safe position when the subscapularis muscle is divided. The subscapularis muscle fibers are horizontally divided, not cut, at a point between the upper two-thirds and lower one-third of the muscle.

The underlying glenohumeral joint capsule is carefully dissected from the subscapularis muscle. A capsulotomy is performed with two incisions placed in the shape of a "sideways T" (Fig. 21-1). Capsular flaps are created as the capsule is dissected from the anterior scapular neck and glenoid rim. The position of capsular dissection depends on which shoulder the surgery is performed. A left shoulder will have incisions at the 10-o'clock and 6-o'clock positions. The right shoulder will have incisions at the 2-o'clock and 6-o'clock positions.

Three drill holes are used to create a secure bony fixation site along the anterior glenoid rim. Using Mitek sutures, the inferior capsular flap is shifted superiorly. This position allows the inferior flap to be inverted within the joint, thereby recreating the bumper effect of the glenoid labrum.

The superior capsular flap is advanced inferiorly, overlapping the inferior capsular flap and secured with Mitek sutures. This establishes a double-thickness anterior capsule at the site of the previous instability (Fig. 21-2). The degree of capsular tightness is then checked by performing passive range of motion (ROM) to ensure at least 90 degrees of abduction and 45 degrees of external rotation before tension is noted at the suture sites. The capsule is then closed and the subscapularis reapproximated.

Postoperatively, the patient's arm is placed in an abduction pillow at 90 degrees abduction, 45 degrees external rotation, and 30 degrees forward flexion. This position is chosen to allow for capsular healing without additional capsular shortening.

The rehabilitation program is designed to allow for protection of the surgically reconstructed capsulola-

221

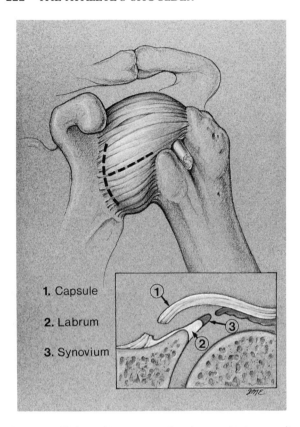

**Fig. 21-1.** T-shaped incision in glenohumeral joint capsule and synovial lining. (From Jobe et al,[1] with permission.)

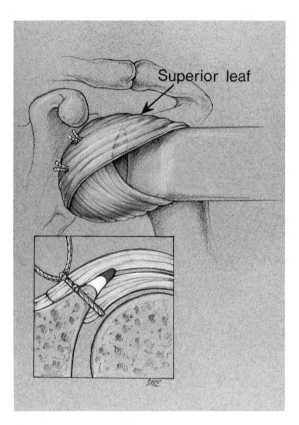

**Fig. 21-2.** Superior shift of inferior capsular flap and inferior shift of superior capsular flap. (From Jobe et al,[1] with permission.)

bral complex, to achieve full ROM with emphasis on regaining external rotation and enhancing strength and endurance to promote normal shoulder biomechanics (Table 21-1). The initial phase focuses on decreasing postoperative pain and swelling and achieving full ROM. Postoperatively, discomfort may be expected in the deltopectoral groove and the split subscapularis. Strengthening exercises are progressively added to the program, with an emphasis on the rotator cuff musculature during the early phase. The anterior deltoid is probably the most resistant to a strengthening program after this surgery. The final phase incorporates a throwing program with special consideration on returning normal scapulothoracic rhythm and throwing mechanics. The timing and sequential firing of the shoulder complex muscles are essential to return the athletes to their previous throwing ability and effectiveness.

# PHASE I

## Initial Phase (0 to 2 Months Postoperation)

Initially, the patient is immobilized for 1 week in an abduction pillow or brace with the glenohumeral joint positioned in approximately 30 degrees forward flexion, 70 to 80 degrees abduction, and 30 to 45 degrees external rotation (Fig. 21-3). Depending on the patient's tissue extensibility and any concurrent pathologies, select patients may be allowed to use a sling or other type of arm orthosis.

During this early portion of the rehabilitation program, the abduction pillow or brace may be removed for gentle active ROM exercises. Abduction, flexion, external rotation, internal rotation, and adduction are performed twice daily. External rotation, internal rota-

**Table 21-1. Summary of the Rehabilitation Program After Anterior Capsulolabral Reconstruction**

Phase I: Early Phase (0 to 2 Months Postoperation)
Immobilized for 1 week using an abduction pillow or sling
Gentle active assistive ROM exercises: flexion, abduction, adduction, external rotation, internal rotation
Multiangle isometric shoulder strengthening exercises: all planes
Squeeze a soft ball, putty, or sponge 20 to 30 times daily
Soft tissue mobilization and /or stretching exercises as needed (e.g., rhomboids, levator scapulae, infraspinatus)
Progress to active resisted strengthening exercises: supraspinatus, external rotation, internal rotation, flexion to 90 degrees, abduction to 90 degrees, shoulder shrugs
Progress to sidelying external rotation
Add horizontal adduction
Begin upper body ergometer

Phase II: Intermediate Phase (2 to 4 Months Postoperation)
Attain full ROM
Continue progressive strengthening exercises
Shoulder flexion to 180 degrees
Should abduction to 180 degrees
Add horizontal abduction (sidelying)
Progress to sidelying internal rotation with free weights
Begin isokinetic strengthening
Begin total body conditioning program

Phase III: Advance Phase (4 to 12 months Postoperation)
May begin tossing (step 1 of throwing program) at 4 months postoperation
First isokinetic strength test at 5 months postoperation
Gradually progress through each step of the throwing program as tolerated. Each phase is performed for a duration of three to four times per week. Note: Throwing at three-quarters speed or more is not permitted until 7 months postoperation. Throwing at full speed is allowed 10 to 12 months postoperation

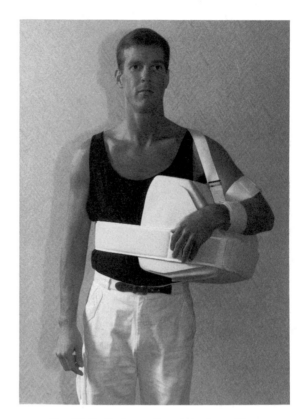

**Fig. 21-3.** Postoperation abduction pillow.

tion, and abduction motions should be conducted in the scapular plane (i.e., 30 degrees horizontal adduction) to protect the capsulolabral reconstruction anteriorly. The movements should not be forced and are performed to the limit of pain. If the patient is using an abduction pillow or brace, the arm should be taken out and passively externally rotated, abducted, adducted, and elevated 10 to 20 times once or twice daily.

Isometric strengthening exercises may be started during the initial 2 weeks postoperation. The exercises are performed in all planes of motion and at multiple angles as tolerated. General hand strengthening exercises are performed daily be squeezing a soft ball, sponge, or putty.

Two weeks postoperation, active assisted exercises are continued to increase ROM. The goal is to attain full ROM by 6 to 8 weeks postoperation. Additional strengthening exercises such as supraspinatus strengthening in the scapular plane (Fig. 21-4) and shoulder shrugs are continued. Also, active resisted shoulder internal and external rotation using elastic or surgical tubing are performed as tolerated. The humerus should be placed at the side of the trunk with the elbow flexed 90 degrees. If discomfort exists with this exercise, modify the arm position by moving the humerus into slight forward flexion. Active shoulder flexion and abduction to 90 degrees may be added to strengthen the anterior deltoid muscle.

At 4 weeks postoperation, the patient may progress to external rotation in a sidelying position with weights (Fig. 21-5). The degree of external rotation is limited to protect the anterior capsule. The starting position is full internal rotation with the humerus externally rotating until the forearm is level with the trunk or in a position of neutral rotation.

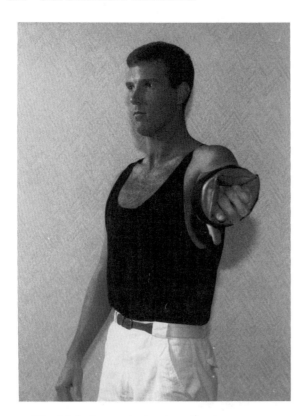

**Fig. 21-4.** Supraspinatus strengthening exercise.

Horizontal adduction within the range of 15 to 90 degrees may be initiated 4 weeks postoperation. The anterior joint capsule is protected in the limited ROM. Upper body ergometer exercises may also begin with emphasis on strength and endurance.

Attention should be given to the glenohumeral motion and scapulothoracic rhythm when assessing normal shoulder mechanics. Tightness of the scapular muscles and shoulder complex musculature will influence both ROM and normal shoulder kinematics. For example, the rhomboids control downward rotation of the scapula, and the latissimus dorsi muscle causes extension of the glenohumeral joint. Restriction by these muscles will inhibit overhead arm motions. In this case, it is important to perform soft tissue mobilization or stretching exercises of these muscles to achieve flexibility allowing proper biomechanics and synchrony of the shoulder complex.

# PHASE II

## Intermediate Phase (2 to 4 Months Postoperation)

During this phase, emphasis is placed on strengthening the rotator cuff muscles and the accompanying shoulder complex and scapular muscles. Full ROM should be attained by the start of this phase. Normal external ROM for an athlete engaged in a throwing sport may exceed the nondominant arm by 10 degrees or more.[4]

The strengthening exercises from phase I are continued, increasing the resistance and progressing in endurance as tolerated. Shoulder flexion and abduction may be performed to 180 degrees and not limited to 90 degrees during overhead motions. Horizontal abduction may be added if full ROM is achieved (Fig. 21-6).

At 2 months postoperation, sidelying internal rotation using free weights may begin. The patient lies on the involved side, allowing for concentric and eccentric strengthening of the internal rotators while protecting the anterior joint capsule. A total body conditioning program is also emphasized in the program at this time.

Isokinetic strength training of the internal and external rotators is added approximately 3 months postoperation, incorporating speeds of 200 degrees and faster. Additional planes of motion may be added as the patients' conditions warrant.

# PHASE III

## Advanced Phase (4 to 12 Months Postoperation)

The patient's first isokinetic test is to measure the strength and endurance of the internal and external rotators. If testing is conducted in more than one plane, each motion is tested on a different day to reduce the influence of fatigue on the other directions. If the patient achieves strength and endurance measures of 90 percent or greater as compared with the uninvolved side, the throwing program may be initiated (Appendix 21-1). The patient may proceed to each step of the throwing program performed three to four times per week provided there is no pain, discomfort, or swell-

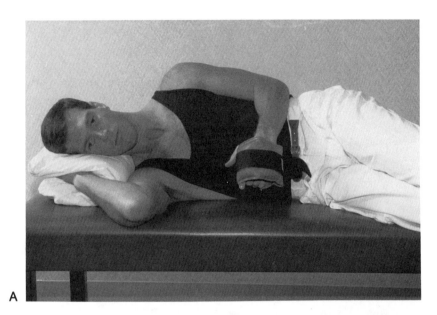

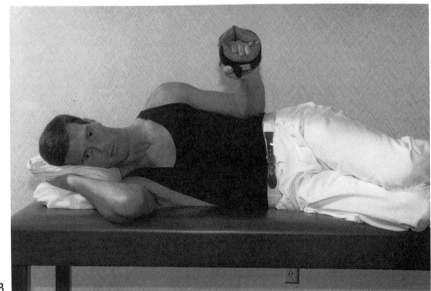

**Fig. 21-5.** External rotation—(**A**) starting position and (**B**) completed position.

ing. Modifications may be required in the number of throws, speed of throwing, distance thrown, and the number of days of throwing, depending on the patient's progress, throwing mechanics, and subjective complaints. Throwing is limited to less than three-fourths speed until 7 months postoperation, with throwing at full speed restricted until 10 to 12 months postoperation. This allows adequate time for the reconstructed tissues to heal and adapt to the high stresses placed on them during the ballistic activity of throwing.

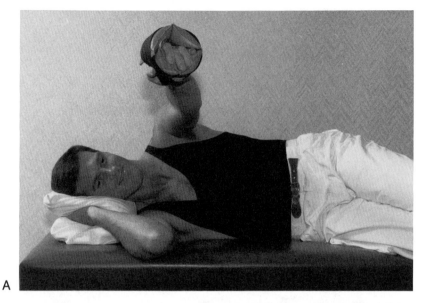

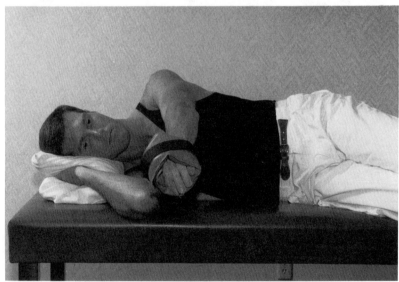

**Fig. 21-6.** Eccentric horizontal abduction—(**A**) starting position and (**B**) completed position.

## SUMMARY

Anterior capsulolabral reconstruction is typically used for throwing athletes who have developed anteriorly unstable shoulders. The rehabilitation program following surgery takes into account protecting the anterior aspect of the joint capsule while restoring normal func-

tion and range of motion. Essential factors considered during the rehabilitation program are

Minimizing anterior translation of the humeral head, thereby reducing the stresses on the joint capsule and anterior joint structures.

Restoring full range of motion, especially external rotation as needed in the throwing athlete (e.g., pitchers).

Promoting strength and endurance of the muscles in the upper quadrant, especially the rotator cuff muscles.

Re-establishing normal joint biomechanics.

## REFERENCES

1. Jobe FW, Giangarra CE, Kvitne RS et al: Anterior capsulolabral reconstruction of the shoulder in athletes in overhand sports. Am J Sports Med 19:428, 1991

2. Jobe FW, Glousman RE: Anterior capsulolabral reconstruction. Techniques Orthop 3:29, 1988

3. Jobe FW, Kvitne RS, Giangarra CE: Shoulder pain in the overhand or throwing athlete: the relationship of anterior instability and rotator cuff impingement. Orthop Rev. 18:963, 1989

4. Brown LP, Niehues SL, Harrah A et al: Upper extremity range of motion and isokinetic strength of the internal and external shoulder rotators in major league baseball players. Am J Sports Med 16:577, 1988

# Appendix 21-1

# Throwing Program

Perform each step and phase of the throwing program at least three times.

STEP 1: Toss the ball (no wind up) against a wall on alternate days. Start with 25 to 30 throws, building up to 70 throws, and gradually increase the throwing distance.

| No. of Throws | Distance (ft) |
|---|---|
| 20 | 20 (warm-up phase) |
| 25–40 | 30–40 |
| 10 | 20 (cool-down phase) |

STEP 2: Toss the ball (playing catch with easy wind-up) on alternate days.

| No. of Throws | Distance (ft) |
|---|---|
| 10 | 20 (warm up) |
| 10 | 30–40 |
| 30–40 | 50 |
| 10 | 20–30 (cool down) |

STEP 3: Continue increasing the throwing distance while still tossing the ball with an easy wind-up.

| No. of Throws | Distance (ft) |
|---|---|
| 10 | 20 (warm up) |
| 10 | 30–40 |
| 30–40 | 50–60 |
| 10 | 30 (cool down) |

STEP 4: Increase throwing distance to a maximum of 60 feet. Continue tossing the ball with an occasional throw at no more than half speed.

| No. of Throws | Distance (ft) |
|---|---|
| 10 | 30 (warm up) |
| 10 | 40–45 |
| 30–40 | 60–70 |
| 10 | 30 (cool down) |

STEP 5: During this step, gradually increase the distance to 150 feet maximum.

*PHASE 5-1:*

| No. of Throws | Distance (ft) |
|---|---|
| 10 | 40 (warm up) |
| 10 | 50–60 |
| 15–20 | 70–80 |
| 10 | 50–60 |
| 10 | 40 (cool down) |

*PHASE 5-2:*

| No. of Throws | Distance (ft) |
|---|---|
| 10 | 40 (warm up) |
| 10 | 50–60 |
| 20–30 | 80–90 |
| 20 | 50–60 |
| 10 | 40 (cool down) |

*PHASE 5-3:*

| No. of Throws | Distance (ft) |
|---|---|
| 10 | 40 (warm up) |
| 10 | 60 |
| 15–20 | 100–110 |
| 20 | 60 |
| 10 | 40 (cool down) |

*PHASE 5-4:*

| No. of Throws | Distance (ft) |
|---|---|
| 10 | 40 (warm up) |
| 10 | 60 |
| 15–20 | 120–150 |
| 20 | 60 |
| 10 | 40 (cool down) |

STEP 6: Progress to throwing off the mound at one-half to three-fourths speed. Try to use proper body mechanics, especially when throwing off the mound:

Stay on top of the ball
Keep the elbow up
Throw over the top
Follow through with the arm and trunk
Use the legs to push

*PHASE 6-1:*

| No. of Throws | Distance (ft) |
|---|---|
| 10 | 60 (warm up) |
| 10 | 120–150 (lobbing) |
| 30 | 45 (off the mound) |
| 10 | 60 (off the mound) |
| 10 | 40 (cool down) |

*PHASE 6-2:*

| No. of Throws | Distance (ft) |
|---|---|
| 10 | 50 (warm up) |
| 10 | 120–150 (lobbing) |
| 20 | 45 (off the mound) |
| 20 | 60 (off the mound) |
| 10 | 40 (cool down) |

*PHASE 6-3:*

| No. of Throws | Distance (ft) |
|---|---|
| 10 | 50 (warm up) |
| 10 | 60 |
| 10 | 120–150 (lobbing) |
| 10 | 45 (off the mound) |
| 30 | 60 (off the mound) |
| 10 | 40 (cool down) |

*PHASE 6-4:*

| No. of Throws | Distance (ft) |
|---|---|
| 10 | 50 (warm up) |
| 10 | 120–150 (lobbing) |
| 10 | 45 (off the mound) |
| 40–50 | 60 (off the mound) |
| 10 | 40 (cool down) |

At this time, if the pitcher has completed successfully phase 6-4 without pain or discomfort and is throwing approximately three-fourths speed, the pitching coach and trainer may allow the pitcher to proceed to step 7: "Up/Down Bullpens." Up/Down Bullpens is used to simulate a game situation. The pitcher rests between a series of pitches to reproduce the rest period between innings.

STEP 7:  Up/Down Bullpens: (one-half to three-fourths speed)

*DAY 1:*

| No. of Throws | Distance (ft) |
|---|---|
| 10 warm-up throws | 120–150 (lobbing) |
| 10 warm-up throws | 60 (off the mound) |
| 40 pitches | 60 (off the mound) |
| REST 10 MINUTES | |
| 20 pitches | 60 (off the mound) |

*DAY 2:* Off

*DAY 3:*

| No. of Throws | Distance (ft) |
|---|---|
| 10 warm-up throws | 120–150 (lobbing) |
| 10 warm-up throws | 60 (off the mound) |
| 30 pitches | 60 (off the mound) |
| REST 10 MINUTES | |
| 10 warm-up throws | 60 (off the mound) |
| 20 pitches | 60 (off the mound) |
| REST 10 MINUTES | |
| 10 warm-up throws | 60 (off the mound) |
| 20 pitches | 60 (off the mound) |

*DAY 4:* Off

*DAY 5:*

| No. of Throws | Distance (ft) |
|---|---|
| 10 warm-up throws | 120–150 (lobbing) |
| 10 warm-up throws | 60 (off the mound) |
| 30 pitches | 60 (off the mound) |
| REST 8 MINUTES | |
| 20 pitches | 60 (off the mound) |
| REST 8 MINUTES | |
| 20 pitches | 60 (off the mound) |
| REST 8 MINUTES | |
| 20 pitches | 60 (off the mound) |

At this point, the pitcher is ready to begin a normal routine, from throwing batting practice to pitching in the bullpen. The program should be monitored and adjusted as needed by the physician, athletic trainer, or physical therapist.

# 22

# Glenoid Labral Lesions

*ERIC J. GUIDI*
*JOSEPH D. ZUCKERMAN*

In recent years, significant attention has been placed on the structure and function of the glenoid labrum. This has enhanced our understanding of different injury patterns that may occur. As our knowledge in this area has expanded and our ability to identify labral injuries has improved, glenoid labral tears are being recognized with greatly increased frequency. It is essential to differentiate asymptomatic labral lesions from those causing significant symptoms. In this chapter we discuss a systematic approach to the evaluation of patients with suspected labral injuries. It is our purpose to provide a method to arrive at an accurate diagnosis so that appropriate and successful treatment can be provided.

## ANATOMY

The glenoid labrum is a narrow, wedged-shaped structure that surrounds the periphery of the glenoid and is intimately associated with the shoulder capsule (Fig. 22-1). Moseley and Overgaard,[1] in an earlier anatomic study, reported that the labrum was primarily composed of fibrous tissue. However, recent histologic studies have clearly shown that in children and adults the labrum is principally fibrocartilaginous tissue and is a distinct anatomical structure.[2] Also, the labrum has been shown to be vascularized throughout its substance, although this vascularity decreases with age, and also to contain rare elastin fibers in adults. Labral tissue from neonates lacks elastin fibers, but in adults, rare elastin fibers are present.

The shoulder capsule, glenohumeral ligaments, and the long head of the biceps tendon are all intimately associated with the glenoid labrum. Because of its shape and location, the labrum increases both the depth and conformity of the glenoid cavity. In an anatomic study designed to show that the labrum and glenoid cavity form a composite socket of significant depth, the labrum was shown to contribute approximately 50 percent of the total depth of the glenoid socket.[3] Besides the capsule, rotator cuff, glenohumeral ligaments, and bony glenohumeral articulation, the labrum also plays a role in glenohumeral stability by increasing the conformity of the glenoid surface and thereby increasing the resistance to translational movements. Further evidence for the relative stability of the glenohumeral joint comes from roentgenographic studies of glenohumeral joint motion in the sagittal (flexion/extension) and coronal (abduction/adduction) plane that showed that the center of the humeral head remained within 1 mm of the center of the glenoid.[4] This degree of stability is provided, in part, by the integrity of the labrum. Detachment of the anterior labrum from the glenoid—the so-called Bankart lesion[5]—is an important factor in anterior shoulder instability. Howell and Galinat[3] have shown that detachment of the labrum anteriorly reduces the depth of the glenoid socket by approximately 50 percent in the anteroposterior direction. They use the analogy of a chock block, wedged between the wheel and the road surface, preventing a tractor trailer from rolling down hill to illustrate the buttress effect of the labrum on glenohumeral translation.

There is considerable variation in the size and shape of the normal glenoid labrum. The labrum ranges in width from 5 mm to 1 mm. Typically, in cross section, the anterior labrum is triangular, or sometimes

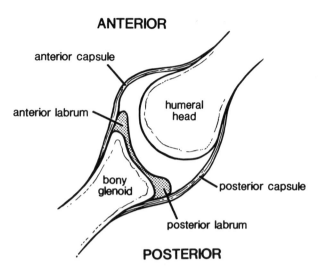

**ANTERIOR**

anterior capsule

anterior labrum

humeral head

bony glenoid

posterior capsule

posterior labrum

**POSTERIOR**

**Fig. 22-1.** Axial view of left shoulder showing cross-sectional anatomy. Note relationship of labrum to shoulder capsule and bony glenoid.

rounded. The posterior labrum is generally rounded in appearance, lacking the triangular shape of the anterior labrum (Fig. 22-1). The labrum is thin superiorly and thicker inferiorly. Detrisac and Johnson[6] described five variations in labral anatomy and classified them as types A through E. The type A labrum has a meniscus-type labrum located only at the superior portion of the glenoid rim. The type B labrum has a large meniscus-type labrum located only at the posterior portion of the glenoid rim. The type C labrum appears to have a meniscus shape in the anterior portion only. The type D labrum is a combination of types A and C and consists of a large labrum that extends from the posterosuperior to the anteroinferior portion of the glenoid rim. A type E labrum is shaped like a circumferential meniscus extending around the entire circumference of the glenoid cavity. Other anatomic studies have identified the presence of a labral sulcus as a normal variant in approximately 20 percent of individuals.[6] This sulcus is present anteriorly, above the equator of the glenoid, and is differentiated from the Bankart lesion by its smooth, well-rounded borders.

## PATHOLOGY (INJURIES)

Injuries to the glenoid labrum are relatively common. They are usually classified into two main categories: degenerative and traumatic. It is important to differenti-

ate these two types because of their different clinical significance. In a study of the macroscopic appearance of the glenoid labrum in 106 unselected shoulder autopsy specimens ranging in age from 1 month to 95 years, Kohn[7] observed lesions in 84 percent of specimens. In many of the shoulders, more than one lesion was present: fissuring (74 percent), posterosuperior detachment from the glenoid (50 percent), rupture or absence of the anterosuperior labrum (35 percent), and ossification (21 percent), which occurred mostly in older patients. The authors concluded that most of the lesions identified represented either age-related degenerative changes or anatomic variations.

Injury to the anterior glenoid capsulolabral complex is known to occur with anterior glenohumeral subluxations or dislocations. A spectrum of injuries can occur including a tear through the labrum, detachment of the labrum from the glenoid, detachment of the labrum from the capsule, or a combination of these lesions. Typically, the disruption of the anterior capsulolabral buttress results in recurrent anterior instability. Pappas et al[8] described a "functional" type of glenohumeral instability that results from a flap—or bucket-handle-type tear of the labrum—that intermittently becomes interposed between the articular surfaces of the shoulder. This mechanical obstruction results in a sensation of catching, slipping, or even locking. Although the shoulder does not truly sublux or dislocate, the patient experiences "apprehension" in the positions that produce the symptoms. In these situations, some degree of true instability may be present, but it may not be evident until the mechanical problem is corrected.

In the throwing athlete, the shoulder is subjected to repetitive stresses of great magnitude, particularly in the position of abduction and external rotation. Andrews et al[9] described an anterosuperior glenoid labral tear near the origin of the long head of the biceps. They postulated that this lesion is secondary to the repetitive, forceful contraction of the biceps during the follow-through phase of throwing when the muscle acts to decelerate the elbow and provide compressive forces to the glenohumeral joint. In their series of 73 throwing athletes evaluated arthroscopically, 83 percent of the cases showed anterosuperior labral tears (60 percent isolated, 23 percent involving both the anterosuperior and posterosuperior labrum). They observed that the tendon of the long head of the biceps appeared to originate through and be continuous with the superior glenoid labrum. With electrical stimulation of the biceps, the superior glenoid labrum was lifted off the glenoid, indicating an area of detachment. The most common presenting symptoms in these patients were pain during throwing (95 percent) and popping or catching during throwing (47 percent). Subjective instability (5 percent) was uncommon.

Recently, an additional anterosuperior labral-biceps complex lesion has been described. This superior labrum, anterior and posterior (SLAP) lesion begins posteriorly and extends anteriorly and involves the "anchor" of the biceps tendon to the labrum.[10] It has been postulated that these lesions can result from two different mechanisms. The first is a compression force applied directly to the shoulder, usually as the result of a fall onto the outstretched arm with the humerus positioned in abduction and slight forward elevation. The second mechanism of injury involves traction on the arm often caused by an overhead sports-type motion. The mechanisms described generally result in the superior labrum and biceps tendon being pinched between the humeral head and the glenoid, resulting in the injury.[10] In contrast to the lesion described by Andrews et al in throwing athletes, the SLAP lesion is felt to be secondary to a single traumatic event rather than repetitive stresses. In the series of Snyder et al[10], SLAP lesions were arthroscopically identified in only 27 of 700 cases (3.8 percent). SLAP lesions have been classified into four types by Snyder et al (Fig. 22-2). In the type I lesion, the superior labrum is markedly frayed, but the attachments of the labrum and biceps tendon remain intact. The type II lesion is similar in appearance, except that the attachment of the superior labrum is compromised, resulting in instability of the labral-biceps complex. The type III lesion consists of a bucket-handle tear of the labrum, which can be displaced into the joint; however, the labral-biceps attachment remains intact. Type IV lesions are similar to type III lesions except that the labral tear extends into the biceps tendon, allowing it to sublux into the joint. Eleven of the 27 cases (41 percent) in the series of Synder et al were type II lesions.

## EVALUATION

The evaluation of suspected labral injuries should follow the same systematic approach used for all shoulder disorders: history, physical examination, standard radiographic studies, special imaging procedures, and arthroscopy. However, in general a definitive diagnosis of glenoid labral pathology is usually difficult without the benefit of specialized studies. Nonetheless, it is important to follow a systematic, meticulous diagnostic approach.

Patients may often describe a single traumatic event: an episode of instability (subluxation or dislocation) in the abducted and externally rotated position or a fall on the outstretched arm. Throwing athletes are also at risk because of the repetitive microtrauma in contrast to the macrotrauma of a fall. Patients often complain of pain with activity, particularly overhead throwing-type activity. A "popping" or "clicking" sensation may be described. In some cases, locking may occur when a large labral tear becomes interposed between the articular surfaces. Pain with overhead use of the arm can be suggestive of impingement-type pain or subtle degrees of instability. This area of confusion becomes more significant when one considers that this patient population often manifests the "instability-impingement syndrome" described by Jobe et al.[11]

Examination should include inspection, palpation, assessment of range of motion, muscle strength, and

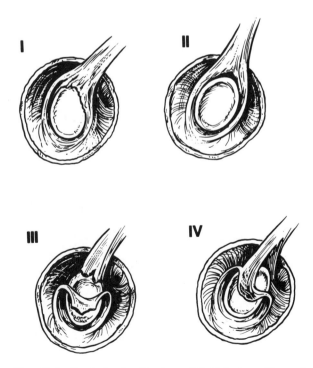

**Fig. 22-2.** Synder's classification of SLAP lesions (Types I-IV). (See text for description of lesions.)

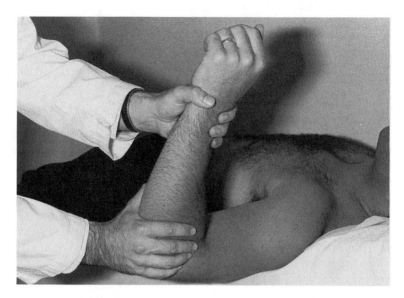

**Fig. 22-3.** Compression-rotation test. (See text for description of maneuver.)

neurologic function. These portions of the examination may be completely unremarkable. As a result, provocative tests and maneuvers should be performed. Standard maneuvers such as the impingement position, cross-chest adduction, and stress testing for anterior, posterior, and inferior laxity should be performed. Stress testing for anterior instability may show significant findings if anterior instability is present. However, two specific clinical tests—the compression-rotation test and the biceps tension test—may be very helpful in the diagnosis of labral lesions.

1. Compression-rotation test (Fig. 22-3): This maneuver compresses the humeral head against the glenoid in an attempt to trap the torn labrum between the articular surfaces. Labral tears will often produce a snapping or catching sensation as the humeral head is rotated.
2. Biceps tension test (Fig. 22-4): Forward flexion of the shoulder is resisted with the elbow extended and the forearm supinated. This maneuver may lift the torn superior labrum off the glenoid rim, thereby reproducing the patient's symptoms.

We have found that assessment of humeral head excursion on the glenoid can also be a helpful maneuver. With the arm at the side, the humeral head is grasped with one hand as the other hand is used to

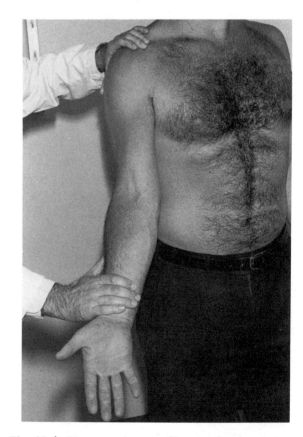

**Fig. 22-4.** Biceps-tension test. (See text for description of maneuver.)

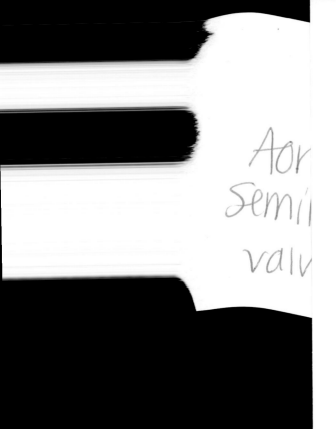

stabilize the scapula (by holding the coracoid process and scapular spine). Translation of the humeral head anteriorly and posteriorly may often result in crepitus or a catching sensation. This often represents a labral tear. However, crepitus may be secondary to anterior labral deficiency from associated instability or from articular surface irregularities. Because it is sensitive but somewhat nonspecific, these findings should be interpreted in conjunction with the other components of the examination.

Standard radiographic studies are not helpful in the diagnosis of glenoid labral pathology, but they can be helpful in identifying or excluding other causes of shoulder pain. The diagnosis of labral tears usually requires special imaging studies including computed tomography (CT)-arthrography and magnetic resonance imaging (MRI). Arthrotomography of the shoulder has been effectively used in the past, but the development of CT-arthrography and MRI obviated the benefits of this approach.

CT-arthrography has been shown to be an accurate and reliable technique for evaluating the glenoid labrum (Fig. 22-5). Wilson et al[12] demonstrated a sensitivity of 100 percent and specificity of 97 percent in the diagnosis of anterior labral tears using this technique. Other investigators reported similar results.[12-14] The primary disadvantages of CT-arthrography are its invasive nature and the radiation exposure to the patient. This is one of the reasons why MRI was believed to be an attractive alternative to CT-arthrography. With the initial use of MRI, it was not evident whether it could provide the same information that could be obtained from CT-arthrography. In an earlier study that compared CT-arthrography and MRI in patients with recurrent anterior shoulder instability, both modalities showed the anterior glenoid labral anatomy equally well.[13] Information about the anterior joint capsule was more difficult to obtain with MRI unless a joint effusion was present that could highlight an area of capsular detachment. However, recently, the development of contrast media (gadolinium) that can be used with MRI has further increased the information that can be obtained. Several reports in the literature document the efficacy of MRI for the diagnosis of glenoid labral lesions. In a review of 48 patients comparing MRI diagnosis with surgical findings, MRI showed a sensitivity of 90.6 percent, a specificity of 68.8 percent, and an accuracy of 83.3 percent for labral abnormalities.[15] An-

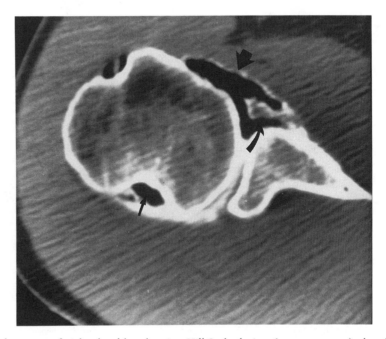

**Fig. 22-5.** CT-arthrogram of right shoulder showing Hill-Sachs lesion (*narrow arrow*), detachment of anterior labrum (*curved arrow*), and redundancy of anterior capsule (*wide arrow*).

other study by Legan et al[16] reviewed 88 shoulders in a similar manner; they specifically evaluated the role of MRI in diagnosing tears of specific areas of the labrum. They reported a sensitivity of 95 percent, a specificity of 86 percent, and an accuracy of 92 percent for anterior labral tears; superior labral tears had a sensitivity of 75 percent, specificity of 99 percent, and an accuracy of 95 percent.[16] In this study, MRI was found to be generally unreliable in the diagnosis of posterior or inferior labral lesions. The authors also noted that axial images were most helpful for assessing the anterior or posterior glenoid labrum (Fig. 22-6) and that coronal oblique images were best to demonstrate the superior and inferior labrum (Fig. 22-7). Based on these results and those of others, MRI has been shown to be a sensitive noninvasive method for identifying labral abnormalities that otherwise could only have been identified using invasive studies.

Shoulder arthroscopy has become a valuable method for the diagnosis and, more recently, the treatment of several shoulder disorders. However, it is im-

portant that arthroscopy main͏_____
the evaluation of suspected lab͏_____
physical examination, and sp͏_____
should always proceed arthrosco͏_____
Diagnostic arthroscopy can be co͏_____
vasive tests fail to establish a diag͏_____
the clinical findings. At the time _____
examination under anesthesia sh͏_____
formed. This may be helpful in ide͏_____
grees of instability that may not be ͏_____
anesthetized patient. Arthroscopic ͏_____
shoulder provides direct visualizatio͏_____
labral complex, glenoid labrum, and _____
capsular structures. It has been shown _____
portant diagnostic information that may _____ ͏_____
identified by other studies. Hurley and Anderson[17] reviewed 100 diagnostic arthroscopies and found that 72 percent of patients had glenoid labral tears, although only 15 percent were suspected preoperatively. They found that 92 percent of patients who had a diagnosis of recurrent anterior instability demonstrated a tear of

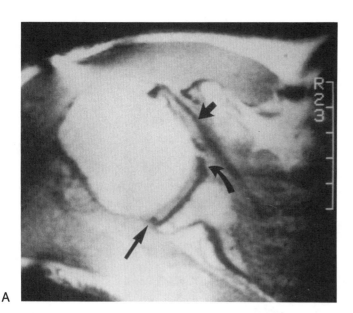

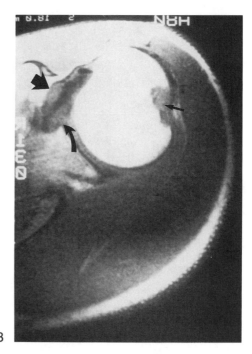

A

B

**Fig. 22-6.** **(A)** Axial MRI of right shoulder showing normal posterior labrum (*narrow arrow*), normal anterior labrum (*curved arrow*), and anterior capsule with subscapularis tendon (*wide arrow*). **(B)** Axial MRI of left shoulder demonstrating Hill-Sachs lesion (*narrow* arrow), absence of anterior labrum (*curved arrow*), and redundancy of anterior capsule (*wide arrow*).

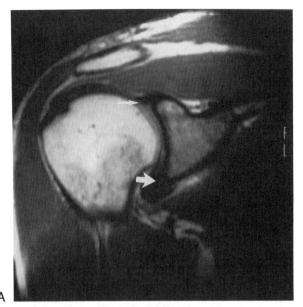 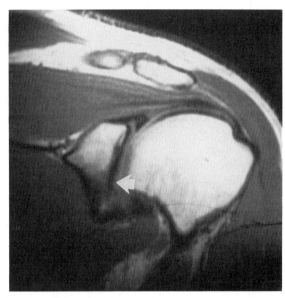

**Fig. 22-7. (A)** Coronal oblique MRI of right shoulder showing normal superior labrum (*narrow arrow*) and normal inferior labrum (*wide arrow*). **(B)** Coronal oblique MRI of left shoulder demonstrating absence of inferior labrum.

the anteroinferior labrum. They also found that 68 percent of patients with a diagnosis of impingement demonstrated tears of the superior labrum. Although the finding of anteroinferior labral tears in patients with instability would be anticipated, the relatively high incidence of superior labral tears in patients with impingement were somewhat surprising. More than 50 percent of these patients were throwing athletes, which may represent more of a "instability-impingement" syndrome.

Others have also shown the accuracy of arthroscopy for the diagnosis of labral lesions.[7,9,10] In many studies that assess the sensitivity and specificity of MRI or CT-arthrography, findings of diagnostic arthroscopy are used as the "reference standard." Arthroscopy also provides different treatment options that are discussed in the following section.

## TREATMENT

The treatment of glenoid labral lesions must first be addressed in the context of the basic principles of shoulder diagnosis and treatment. If diagnostic evalua-

tion indicates the presence of a labral tear, three basic questions must be answered:

1. Is the labral tear responsible, in whole or in part, for the patient's symptoms?
2. Is the labral tear an isolated lesion, or is it a component of a larger problem (i.e., instability)?
3. Can resection of the labral tear be expected to resolve symptoms or is a more extensive procedure necessary?

The surgeon's ability to answer these questions accurately will be a significant factor in determining successful treatment outcomes.

When labral tears are identified in a patient with clicking, snapping, or a locking sensation, arthroscopic resection is generally indicated. In these patients, resection of the labral tear usually results in symptomatic improvement. However, if the labral tear is associated with glenohumeral instability, excision of the torn labrum will probably result in resolution of the pain and mechanical symptoms but may unmask the instability. In these cases, the initial examination under anesthesia and arthroscopic evaluation may provide evidence consistent with instability. However, in some cases, the manifestation of instability symptoms only occurs after excision of the torn labrum. This is a consideration that should be discussed with patients before surgery so that they will be aware of the potential for additional problems.

Symptomatic glenoid labral lesions in which there was no evidence of associated instability can be treated by arthroscopic resection. The results of this approach have been variable. Pappas et al[8] excised all partially detached labral tears that were believed to be causing mechanical symptoms in their patients with excellent results. They did not report any evidence of instability at follow-up evaluation. In the series of Andrews and Carson[18] of 73 throwing athletes, debridement of anterosuperior labral tears (as well as partial tears of the supraspinatus and biceps tendons when present) resulted in symptomatic improvement with return to throwing in 88 percent of patients at 1-year follow-up. However, Altchek et al[19] reported distinctly different results in 40 competitive athletes who underwent arthroscopic labral debridement and were followed for at least 2 years (mean follow-up, 43 months). They differentiated the labral injuries with respect to location (anterosuperior, anteroinferior, posteroinferior) and character (tears versus detachments). Eighty-five percent of patients with labral tears had a good initial relief of pain and return to athletics. However, by 2 years postoperatively, the pain had recurred and function was compromised in 90 percent of these patients.[19] All patients with labral detachments that were debrided had minimal improvement in symptoms. The authors concluded that labral tears were generally indicative of increased translation of the humeral head on the glenoid and that debridement did not treat the underlying problem. This questions whether labral tears can truly represent an isolated injury, a question that has not been definitely answered at present. In our opinion, labral tears (particularly anteroinferior tears) are not isolated injuries but result from some degree of glenohumeral instability. However, the degree of instability may be limited enough so that a structured, directed rehabilitation program after excision may provide adequate compensation. However, we agree with Altchek et al that labral detachment, particularly in the presence of compromise of the attachment of the capsule to the anterior glenoid, should not be treated by isolated excision but rather represents underlying

instability that will require operative treatment for resolution of symptoms.

In patients with preoperative symptoms consistent with instability and evidence of a labral tear, the examination under anesthesia and arthroscopic evaluation become important diagnostically. If the findings during the examination under anesthesia and arthroscopic evaluation further support the presence of significant instability, a stabilization should be performed at the time of treatment of the labral tear. Anterior shoulder repairs can be performed as either an open or arthroscopic procedure. The largest experience has been with open repairs. The results documented have shown up to a 97 percent success rate for anterior capsular-type repairs.[20] The recent development of arthroscopic stabilization techniques have been promising. Although recurrence rates have been reported to be from 10 percent to 20 percent, improvements in experience, technique, and technology have resulted in improved results.[21, 22] The important principle to follow is that patients with labral tears in association with definite instability will not improve after simple excision of the labral tear. In these patients, a stabilization procedure should be considered using the surgeon's preferred method.

Recent recognition of the SLAP lesions has also brought specific treatment recommendations. Snyder et al[10] reported that treatment should depend on the type of lesion identified. In type I lesions, the frayed labral tissue should be debrided back to the intact labrum, being careful to preserve the attachment of the remaining labrum and biceps tendon to the superior glenoid. In type II lesions, a similar debridement should be performed and the superior glenoid labrum should be reattached to the superior glenoid using an absorbable tack or similar device. The bone of the superior glenoid should be abraded to promote healing. In type III lesions, excision of the bucket-handle-type tear has been recommended. Type IV lesions can be treated in a similar fashion, but the split portion of the biceps tendon should either be excised or tenodesed if it involves greater than 50 percent of the tendon. The clinical results in the small series reported in Snyder et al have been encouraging. However, a much larger number of patients and longer follow-up will be needed to determine the accuracy of these treatment recommendations.

It is important to emphasize that the treatment after

arthroscopic debridement or excision of labral tears must include a structured, supervised rehabilitation program. Initially, this should include active and active assisted range of motion to restore the complete range. Strengthening exercises should be directed to the deltoid, rotator cuff (internal/external rotators), and scapular stabilizers and should progress from early isometrics to a progressive resistance and isokinetic program. The goal of the program should be to restore patients to their previous type and level of activity. Therefore, each rehabilitation program should be tailored to meet the specific needs of the patient being treated.

# REFERENCES

1. Moseley HF, Overgaard B: The anterior capsular mechanism in recurrent anterior dislocation of the shoulder. J Bone Joint Surg 44B:913, 1962
2. Prodromos CC, Ferry JA, Schiller AL, Zarins B: Histological studies of the glenoid labrum from fetal life to old age. J Bone Joint Surg 72A:1344, 1990
3. Howell SM, Galinat BJ: The glenoid-labral socket. A constrained articular surface. Clin Orthop 243:122, 1989
4. Howell SM, Galinat BJ, Renzi AJ, Marone PJ: Normal and abnormal mechanics of the glenohumeral joint in the horizontal plane. J Bone Joint Surg 70A:227, 1988
5. Bankart ASB: The pathology and treatment of recurrent dislocation of the shoulder. Br J Surg 26:23, 1938
6. Detrisac DA, Johnson LL: Arthroscopic Shoulder Anatomy. Pathologic and Surgical Implications. Slack, Thorofare, NJ, 1986
7. Kohn D: The clinical relevance of glenoid labrum lesions. Arthroscopy 3:223, 1987
8. Pappas AM, Goss TP, Kleinman PK: Symptomatic shoulder instability due to lesions of the glenoid labrum. Am J Sports Med 11:279, 1983
9. Andrews JR, Carson WG, McLeod WD: Glenoid labrum tears related to the long head of the biceps. Am J Sports Med 13:337, 1985
10. Snyder SJ, Karzel RP, Del Pizzo W et al: SLAP lesions of the shoulder. Arthroscopy 6:274, 1990
11. Jobe FW, Kvitne RS, Giangarra CE: Shoulder pain in the overhand or throwing athlete. The relationship of anterior instability and rotator cuff impingement. Orthop Rev 18:963, 1989
12. Wilson AJ, Totty WG, Murphy WA et al: Shoulder joint: arthrographic CT and long-term follow-up with surgical correlation. Radiology 173:329, 1989
13. Kieft GJ, Bloem JL, Rozing PM, Obermann WR: MR imaging of recurrent anterior dislocation of the shoulder: comparison with CT arthrography. AJR 150:1083, 1988
14. Bigliani LU, Singson R, Feldman F, Flatow EL: Double contrast CT arthrography in the evaluation and treatment of shoulder instability. Surg Rounds Orthop 1:37, 1987
15. Gross ML, Seeger LL, Smith JB et al: Magnetic resonance imaging of the glenoid labrum. Am J Sports Med 18:229, 1990
16. Legan JM, Burkhard TK, Goff WB et al: Tears of the glenoid labrum: MR imaging of 88 arthroscopically confirmed cases. Radiology 179:241, 1991
17. Hurley JA, Anderson TE: Shoulder arthroscopy: its role in evaluating shoulder disorders in the athlete. Am J Sports Med 18:480, 1990
18. Andrews JR, Carson WG: The arthroscopic treatment of glenoid labrum tears in the throwing athlete. Orthop Trans 8:44, 1984
19. Altchek DW, Ortiz G, Warren RF, Wickiewicz T: Arthroscopic labral debridement—a three year follow-up study. Orthop Trans 14:258, 1990
20. Rowe CR, Patel D, Southmayd WW: The Bankart procedure. A long-term end-result study. J Bone Joint Surg 60A:1, 1978
21. Hawkins RB: Arthroscopic stapling repair for shoulder instability. A retrospective study of 50 cases. Arthroscopy 5:122, 1989
22. Morgan CD, Bodenstab AB: Arthroscopic Bankart suture repair: technique and early results. Arthroscopy 3:111, 1987

# 23

# Soft Tissue Injuries of the Shoulder

*JUDSON W. OTT*
*WILLIAM G. CLANCY, JR.*
*KEVIN E. WILK*

There are a multitude of painful soft tissue injuries about the shoulder. Most of these injuries are a result of primary injury to the tendon sheath or primary fatigue failure within the tendon. Additional injuries may result from either complete or partial rupture of either a tendon or the muscle tendon complex, whereas other painful conditions are due to acute or chronic bursitis or bony impingement.

## TENDONITIS, BURSITIS, AND THE INFLAMMATORY RESPONSE

Most soft tissue injuries about the shoulder occur as a result of primary failure within a tendon, with pain emanating from the inflammatory repair response within the tendon sheath. Inflammation can be thought of as a series of step-like processes, beginning with vasal dilatation mediated by histamine, serotonin, and kinins followed by the appearance of gaps in the endothelial cells, resulting in increased vascular permeability and subsequently local tissue inflammation. Inflammatory cells, such as leukocytes, are drawn to a specified area by a process known as chemotaxis.[1,2] Acute inflammation typically lasts hours to days. If the initiating stimuli continues, the inflammatory response will produce a thickened, chronically inflamed tendon sheath. The process of inflammation is perceived as pain through the detection of noxious stimuli by afferent nerve fibers.[3] These consist primarily of two fiber types: the unmyelinated, slow-conducting C fibers, which are responsible for dull, aching, or burning-type pain, and the finely myelinated, fast-conductive A-γ fibers, which are important in perception of joint pain.[3] These nerve endings become sensitized to the release of tissue mediators and prostaglandins; inflammatory mediators may moderate the release of neural peptides, all of which are ultimately perceived through peripheral nerves, transported to the central nervous system, and perceived as pain.

Tendonitis as described by Clancy[4,5] and Clement et al[6] is believed to represent devitalization and disruption of tendon fascicles caused by repetitive microtrauma. Some unknown mechanism stimulates an inflammatory response within the tendon sheath; however, no observable inflammatory response appears to be initiated within the tendon. To our knowledge, there have been no biopsy reports of any tendon in patients with a first episode of acute tendonitis. All published pathologic studies have dealt with biopsies of those with chronic tendonitis or biopsies of only the tendon sheath in those with acute tendonitis. Biopsies of patients with chronic tendonitis reported by Clancy[5] and Nirschl[7,8] noted a complete absence of inflammatory cells in the tendinous tissue itself, particularly in areas of tendon degeneration. Clancy noted that inflammatory cells were found only in those cases with gross partial ruptures. This lack of inflammatory cells was noted in histologic examination of the biceps tendon by Becker and Cofield.[9] These areas are charac-

241

teristic in that there is a loss of the normal collagen architecture and a paucity of tenocytes. Degenerative changes within a tendon in patients who were asymptomatic and on histologic examination showed no signs of inflammation have been described by Puddu et al[10] as representing a condition called *tendenosis*. Clancy[5] more appropriately used the term *paratenonitis* with tendinosis to describe more accurately the clinical and histologic findings in those patients with "classic symptomatic tendonitis."

Bursitis is an inflammation of the synovial sac, which is generally present at any site where increased friction may occur. The olecranon, greater trochanter, and patella are three of the common areas in which bursal inflammation may occur. A bursa is located between the superomedial angle of the scapula and the underlying rib cage that may become inflamed as a result of mechanical irritation. Even though bursal tissue is usually located in areas of friction, a bursa may also act as a tendon sheath in some locations. The subacromial and subdeltoid bursa are we feel the tendon sheath of the rotator cuff and, as such, may be primarily inflamed because of mechanical irritation by the coracoacromial ligament or by anterolateral impingement of the acromion. It may be secondarily inflamed when there is failure within the tendon manifested as a partial or complete rupture of any of the cuff tendons. Indeed, it is almost impossible to differentiate clinically rotator cuff bursitis as primary or secondary unless there is adequate biopsy material from the rotator cuff tendon. It is the authors' opinion that in the young throwing athlete, the primary entity is a bursitis caused by mechanical impingement from the coracoacromial ligament without rotator cuff pathology.

# BICEPS TENDON

Lesions of the biceps tendon are not infrequent about the shoulder whether related to a single traumatic incident, repetitive microtrauma, or impingement. These lesions can be divided into three main categories: bicipital tendonitis, whether primary or secondary, instability of the biceps tendon (subluxation or dislocation), and biceps tendon rupture. DePalma and Callery[11] reported biceps tenosynovitis as the most common cause of shoulder pain and found it to commonly coexist with frozen shoulder. Barnes and Tullos[12] reported five cases of bicipital tendonitis and three cases of subluxation of the biceps long-head tendon in 56 painful shoulders among baseball players, reiterating its common cause of the painful shoulder.

## Functional Anatomy of the Biceps

The long head of the biceps tendon arises from the supraglenoid tubercle of the scapula and from the superior glenoid labrum of the shoulder joint. The tendon traverses the glenohumeral joint through a synovial extension of the shoulder and leaves the joint in the intertubercular groove deep to the transverse humeral ligament. The muscle then joins the short head arising from the caracoid process and extends down the humerus before reaching a common insertion on the bicipital tuberosity of the radius.[13,14] The nervous supply emanates from the musculocutaneous nerve derived from a coalescence of the fifth and sixth cervical nerve roots.[13,14] Although the exact role of the long head remains somewhat controversial, it appears to assist in depression of the humeral head and further aid in the stabilization of the humeral head in the glenoid. The biceps muscle is important in both flexion and supination of the forearm, performing maximally with the elbow flexed at 90 degrees.[14] Cadaveric studies[15] have shown the long head is important in preventing upward migration of the humeral head when the short head is contracted. Kumar et al[15] believed that an absent long-head tendon would allow upward migration of the humeral head when the short head is stimulated, and it was believed to be important in fine positioning of the head in the glenoid to improve elbow flexion and supination power. Studies by Rodosky et al[16] noted the biceps contribution to shoulder stability by resisting external rotation forces that occur in the abducted, externally rotated position that occurs during the late cocking phase of throwing. Electromyographic studies by Jobe et al,[17,18] in throwers noted modest intensity during the cocking phase, with a lessening of activity until ball release and peak activity occurring during the follow-through phase. The activity was believed to be closely associated with elbow motion (deceleration and forearm pronation) during follow-through and was believed to be important in preventing hyperextension of the elbow.[17–20]

## Biceps Tendonitis

Although biceps tendonitis is not uncommon, controversy exists as to whether this is an entity in and of itself or whether it exists only secondary to some other shoulder pathology. DePalma and Callery[11] reported biceps tendonitis as the most common cause of shoulder pain, and early literature is replete with articles on the diagnosis and treatment of the primary entity. Neer[21-23] noted the potential for biceps tendonitis in those with impingement and believed that biceps tendonitis may be an early sign of impingement. It is our experience that both conditions exist, and we concur with Post and Benca[24] that primary biceps tendonitis represents about 5 percent of all clinical cases. In most cases the biceps tendonitis appears secondary to mechanical or chemical irritation.

## Clinical Presentation

Typically, the patient will complain of anterior shoulder pain, usually with activity. This may be insidious in onset, follow a single traumatic incident, or (as usually occurs in the athletic population) frequently occurs as an overuse phenomenon as a consequence of repetitive microtrauma or secondary to impingement. It may occur as an isolated entity but more commonly is secondary to some other pathologic process. It is important to note the presence of other shoulder pathology, particularly rotator cuff pathology, glenohumeral instability,[25] impingement, or generalized inflammatory conditions of the shoulder as the cause. The authors believe that in those patients with chronic rotator cuff tendonitis, the long head of the biceps acts in a prolonged fashion to depress and steer the humeral head and provide more room for the inflamed bursa and cuff and thus be more susceptible to development of a painful tendonitis-type syndrome.

The most common physical examination finding is tenderness to palpation over the bicipital groove.[11,24,26,27] Speed's test[26,28] is performed by flexing the shoulder against resistance while the elbow is extended and forearm supinated. A positive test localizes pain to the bicipital groove. Yergason's sign[28,29] is positive when biceps pain results from supination against resistance with the elbow flexed. Both tests can be helpful but are often nonspecific.[23] The relationship of bicipital tendinitis and frozen shoulder has been described[11,26] and must be remembered during the examination. Also, one must always remember the possibility of cervical pathology in the patient with shoulder pain and a paucity of physical examination findings.

## Radiographic Evaluations

Although radiographs are believed to be of little value,[24] several abnormalities have been reported to be associated with biceps tendinitis, including the presence of a supratubercular ridge and shallow bicipital grooves,[27,30] as well as noting the presence of any osteophyte or spur formation in or near the groove.[11,29] Ahovuo et al[31] noted plain radiographs revealed degenerative changes in the walls of the groove in one-half the patients with bicipital tendinitis. They also noted that arthrography was helpful in those with dislocated biceps tendons, but there was no difference in filling of the tendon sheath between those with surgically verified tendinitis or normal tendons. They also reported on the accuracy of sinography in discerning biceps tendon position and believed this was a useful technique when the sheath was not visualized by arthrography.[32] Magnetic resonance imaging (MRI) has proved useful in delineating the different pathologic entities that may be present in those patients with rotator cuff symptoms.[33,34] It has proved as accurate as ultrasound for evaluating rotator cuff tendinitis and tendon disruption but more accurate in diagnosing biceps tendon dislocation.[35]

## Pathology

DePalma and Callery[11] reported on the gross and microscopic pathology in 86 symptomatic shoulders, noting isolated biceps tendon involvement in 62 percent, and in 38 percent this was found to be secondary to a more generalized inflammatory process. The essential pathology was of varying intensity and involved the tendon sheath complex. Grossly, the outer synovial sheath was hemorrhagic and constricted on either side of the transverse humeral ligament. Microscopically, edema, collagen degeneration, increased vascularity, and round cell infiltration were noted.[11] In his operative procedure for refractory bicipital tenosynovitis, Michele[29] noted an adhesive inflammatory process may actually attach the tendon to the groove, diminishing the effect of the gliding mechanism. In patients with the diagnosis of bicipital tenosynovitis, Crenshaw and Kilgore[26] noted capillary dilatation, edema, and cellular infiltration in acute cases, with tendon fraying, narrowing, and fibrosis in chronic cases. In general, the pathologic processes were believed to parallel the duration and severity of clinical symptoms.[11,29] More recently, in 13 inflammatory tendons in which tenodesis was performed, Dines et al[36] noted varying degrees of inflammation; adhesions and synovitis were noted in all, with only one grossly irregular groove. In patients with chronic tendonitis, Becker and Cofield[9] noted gross tendon abnormalities in 32 of 38 tendons; but in contrast to other studies histologically, most tendons were normal, and only one had evidence of tendon inflammation.

## Biceps Tendon Subluxation and Dislocation

Biceps tendon dislocation typically occurs medially as originally described by Meyer.[30] The presentation may be after a specific traumatic incident, such as a tuberosity fracture, or on a chronic basis associated with rotator cuff pathology. Neer[23] believed this entity to be unusual in patients younger than 40 years unless in association with a fracture. Clinically, there is no pathognomonic sign,[37] but the test of Abbott and Saunders[38] may help to differentiate biceps tendon dislocation from tendonitis. The test is performed by placing the arm in full abduction and external rotation; then it is slowly brought down to the side. A palpable, audible, or painful click may be felt or heard, which strongly suggests the diagnosis. Frequently, however, the patient will complain of pain and a feeling of snapping in the anterior shoulder. The ultimate diagnosis of a subluxating biceps tendon is difficult to make based on examination; but arthrography, ultrasound, and MRI are all helpful in identifying the chronically dislocated tendon. DePalma and Callery[11] reported seven cases of subluxation and dislocation. They discerned the tendon slipping in and out of the groove with abduction and external rotation. Dines et al[36] also reported seven cases diagnosed at the time of biceps tenodesis for localized anterior shoulder pain over the bicipital groove. In cadaveric studies, Slatis and Aalto[37] found the most important ligament for stabilization was not the transverse humeral ligament but the medial portion of the coracohumeral ligament. Transection of the transverse humeral liga-

ment did not affect stability of the biceps tendon. They also reported five cases of medial dislocation and four cases of subluxation in live patients. In the cases of dislocation, the biceps tendon was found displaced medially, laying on the superficial aspect of the subscapularis. These patients were noted to have associated supraspinatus tears with involvement of the coracohumeral ligament. The tendon was located in a fascial sling on the ventral aspect of the subscapularis tendon. The four patients with subluxating tendons had limited cuff lesions, and these tendons were located in the groove. Good results were obtained in eight of nine patients when treated by tenodesis and rotator cuff repair when indicated.[37] Petersson[39] reported an incidence of medial dislocation of 6.5 percent in 77 autopsy dissections. He found dislocation always associated with full-thickness supraspinatus tendon ruptures and with partial- or full-thickness subscapularis tears, allowing the tendon to dislocate deep to the subcapularis muscle. Paulos et al[40] more recently reported on three unstable tendons after shoulder injuries that were described usually to consist of a combined distal arm traction, and biceps contraction, or a forceful biceps contraction alone in athletic activity. Two dislocated superficial to an intact subscapularis and one deep to a partially ruptured subscapularis.

Two main mechanisms of dislocation have been described, and they typically occur in concert with rotator cuff pathology. Either the tendon dislocates medially and lies superficial to the subscapularis after coracohumeral ligament rupture or after undersurface subscapularis rupture in which the superficial fibers stay attached to the transverse humeral ligament, allowing the tendon to dislocate medially and deep to the subscapularis muscle. Tenodesis is believed to be the treatment of choice, combined with rotator cuff reconstruction when indicated.

## Long-head Tendon Ruptures

Petersson[39] reported six cases of long-head tendon rupture in 153 cadaver shoulders. In most cases, this is believed to occur in patients older than 40 years[23] with a history of shoulder pain suggesting a pre-existing rotator cuff lesion. Carroll and Hamilton[41] reported an average age of 51 years in their series of 54 long-head ruptures. Rarely do long-head ruptures occur in an individual before the fourth decade. If this does occur, it is frequently the result of a single traumatic incident and may occur at the musculotendinous junction.[25] A mechanism of traumatic injury has been described as a forceful biceps contraction during athletic maneuvers with biceps contraction combined with arm traction (gymnastics),[40] or the result of a sudden biceps contraction with the arm in external rotation abduction.[25] Neer[23] described three types of biceps long-head ruptures usually occurring at the cephalad aspect of the groove. Those consist of rupture with retraction in which the diagnosis is often easy, based on swelling, pain, and the sudden appearance of a "popeye" muscle. Rupture may also occur with partial recession or self-attaching to the groove or transverse ligament, which makes the diagnosis more difficult because of lack of deformity. We have noted an occasional patient with chronic rotator cuff tendinitis in whom the symptoms are relieved, at least initially, after rupture of the long head.

Isokinetic strength testing at 2 years after rupture in 10 patients revealed no significant loss of elbow flexion strength and only a 10 percent decrease in elbow supination strength.[25] Sturzeneggar et al[42] used isokinetic testing to compare strength in the conservatively treated versus surgically treated long-head biceps tendon rupture (tenodesis) and found strength decreased by 16 percent in elbow flexion in the nonoperative group versus 8 percent in the surgical group. Comparing supination, strength was decreased 11 percent in the conservative group and 7 percent in the surgical group. Interestingly, a slight strength loss (4 percent) of shoulder abduction was noted in the surgical group. There have been reports of rotator cuff tears coexisting with biceps ruptures.[22,25] Usually the supraspinatus tear precedes the biceps rupture. As previously reported,[23,25] the treatment is based on several factors, the most important of which is the presence of preexisting shoulder pain. If pain is present prerupture, an arthrogram is indicated to rule out associated rotator cuff tear. If the arthrogram reveals a tear and pain persists, cuff repair, acromioplasty, and biceps tenodesis are performed. If the arthrogram is negative and the patient accepts the "popeye" muscle, nonoperative treatment is indicated. If the patient does not like the cosmetic deformity, tenodesis, acromioplasty, and exploration of the rotator cuff are indicated. Early tenodesis is usually considered only in the young athletic individual after an acute traumatic incident. Burkhart

and Fox[43] reported two cases of long-head tendon rupture in young patients associated with significant intra-articular pathology, including labral tears. A loose body and retained biceps tendon stump resulting in grade IV chondromalacia of the glenoid were noted in one. Arthroscopy was recommended after acute ruptures when surgical tenodesis is chosen or in those patients with persistent symptoms after nonoperative management to rule out significant intra-articular pathology.

## Author's Preferred Method of Treatment

It is our contention that the true cases of primary bicipital tendonitis are rare and that most cases are secondary to underlying shoulder pathology, usually chronic rotator cuff tendonitis. Although the biceps tendonitis may be the most prominent symptom at any time during the disease course, careful evaluation of the rotator cuff is mandatory. Conservative treatment consists of a comprehensive exercise program and a short course of oral nonsteroidal anti-inflammatory agents. Selective injections with 1 percent lidocaine and Decadron mixture are helpful from both a therapeutic and diagnostic standpoint. These may be delivered in the subacromial space or into the biceps tendon sheath, or groove, avoiding direct injection of the tendon. Performing isolated biceps tenodesis is rarely indicated, with the exception of the previously operated shoulder in which the patient has failed an adequate decompression and continues to have pure shoulder pain consistent with biceps tendonitis.

It may be indicated to perform a biceps tenodesis or to make several longitudinal incisions in the long-head tendon in the hope of stimulating a healing response in those with persistent symptoms suggestive of biceps tendonitis despite being adequately treated for rotator cuff tendonitis with a nonoperative regimen or in those patients who are undergoing arthroscopic decompression.

Subluxating or dislocating long-head biceps tendons are not common clinically, particularly in the young, active, athletic population. As reported, this usually occurs in combination with rotator cuff tears, and if tenodesis becomes necessary, it is usually combined with decompression and rotator cuff reconstruction. Although long-head ruptures are also rare in the young athlete, an aggressive surgical approach is indicated in some of these patients. In the older athlete, long-head ruptures are usually treated early with oral, nonsteroidal anti-inflammatory agents and an aggressive functional rehabilitation program. However, in patients with persistent shoulder pain or weakness an arthrogram or MRI should be obtained; if a rotator cuff tear or partial tear exists, an arthroscopic evaluation, rotator cuff repair, tenodesis, and acromioplasty should be considered.

## PECTORALIS MAJOR RUPTURES

### Anatomy and Function

The pectoralis major originates from both the clavicle and sternum, courses laterally, invested by the pectoral fascia as it forms the anterior axillary fold. It has clavicular, sternocostal, and abdominal portions, of which the sternocostal is the largest. The fibers converge to insert on the crest of the greater tuberosity of the proximal humerus.[13,14] The muscle functions in both flexion and adduction and assists in internal rotation of the humerus and, to a lesser extent, both elevation and depression of the shoulder.[13,14] Marmor et al[44] studied strength differences between arms in a patient with a congenital absence of the pectoralis major, noting the primary strength loss in adduction and internal rotation of the humerus. Innervation is by the lateral and medial pectoral nerves.[13,14] Electromyographic studies of the throwing shoulder[17,18,45] report the pectoralis major becoming active in the late cocking phase when external rotation reaches its maximum. Activity continues in the muscle in concert with the latissimus dorsi during the acceleration phase (internal rotation and adduction); activity decreases during follow-through. The pectoralis major is of primary importance in producing ball velocity.[45]

### Etiology

Marmor et al[44] stated that pectoralis major ruptures were rare. They postulated that because of its unique anatomy, rupture must be a result of trauma to a normal tendon. They studied load velocity curves in healthy muscles and found muscle could hold four times as much as it can lift. They postulated that rupture in a healthy athlete is due to application of excessive weight when the muscle is already holding at its maximum power. As reported by McMaster,[46] under heavy loads rupture would occur at the tendon insertion or musculotendinous junction and not through a healthy tendon.

The age range reported is from infancy to 72 years.[47] The median age, excluding infants, was 30 years, with a peak age between 20 and 30 years.[48] The most common cause of rupture is improper muscle coordination during heavy lifting,[47] as occurs during violent involuntary contractions[48] as a result of excessive muscle tension.[49] All patients were male.[47,48] Complete ruptures usually occur at the tendinous insertion.[48] Partial ruptures may occur at the musculotendinous junction or within the muscle belly itself.[48] Tendinitis of the pectoralis major insertion is no doubt more common than rupture, but because of the benign nature of the injury and excellent response to nonoperative treatment, little has been written about the subject. Chadwick[50] reported two cases of insertional tendinitis presenting as a suspicious humeral lesion at the insertion site, necessitating biopsy. Pathology was consistent with benign inflammation and tendon degeneration, indicating that the diagnosis does exist. Whether insertional tendinitis or tendenosis is a common precursor to rupture is a matter of conjecture.

### Presentation

The typical presenting complaint is a sudden sharp pain in the upper arm or shoulder[47] during an exertional athletic maneuver or a fall. An audible snap or pop may be heard.[48] On examination, ecchymosis is common over the lateral chest wall, axilla, or proximal humerus (Fig. 23-1). Indeed, hemorrhage may occur almost entirely over the area of the biceps muscle, suggesting a possible proximal biceps rupture, particularly when the individual has pain with resisted arm flexion. A bulge of the anterior chest wall on flexion and pain and weakness on adduction internal rotation are present. Effort to contract against resistance is painful and accentuates the defect. A visible, palpable defect in the lower fibers of the pectoralis muscle adjacent to the deltopectoral interval may be present, but this is not believed to be a reliable sign, as a fascial covering may remain intact and feel remarkably similar to an intact tendon.[49] The most reliable clinical test is to have the patient place both hands on his or her lateral iliac crest and then push inward (Fig. 23-2). One can then

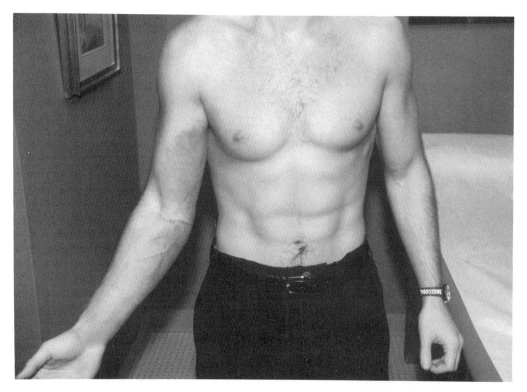

**Fig. 23-1.** This patient was referred with presumed diagnosis of proximal long head of biceps rupture based on location of eccyhmosis. This location is commonly seen in pectoralis major ruptures.

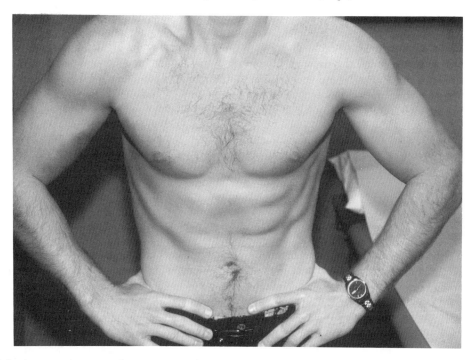

**Fig. 23-2.** Asymmetric pectoralis major muscles consistent with partial rupture. A complete rupture usually shows a more dramatic assymetry.

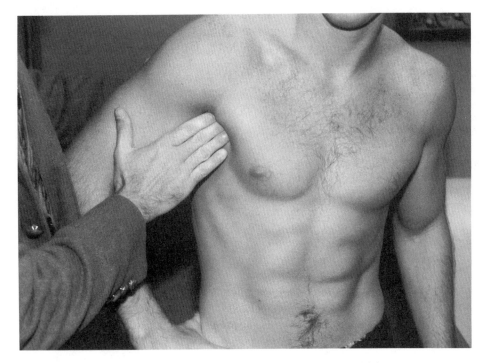

**Fig. 23-3.** Palpation of pectoralis major tendon, a key to successful examination.

readily palpate the combined tendon of the sternal and calvicular portions and compare it with the opposite noninjured side (Fig. 23-3). Partial ruptures, although not common, appear in the authors' experience to be equal to complete ruptures in incidence. This later entity is often missed or misdiagnosed, but with the above clinical tests, it is more easily discovered. Chest x-ray may show a loss of the normal axillary tendon shadow.[44,47,49] MRI may prove to be the best available diagnostic test in the future.

## Treatment

Although satisfactory results can be obtained in the non-high-profile, non-weight lifting athlete with nonoperative treatment, surgical repair is otherwise necessary and has been proven very successful.[47–49] The chosen method of treatment depends not only on the activity level and age of the individual but also on the location of the tear and the ability of the patient to accept a cosmetic defect. Proximal injuries at the muscle tendon junction (probably rare) respond favorably to nonoperative treatment, but distal lesions are best treated surgically.[48,49] Zeman et al[49] reported on nine

ruptures. The average age was 30 years. Seven were believed to be caused by excessive muscle tension. The five patients treated nonoperatively could not return to their previous athletic activity levels. The four patients treated surgically had excellent results, and all were able to return to their prior activity levels. Kretzler and Richardson[51] reported operative treatment of 16 ruptures treated up to 5.5 years postinjury. All 16 had good pain relief. Thirteen of the 16 reported full, subjective strength return.

## Authors' Preferred Method of Treatment

Our experience is consistent with that of other authors in that most ruptures occur during violent muscle contraction, such as bench press or the lifting of heavy objects. The diagnosis can usually be made on the basis of a typical history and the aforementioned physical examination findings, although MRI may prove helpful in difficult cases. We are aggressive in recommending repair in the young athletic population. Most tears have occurred at the tendinous insertion and are readily repaired to the original insertion sites through a bony trough with consistently good results. Bone implanted suture devices can facilitate the repair process.

# SNAPPING SCAPULA SYNDROME

This uncommon but significant disorder affecting the shoulder region is frequently confused with myofascitis and seldom recognized. The scapula is the site of origin of rotator cuff musculature, and the scapulothoracic joint is an important contributor to shoulder motion. As noted by Milch,[52] the snapping scapula is far from rare but is commonly neglected; the patients are often described as neurotic and rarely referred to an orthopaedist for evaluation. The etiology of the snapping scapula is believed to include an abnormal superior scapular angle; tumorous conditions, particularly osteochondromas; and changes consistent with interstitial fibrosis in the surrounding musculature.[52] A series of five cases resulting from subscapular exostoses have been reported.[53] Recently, four cases resulting from scapulothoracic bursitis at the inframedial scapular border in professional baseball pitchers were reported.[54] Three subsequent cases at the superior medial angle were described in manual laborers, citing repetitive trauma as a possible etiology.[55] It has been the authors' experience that the undersurface of the superior medial angle may be more rounded and somewhat thicker than normal, subsequently rubbing over the posterior upper thoracic ribs and producing a painful bursitis and perhaps a periostitis.

## Clinical Presentation

The patient usually presents with "neck pain" but on questioning can pinpoint the pain to the general area of the insertion of the trapezius and rhomboid muscles at or near the superior angle of the scapula. Often times, the patient may also complain of a painful snapping or grating over the superior medial scapular angle. These symptoms are made worse with overhead rotation of the arm, which produces scapular compression over the posterior ribs. On physical examination, the painful area can usually be localized to this area, and often a palpable, audible snapping or popping sensation can be elicited, particularly when the examiner applies compression to the superior scapula during the overhead motion. This frequently will produce a grating sound, which may be caused by compression of the bursa or by the scapula grating over the ribs. This entity can usually be differentiated from myofascitis (trigger point) in that the maximal area of tenderness is not at the scapular angle but well localized to a small area in the trapezius muscle in the case of myofascitis. A local injection of Xylocaine or Marcaine under the superior medial edge of the scapula should render the area almost completely asymptomatic, even with overhead motion and compression applied to the superior medial angle of the scapula. Plain radiographs are usually normal.[54] The importance of obtaining oblique views[53] and a computed tomography (CT) scan[55] have been reported, and CT scan is now the procedure of choice, particularly when bony lesions are suspected.

## Treatment

This entity is occasionally seen in pitchers, throwers, and golfers in the acute or subacute state. Initial treatment consists of differentiating the entity from the far more common entities of muscle strain and myofascitis. If the diagnosis is consistent with "snapping scapula," the primary entity is probably a bursitis, and treatment consists of active rest, combined with oral anti-inflammatory medications, and occasional injections. In resistant pain, and particularly if the problem is secondary to an exostosis, surgical treatment is offered. Milch[52] reported that simple removal of small parts of the scapula will predictably result in a cure.

Parsons[53] reported four cases resulting from exostoses that were successfully treated surgically. Sisto and Jobe[54] reported four bursal excisions at the inferomedial angle, allowing four professional pitchers to return to their prior levels of competition. Richards and McKee[55] reported three successful outcomes after resection of the superior medial angle of the scapula in laborers, and Arntz and Matsen[56] reported satisfactory outcome in 12 of 14 patients after superior medial angle resection.

## Authors' Preferred Method of Treatment

We have seen several cases, usually of a chronic nature, within the past several years. None of these patients have had an exostosis or osteochondroma. Initial treatment consists of rest, oral anti-inflammatory medications, and injections. Proper injection technique is important because of the proximity to the posterior thoracic wall and pleural cavity. After applying a sterile preparation, a 22-gauge 1.5-in. needle with 1 percent lidocaine and Decadron is introduced, angling from cephalad to caudad at a 45-degree angle just off the superior medial tip of the scapula, as the bursa usually resides approximately 2 cm lateral to the superior medial angle. Conservative treatment consists of gentle active assisted range of motion exercises, isometric shoulder and scapular strengthening, progressing to isotonic strengthening. Once the patient has accomplished full nonpainful motion and strength equal to the opposite side, a return to sport is allowed. If conservative treatment fails, surgery is indicated if so desired by the patient. The surgical technique[55] consists of a curved 4-cm incision over the superior medial angle. The fascia is divided longitudinally, and the trapezius is split in line with its fibers. The levator and subscapularis attachments are elevated in subperiosteal fashion off the angle. A large, malleable retractor is placed beneath the tip to protect the posterior chest wall. A 1-in. osteotome is used to remove the tip, which consists of a $3 \times 1.5$-cm area of bone. The edges are trimmed with a rongeur, and the bursal tissue is excised. The wound is closed in routine fashion. The results are predictably good in our limited experience. Early functional rehabilitation is begun immediately postsurgery, and it is essentially similar to that used for an arthroscopic shoulder decompression.

## QUADRILATERAL SPACE SYNDROME

The quadrilateral space is defined as the area bounded medially by the long head of the triceps, laterally by the humerus, superiorly by the teres minor, and inferiorly by the teres major, through which pass the axillary nerve and the posterior circumflex humeral artery.[14] Quadrilateral space syndrome was originally described by Cahill and Palmer[57] in 1983. The syndrome typically occurs in young, active adults between the ages of 22 and 35 years. It usually is not associated with any history of shoulder trauma. A patient complains of insidious onset of pain and nondermatomal, nonradiating paresthesias in the involved shoulder. A throwing athlete may complain of early fatigue, weak abduction, a numb shoulder, or dead arm-type syndrome.[58] Physical examination reveals tenderness consistently over the involved quadrilateral space, and symptoms may be reproduced with abduction and external rotation of the arm.

The etiology as described by Cahill and Palmer[57] is believed to be tethering of the neurovascular structures by obliquely oriented fiber bands in the quadrilateral space. Electromyographic/nerve conduction velocity studies are not helpful in making the diagnosis and are typically normal. Arteriographic evidence of posterior circumflex arterial occlusion, and the associated axillary nerve compression combined with a typical history and physical examination findings, is believed to be diagnostic. The importance of proper angiographic technique to visualize the posterior circumflex humeral artery with the arm at the side and also in the abduction, external rotation position has been stressed.[58] As stated by Cahill and Palmer,[57] 70 percent of the patients in their series had symptoms that did not warrant surgery, and alteration of pitching mechanics may prove beneficial in symptom relief.[58] In those patients resistant to nonoperative treatment methods, Cahill and Palmer[57] reported a series of 18 cases treated surgically. In their series, 16 of 18 patients improved with surgical decompression.

## FROZEN SHOULDER

The term *frozen shoulder* is used to refer to a condition of the shoulder consisting of gradual onset of pain, which may be severe, and is associated with limitations in shoulder range of motion, particularly overhead motion. The term *adhesive capsulitis* has been adapted more recently,[59] and its use persists despite several recent studies that have failed to reveal evidence of intra-articular adhesions.[60,61] Although the pathology has become better defined in recent years, considerable controversy remains concerning the etiology and what constitutes effective treatment. The following is an attempt to discuss the clinical presentation and the use of diagnostic aids, pathology, etiology, and different modes of proven effective treatment.

### Clinical Presentation

A frozen shoulder may present primarily or as a consequence of some other pathologic process.[61,62] The condition is typically more common in women and typically occurs during the sixth and seventh decade.[63–65] However, the authors' experience has been somewhat different in that most presenting patients are in their 40s and early 50s. In a study of more than 1,000 patients, the incidence in the nondiabetic population was reported as 2.3 percent.[66] Seventeen percent may have bilateral involvement, and five percent occur after a period of forced inactivity.[62] Associated conditions are multiple and include rotator cuff tendonitis, rotator cuff tears, cervical spine degenerative disease, arthritic changes, avascular necrosis, unreduced shoulder dislocations, epilepsy, chest wall tumors, diabetes mellitus, thyroid disease, intracranial disorders, and different central nervous system abnormalities.[61,62,67,68] The onset is usually insidious and may occur without any preceding traumatic event. Frequently, the problem is seen by the primary care physician with only the most resistant cases being referred to the orthopaedist. Inability to comb the hair or reach behind their back are common complaints at presentation, particularly among the female population. It is important to rule out other conditions as noted in Wiley's series,[61] in which 113 of 150 patients referred for manipulation were found to have other abnormalities. The process consists of four stages as described by Neviaser.[69,70] Stage 1, or the preadhesive stage, is uncommon to diagnose with its mild symptoms and insidious onset. Stage 2, or the adhesive stage, is considered to be the most painful stage. During this stage, the patient first notices motion loss. The third stage, or the maturation stage, is the time at which the capsule and synovium appear to be most angry. This is also the stage when the pain begins to decrease. In the fourth stage, the pain and synovitis is minimal; however, the range of motion is very restricted. Therefore, in stage 1 and 2, pain restricts the motion, whereas in the latter stage, motion is restricted by the capsular changes. It is important to realize the tremendous variability in the severity of the process. The course may consist of minimal pain and motion limitation of short duration with essentially no functional loss or range to a protracted course of severe pain and motion restriction resulting in severe disability. The pain is usually centered over the shoulder but may radiate proximally into the trapezius or distally to the elbow. McLaughlin[71] noted limb disuse and dependency combined with chronic muscle spasm may produce many different symptoms and clinical presentations. Ozaki et al[72] reported a presentation mimicking chronic fatigue as a result of sleep loss

secondary to pain or emotional depression, which in our experience is probably far more common than realized.

On physical examination, the shoulder may be globally tender to examination. The most distinguishing feature, however, is the motion limitation involving primarily abduction and external rotation, followed by flexion and internal rotation to a lesser extent. Fareed and Gallivan[67] believed exquisite pain on external rotation was the most sensitive indicator. Again, the importance of ruling out associated conditions is stressed, and a high index of suspicion is necessary to make the diagnosis in the milder cases.

## Radiology

Lundberg and Nilsson[73] reported 50 percent loss of mineral content in shoulder radiographs of patients with frozen shoulder, which may result in significant osteopenia; however, plain films are usually negative.[64,74] Significant degenerative changes are rare; however, if present, such as at the acromioclavicular joint, they may be a potential source of pain, resulting in a secondary frozen shoulder. Binder et al[74] reported increased uptake on bone scan in 35 of 38 patients; however, it did not correlate with arthrographic findings, and neither bone scan nor arthrography in that series proved diagnostic or useful in predicting ultimate outcome. In another series, arthrography has proven to be a helpful diagnostic tool. Typically, the synovial recesses do not fill with contrast medium, and the radiologist notes significant back pressure on injecting dye. A normal glenohumeral joint can easily accommodate between 20 and 35 ml normal saline. The ability to inject only a few ml with significant back pressure usually indicates capsular restriction and loss of glenohumeral joint space volume.

## Etiology/Pathology

Frozen shoulder may be associated with a multitude of medical conditions, including thyroid disorders, diabetes, autoimmune diseases, coronary artery disease, cervical arthrosis, epilepsy, pulmonary disorders, gastrointestinal disorders, ankylosing spondylitis, and central nervous system abnormalities.[61,62,67,68,75] Also, an increase in immune complex levels and changes in glycosaminoglycan content in frozen shoulder tissues have been found.[76,77] Onset may be related to initial trauma or the result of a forced period of immobilization,[62] but in most cases it appears to be insidious.

The pathology was described by Neviaser[59] on open exploration of 10 shoulders, noting the essential pathology to consist of thickening and contraction of the capsule, ultimately becoming adhered to the humeral head—thus the term *adhesive capsulitis*. Microscopically, reparative and inflammatory changes were noted in the capsule. Simmonds[78] later reported an increase in vascularity and thickening of the subacromial bursa and rotator cuff but found no intra-articular adhesions. He did not find any evidence of biceps tendinitis and believed the joint itself was normal. He believed the frozen shoulder was caused by a chronic inflammatory reaction in the supraspinatus tendon, brought on by local tendon degeneration that may be related to an impingement-type syndrome. McLaughlin[71] believed that intra-articular adhesions were more the result and not the cause of the symptoms. Nobuhara et al[65] believed it was associated with impingement of the greater tuberosity on the acromion and coracohumeral ligament contracture, limiting external rotation. Other recent etiologies were believed to result from localized synovitis, involving the triangle area between the long head of the biceps and the subscapularis tendon, with loss of coracoid and axillary recesses,[67] and Ozaki et al[72] believed the contracted coracohumeral ligament and rotator interval was the key. Electron microscopic studies by Lundberg[62] did not reveal any changes in the collagen ultrastructure of the capsule.

Recent arthroscopic studies noted absence of intra-articular adhesions and degenerative changes.[60,79] Two recent studies[60,61] emphasize the subscapularis bursa as a primary abnormality with a less frequent vascular reaction around the rotator cuff and biceps tendon. This is believed to be the key element in the etiology. Despite the recent attention to the subscapularis bursa and contracted coracohumeral ligaments as the initiating pathology, it is most probable that the etiology is multifactorial, whether related to pericapsular soft tissues or a more generalized, systemic process.

## Natural History

Natural history studies have documented spontaneous resolution of symptoms during an 18- to 24-month period[80]; however, the ultimate return to preinvolvement range of motion has been inconsistent, and the patient is often left with some motion limitations that may be significant although usually functionally improved.[81,82] Simmonds[78] reported only six of 21 regained normal function at 3 years. Reeves[82] followed 41 shoulders, using only rest and encouraging use of the extremity. At a mean of 30 months, 16 gained full recovery, 22 had mild clinical limitations, and only three had functional limitations. Binder et al[81] followed 40 shoulders for 44 months. Forty percent had residual symptoms at 3 years, but in only one were symptoms considered severe. They noted a tremendous discrepancy between subjective and objective results, concluding that residual motion loss rarely led to persistent functional deficits as the patients adapted to their disabilities.

## Treatment

Many treatment modalities have been used, although prevention remains the primary goal.[63] It remains difficult, however, to prevent the problem when the precipitating etiology remains unclear. Initial treatment during the painful inflammatory phase should be directed at pain relief by use of anti-inflammatory medications, occasional injections, and different physical therapy modalities, such as ice, ultrasound, and transcutaneous electrical nerve stimulation (TENS) units. Aggressive range of motion during this stage can result in an increased level of discomfort, ultimately prolonging this phase. We do believe that it is important to begin early, gentle range of motion, such as gentle Codman's exercises and active assisted range of motion exercises, as soon as tolerated by the patient. The range of motion program is advanced as the symptoms evolve from the inflammatory stage to the less painful maturation phase. Each patient, however, has a different pain threshold and does not always progress between clearly defined stages; the physical therapy program must be tailored to each individual. Also, the patient must receive proper education regarding his or her condition and he or she must be strongly encouraged to perform motion exercises frequently.

The main treatment groups are divided between manipulation and nonmanipulation treatment modalities. Not only is manipulation somewhat controversial,[68,83] but the manipulation technique varies from author to author, and there is not a definite agreement on the most appropriate time to manipulate.[68] Parker et al[83] reported on the manipulation of 22 shoulders, manipulating the arm into external rotation first, followed by abduction, grasping the arm near the axilla to decrease lever arm. At follow-up at 6 years, 91 percent good and excellent results were noted with a single complication consisting of a transient posterior-axillary nerve palsy and a 7.5 percent recurrence rate within 1 year. Neviaser's[70] technique differed, manipulating into abduction first, followed by external rotation, then internal rotation, and if unsuccessful, performing an open release. Lundberg[62] applied force at the elbow to increase the lever arm in comparing a manipulation group with a hydroinjection group and a control group. He noted the main advantage of manipulation was a shortening of the time course, and patients with the stiffest shoulders seemed to benefit most. Joint distention improved the restoration of motion but did not affect the overall treatment course.

Successful open treatment has been reported by Ozaki et al,[72] Kieras and Matsen,[84] and Nobuhara et al.[65] Ozaki et al[72] reported successful results in 17 patients after open release of the coracohumeral ligament and rotator interval, which they found to be the primary cause of the restricted motion. Sixteen of 17 were pain-free and had achieved full range of motion by 3 months. Nobuhara et al[65] reported successful treatment with coracohumeral ligament resection combined with freeing of the subdeltoid and subcoracoid adhesions and partial acromionectomy, when necessary, combined with gentle manipulation.

Treatment with hydraulic distention therapy has also proved successful. Fareed[67,85] reported successful results using intra-articular lidocaine, followed by injection of cool saline, and 1 ml celestone on an outpatient basis. He reported immediate pain resolution and normal motion in all patients by 4 weeks. There were no complications in this series, and he believed this should be the first choice in treatment and management of the frozen shoulder. Loyd and Loyd[86] reported on 33 shoulders treated by injection of lidocaine and long-lasting corticosteroid at the time of arthrography, followed by gentle manipulation. At 8 months, excellent pain relief and restoration of function were reported in 94 percent of the patients. Bulgen et al[87] randomly assigned 42 patients into four treatment groups: intra-articular lidocaine and methylprednisolone; 6 weeks of physical therapy; ice therapy after proprioceptive neuromuscular facilitation and a control group receiving no treatment. Little long-term advantage was noted in any treatment group, but steroid injection may improve pain and range of motion in

the early stages. Different physical therapy modalities have been used. Rizk et al[88] divided 56 shoulders into two treatment groups, noting 90 percent improved range of motion in the group treated by prolonged pulley traction and transcutaneous nerve stimulation and less satisfactory results in the group treated with different heat modalities, Codman's exercises, and wall-climbing exercises followed by a general rhythmic joint manipulation. Nicholson[89] compared two physical therapy treatment groups, the first receiving joint mobilization and active exercise versus a group doing only active motion exercise. He reported no significant difference between the two groups regarding pain; however, the mobilization group did exhibit greater passive shoulder abduction.

The role of arthroscopy in the treatment of the frozen shoulder appears to be expanding. Ha'eri and Maitland[79] first reported arthroscopic findings in 24 patients, and Neviaser[69,70] later divided arthroscopic findings into four stages, reporting an advanced synovitis by stage 2 and loss of the dependent fold by stage 4. Two subsequent series[60,61] have been published consisting of arthroscopy either preceded or followed by manipulation. These series report a rapid pain relief and return to motion at variable postoperative times.

## Authors' Preferred Method of Treatment

Perhaps the term *frozen shoulder syndrome* is more appropriate to describe the condition that appears to be multifactorial in etiology and responds to many different treatment modalities. It has been our experience that frozen shoulder is extremely common, and a high index of suspicion is needed to make the diagnosis in the mild cases. As previously reported,[70] perhaps the most difficult case is the very early case with mild motion loss that presents with signs and symptoms similar to an impingement-type syndrome. It is important to avoid early operative decompression in these patients, as this may facilitate a full-blown frozen shoulder syndrome and a protracted, postoperative course in a patient when the symptoms would otherwise have quickly resolved. Often the patient will have significant weakness of the rotator cuff muscles secondary to pain, bringing up the possibility of rotator cuff tear. When the diagnosis is unclear, we have found the use of arthrography to be helpful, not only to diagnose the frozen shoulder syndrome but also to rule out any associated rotator cuff tear. Initial treatment consists of an individually tailored physical therapy program, using oral anti-inflammatory medications and occasional subacromial or intraarticular injections for pain relief. The patient must be placed on an early range of motion exercise program consisting of active assisted shoulder flexion, external/internal rotation, and pendulum exercises. The range of motion program becomes more aggressive as the patient's pain subsides.

The physical therapy program we use is designed to relieve the patient's discomfort, restore shoulder motion, and most important, improve the function of the arm. An outline of our treatment program can be found in Table 23-1. The program begins with an extensive patient education session. We believe it is essential for the patient to understand what has happened to his or her shoulder and to explain the importance of the exercise program. Binder et al[74] reported in their series that only 50 percent of the patients seen received information regarding their shoulder condition and that only 25 percent of those who did receive advice were told to perform motion exercises, whereas the others were instructed to rest.

When first seen in physical therapy, the patient typically exhibits a painful stiff shoulder. Motion is severely restricted because of pain. A capsular pattern is observed[90] (external rotation limited more than elevation limited more than internal rotation), and a pain before resistance spasm end feel is perceived.[91] During this phase, the patient is initiated on gentle motion exercises with an L-bar (Breg Corp., Vista, CA) (flexion, external rotation, internal rotation, pendulum exercises, and occasionally a rope and pulley flexion motion). Gentle joint mobilization techniques are used (grades I, II, and possibly III) to neuromodulate the patient's pain, and additional modalities can be used. The patient is strongly encouraged to perform these motion exercises eight to 10 per day. The patient is instructed that if night pain occurs, a short exercise program should be initiated; this will facilitate a return to sleep. Several authors[74,92] have recommended motion exercises 3 to 5 minutes every 2 hours the patient is awake.

Phase 2 of the physical therapy program is marked by an improvement in the patient's motion (still restricted); pain occurs at end-range resistance, and a capsular end feel is present. The motion exercises are progressed, and the joint mobilization techniques are increased to stretching the capsule with grade III and

**Table 23-1. Program for the Shoulder with Loss of Motion**

*Phase 1—Painful Stage*
Patient exhibits
    Pain before resistance
    Decreased motion (capsular pattern)
    Spasm end feel
Treatment plan
    Pain medication
    Pendulum exercises
    Active assisted range of motion exercises (flexion, external rotation, internal rotation)
    Gentle joint mobilization (grades I, II, and possibly III)
        Modalities: heat, ultrasound, TNS, etc.
    Home program 8–10 times a day

*Phase 2—Transitional Stage*
Patient exhibits
    Improvement in motion, still restricted
    Pain with resistance
    Capsular end feel
Treatment plan
    Pain medication (weaned)
    Active range of motion exercises
    Active assisted range of motion exercises (L-bar)
    Joint mobilization techniques (grade III and IV)
    End-range isometrics for stretching capsule
    Self joint mobilization
    Home program 4–6 times a day

*Phase 3—"Almost There" Stage*
Patient exhibits
    Minimal to moderate loss of motion
    Decreased strength
    Resistance before pain
    Capsular end feel
Treatment plan
    Active assisted range of motion exercises
    Joint mobilization
        Single plane glides (aggressive) (grade III/IV)
        Multiplane glides
    Gentle strengthening program
    Home program

*Phase 4—Maintenance Stage*
Patient continues exercises for the next 6 to 12 months

possibly grade IV techniques.[91] End-range isometrics are used (Fig. 23-4) to stretch the capsule. Also, self-capsular stretches are initiated by the patient performing self-mobilization techniques at home[93] (Fig. 23-5). Often the patient exhibits a subscapularis trigger point.[94] Release of this trigger point often results in an immediate increase in external rotation motion, from 5 to 15 degrees.

The last phase of rehabilitation is often the most difficult. Typically, this marks the period of time when motion progression has reached a plateau. The patient exhibits a mild decrease in motion; the end feel is one of a hard end feel, and the end point is no longer

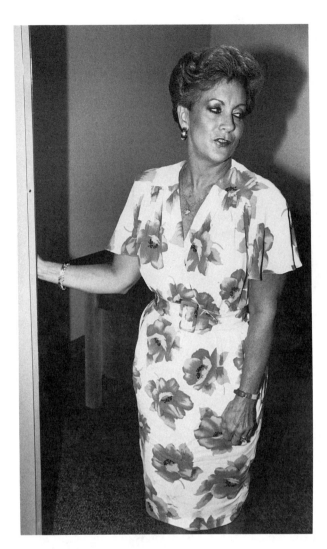

**Fig. 23-4.** End-range isometrics for internal rotators, used to stretch anterior capsule.

multiplane glide is occurring with a glide being applied anteriorly as the shoulder is distracted and the capsule is rotated posteriorly. This form of joint mobilization technique has proved extremely beneficial in our hands and has allowed the progression of motion through the motion restricted plateau. Additionally, low load long duration stretches have been shown more efficient in the elongation of soft tissue compared with high load short duration.[100,101] Lentell has shown that heat in conjunction with low load long duration facilitates long term improvements in shoulder flexibility.[102] Thus, the patient can be put in a comfortable elongated position (abduction and external rotation) with a slight load applied with heat for 40 minutes or longer. This technique can be used clinically or as part of the home program. The patient is encouraged to continue his or her exercise program at home for the next 6 to 12 months, usually twice a day. This prevents

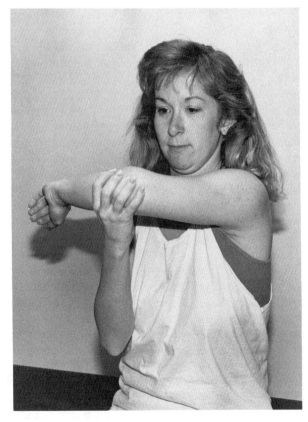

**Fig. 23-5.** Posterior capsule self-mobilization technique.

painful. Treatment consists of grade III and IV joint mobilization techniques to the anterior, inferior, and posterior capsule. However, often in this phase these single plane glides are ineffective in stretching the collagen tissue. Therefore, we initiate multiplane glides to provide an aggressive stretch to the joint capsule.[95] This joint mobilization technique uses the decreased capability of the ligamentous capsule to restrain force in multiple directions simultaneously.[96,97] Also, these multiplane glides are applied at moderate force for longer duration (30 seconds).[98,99] A technique to stretch the anterior capsule is seen in Figure 23-6. The

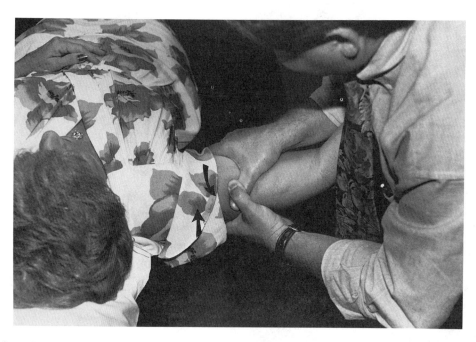

**Fig. 23-6.** Multiplane joint mobilization technique to stretch anterior glenohumeral joint capsule. Glide is applied anteriorly as a distraction, and posterior rotation force is applied.

the return of the motion restriction. The authors believe that with early intervention, patient education, and early motion, most adhesive capsulitis conditions can be treated successfully.

If the patient proves nonresponsive, manipulation and surgical treatment are discussed. The actual time course depends on the discomfort level and specific demands of the patient, but rarely is it ever considered before 3 months of nonoperative treatment.

Generally, we combine manipulation under anesthesia with arthroscopy. Our technique of manipulation consists of grasping the humerus close to the axilla to decrease the lever arm and obtaining abduction initially before proceeding with external rotation and internal rotation. The joint is then prepared and draped, and the arthroscope is introduced. After a successful manipulation, actual tears in the capsule are usually noted inferiorly and will be seen arthroscopically. On occasion, the arthroscopic bovie may be used to release the inferior capsule (Fig. 23-7). The cuff is evaluated, and in patients with a history suggestive of impingement (i.e., a history of chronic shoulder pain proceeding the onset of a frozen shoulder syndrome), a sub-

acromial decompression and bursal debridement will be used. It is important to perform minimal surgery as larger procedures may predispose to an increase in scarring and postoperative pain. Manipulation then is repeated, after arthroscopy, and the joint is injected with a 0.25 percent Marcaine without epinephrine solution for postoperative pain relief. Rarely has open debridement been necessary, only perhaps in the resistent diabetic patient. We have no experience with hydraulic distention therapy, but perhaps joint distention by arthroscopy may partly accomplish a similar result. Immediately after this procedure, the patient is placed on a continuous passive motion machine to facilitate shoulder motion and to neuromodulate the patient's pain. Also, active assisted motion exercises are performed with an L-bar, and passive gentle motion is performed by the physical therapist. As the patient improves and motion increases, the patient is placed on an aggressive motion exercise program for the home. This program should be performed six to eight times a day. We believe that it is essential for the patient to continue a motion exercise program for 9 to 12 months after this surgical procedure.

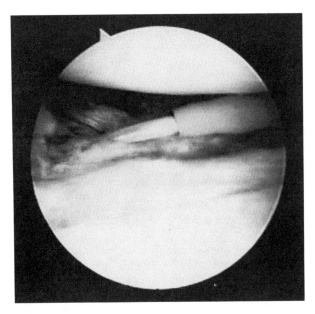

**Fig. 23-7.** Arthroscopic release of inferior capsule performed arthroscopically for frozen shoulder.

# REFERENCES

1. Ryan GB: Inflammation—A Scope Publication. Upjohn Publishing, Kalamazoo, MI, 1977
2. Schurman DJ, Goodman SB, Smith RL: Inflammation and tissue repair. p. 277. In Leadbetter WB, Buckwalter JA, Gordon SL (eds): Sports-induced Inflammation. American Academy of Orthopaedic Surgeons, Chicago, 1990
3. Hargreaves KM: Mechanisms of pain sensation resulting from inflammation. p. 383. In Leadbetter WB, Buckwalter JA, Gordon SL (eds): Sports-induced Inflammation. American Academy of Orthopaedic Surgeons, Chicago, 1990
4. Clancy WG Jr: Specific rehabilitation for the injured recreational runnter. Instr Course Lect 38:483, 1989
5. Clancy WG Jr: Tendon trauma and overuse injuries. p. 609. In Leadbetter WB, Buckwalter JA, Gordon SL (eds): Sports-induced Inflammation. American Academy of Orthopaedic Surgeons, Chicago, 1990
6. Clement DB, Taunton JE, Smart GW: Achilles tendinitis and peritendinitis: etiology and treatment. Am J Sports Med 12:179, 1984
7. Nirschl RP: Patterns of failed healing in tendon injury. In Leadbetter WB, Buckwalter JA, Gordon SL (eds): Sports-induced Inflammation. American Academy of Orthopaedic Surgeons, Chicago, 1990
8. Nirschl RP: Rotator cuff tendinitis: basic concepts of pathoetiology. Instr Course Lect 38:439, 1989
9. Becker DA, Cofield RH: Tenodesis of the long head of the biceps brachii for chronic bicipital tendinitis. J Bone Joint Surg 71A:376, 1989
10. Puddu G, Ippolito E, Postacchini F: A classification of achilles tendon disease. Am J Sports Med 4:145, 1976
11. DePalma AF, Callery GE: Bicipital tenosynovitis. Clin Orthop 3:69, 1954
12. Barnes DA, Tullos HS: An analysis of 100 symptomatic baseball players. Am J Sports Med 6:62, 1978
13. Netter F: Anatomy of the Musculoskeletal System. The Ciba Collection of Medical Illustrations. Vol. 8, Part 1. Ciba-Geigy, West Caldwell, NJ, 1987
14. Romanes GJ: Cunningham's Textbook of Anatomy. Oxford University Press, New York, 1981
15. Kumar VP, Satku K, Balasubramaniam P: The role of the long head of biceps brachii in the stabilization of the head of the humerus. Clin Orthop 244:172, 1989
16. Rodosky MW, Harner CD, Rudert MJ et al: The role of the biceps-superior glenoid labrum complex in anterior stability of the shoulder. Orthop Trans 15:58, 1991
17. Jobe FW, Tibone JE, Perry J, Moynes D: An EMG analysis of the shoulder in throwing and pitching. Am J Sports Med 11:3, 1983
18. Jobe FW, Moynes DR, Tibone JE, Perry J: An EMG analysis of the shoulder in pitching—a second report. Am J Sports Med 12:218, 1984
19. Abrams JS: Special shoulder problems in the throwing athlete: pathology, diagnosis, and nonoperative management. Clin Sports Med 10:839, 1991
20. Andrews JR, Carson WG Jr, McLeod WD: Glenoid labrum tears related to the long head of the biceps. Am J Sports Med 13:337, 1985
21. Neer CS II: Anterior acromioplasty for the chronic impingement syndrome in the shoulder. J Bone Joint Surg 54A:41, 1972
22. Neer CS II: Impingement lesions. Clin Orthop 173:70, 1983
23. Neer CS II: Cuff tears, biceps lesions, and impingement. p. 62. In: Shoulder Reconstruction. WB Saunders, Philadelphia, 1990
24. Post M, Benca P: Primary tendinitis of the long head of the biceps. Clin Orthop 246:117, 1989
25. Warren RF: Lesions of the long head of the biceps tendon. Instr Course Lect 34:204, 1985
26. Crenshaw AH, Kilgore WE: Surgical treatment of bicipital tenosynovitis. J Bone Joint Surg 48A:1496, 1966
27. Hitchcock HH, Bechtol CO: Painful shoulder—observations on the role of the tendon of the long head of the biceps brachii in its causation. J Bone Joint Surg 30A:263, 1948

28. Simon WH: Soft tissue disorders of the shoulder—frozen shoulder, calcific tendinitis, and bicipital tendinitis. Orthop Clin North Am 6:521, 1975

29. Michele AA: Bicipital tenosynovitis. Clin Orthop 18:261, 1960

30. Meyer AW: Spontaneous dislocation of the tendon of the long head of the biceps brachii. Arch Surg 13:109, 1926

31. Ahovuo J, Paavolainen P, Slatis P: Radiographic diagnosis of biceps tendinitis. Acta Orthop Scand 56:75, 1985

32. Ahovuo J, Paavolainen P, Slatis P: Diagnostic value of sonography in lesions of the biceps tendon. Clin Orthop 202:184, 1986

33. Iannotti JP, Zlatkin MB, Esterhai JL et al: Magnetic resonance imaging of the shoulder. J Bone Joint Surg 73A:17, 1991

34. Nelson MC, Leather GP, Nirschl RP et al: Evaluation of the painful shoulder. J Bone Joint Surg 73A:707, 1991

35. Vellet AD, Munk PL, Marks P: Imaging techniques of the shoulder: present perspectives. Clin Sports Med 10:721, 1991

36. Dines D, Warren RF, Inglis AE: Surgical treatment of lesions of the long head of the biceps. Clin Orthop 164:165, 1982

37. Slatis P, Aalto K: Medial dislocation of the tendon of the long head of the biceps brachii. Acta Orthop Scand 50:73, 1979

38. Abbott LC, Saunders JB: Acute traumatic dislocation of the tendon of the long head of the biceps brachii. A report of six cases with operative findings. Surgery 6:817, 1939

39. Petersson CJ: Spontaneous medial dislocation of the tendon of the long biceps brachii—an anatomic study of prevalence and pathomechanics. Clin Orthop 211:224, 1986

40. Paulos LE, Grauer JD, Smutz WP: Traumatic lesions of the biceps tendon, rotator cuff interval, and superior labrum. Orthop Trans 15:85, 1991

41. Carroll RE, Hamilton LR: Rupture of biceps brachii—a conservative method of treatment. J Bone Joint Surg 49A:1016, 1967

42. Sturzeneggar M, Beguin D, Grunig B, Jakob RP: Muscular strength after rupture of the long head of the biceps. Arch Orthop Trauma Surg 105:18, 1986

43. Burkhart SS, Fox DL: SLAP lesions in association with complete tears of the long head of the biceps tendon: a report of two cases. J Arthroscopic Rel Surg 8:31, 1992

44. Marmor L, Bechtol CO, Hall CR: Pectoralis major muscle—function of sternal portion and mechanism of rupture of normal muscles: case reports. J Bone Joint Surg 43A:81, 1961

45. Bradley JP, Tibone JE: Electromyographic analysis of muscle action about the shoulder. Clin Sports Med 10:789, 1991

46. McMaster PE: Tendon and muscle ruptures. Clinical and experimental studies on the causes and location of subcutaneous ruptures. J Bone Joint Surg 15:705, 1933

47. Park JY, Espiniella JL: Rupture of pectoralis major muscle—a case report and review of literature. J Bone Joint Surg 52A:577, 1970

48. McEntire JE, Hess WE, Coleman SS: Rupture of the pectoralis major muscle—a report of eleven injuries and review of fifty-six. J Bone Joint Surg 54A:1040, 1972

49. Zeman SC, Rosenfeld RT, Lipscomb PR: Tears of the pectoralis major muscle. Am J Sports Med 7:343, 1979

50. Chadwick CJ: Tendinitis of the pectoralis major insertion with humeral lesions—a report of two cases. J Bone Joint Surg 71B:816, 1989

51. Kretzler HH Jr, Richardson AB: Rupture of the pectoralis major muscle. Am J Sports Med 17:453, 1989

52. Milch H: Partial scapulectomy for snapping of the scapula. J Bone Joint Surg 32A:561, 1950

53. Parsons TA: The snapping scapula and subscapular exostoses. J Bone Joint Surg 55B:345, 1973

54. Sisto DJ, Jobe FW: The operative treatment of scapulothoracic bursitis in professional pitchers. Am J Sports Med 14:192, 1986

55. Richards RR, McKee MD: Treatment of painful scapulothoracic crepitus by resection of the superomedial angle of the scapula—a report of three cases. Clin Orthop 247:111, 1989

56. Arntz CT, Matsen FA: Partial scapulectomy for disabling scapulo-thoracic snapping. Orthop Trans 14:552, 1990

57. Cahill BR, Palmer RE: Quadrilateral space syndrome. J Hand Surg 8:65, 1983

58. Redler MR, Ruland LJ III, McCue FC III: Quadrilateral space syndrome in a throwing athlete. Am J Sports Med 14:511, 1986

59. Neviaser JS: Adhesive capsulitis of the shoulder. J Bone Joint Surg 27:211, 1945

60. Uitvlugt G, Detrisac DA, Johnson LL: The pathology of the frozen shoulder: an arthroscopic perspective. Arthroscopy 4:137, 1988

61. Wiley AM: Arthroscopic appearance of frozen shoulder. Arthroscopy 7:138, 1991

62. Lundberg BJ: The frozen shoulder. Acta Orthop Scand Suppl 119:3, 1969

63. Murnaghan JP: Adhesive capsulitis of the shoulder: current concepts and treatment. Orthopedics 11:153, 1988

64. Parker RD, Froimson AI, Winsberg DD, Arsham NZ: Frozen shoulder—part I: chronology, pathogenesis, clinical picture, and treatment. Orthopedics 12:869, 1989

65. Nobuhara K, Sugiyama D, Ikeda H, Makiura M: Contracture of the shoulder. Clin Orthop 254:105, 1990

66. Bridgman JF: Periarthritis of the shoulder and diabetes mellitus. Ann Rheum Dis 31:69, 1972
67. Fareed DO, Gallivan WR Jr: Office management of frozen shoulder syndrome. Clin Orthop 242:177, 1989
68. Leffert RD: The frozen shoulder. Inst Course Lect 34:199, 1985
69. Neviaser TJ: Adhesive capsulitis. In: McGinty Operative Arthroscopy. Raven Press, New York, 1991
70. Neviaser TJ: Adhesive capsulitis. Orthop Clin North Am 18:439, 1987
71. McLaughlin HL: The "frozen shoulder." Clin Orthop 20:126, 1961
72. Ozaki J, Nakagawa Y, Sakurai G, Tamia S: Recalcitrant chronic adhesive capsulitis of the shoulder. J Bone Joint Surg 71A:1511, 1989
73. Lundberg BJ, Nilsson BE: Osteopenia in the frozen shoulder. Clin Orthop 60:187, 1968
74. Binder AI, Bulgen DY, Hazleman BL et al: Frozen shoulder: an arthrographic and radionuclear scan assessment. Ann Rheum Dis 43:365, 1984
75. Emery RJH, Ho EKW, Leong JCY: The shoulder girdle in ankylosing spondylitis. J Bone Joint Surg 73A:1526, 1991
76. Lundberg BJ: Glycosaminoglycans of the normal and frozen shoulder-joint capsule. Clin Orthop 69:279, 1970
77. Bulgen DY, Binder A, Hazleman BL, Park JR: Immunological studies in frozen shoulder. J Rheumatol 9:893, 1982
78. Simmonds FA: Shoulder pain with particular reference to the "frozen" shoulder. J Bone Joint Surg 31B:426, 1949
79. Ha'eri GB, Maitland A: Arthroscopic findings in the frozen shoulder. J Rheumatol 8:149, 1981
80. Grey RG: The natural history of "idiopathic" frozen shoulder. J Bone Joint Surg 60A:564, 1978
81. Binder AI, Bulgen DY, Hazleman BL, Roberts S: Frozen shoulder: a long-term prospective study. Ann Rheum Dis 43:361, 1984
82. Reeves B: The natural history of the frozen shoulder syndrome. Scand J Rheumatol 4:193, 1975
83. Parker RD, Froimson AI, Winsberg DD, Arsham NZ: Frozen shoulder—part II: treatment by manipulation under anesthesia. Orthopedics 12:989, 1989
84. Kieras DM, Matsen FA: Open release in the management of refractory frozen shoulder. Orthop Trans 15:801, 1991
85. Fareed DO: Letter to the editor. Orthopedics 13:506, 1990
86. Loyd JA, Loyd HM: Adhesive capsulitis of the shoulder: arthrographic diagnosis and treatment. South Med J 76:879, 1983
87. Bulgen DY, Binder AI, Hazleman BL et al: Frozen shoulder: prospective clinical study with an evaluation of three treatment regimens. Ann Rheum Dis 43:353, 1984
88. Rizk TE, Christopher RP, Pinals RS et al: Adhesive capsulitis (frozen shoulder): a new approach to its management. Arch Phys Med Rehabil 64:29, 1983
89. Nicholson G: The effects of passive joint mobilization on pain and hypomobility associated with adhesive capsulitis of the shoulder. J Orthop Sports Phy Ther 6:238, 1985
90. Cyriax J: Textbook of Orthopaedic Medicine. Vol. II: Treatment by Manipulation, Massage and Injection. 9th Ed. Balliere Tindall, London, 1977
91. Maitland G: Peripheral Manipulation. 2nd Ed. Butterworth, London, 1978
92. Watson Jones R: Simple treatment of stiff shoulders. J Bone Joint Surg 45:207, 1963
93. Wilk KE, Arrigo CA, Courson RE et al: Preventive and rehabilitative exercises for the shoulder and elbow. American Sports Medicine Institute, Birmingham, AL, 1991
94. Travell JG, Simmons DG: Myofascial pain and dysfunction, the trigger point manual. Williams & Wilkins, Baltimore, 1983
95. Mangine RE: Alternative treatments for the restricted shoulder. Presented at Current Concepts in the Evaluation of the Knee and Shoulder, Chicago, IL, Aug 28, 1991
96. Arem AJ, Madden JW: Effects of stress on healing wounds: intermittent non-cyclical tension. J Surg Res 20:93, 1976
97. Enneking W, Horowitz M: The intra-articular effects of immobilization on the knee. J Bone Joint Surg 54A:973, 1972
98. Kottke FJ, Pauley DL, Ptak RA: The rationale for prolonged stretching for correction of shortening of connective tissue. Arch Phys Med Rehabil 47:345, 1966
99. Tabarg JC, Tabarg C, Tardiev C: Physiological and structural changes in the cat's soleus muscle due to immobilization at different lengths by plaster casts. J Physiol (Hand) 224:231, 1972
100. Light LE, Nuzik S, Personius W, Barstrom A: Low-load prolonged stretch vs high load in treating knee contractures. Phys Ther 64:330, 1984
101. Warren CG, Lehman JF, Koslonski NJ: Elongation of rat tail tendon: Effect of load and temperature. Arch Phys Med Rehabil 52:465, 1971
102. Lentell G, Hetherington T, Eagan J et al: The use of thermal agent to influence the effectiveness of a low-load prolonged stretch. Ortho Sports Phys Ther 5:200, 1992

# 24

# Neurovascular Compression Syndromes of the Shoulder

CHAMP L. BAKER
STEPHEN H. LIU
T.A. BLACKBURN

Shoulder injuries in the throwing athlete most often involve soft tissue structures and may sometimes result in compression of neurovascular structures in the shoulder and arm. The signs and symptoms of neurovascular compression of the shoulder, however, are often vague and, as a result, frequently overlooked. Diagnosis and treatment are commonly delayed. Recent interest in injuries of the throwing athlete has led to better definition of neurovascular compression syndromes, resulting in increased awareness of causative factors and effective treatments.

## HISTORY

The earliest reports on neurovascular compression in the shoulder focused on thoracic outlet syndromes. In 1743, Hunald[1] was the first to describe cervical ribs as the anatomic anomaly causing thoracic outlet compression. Similar findings were reported by Coote[2] in 1861 when he performed a successful decompression by removing the cervical rib. In 1919, Stopford and Telford[3] showed that thoracic outlet structures could be compressed by the first thoracic rib and that surgical removal of the rib alleviated associated symptoms. These findings were further described by Wheeler in 1920,[4] Brickner and Milch in 1927,[5] and Telford and Mottershead in 1948.[6] In 1927, Adson and Coffey[7] reported successful relief of thoracic outlet compression by sectioning the scalenus anticus muscle. Their results were later confirmed by Ochsner et al in 1935[8] and Naffziger and Grant in 1938.[9]

Compression of neurovascular structures at the costoclavicular level, secondary to hyperabduction of the arm, was first described by Lewis and Pickering in 1934[10] and later by Eden in 1939.[11] Vascular compression in this region was defined as costoclavicular syndrome by Falconer and Weddel in the 1940s.[12] In 1945, Wright[13] reported on a hyperabduction syndrome in which the second part of the axillary artery was occluded by external pressure exerted by the pectoralis minor muscle when the arm was brought overhead. Tullos et al[14] related occlusion of the axillary artery during the pitching act as secondary to this hyperabduction maneuver.

The first report in the American literature on the existence of subclavian vein thrombosis was by Matas in 1934.[15] This condition, previously described by Sir James Paget in 1875[16] and Von Schroetter in 1884,[17] was known as the Paget-von Schroetter syndrome. The current description of subclavian vein thrombosis as effort thrombosis is due to the associated physical activity that produces direct or indirect injury to the vein.

In 1967, Cahill attributed a high percentage of treatment failure of thoracic outlet syndrome to occlusion of the posterior humeral circumflex artery. Further investigation by Cahill and Palmer[18,19] led to the recognition of the quadrilateral space syndrome.

261

## ANATOMY

The space through which the great vessels traverse from the neck to the chest is referred to as the throacic outlet. The floor is formed by the superior border of the first rib, and the roof is formed by the inferior border of the clavicle. The space is partitioned by the scalene muscles. The anterior scalene muscle originates from the transverse process of the third, fourth, fifth, and sixth cervical vertebrae and inserts posterior to the subclavian vein into the first rib. The middle scalene muscle originates from the transverse process of the second through the seventh cervical vertebrae and inserts behind the subclavian artery into the first rib. The subclavian artery and the brachial plexus enter between the anterior and middle scalene muscles (Fig. 24-1). The neurovascular bundle (including the axillary artery) traverses more distally underneath the pectoralis minor muscle.

Lateral to the first rib, the subclavian artery becomes the axillary artery. The axillary artery has six primary branches: the superior thoracic artery, medial to the pectoralis minor muscle; the thoracoacromial artery and lateral thoracic artery, at the level of the pectoralis minor muscle; and the subscapular artery and posterior and anterior circumflex humeral arteries, before the origin of the brachial artery. Lateral to the border of the first rib, the axillary vein becomes the subclavian vein, which follows the same general path as the subclavian artery. Near its insertion into the first rib, the anterior scalene muscle separates the subclavian artery and subclavian vein.

Based on these anatomic relationships, there are several locations where compression of the neurovascular structures can occur. These include (1) proximal compression of the brachial plexus and subclavian artery as they pass between the anterior and middle scalene muscle; more distally, compression through the costoclavicular space; and most distally, compression proximal to the axilla as they pass underneath the pectoralis minor muscle; (2) compression of the subclavian vein between the anterior scalene muscle, clavicle, and first rib; and (3) compression of the posterior circumflex humeral artery and axillary nerve as they exit through the quadrilateral space bordered by the teres minor and major muscles, the humerus, and the medial head of the triceps.

## CLINICAL PRESENTATIONS

The diagnosis of neurovascular compression syndrome of the shoulder is most often made after a detailed history, physical examination, and ancillary diagnostic studies. Athletes suffering from compression of neurovascular structures of the shoulder can present with subtle and diverse symptoms and signs, making the diagnosis difficult.

### Symptoms

Symptoms vary depending on the anatomic structures (nerve, artery, or vein) being compromised and on the site of the compression. Primary compression of the lower trunk of the brachial plexus in the thoracic outlet frequently results in pain and paresthesia from the neck and shoulder down to the medial aspect of the hand, with associated weakness of grasp and difficulty with fine finger movements. Compression of the upper

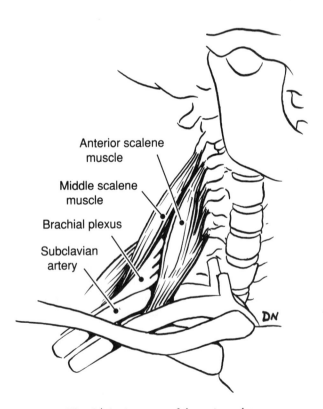

Anterior scalene muscle

Middle scalene muscle

Brachial plexus

Subclavian artery

**Fig. 24-1.** Anatomy of thoracic outlet.

trunk of the brachial plexus results in more obscure symptoms, with pain more proximal in the neck and shoulder region. The symptoms are frequently similar to those of cervical disc herniation.

Patients with vascular compression often present with complaints of upper limb heaviness, fatigability, and claudication. Swelling, discoloration, ulceration, and infrequently, symptoms of Raynaud syndrome may be present.[20] The symptoms will reflect to what degree the vascular compromise is arterial and to what degree venous. Arterial insufficiency usually produces symptoms of coolness, numbness, and exertional fatigue. Venous obstruction causes upper limb edema, heaviness, and cyanosis.

If both nerves and vessels are being compressed, a mixed pattern of neurologic and vascular symptoms may be present. Thus, one must be aware of the symptoms of neurologic compression and vascular compromise and alert to a possible association when they are present at the same time.

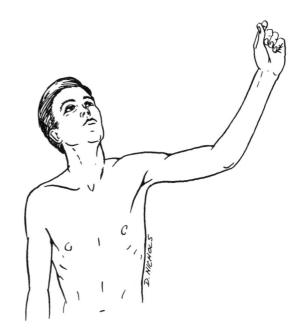

**Fig. 24-2.** Adson's test.

## Signs

A thorough clinical examination, with emphasis on the cervical spine and shoulder girdle, and the use of three specific tests (Adson's test, costoclavicular maneuver, and hyperabduction maneuver) are essential in localizing the anatomic site of compression.

During inspection of the shoulder complex, particular attention should be paid to shoulder asymmetry, unusually larger breasts, and poor muscular development. These findings may indicate developmental or postural abnormalities that can predispose a patient to neurovascular compression syndromes.[21]

Several additional physical findings may be helpful in establishing the diagnosis of neurovascular compression syndrome. Firm pressure on or percussion over the brachial plexus in the supraclavicular fossa may produce pain or paresthesias caused by nerve irritation at the site of compression. The presence of bruits during provocative testing is a sign of vascular compromise. The overhead exercise test, performed with the patient sitting down, rapidly flexing and extending the fingers while keeping the arms elevated overhead, is considered positive when the symptoms are reproduced.[21]

Adson's test, as described by Alford Adson in 1927, is used to demonstrate compression of the subclavian artery by the scalene anticus muscle.[7] The test is performed by having the patient inhale deeply, extend his or her neck, and turn his or her chin toward the affected shoulder (Fig. 24-2). Diminution or obliteration of the radial pulse or change in blood pressure indicates scalene anticus syndrome.

The costoclavicular maneuver is performed by having the patient thrust the shoulders backward and downward, similar to a military brace position[22] (Fig. 24-3). This maneuver decreases the space between the clavicle and the first rib, thus compressing the neurovascular structures located in that area.

The third test is the hyperabduction maneuver as described by Wright in 1945.[13] The patient is asked to take a deep breath and then turn his or her head to the opposite side as the affected arm is abducted and externally rotated. (Fig. 24-4). This test is most specific for neurovascular compression in the subcoracoid region, particularly compression of the second part of the axillary artery under the pectoralis minor muscle.

Each of these tests, however, can result in false-positive and false-negative findings. Several authors have reported that 50 percent of normal asymptomatic individuals will have a positive Adson's test.[23,24] Thus, a test should be considered truly positive only

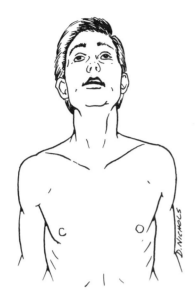

**Fig. 24-3.** Costoclavicular maneuver.

when the maneuver reproduces the patient's symptoms.

## ANCILLARY DIAGNOSTIC STUDIES

Besides the history and physical examination, several ancillary studies can be performed to help confirm the diagnosis of a neurovascular compression syndrome.

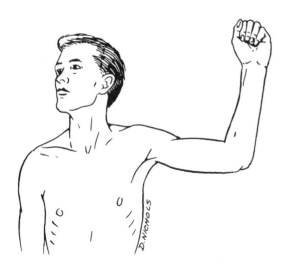

**Fig. 24-4.** Hyperabduction maneuver.

Plain radiographs of the cervical spine should be taken to determine the presence of cervical or first thoracic ribs or irregularities of the clavicle or first rib. Although cervical ribs are the most common bony abnormalities associated with neurovascular compression, less than 10 percent of these patients have symptoms.[25] The ribs, originating from the transverse process of C7, usually attach directly or by ligaments to the first rib (Fig. 24-5). An anteroposterior view may reveal abnormalities or fractures of the clavicle or first rib, which can produce constriction of neurovascular structures depending on the position of the bones. Arthritic changes of the cervical spine may result in nerve root compression, which can produce symptoms similar to those found in neurovascular compression syndromes. Chest radiographs can rule out conditions that may refer pain to the shoulder, such as a Pancoast's tumor,

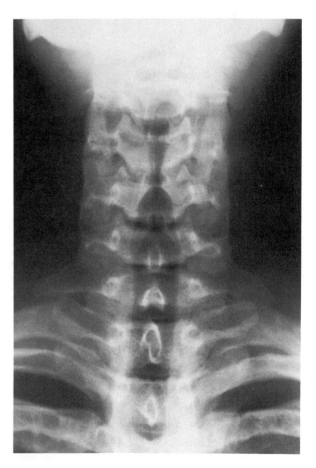

**Fig. 24-5.** Radiographic demonstration of cervical rib.

although this is a rare finding in the young athletic population.

Some authors have reported the usefulness of electrodiagnostic studies in confirming the diagnosis of neurovascular compression syndromes.[26,27] Others, however, have shown that neither nerve conduction studies nor evoked potential stimulation is reliable in establishing the diagnosis of neurovascular compression syndromes.[23,24,28,29] These tests, however, can be useful in ruling out more peripheral lesions at the elbow or wrist (e.g., carpal tunnel syndrome or ulnar nerve neuropathy) or in the differential diagnosis of cervical radiculopathy with referred shoulder pain.[22]

Noninvasive and invasive vascular studies also can be used to help in the diagnosis of neurovascular compression syndromes.[13,14,18,22] Doppler sonography, an effective technique for measuring arterial flow in the arm, has been used successfully by physicians in screening throwing athletes.[30] Digital subtraction angiography may be used in place of arteriograms in certain patients. However, definitive diagnosis of vascular compromise requires venogram and angiogram studies of the subclavian and axillary vessels. When performing these studies, it is important to do them with the affected arm in both the normal anatomic position and in the position in which the symptoms are produced.

## SPECIFIC SYNDROMES
### Thoracic Outlet Syndrome

Thoracic outlet syndrome is an ill-defined term that encompasses the signs and symptoms attributed to compression of the nerves and vascular structures as they traverse from the neck to the axilla. Because of the proximity of nerves and vessels to one another in the thoracic outlet, varying degrees of compression of the brachial plexus and subclavian vessels can exist. First described by Hunald[1] more than 200 years ago, this syndrome has recently been associated with throwing injuries in athletes.[30–32]

There are many causes of thoracic outlet syndrome. Early reports of thoracic outlet compression are rich in their description of congenital and structural abnormalities. Although cervical ribs are present in less than 1 percent of the population, they are the most common bony abnormality associated with thoracic outlet syndrome. However, less than 10 percent of patients with cervical ribs have symptoms related to thoracic outlet

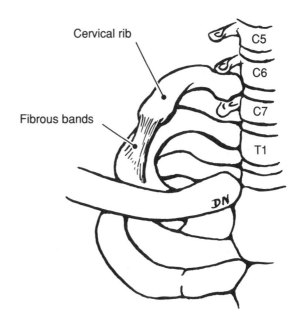

**Fig. 24-6.** Cervical rib fibrous bands.

compression.[25] Another aberrant structure that can cause mechanical compression within the thoracic outlet is fibrous bands originating from the end of a prominent C7 transverse process or from the end of a short cervical rib.[21] (Fig. 24-6). Abnormal scalene muscle development has also been associated with thoracic outlet syndrome. Frequently, anomalous fibromuscular bands that can entrap the upper trunk of the brachial plexus are present in these muscles.[28,29]

In recent years, trauma and dynamic changes in the shoulder secondary to throwing mechanics have come to be recognized as common causes of thoracic outlet syndrome.[21,30] Injury to the shoulder muscles may result in hemorrhage and abnormal shoulder mechanics, which can cause functional impairment and secondary neurovascular compression. Also, excessive callus formation or malunion after a clavicle fracture may result in reduction of the costoclavicular space and subsequent signs and symptoms of thoracic outlet syndrome.[33]

Signs and symptoms depend on the degree to which particular nerves and vascular structures are compromised and are similar to those of any compression of the nerves, arteries, or veins in the thorax. These include venous engorgement, coolness, numbness, and tingling in the affected extremity. Also, the extremity may feel weak or heavy or be easily fatigued. In athletes, the neurologic and vascular symptoms of thoracic outlet compression are usually associated with specific athletic activities. The symptoms can be elicited by reproducing the activity and often are relieved by abstaining from the activity.

Initial treatment of thoracic outlet syndrome is nonoperative. Most patients can be treated successfully with nonsteroidal anti-inflammatory medications and local trigger-point injections and by abstaining from the precipitating activity until the symptoms resolve. Patients with complicating vascular problems should have appropriate invasive studies and follow-up treatment.

As the pain subsides, an exercise program should be implemented that includes correcting any postural abnormalities (rounded shoulders and a head-forward position can contribute to neurovascular compression) and strengthening the shoulder girdle and scapular musculature.[34] It is important, though, not to aggravate symptoms with any of the exercises.

Shoulder shrugs with scapular abduction exercises will help firm up the trapezius muscle group, which is the suspension structure for the shoulder girdle, and the parascapular muscles, which aid in proper alignment of the shoulder. Abduction in the plane of the scapula, sitting dips, bent rows, and push-ups with protraction of the shoulder girdle are best for strengthening the scapular rotators. The exercise program should consist of three to five sets of 10 repetitions at 0 to 5 lb at least two times a day. If the levator scapulae is tight, a good stretching program consists of pulling the patient's head forward and to the opposite side while rotating toward the tight side. If the scalene muscles are involved, it may be possible to alleviate symptoms by stretching the anterior muscles by moving the patient's head and neck into extension and rotating toward the involved side; and the posterior muscles by lateral flexion and rotation away from the involved side. Stretching routines should be performed 15 to 25 times at least three times a day. Besides these exercises, having the patient sleep supine or in the semi-sidelying position with a small pillow supporting the thoracic spine may help to "open" the thoracic outlet. Congenital abnormalities, such as cervical ribs or fibrous bands at C7, are difficult to treat with exercises. However, increasing cervical spine flexibility with different cervical stretches may help decrease compression.

Surgical intervention is reserved for patients who continue to have pain and functional impairment despite a well-directed rehabilitation program. Occasionally, surgical decompression is indicated for acute vascular insufficiencies or progressive neurologic symptoms. Surgical treatment depends on the particular condition causing the syndrome and can be excision of a cervical rib, scalenotomy of the scalene anticus muscle, or release of fibromuscular bands located in the thorax at the site of occlusion.[22] Many authors have reported good to excellent results with surgery. Unsatisfactory outcomes have been attributed to either poor patient selection or association with a different neurovascular syndrome.[18,35]

## Axillary Artery Occlusion

Anatomically, the axillary artery is the main artery of the upper extremity and originates as a continuation of the subclavian artery at the outer border of the first rib. It is divided into three sections. The first is proximal to the pectoralis minor muscle, the second is deep to the muscle, and the third is distal (Fig. 24-7).

In 1945, Wright[13] described a hyperabduction syndrome in which the second part of the axillary artery was occluded by pressure from the overlying pectoralis minor muscle when the arm was brought overhead. This hyperabduction of the arm became a classic ma-

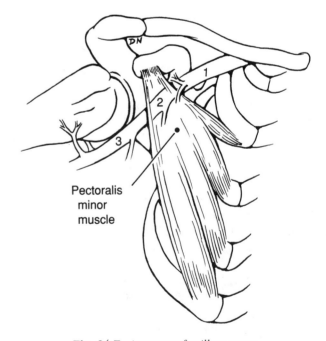

**Fig. 24-7.** Anatomy of axillary artery.

neuver of Wright. Tullos et al[14] were the first to describe this mechanism of occlusion of the axillary artery in professional baseball pitchers. During the cocking phase, the arm is brought into hyperabduction, extension, and external rotation. With each pitch, transient occlusion of the artery likely occurs secondary to pressure from the pectoralis minor muscle. Axillary artery occlusion also has been reported by others in throwing athletes and in a windsurfer.[30,32,36] The mechanism of the injuries was repetitive overhand activity requiring hyperabduction and external rotation of the shoulder.

Symptoms associated with axillary artery occlusion include pain, tenderness over the supraclavicular space, claudication, fatigue, diminished skin temperature, decreased or absent distal pulses, and cyanosis. These symptoms can be elicited when the arm is hyperabducted and externally rotated. Definitive diagnosis usually requires angiographic demonstration of thrombosis with complete arterial occlusion or aneurysmal dilatation of the artery secondary to partial occlusion.

When the pectoralis minor is causing the compression, flexibility of the muscle is important. An overhead stretch may help loosen the pectoralis minor, and light strengthening such as sitting dips may alleviate spasms in the muscle. However, because hyperabduction and external rotation cause the compression, this stretching may not be effective. Strengthening the posterior rotator cuff may protect against added stress on the anterior shoulder neurovascular structures by minimizing subluxation of the humeral head during the acceleration phase of throwing. Exercises include prone horizontal abduction, prone external rotation, and external rota-

tion with the arm at 0 degrees abduction. Strengthening of scapular muscles may enhance the posture of the scapulae.

Surgical intervention is usually necessary for treating axillary artery occlusion. Commonly used procedures include thrombectomy, sympathectomy, segmental excisions, bypass with vascular graft, and anastomosis or angioplasty.[14,30,32,37]

## Effort Thrombosis

The axillary vein lies on the medial side of the axillary artery. It originates at the lower border of the teres major muscle as a continuation of the basilic vein and becomes the subclavian vein at the lateral margin of the first rib. Compression of the axillary vein can happen at different locations along its anatomic course. The most significant compression occurs in the costoclavicular space (Fig. 24-8), especially after a combined maneuver of hyperextension of the neck and hyperabduction of the arm, or the assumption of the military brace position with a backward thrust of the shoulders. Compression also can occur between the costocoracoid ligament and the first rib, the subclavian muscles and the first rib, or more commonly, between the clavicle and the first rib.

This condition is called effort thrombosis because of its frequent association with repetitive vigorous activities or blunt trauma that produces direct or indirect injury to the vein.[38] Effort thrombosis, however, can occur in healthy individuals with no apparent predisposing causes.[37] Although this clinical entity may be

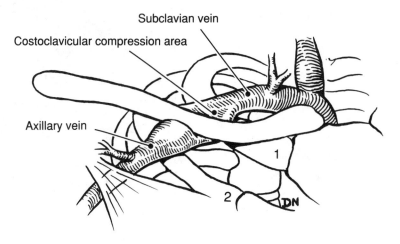

**Fig. 24-8.** Anatomy of subclavian and axillary vein.

the most common vascular problem in athletes, effort thrombosis is rare. It accounts for less than 2 percent of the total venous thromboses,[39] and only 53 cases of sports-related effort thrombosis have been reported.[40] Associated athletic activities include swimming, basketball, tennis, golf, rowing, handball, volleyball, weight lifting, football, baseball, gymnastics, and hockey.[30,32,37,38,40–44]

Symptoms usually manifest themselves within the first 24 hours after the preceding trauma or activity. Symptoms are limited to the affected upper extremity and most often consist of a dull aching pain and swelling. The pain is associated with numbness and heaviness of the upper extremity and activity-related fatigue.

Examination reveals edema involving the entire upper extremity. The skin may be mottled and cool, and prominent superficial veins (Fig. 24-9) may be present.

Pulses are usually normal. Neurologic examination is most often normal but may reveal hyperesthesia in a nondermatomal pattern. Occasionally, a tender cord-like structure is palpable in the axilla. These physical findings may become pronounced during overhead arm activities. The use of exercise tests may be helpful in the diagnosis.[43]

The diagnosis of effort thrombosis is often made by detailed history and physical examination and confirmed with venography. The presence of thrombi occluding the axillary or subclavian veins is the typical finding (Fig. 24-10). Collateralization and recanalization of the thrombosed vein may be extensive.[37,38]

Initial treatment should be directed toward alleviating symptoms, with the ultimate goal of returning the athlete to his or her previous level of activity. Although rest and elevation of the arm usually resolve the acute pain and swelling within 3 to 4 days in most cases, 60

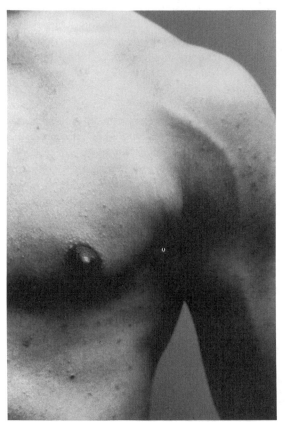

A

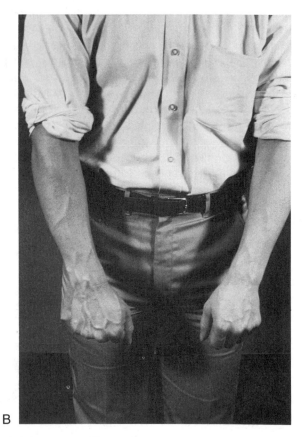

B

**Fig. 24-9.** (**A**) Shoulder and (**B**) arm vein dilatations.

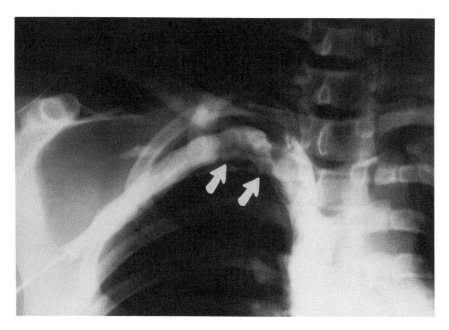

**Fig. 24-10.** Venogram demonstration of effort thrombosis.

to 85 percent of conservatively treated patients may experience residual symptoms caused by continuing occlusion of the vein with inadequate collateral flow, resulting in possible chronic disability.[41]

Anticoagulation therapy with heparin, followed by warfarin, is often used in the acute phase to prevent progression of the thrombus.[37–39] Adams and DeWeese,[39] however, found that 50 percent of their patients treated with anticoagulation continued to have symptoms. Also, both Adams and DeWeese[39] and Campbell et al[45] noted patients who developed pulmonary embolism despite anticoagulation. Recently, streptokinase has been indicated for the lysis of intravenous clots.[42,46] This fibrinolytic therapy is very effective with acute clots but ineffective with chronic clots.

Several authors have reported long-term results with surgical treatment.[39,45,47] Both Adams and DeWeese[39] and Aziz et al[47] reported good results and no residual symptoms with early thrombectomy and simultaneous decompression of the thoracic outlet. Taylor et al[42] reported that patients treated with fibrinolytic therapy followed by first-rib resection remained asymptomatic after treatment.

Although athletic activities requiring repetitive and vigorous shoulder activities have been implicated as causes of effort thrombosis, very little has been written regarding the level of athletic activity after treatment. Several authors reported on effort thrombosis related to athletic activities but did not mention the return-to-play status of their patients.[38,39,43,48] Butsch[49] reported on effort thrombosis with hockey players, one of whom developed both subclavian vein thrombosis and pulmonary embolism. The patient was treated nonoperatively with anticoagulation therapy. He returned to professional hockey in 8 weeks and was still playing 4 years after treatment. Donayre et al[44] reported on a quarterback and a swimmer, both of whom returned to college competition after thrombolytic treatment and first-rib resection. Skerker et al[40] cited a high school athlete (football quarterback and baseball pitcher) who returned to pitching after anticoagulation therapy but rethrombosed the subclavian vein 5 months later.

Even though the syndrome is rare, athletes who perform repetitive and vigorous upper extremity activities are clearly at risk of developing effort thrombosis. Physicians, therefore, should be familiar with the signs and symptoms associated with this condition so that vascular occlusion in the proximal upper extremity can be diagnosed promptly and not be overlooked.

## Quadrilateral Space Syndrome

The quadrilateral space, located over the posterior scapular and subdeltoid region, consists of the teres minor superiorly, the long head of the triceps medially, the teres major inferiorly, and the surgical neck of the humerus laterally (Fig. 24-11). The axillary nerve and posterior humeral circumflex artery pass through this space.

Quadrilateral space syndrome, first described by Cahill and Palmer in 1967, involves compression of the axillary nerve (or one of its main branches) and the posterior humeral circumflex artery in the quadrilateral space.[18,19] Fibrous bands within this space also can cause compression of the neurovascular structures when the arm is abducted and externally rotated. Recently, this syndrome has been noted in the throwing athlete.[30,32,41]

Symptoms usually include pain and paresthesia in the upper extremity not associated with a history of trauma. The pain is poorly localized, aggravated by abduction and external rotation of the humerus, and often interferes with specific athletic activities.

Physical examination is essentially normal, although discrete point tenderness may be noted over the affected quadrilateral space. Neurologic examination, as well as nerve conduction and electromyogram studies, is normal.

The diagnosis is based on a subclavian arteriogram performed with the arm both held at the patient's side

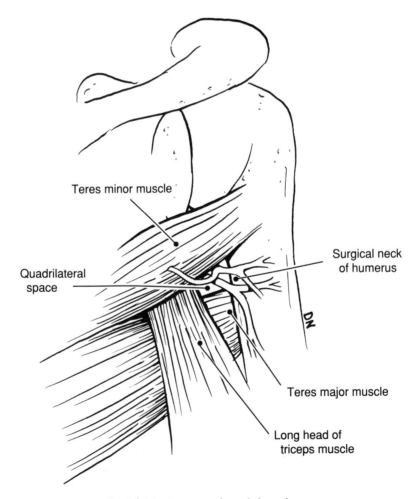

**Fig. 24-11.** Anatomy of quadrilateral space.

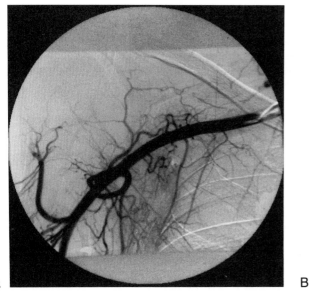
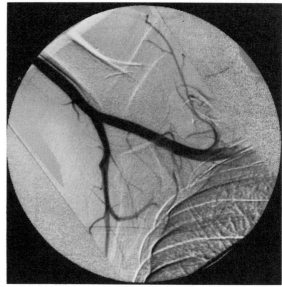

**Fig. 24-12.** Arteriograms showing compression of posterior humeral circumflex artery. (**A**) Arm at side; (**B**) arm abducted.

and in an abducted, externally rotated position. In affected patients, the subclavian arteriogram will show a patent posterior humeral circumflex artery with the humerus at its side, but occlusion of the artery when the humerus is hyperabducted and externally rotated (Fig. 24-12).

Treatment of quadrilateral space syndrome includes symptomatic care, reassurance, and surgical decompression. Gentle internal rotation stretching of the glenohumeral joint, horizontal stretching into adduction, and posterior cuff strengthening may help alleviate symptoms. Redler et al[41] reported on a baseball pitcher who experienced symptomatic relief and continued pitching after changing his pitching delivery from overhead to three-quarters. Cahill[18] recommended surgical decompression of the quadrilateral space through a posterior approach for symptomatic patients.

## DIFFERENTIAL DIAGNOSIS

Besides the neurovascular syndromes described, other conditions of the shoulder and arm can produce symptoms similar to those resulting from compression of neurovascular structures. These include (1) diseases of the cervical spine, (2) acute brachial neuropathy, (3) carpal tunnel syndrome, (4) cubital tunnel syndrome, and (5) peripheral nerve injuries of the shoulder involving the suprascapular nerve, axillary nerve, long thoracic nerve, musculocutaneous nerve, spinal accessory nerve, or dorsal scapular nerves. These lesions, well described in the literature, may occur as isolated entities. Increased awareness, along with a complete history, careful physical examination, and electromyography and nerve conduction studies, can clarify the diagnosis of these lesions and help differentiate them from neurovascular compression syndromes.

## SUMMARY

Compression of the neurovascular structures of the shoulder and upper extremity can occur as a result of local trauma or repetitive activity such as found in the throwing athlete. Because of the unusual demands placed on the shoulder of the throwing athlete, normal anatomic structures can become pathologic and can cause compression of nerves and vessels, producing symptoms that are neurologic or vascular. Symptoms depend on the nerves or vessels being compressed and on the site of the occlusion. These symptoms often are vague and obscure, ranging from exertional fatigue to frank anesthesia and loss of blood supply.

Specific syndromes occur because of compression of specific anatomic structures and include (1) thoracic outlet compression of adjacent neurovascular structures by the clavicle, first rib, or scalene anticus muscle, (2) axillary artery occlusion by the pectoralis minor muscle, (3) venous thrombosis of the subclavian or axillary vein as a result of constriction by the clavicle or first rib, and (4) occlusion of the posterior humeral circumflex artery or axillary nerve in the quadrilateral space.

Because neurovascular compression syndromes are rare in athletes, diagnosis of these conditions requires (1) a thorough history and detailed physical examination with emphasis on Adson's test, the costoclavicular maneuver, and Wright's hyperabduction maneuver, and (2) ancillary diagnostic studies including cervical radiographs, chest films, Doppler measurements, venography, arteriography, and possibly electromyograms and nerve conduction studies.

Once the diagnosis is established, initial treatment usually is nonoperative, including postural and shoulder girdle strengthening exercises and avoidance of precipitating events. Surgical decompression to enlarge the floor of the thoracic outlet is indicated for chronic symptomatic patients. Vascular occlusion can be treated with anticoagulation or thrombolytic therapy. Surgical intervention includes thrombectomy, sympathectomy, segmental excisions, and vascular bypass grafts.

When the throwing athlete presents with upper extremity pain, neurovascular compression syndromes of the shoulder should be considered in the differential diagnosis. Awareness of these clinical syndromes will facilitate the diagnosis and treatment. As a result, the athlete will be able to return to his or her sport without prolonged delay or unnecessary disability.

# REFERENCES

1. Hunald (cited by Tyson RR, Kaplan GF): Modern concepts of diagnosis and treatment of the thoracic outlet syndrome. Orthop Clin North Am 6:507, 1975
2. Coote H: Pressure on the axillary vessels and nerve by an exostosis from a cervical rib; interference with the circulation of the arm, removal of the rib and exostosis; recovery. Med Time 2:108, 1861
3. Stopford JSB, Telford ED: Compression of the lower trunk of the brachial plexus by a first dorsal rib. Br J Surg 7:168, 1919
4. Wheeler WI: Compression neuritis due to the normal first dorsal rib. Practitioner 104:409, 1920
5. Brickner WM, Milch H: First dorsal, simulating cervical rib by maldevelopment or by pressure symptoms. Surg Gynecol Obstet 40:38, 1925
6. Telford ED, Mottershead S: Pressure at the cervicobrachial junction. J Bone Joint Surg 30:249, 1948
7. Adson AW, Coffey JR: Cervical rib: method of anterior approach for relief of symptoms by division of scalenus anticus. Ann Surg 85:839, 1927
8. Ochsner A, Gage M, DeBakey M: Scalenus anticus (Naffziger) syndrome. Am J Surg 28:669, 1935
9. Naffziger HC, Grant WT: Neuritis of the brachial plexus, mechanical in origin: the scalenus syndrome. Surg Gynecol Obstet 67:722, 1938
10. Lewis T, Pickering G: Observations upon maladies in which the blood supply to the digits ceases intermittently or permanently. Clin Sci 1:327, 1934
11. Eden JC: Vascular complications of cervical ribs and first thoracic rib abnormalities. Br J Surg 27:105, 1939
12. Falconer MA, Weddel G: Costoclavicular compression of the subclavian artery and vein. Relation to the scalenus anticus syndrome. Lancet 2:539, 1943
13. Wright IS: The neurovascular syndrome produced by hyperabduction of the arms. Am Heart J 29:1, 1945
14. Tullos HS, Erwin WD, Woods GW et al: Unusual lesions of the pitching arm. Clin Orthop 88:169, 1972
15. Matas R: Primary thrombosis of the axillary vein caused by strain. Am J Surg 24:642, 1934
16. Paget J: Clinical Lectures and Essays. Longman's Green Co., London, 1875
17. Von Schroetter L: Erkrankungen der Gefasse. In: Nothnagel Handbuch der Pathologie und Therapie. Holder, Vienna, 1884
18. Cahill BR: Quadrilateral space syndrome. p. 602. In Omer GE, Spinner M (eds): Management of Peripheral Nerve Problems. WB Saunders, Philadelphia, 1980
19. Cahill BR, Palmer RE: Quadrilateral space syndrome. J Hand Surg 8:65, 1983
20. Lord JW, Rosati LM: Thoracic-outlet syndromes. Clin Symp 23:3, 1971
21. Karas SE: Thoracic outlet syndrome. Clin Sports Med 9:297, 1990
22. Baker CL, Thornberry R: Neurovascular syndromes. p. 176. In Zarins B (ed): Injuries to the Throwing Arm. WB Saunders, Philadelphia, 1985
23. Riddell DH, Smith BM: Thoracic and vascular aspects of

the thoracic outlet syndrome, 1986 update. Clin Orthop 207:31, 1986

24. Sellke FW, Kelly TR: Thoracic outlet syndrome. Am J Surg 156:54, 1988
25. Brown C: Compressive, invasive referred pain to the shoulder. Clin Orthop 173:55, 1983
26. Huffman JD: Electrodiagnostic techniques for and conservative treatment of thoracic outlet syndrome. Clin Orthop 207:21, 1986
27. Urschel HC Jr, Razzuk MA: Management of thoracic outlet syndrome. N Engl J Med 286:1140, 1972
28. Roos DB: The place for scalenectomy and first rib resection in thoracic outlet syndrome. Surgery 92:1077, 1982
29. Stallworth JM, Horne JB: Diagnosis and management of thoracic syndrome. Arch Surg 119:1149, 1984
30. Nuber GW, McCarthy WJ, Yao JST et al: Arterial abnormalities of the shoulder in athletes. Am J Sports Med 18:514, 1990
31. Strukel RJ, Garrick JG: Thoracic outlet compression in athletes. A report of four cases. Am J Sports Med 6:35, 1978
32. Rohrer MJ, Cardullo PA, Pappas AM et al: Axillary artery compression and thrombosis in throwing athletes. J Vasc Surg 11:761, 1990
33. Bateman JE: Nerve injuries about the shoulder in sports. J Bone Joint Surg 49A:785, 1967
34. Britt LP: Nonoperative treatment of thoracic outlet syndrome symptoms. Clin Orthop 51:45, 1967
35. Hawkes CD: Neurosurgical considerations in thoracic outlet syndrome. Clin Orthop 207:24, 1986
36. Sadat-Ali M, Al-Awami SM: Wind-surfing injury to the axillary artery. Br J Sports Med 19:165, 1985
37. Sotta RP: Vascular problems in the proximal upper extremity. Clin Sports Med 9:379, 1990
38. Vogel CM, Jensen JE: "Effort" thrombosis of the subclavian vein in a competitive swimmer. Am J Sports Med 13:269, 1985
39. Adams JT, DeWeese JA: "Effort" thrombosis of the axillary and subclavian veins. J Trauma 11:923, 1971
40. Skerker RS, Flandry FC, Henderson JM: Painless arm swelling in a high school football player. Med Sci Sports Exerc, suppl. 23:S133, 1991
41. Redler MR, Ruland LJ, McCue FC: Quadrilateral space syndrome in a throwing athlete. Am J Sports Med 14:511, 1986
42. Taylor LM, McAllister WR, Dennis DL, Porter JM: Thrombolytic therapy followed by first rib resection for spontaneous "effort" subclavian vein thrombosis. Am J Surg 149:644, 1985
43. Kleinsasser LJ: Effort thrombosis of the axillary and subclavian vein. Arch Surg 59:258, 1949
44. Donayre CE, White GH, Mehringer SM, Wilson SE: Pathogenesis determines late morbidity of axillosubclavian vein thrombosis. Am J Surg 152:179, 1986
45. Campbell CB, Chandler JG, Tegtmeyer CJ et al: Axillary, subclavian and brachiocephalic vein obstruction. Surgery 82:816, 1977
46. Smith-Behn J, Althar R, Katz W: Primary thrombosis of the axillary/subclavian vein. South Med J 79:1176, 1986
47. Aziz S, Straehley CJ, Whelan TJ: Effort related axillosubclavian vein thrombosis. A new theory of pathogenesis and a plea for direct surgical intervention. Am J Surg 152:57, 1986
48. Tilney NL, Griffiths HJG, Edwards EA: Natural history of major venous thrombosis of the upper extremity. Arch Surg 101:792, 1970
49. Butsch JL: Subclavian thrombosis following hockey injuries. Am J Sports Med 11:448, 1983

# 25
# Brachial Plexus Injuries

*TANDY R. FREEMAN*
*WILLIAM G. CLANCY, JR.*

Injuries to the brachial plexus and peripheral nerves about the shoulder are uncommon in sports other than American football. Hirasawa and Sakakida[1] reported that among 1,176 cases of peripheral nerve and brachial plexus injuries treated over an 18-year period, only 66 were related to sports. Sixteen of these were compression injuries to the brachial plexus. They also noted a report by Takazawa et al[2] of only 28 peripheral nerve injuries among 9,550 sports injuries seen over 5 years. In contrast to these Japanese studies, Clarke[3] reported the incidence of brachial plexus injury among U.S. high school and college football players over a 4-year period to be 2.2 injuries per 100 players per year, and Clancy et al[4] noted a 30 to 50 percent incidence of transitory brachial plexus injury over the course of high school or college career. Peripheral nerve injuries, although rare, tend to be more prevalent than brachial plexus injuries in sports other than football and wrestling, especially noncontact sports.[1] Prompt recognition, appropriate assessment, and proper treatment are essential for the safe and timely return of the injured athlete to participation.

## CLASSIFICATION OF NERVE INJURIES

Seddon[5] classified peripheral nerve injuries based on the degree of injury correlating histologic and clinical findings with prognosis. Injury may result in different amounts of damage to neural fibers within a given nerve producing a mixed clinical picture based on this classification system.

Neurapraxia represents a physiologic interruption of nerve function without anatomic axonal disruption. Demyelination may occur,[6-8] but repair is rapid. Function returns from within minutes to 3 weeks of injury, and neurophysiologic studies are normal at that time. Axomotmesis is an injury resulting in axonal disruption without significant injury to the supporting stroma, including the endoneurium, perineurium, and epineurium (Fig. 25-1). Wallerian degeneration of the axon occurs distal and, to some extent, proximal to the level of injury, but the neural tube remains intact. Return of function requires complete regeneration of the axon, which is facilitated by intact fascicles. Electromyogram (EMG) studies at 3 weeks reveal fibrillations and positive sharp waves with loss of motor unit potentials in the denervated muscles. After recovery, the EMG may show large motor unit potentials.

Neurotmesis is an injury in which not only is the axon disrupted but there is also loss of the integrity of the supporting stroma of the nerve including the endonerium. Nonoperative recovery is unlikely because of loss of continuity of the neural tube; and, even with surgical repair or reconstruction, complete return of function is unlikely. EMG studies show denervation patterns at 3 weeks and at 1 year or later.

## ANATOMY

An understanding of the anatomy of the brachial plexus is essential for establishing an accurate diagnosis and prognosis in brachial plexus injuries. The brachial plexus is formed in the neck from the ventral rami of cervical nerve roots V through VIII and the first thoracic nerve root and lies between the anterior and middle scalene muscles. It passes over the first rib and deep to the sternocleidomastoid and the clavicle in its course. It may receive contributions from C4 (prefixed plexus) or T2 (postfixed plexus).

The ventral (motor) and dorsal (sensory) roots at each level unite near or within the vertebral foramen to form the nerve roots (Fig. 25-2). The cell bodies of the sensory nerves in the dorsal root are located within the dorsal root ganglia situated just proximal to the confluence of the ventral and dorsal roots and outside the spinal cord. Injury proximal to the dorsal ganglion (preganglionic lesion or root avulsion) is, at this time, irreparable and has a hopeless prognosis. Injury distal to the dorsal ganglion (postganglionic lesion) represents a peripheral nerve injury with the potential for recovery spontaneously or with surgical repair or reconstruction.

Just distal to the confluence of the ventral and dorsal roots and as the nerve root exits the vertebral foramen,

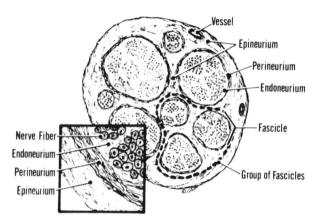

**Fig. 25-1.** Cross-sectional anatomy of a peripheral nerve. (From Wilgis and Brushart,[27] with permission.)

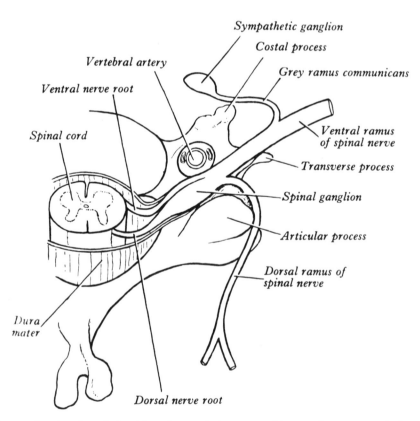

**Fig. 25-2.** Scheme showing the relationships of a cervical nerve and its ganglion to a cervical vertebra. (From Williams et al.,[26] with permission.)

the root divides into ventral and dorsal rami. The ventral rami are larger and form the brachial plexus. The smaller dorsal rami innervate the paraspinal musculature and provide sensation dorsally.

The ventral rami unite just above the clavicle to form the three trunks—upper (C5 to C6), middle (C7), and lower (C8 to T1) (Fig. 25-3). The site of confluence of C5 and C6 is known as Erb's point. Between the takeoff of the dorsal rami and Erb's point, the long thoracic nerve (serratus anterior) arises from C5 through C7 and the dorsal scapular nerve (rhomboids) arises from C5. The suprascapular nerve (supraspinatus, infraspinatus) arises distal to Erb's point from the upper trunk. Postganglionic injury of C5 to C6 proximal to Erb's point represents a peripheral nerve root injury with loss of C5 to C6 paraspinous, serratus anterior, and rhomboid function. This distinguishes nerve root injuries from upper trunk injuries, which leave dorsal rami, long thoracic, and dorsal scapular nerve functions intact.

Below the clavicle, the trunks divide into anterior and posterior divisions, which then form the lateral (C5 to C7), posterior (C5 to T1), and medial (C8 to T1) cords, named for their relationships to the axillary artery. The upper and lower subscapular, medial and lateral pectoral, thoracodorsal, medial brachial cutaneous, and medial antibrachial cutaneous nerves arise from the cords. The cords terminate in the five terminal branches—the musculocutaneous, axillary, radial, ulnar, and median nerves.

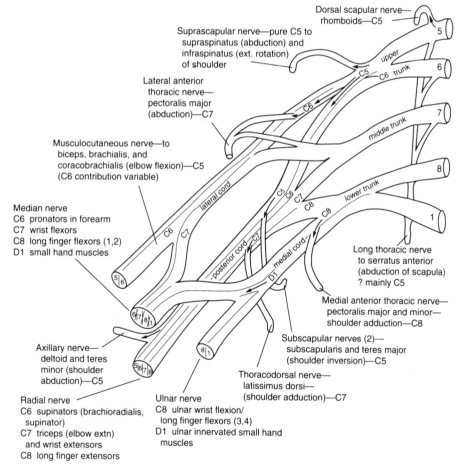

**Fig. 25-3.** Brachial plexus with site of upper trunk plexus injury and distribution highlighted. (From Patten,[28] with permission.)

## HIGH-VELOCITY INJURIES

High-velocity injuries are rare in sports, typically occurring as a result of motorcycle or motor vehicle accidents or falls from a height. These injuries are the result of severe traction on the plexus caused by forcible displacement of the head and shoulder away from one another. High-velocity traction injuries are usually root avulsions, with the involved levels determined by the position of the upper extremity at the time of impact. Adduction results in injury to the upper roots. Abduction and extension results in injury to the entire plexus, and overhead abduction results in lower root injury.

Clinically, root avulsions are often accompanied by other significant injuries, including head injuries. Examination reveals motor and sensory deficits attributable to the involved roots. Cervical spine films may show transverse process fractures. Myelography and magnetic resonance imaging may be used to show evidence of root avulsion such as traumatic meningoceles.

Histamine skin testing produces a normal three-phase response. The injection of a 1 percent solution of histamine acid phosphate intradermally results in local vasodilatation, whealing, and flare formation in the normal state. The vasodilatation and whealing are due to local effects of the histamine. The flare reaction is due to vasodilatation mediated through the sensory root ganglion and its distal afferent axons. Postganglionic injury disrupts the distal afferent axons, and the flare response is blocked. In preganglionic lesions, the distal afferent axons are intact, and the flare response is present. A normal three-phase response by identifying a preganglionic lesion suggests a poor prognosis. This test is seldom used clinically.

Sensory nerve conduction velocities and sensory nerve action potentials to the anesthetic regions are normal in these preganglionic lesions as the dorsal root ganglion and distal afferent axons are intact. The EMG of the posterior cervical muscles as well as serratus anterior and rhomboids will reveal denervation patterns.

Recovery of function does not occur in root avulsions. Present surgical treatment consists primarily of muscle transfers with or without arthrodesis, although attempts at microsurgical repair may prove beneficial in the future. Associated postganglionic injury that may recover and reduce the extent of reconstruction required to obtain optimal function is the primary reason for delaying reconstruction. Early aggressive rehabilitation to maintain joint motion is important for obtaining optimal results.

## BURNERS

Burners, often referred to as stingers or cervical nerve pinch injuries, and upper-trunk brachial plexus injuries are among the most common injuries in American football[4] and are seen, to a lesser degree, in wrestling and other contact sports. Clarke[3] reported an incidence of 2.2 brachial plexus injuries per 100 players per year from 1975 to 1978. Clancy et al[4] reported that, at the collegiate level, approximately 50 percent of football players have sustained a burner at some time during their career. Of these, approximately 30 percent sustain their first injury in high school. Warren[9] noted a similar incidence in professionals on one team. Injury most commonly occurs while tackling, thus most often affecting defensive and specialty team players.

The mechanism of injury initially is a downward or backward blow to the ipsilateral shoulder with the neck flexed laterally away from the side of injury. This results in an increase in the acromiomastoid distance, stretching of the brachial plexus, and damage to the plexus, the degree of which depends on the force applied.[10] The mechanism of initial injury is similar to that resulting in acromioclavicular sprain with the difference being the site of application of force—the acromium in acromioclavicular joint injuries and the clavicle in brachial plexus injuries.[11] Concomitant burners and acromioclavicular joint injuries are therefore rare. Subsequent injuries may occur with the neck laterally flexed toward the side of injury or hyperextended. This may be the result of scarring and fixation of the plexus to the scalene muscles[12] or foraminal narrowing.[13] Cadaver study,[4] however, has shown that the tension in the upper trunk of the brachial plexus can be increased with a posterior force on the shoulder girdle while the neck is ipsilaterally flexed or ipsilaterally rotated and hyperextended. In a previously injured brachial plexus, this mechanism may produce adequate tension to result in reinjury without the presence of scarring or foraminal narrowing.

When the injury occurs, the athlete feels a sharp, burning or stinging pain (hence the common names "burner" or "stinger") radiating from the supraclavicular area down the arm to the hand. This is accompanied by numbness or tingling of the upper extremity. The pain and paresthesia are not dermatomal in distribution and usually resolve within 1 to 2 minutes. The athlete will usually try to "shake off" the injury to restore feeling. True neck pain is not associated with brachial plexus injury and, when present, should raise concern about a possible cervical spine injury.

Weakness may be present at the time of injury, with the athlete supporting the slightly dangling extremity with the uninjured hand while leaving the field. Weakness present at the time of injury usually resolves within minutes. Conversely, weakness may not develop for hours or several days after the injury, necessitating repeated neurologic examination postinjury. Weakness involves the deltoid, supraspinatus, infraspinatus, biceps, and on rare occasions, also the supinator, brachioradialis, and/or pronator teres. Tenderness over the trapezius in the supraclavicular region may be found on examination up to several days after injury. Chrisman et al[14] reported a 9 percent decrease in lateral neck flexion. This is probably related to the trapezial tenderness and is frequently too small to detect clinically.

The site of injury has variously been postulated as the upper trunk[4,14–19] versus the upper nerve roots.[14,18–21] Based on clinical evidence and electrophysiologic studies showing involvement of muscles in the distribution of the upper trunk but no involvement of the cervical paraspinal muscles, serratus anterior, or rhomboids, which received their innervation from proximal to Erb's point, Clancy et al[4] identified the upper trunk as the site of injury. Subsequent studies[16,17] have confirmed these findings. Other authors[18,19,21] have identified some athletes with involvement of posterior cervical musculature, indicating injury at the root level; however, included in these studies[18] are athletes with abnormal spine films, which are not associated with burners. These root injuries appear to be more severe in terms of duration of symptoms and disability.

Clancy[22] classified brachial plexus injuries based on the duration of motor weakness and, roughly, parallel-

ing Sunderland's[23] classification of nerve injury. Grade I injuries are the most common brachial plexus injuries with a transitory loss of motor and nerve function, lasting from minutes to hours and completely resolving within 2 weeks. This represents a neurapraxia or physiologic interruption of nerve function. This may be due to edema or demyelination of the axon without intrinsic axonal disruption leading to a conduction block at the site of injury. Function returns as the edema resolves or when remyelination is completed, usually within 2 to 3 weeks of injury. There is complete return of strength. EMG studies at 2 to 3 weeks do not show any findings.

Grade II injuries exhibit motor weakness lasting more than 2 weeks but with eventual full clinical recovery. Some have significant weakness from the time of injury, whereas others may not exhibit weakness for several days. This is consistent with the work of Denny-Brown and Brenner.[6,7] There appears to be a two-phase recovery, with the return of 80 to 90 percent of strength and endurance in 6 weeks and full recovery by 6 months. This pattern suggests a combined neurapraxia and axonotmesis. Wallerian degeneration of the distal axon is responsible for the delay in complete recovery, as axon regeneration requires as long as 6 months in this region. EMG changes at 3 weeks postinjury reveal classic evidence of muscle denervation with decreased motor unit potentials, fibrillations, and sharp positive waves. After complete clinical recovery, there may continue to be EMG changes, most commonly large motor unit potentials.

Grade III injuries are the rarest. These athletes continue to exhibit motor and sensory loss at 1 year without clinical improvement. This represents a neurotmesis with axonal regeneration frequently impossible because of the extent of injury. EMGs show evidence of denervation at 3 weeks and, subsequently, at 3 months without evidence of recovery. Differentiation of axonotmesis from neurotmesis is important in determining the prognosis of the injury and the course of treatment. A grade III injury may benefit from operative intervention at or before 3 months.

Management of the athlete with brachial plexus injury is based on clinical presentation. On-the-field evaluation includes motor and sensory examination. Weakness and anesthesia will persist while the pain is present but will usually resolve rapidly after the pain subsides. The supraspinatus, infraspinatus, deltoid, and biceps are the muscles most often involved. Elbow flexion and shoulder flexion usually return first, followed by shoulder external rotation and abduction. Sensory deficits are usually patchy and are most often present over the lateral shoulder. Persistent anesthesia is uncommon. Also uncommon in brachial plexus injuries are neck pain or loss of neck motion, and the presence of either should raise concern about a cervical spine injury with the athlete appropriately managed. Bilateral upper extremity burning dysesthesias may also represent a significant cervical spine injury.[24]

On the field, if the athlete has no evidence of neck injury, testing of the shoulder rotators, deltoid, biceps, and triceps against resistance is performed. If the athlete's pain and subjective weakness have resolved and if no weakness is shown on examination, he may return to play. The athlete must be examined again after the game and during the following week, as weakness may appear on a delayed basis. Routine cervical spine films are recommended for athletes sustaining their first brachial plexus injury. Athletes with persistent pain or weakness beyond 2 weeks (grade II injury) should have routine cervical spine films and an EMG at 3 weeks to identify the sight of lesion. Evidence of nerve root injuries should prompt further study to rule out a disc herniation.

Treatment of grade I and II injuries involves removal of the athlete from participation as long as symptoms or weakness to manual testing persist. The athlete is placed on a neck and shoulder strengthening program as soon as tolerated. Return to contact sports is based on a return of strength and endurance of the shoulder muscles to normal as compared with the opposite side. EMG studies in grade II injuries may show persistent changes, even after return of strength, and are not useful for determining return to sport.[17–19,25] With return to football, a neck roll to prevent lateral flexion and posterior extension and built-up shoulder pads may reduce the incidence of recurrence of burners.[9,13,16,18] Athletes with multiple burners may continue to participate as long as there is no loss of strength. Weakness should preclude participation until strength returns to normal. Neck and shoulder strengthening and the use of neck rolls and built-up shoulder pads may reduce the frequency of burners. Stopping contact sports will eliminate further burners, but a return even after a prolonged period of nonparticipation is frequently associated with recurrence.

Treatment of grade III injuries parallels treatment of the lesser injuries early on. Return to contact sports is prohibited because of the continued weakness.

## PACK PALSY OR BACKPACK PARALYSIS

Pack palsy or backpack paralysis represents an injury to the brachial plexus or its branches and is generally believed to be due to extrinsic compression of the plexus. The shoulder straps on a heavy pack create a compressive force on the plexus against the clavicle or first rib. The backward pull of a heavy pack on the shoulder girdle placing traction on the plexus has also been postulated as a contributing factor. Either mechanism is consistent with the studies of Denny-Brown,[6–8] which showed that prolonged compression or low-grade traction can disrupt nerve function, which can subsequently be recovered.

Pack palsy typically results in weakness involving a significant portion of the brachial plexus but may be restricted to the axillary or radial nerves. The clinical picture is one of profound weakness in the muscle groups involved. The condition is rarely painful, and sensory changes are not prominent.

Treatment of pack palsy is nonoperative with an excellent prognosis. Hirasawa and Sakakida[1] described the "complete recovery" of all 19 patients in their review, with "good results" using range of motion and strengthening exercises.

Fractures of the clavicle may cause injury to the brachial plexus by compression from a displaced fragment acutely or from excessive callous formation or hypertrophic nonunion in a delayed fashion. Treatment of an acute clavicle fracture with a figure-eight bandage may also result in compression of the brachial plexus.

Hypertrophic nonunions producing brachial plexus symptoms generally involve the middle one-third of the clavicle compressing the plexus between the clavicle and the first and second rib. The medial cord is usually involved, producing ulnar nerve symptoms. Treatment consists of open reduction and internal fixation with bone grafting or partial excision of the clavicle. Exuberant callous formation may result in brachial plexus compression, with gradual onset of symptoms about the third week. Treatment is resection of the excessive callous.

Cervical ribs have been implicated in brachial plexus compression, as well. This phenomenon is discussed in Chapter 24.

## ACUTE BRACHIAL NEUROPATHY

Acute brachial neuropathy is a clinical entity of unknown etiology that must be considered in the differential diagnosis of shoulder pain in the athlete. Acute brachial neuropathy is described in the literature by the names serum brachial neuritis, multiple neuritis, localized neuritis of the shoulder girdle, acute brachial radiculitis, neuralgic amyotrophy, shoulder girdle syndrome, paralytic brachial neuritis, Parsonage-Turner syndrome, and brachial plexus neuropathy. Acute brachial neuropathy has variously been related to trauma, exercise, surgery, infection, immunization, and genetics. Acute brachial neuropathy is characterized by constant, severe shoulder pain that is present at rest and responds poorly to analgesics. The onset of pain is sudden, frequently waking the patient, may occur acutely or subacutely in association with sports, and is typically not related to a specific traumatic event. The pain may last for several hours to weeks. Shoulder and elbow motion aggravate the pain. Shoulder adduction with elbow flexion is the most comfortable resting posture. Radiation of pain below the elbow suggests diffuse involvement of the brachial plexus or involvement of the lower plexus.

Weakness or paralysis usually appear within 2 weeks of pain onset. Weakness or paralysis may accompany the onset of pain but is more commonly noted as the pain is resolving and may become apparent during athletic activity. Weakness or paralysis is characteristically patchy in distribution and involves lower motor neurons without a precise motor nerve, radicular, or nerve trunk pattern. The most commonly affected muscles are the deltoid, followed by the supraspinatus and infraspinatus, serratus anterior, biceps, triceps, and wrist and finger extensors. Sensory deficits are minimal, usually limited to a small area over the lateral shoulder or radial surface of the forearm, and do not parallel the motor changes. Changes in deep tendon reflexes depend on the severity of muscle weakness, and decreased biceps and triceps reflexes are most common. Bilateral involvement is common and is usually asymmetric with subclinical involvement of one side requiring EMG evaluation for diagnosis.

EMG yields variable data with involvement of a single muscle to diffuse involvement of the brachial plexus. The EMG findings are primarily fibrillation potentials in affected muscles, and nerve conduction changes consist of decreases in amplitudes of motor and sensory nerve conduction in involved nerves. Nerve conduction velocities and motor distal latencies are not affected to any significant degree. The principal findings in EMG studies in acute brachial neuropathy that differ from traumatic upper trunk injuries are involvement of muscles not innervated by the upper trunk (trapezius, serratus anterior, diaphragm), involvement of muscles enervated by a single or two peripheral nerves, involvement of a single muscle or sparing of other muscles enervated by the same portion of the trunk or plexus, severe motor involvement with sparing of sensory functions in the same portion of the plexus, and unequal involvement of sensory nerves in the same portion of the plexus. These findings have led some to consider acute brachial neuropathy to be a multiple axon loss mononeuropathy multiplex rather than a brachial plexopathy.

The treatment of acute brachial neuropathy is divided into two phases. Phase 1 is from onset to resolution of pain with treatment consisting of rest, support with a sling, and analgesia. Activity may exacerbate the pain, but if tolerated, general range of motion exercises are performed to maintain joint motion. The second phase begins after the resolution of pain and consists of bilateral complete upper body strengthening, including scapular rotators. This total upper extremity approach is important because of the frequent subclinical involvement of muscles.

Return to normal function occurs in 75 percent of patients within 2 years and 90 percent of patients within 3 years. Recovery usually begins within 1 to 2 months, with upper trunk lesions, unilateral lesions, and incomplete lesions progressing more rapidly than lower trunk lesions, bilateral lesions, or complete lesions. Mild residual deficits are relatively frequent, and scapular winging when present initially is likely to persist.

Return to sport is considered when strength has reached a plateau that is adequate for safe participation. This requires consideration of each case individually. Recurrences are rare and are characterized by less severe symptoms of shorter duration.

## SUMMARY

Brachial plexus injuries, although rare in noncontact sports, are common in American football and wrestling. Although severe, permanent disabilities may result, complete clinical recovery from sports-related brachial plexus injuries is the rule. During the recovery period, protection from further injury by avoidance of contact sport and rehabilitation through range of motion and strengthening exercises are the cornerstones of treatment. Safe return to sport may be allowed when clinical recovery (normal sensation and strength parity) is achieved despite mild changes in neurophysiologic studies.

## REFERENCES

1. Hirasawa Y, Sakakida K: Sports and peripheral nerve injury. Am J Sports Med 11:420, 1983
2. Takazawa H, Sudon, Aoki K et al: Statistical observation of nerve injuries in athletics. (In Japanese) Brain Nerve Injuries 3:11, 1971
3. Clarke K: An epidemiologic view. In Torq JS (ed): Athletic Injuries to the Head, Neck, and Face. 2nd Ed. Mosby Year Book, St Louis, 1991
4. Clancy W, Brand R, Bergfeld J: Upper trunk brachial plexus injuries in contact sports. Am J Sports Med 5:209, 1977
5. Seddon H: Surgical Disorders of the Peripheral Nerves. Churchill-Livingstone, Edinburgh, 1972
6. Denny-Brown D, Brenner C: Paralysis of nerve induced by direct pressure and by tourniquet. Arch Neurol Physiol 51:1, 1944
7. Denny-Brown D, Brenner C: Lesion in peripheral nerve resulting from compression by spring clip. Arch Neurol Physiol 52:1, 1944
8. Denny-Brown D, Doherty M: Effects of transient stretching of the peripheral nerve. Arch Neurol Psychiatry 54:116, 1945
9. Warren R: Neurologic injuries in football. In Jordan BD, Tsairis P, Warren RF (eds): Sports Neurology. Aspen Publishers, Rockville, MD, 1989
10. Barnes R: Traction injuries of the brachial plexus in adults. J Bone Joint Surg 31B:10, 1949
11. Bergfeld J: Brachial Plexus Injuries. Presented at the American Association of Orthopedic Surgeons Winter Sports Injuries Course. Steamboat Springs, CO, March 27, 1987
12. Rockett F: Observations on the "burner": traumatic cervical radiculopathy. Clin Orthop 164:18, 1982
13. Marshall T: Nerve pinch injuries in football. J Ky Med Assoc 68:648, 1970
14. Chrisman O, Snook G, Stanitis J et al: Lateral-flexion neck injuries in athletic competition. JAMA 192:117, 1965
15. Archambault J: Brachial plexus stretch injury. J Am Coll Health 31:256, 1983
16. DiBenedetto M, Markey K: Electrodiagnostic localization of traumatic upper trunk brachial plexopathy. Arch Phys Med Rehabil 65:15, 1984
17. Robertson W, Eichman P, Clancy W: Upper trunk brachial plexopathy in football players. JAMA 241:1480, 1979
18. Speer K, Bassett F: The prolonged burner syndrome. Am J Sports Med 18:591, 1990
19. Wilbourn A, Hershman E, Bergfeld J: Brachial plexopathies in athletes, the EMG findings. Muscle Nerve 9:254, 1986
20. Albright J, Moses J, Feldick H et al: Non fatal cervical spine injuries in interscholastic football. JAMA 236:1243, 1976
21. Poindexter D, Johnson E: Football shoulder and neck injury: a study of the "stinger." Arch Phys Med Rehabil 65:601, 1984
22. Clancy W: Brachial plexus and upper extremity peripheral nerve injuries. In Torq JS: Athletic Injuries to the Head, Neck, and Face. 1st Ed. Lea & Febiger, Philadelphia, 1982
23. Sunderland S: Nerve and Nerve Injuries. 2nd Ed. Churchill Livingstone, Edinburgh, 1978
24. Maroon J: "Burning hands" in football spinal cord injuries. JAMA 238:2049, 1977
25. Bergfeld J, Hershman E, Wilbourn A: Brachial plexus injury in sports: a five-year follow-up. Orthop Trans 12:743, 1988
26. Williams PL, Warwick R, Dyson M, Bannister LH: Gray's Anatomy. 37th Ed. Churchill Livingstone, Edinburgh, 1989
27. Wilgis EFS, Brushart TM: Nerve repair and grafting. p. 1315. In Green DP (ed): Operative Hand Surgery. 3rd Ed. Churchill Livingstone, New York, 1993
28. Patten JP: Neurological Differential Diagnosis. Springer-Verlag, New York, 1977

# 26

# Suprascapular Nerve Entrapment

## CLIFFORD J. SCHOB

Suprascapular nerve entrapment syndrome is a constellation of different etiologies leading to dysfunction or neuropathy of the suprascapular nerve. Once only thought of as a rare entity in both the athletic and general population, today it is being recognized more frequently as a cause of shoulder pain. In a large series of 2,520 patients with shoulder pain, 10 cases of suprascapular nerve entrapment were identified, for an incidence of 0.4 percent.[1] In the differential diagnosis of shoulder pain, suprascapular nerve entrapment can mimic each of these entities, especially in its early presentation (Table 26-1). However, a keen "sense of awareness," thorough history and physical examination, and proper use of diagnostic modalities can lead the physician to earlier diagnosis and treatment. Any description of a nerve entrapment syndrome needs to begin with a clear depiction of the anatomy.

## ANATOMY

The brachial plexus is formed in the posterior triangle of the neck, comprising the anterior ramii of the spinal roots C5, C6, C7, C8, and T1. The roots combined to form three trunks. Roots C5 and C6 merge to form the upper trunk. Where C5 and C6 join has been called Erb's point. Relatively fixed, it is found 2 to 3 cm above the clavicle, just behind the posterior edge of the sternocleidomastoid muscle.[2,3] The suprascapular nerve arises from the superior lateral aspect of the upper trunk distal to Erb's point. It remains mobile as it crosses obliquely in the posterior triangle under the trapezius muscle to enter the suprascapular notch of the scapula under the superior transverse scapular ligament (Fig. 26-1). This is the first anatomic site of possible constriction to the nerve. Note that the suprascapular vessels cross over this ligament.[4] The nerve then curves from a horizontal to an upward direction under the ligament and enters the supraspinatus fossa.[5] This angular deformity or tethering of the nerve by the superior transverse scapular ligament has been termed the *sling effect* and may account for traumatic causes of neuropathy (Fig. 26-2).[5]

In the supraspinatous fossa, the suprascapular nerve gives off articular branches to the glenohumeral joint and acromioclavicular joint supplying proprioception and pain. Because it is a "motor nerve," it has no sensory cutaneous branches.[6] The suprascapular nerve then passes around the base of the spine at the spinoglenoid notch and enters the infraspinatus fossa. In half the population, there is a membranous band, the inferior transverse scapular ligament, under which the nerve and artery run together (Fig. 26-3).[4,7,8] This ligament attaches medially to the spine and extends laterally to the glenoid rim and occasionally to the glenohumeral capsule.[9] This is the second anatomic site of possible nerve entrapment. In the infraspinatus fossa, the nerve arborizes in to two or three motor branches to innervate the infraspinatus muscle. Occasionally, it will wind around the spine of the scapula as a single nerve forming a sharp right angle.[7] The infraspinatus branch may also give sensory nerves to the posterior-superior aspect of the glenoid humeral joint.[10]

## FUNCTION

The suprascapular nerve (C5 and C6) innervates the supraspinatus and infraspinatus muscles, two of the four muscles making up the rotator cuff. The function

**Table 26-1. Differential Diagnosis of Shoulder Pain**

Rotator cuff disease
Glenohumeral instability
Adhesive capsulitis
Acromioclavicular joint disease
Cervical radiculopathy
Thoracic outlet syndrome
Diffuse peripheral neuropathy
Neoplasia

of the rotator cuff as a glenohumeral joint stabilizer has been well described.[11] Using selective nerve blocks of the suprascapular nerve and axillary nerve, Howell et al[12] showed that the supraspinatus muscle contributes equally to the deltoid muscle in generating torque about the shoulder, and each is capable of initiating abduction. Strohm and Colachis[13] determined that the infraspinatus is one of the two main external rotators of the humerus and accounts for as much as 60 percent of the external rotation force generated by the shoulder. Thus, suprascapular nerve neuropathy can have a major impact on shoulder function and glenohumeral stability. Subsequent pain and dysfunction not only mimic injuries of the rotator cuff but may actually con-

tribute to secondary rotator cuff disease, such as impingement syndrome and tensile rotator cuff failure.

## ETIOLOGY

Suprascapular nerve entrapment syndrome has multiple etiologies, all of which impair suprascapular nerve function. Andrews (personal communication) classifies them into two major groups: (1) traction injuries, and (2) compression injuries (Table 26-2).

Traction injuries of the suprascapular nerve occurring at the suprascapular notch were first described in 1959 by Thomspon and Kopell.[6] They proposed that the nerve is injured in summation, either by repetitive motion or by a single traumatic incident. With excessive scapular protraction as with the arm in cross-body adduction, the suprascapular nerve can become taut between Erb's point and the edges of the suprascapular notch.[6] The resulting neuropathy is a traction neuropraxia or axonotmesis and not a true nerve compression.[3] An example of cross-body adduction occurs during the follow-through phase of pitching (Fig. 26-4). Rengachary et al[5] further showed that the suprascapular nerve does not slide or translate under the superior

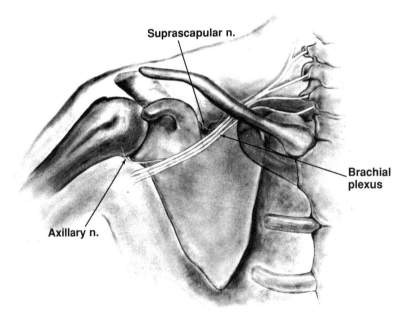

**Fig. 26-1.** Suprascapular nerve and brachial plexus in relation to anterior aspect of the shoulder. (From Butters,[33] with permission.)

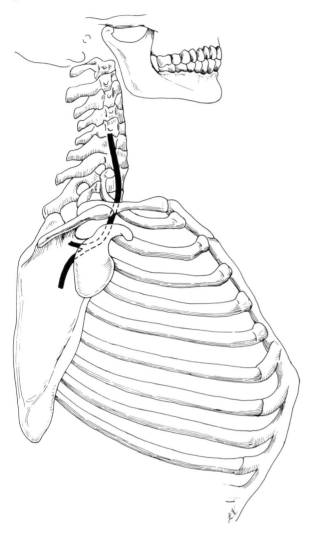

**Fig. 26-2.** Course of suprascapular nerve under superior transverse scapular ligament that accounts for the "sling effect." (From Rengachary et al.,[5] with permission.)

transverse scapular ligament during scapular motion, eliminating friction as a cause of neuropraxia. Neuropathy of the suprascapular nerve at the suprascapular notch would cause involvement of the supraspinatus and infraspinatus muscles.

A second site of potential traction occurs at the spinoglenoid notch, as the fixed nerve wraps around the scapular spine and inserts into the mobile infraspinatus muscle[7,14] (Fig. 26-3). External rotation of the arm would then place tension on the terminal portion of the suprascapular nerve. Constriction of the supra-

scapular nerve at this level would cause selective involvement of the infraspinatus muscle only and sparing of the supraspinatus muscle.

Trauma to the shoulder that results in scapular depression places the suprascapular nerve at risk of injury at the suprascapular notch. The nerve becomes kinked by the superior transverse scapular ligament, known as the sling effect, and results in an axonotmesis of the suprascapular nerve.[5] In similar fashion, these may be multiple repetitive injuries with a cumulative effect (i.e., football linebacker) or a single traumatic blow (i.e., fall).[1,3,5] A single case has been reported that resulted from an anterior shoulder dislocation.[16]

Compression as a cause of suprascapular nerve entrapment occurs at several potential sites along the course of the nerve (Table 26-2). Idiopathic con-

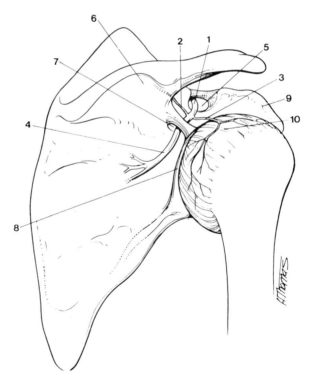

**Fig. 26-3.** Suprascapular nerve and relationship to posterior aspect of shoulder. *1,* suprascapular nerve; *2,* branch to supraspinatus; *3,* branches to joint capsule; *4,* branch to infraspinatus; *5,* suprascapular notch; *6,* scapular spine; *7,* spinoglenoid notch; *8,* glenoid rim; *9,* coracoid process; *10,* posterior joint capsule. (From Liveson et al.,[8] with permission.)

**Table 26-2. Etiology of Suprascapular Nerve Entrapment**

Traction
    Repetitive motion
        Suprascapular notch
            Cross-body adduction
            Hyperabduction
        Spinoglenoid notch
            External rotation
    Traumatic blows
        Suprascapular notch (S.S.N.)
            Scapula depression
            Dislocation glenohumeral joint
Compression
    Anatomic sites of constriction
        Superior transverse scapular ligament
        Inferior transverse scapular ligament
        Congenital stenotic notch
    Extrinsic mass effects
        Ganglionic cyst spinoglenoid notch
        Ganglionic cyst subacromial space
        Fracture base of coracoid or notch
        Neoplasia

striction at the suprascapular notch by the superior transverse scapular ligament has been well documented.[15,17,18] Selective involvement of the infraspinatus muscle as a result of isolated hypertrophy of the inferior transverse scapular ligament has also been reported.[9] Aiello et al[9] theorized that excessive traction on the fibers of these ligaments which insert into the glenohumeral joint, lead to hypertrophy and subsequent nerve compression.

Lastly, a congenital stenotic suprascapular notch (type IV) may be a predisposing factor; Rengachary et al[5] described six types of suprascapular notches classified on morphology and degree of ossification of the superior transverse scapular ligament.

Extrinsic mass effects causing compression of the suprascapular nerve are being recognized more frequently with the advent of magnetic resonance imaging. Ganglion cysts located at the spinoglenoid notch have been implicated in many cases of isolated infraspi-

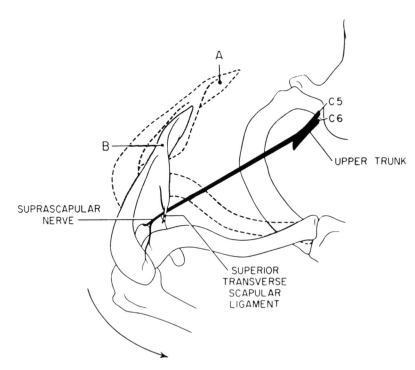

**Fig. 26-4.** Scapular protraction. Note relation of suprascapular nerve at scapular notch to its origin when arm is in anatomic position (shaded area, **A**) and in cross-body adduction (unshaded area, **B**). (From Thompson and Kopell,[6] with permission.)

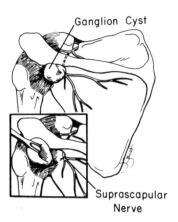

**Fig. 26-5.** Compression of suprascapular nerve by a ganglionic cyst in region of spinoglenoid notch. (From Ganzhorn et al.,[19] with permission.)

natus atrophy[19–21] (Fig. 26-5). These cysts are thought to arise from the shoulder joint but are usually not identifiable by arthrogram.[21] Weight lifting appears to be a predominant factor in most cases reported. Symptomatic spinoglenoid notch cysts by an intact inferior transverse scapular ligament may also be sex-related. An intact inferior transverse scapular ligament is found in 87 percent of the male population but only in 40 percent of the female population.[21]

Other causes of suprascapular nerve entrapment secondary to compression include neoplasia[5] and fractures of the coracoid process and scapular notch.[22] A single case of a subacromial ganglion cyst[23] has also been reported.

## CLINICAL EXAMINATION

The diagnosis of suprascapular nerve entrapment syndrome is frequently overlooked on the initial presentation of shoulder pain. It is often not considered until the patient exhibits marked atrophy of the supraspinatus and/or infraspinatus. A thorough history, physical examination, and diagnostic tests help the examiner distinguish suprascapular nerve entrapment syndrome from other causes of shoulder pain and neuropathy (Table 26-1). Chief complaints are pain poorly localizing to the posterior lateral aspect of the shoulder.[1] It is frequently described as vague and aching. Like other neuropathies, patients may complain of pain radiating into the neck or down the arm.[24] A history of repetitive

motion (e.g., throwing, weight lifting, vigorous exercises) is common; however, it may also be associated with a single traumatic event, such as a severe blow to the shoulder.[6] Many cases have also been insidious in onset and are without any pain.[14]

Physical examination of the upper extremity is performed in a routine systematic fashion. Patients may exhibit different degrees of weakness (i.e., abduction or external rotation). However, the patients' weakness may be greater than it appears, because these motions may be compensated for by synergistic muscle actions.[8] Atrophy is more readily seen in the infraspinatus muscle, which is not covered by the broad trapezius. Supraspinatus and infraspinatus muscle tenderness may also be clinically apparent.

Palpation along the nerve at points of entrapment (suprascapular notch or spinoglenoid notch) or point of origin (Erb's point) may be very painful.[15] Provocative tests to precipitate pain include the "cross-arm adduction test."[6] The examiner adducts the extended arm across the patient's body, causing scapular protraction and subsequent tension on the suprascapular nerve (Fig. 26-3). A positive test reproduces the patient's pain.

It is important to remember that the suprascapular nerve is a motor nerve and carries only pain sensation from the muscles and joints it innervates. It does not have a cutaneous distribution. There can be wide variations in the distribution of these nerve branches[6] and injury to them. This variation explains the great many clinical symptoms and physical findings. Diagnostic tests are important in localizing and confirming the diagnosis of suprascapular nerve entrapment syndrome.[1,3,6]

## DIAGNOSTIC TESTS

Several diagnostic procedures are necessary to facilitate the diagnosis of suprascapular nerve syndrome. Standard radiographs of the shoulder including "outlet view" and lateral scapula view are in order to rule out other causes of shoulder and scapular pain. Radiographs of the scapular notch are useful in cases of suspected fracture of the suprascapular notch or base of coracoid process.[5]

The lidocaine test first described by Thompson and Kopell[6] in 1959 consists of local infiltration of lidocaine at the point of entrapment, usually the superior transverse scapular ligament. A positive test will provide transient but complete relief of pain. In the largest series of suprascapular nerve entrapment, all 27 cases were correctly diagnosed with a positive lidocaine test.[15] A negative test, however, does not exclude the diagnosis because the examiner may have inadvertently missed the nerve.[1]

Electromyography and nerve conduction tests have become fundamental to confirming the diagnosis and localizing the lesion to either the suprascapular notch (supraspinatus and infraspinatus involvement) or the spinoglenoid notch (infraspinatus only).[1,3] Increased latency above the normal 2.7 ms (range, 1.7 to 3.7 ms) indicates impaired conduction.[1] The electromography shows positive fibrillation potentials, positive sharp waves, and polyphasic potentials.[1]

Magnetic resonance imaging is playing a greater role in the diagnosis of typical and atypical ailments of the shoulder. This may be the best test to facilitate diagnosis and identify soft tissue masses causing compression neuropathy in clinically suspected cases of suprascapular nerve syndrome. In a review of 27 masses compressing the suprascapular nerve, there were 21 ganglion cysts, five malignancies, and one fracture hematoma.[21]

## TREATMENT

Treatment of suprascapular nerve entrapment syndrome should be directed toward the relief of pain and restoration of function. After a routine workup, including electromyography, nerve conduction tests, and magnetic resonance imaging scan, one should be able to localize the lesion and determine the etiology. In general, most lesions are secondary to repetitive trauma to the nerve, and the resulting axonotmesis will respond to conservative treatment. It has been our experience that many patient's become asymptomatic within 6 months to 1 year. We stress a vigorous rehabilitative program to strengthen the supraspinatus and infraspinatus musculature along with the scapular stabilizers. A portable electrical stimulator unit has also been advocated and is in our current practice.[3] Some patient's may not regain full motor strength as determined by isokinetic testing (Cybex II or Biodex) and may continue to show signs of muscle atrophy. However, most are able to return to competitive sports.[3,8,14]

Surgical treatment in peripheral nerve surgery does not always result in reversal of muscle atrophy or restoration of strength.[19,25,26]

In contrast, if a symptomatic patient is evaluated and found to have an extrinsic mass, such as a ganglion cyst that is surgically correctable, and fails to respond to conservative measures, it is our feeling that these should be explored and undergo excision.[15] It has been proposed that if magnetic resonance imaging shows a spenoglenoid ganglion cyst, then percutaneous needle aspiration and decompression may be an option over formal exploration.[21] We have no experience with this technique, but this may certainly be considered an alternative before open exploration and excision.

## REFERENCES

1. Post M, Mayer J: Suprascapular nerve entrapment. Clin Orthop 223:126, 1987
2. Jobe CM: Gross anatomy of the shoulder. p. 69. In Rockwood CA, Matsen FA III (eds): The Shoulder. WB Saunders, Philadelphia, 1990
3. Drez D Jr: Suprascapular neuropathy in the differential diagnosis of rotator cuff injuries. Am J Sports Med 4:43, 1976
4. Williams P, Warwick R: p. 456. Gray's Anatomy. 36th Ed. Churchill Livingstone, New York, 1980
5. Rengachary SS, Burr D, Lucas S et al: Suprascapular entrapment neuropathy: clinical, anatomical, and comparative study part 2: anatomical study. Neurosurgery 5:447, 1979
6. Thompson WAL, Kopell HP: Peripheral entrapment neuropathies of the upper extremity. N Engl J Med 260:1261, 1959
7. Black KP, Lombardo JA: Suprascapular nerve injuries with isolated paralysis of the infraspinatus. J Sports Med 18:225, 1990
8. Liveson J, Bronson M, Pollack M: Suprascapular nerve lesions at the spinoglenoid notch: report of three cases and review of the literature. J Neurol Neurosurgery, Psychiatry 54:241, 1991
9. Aiello I, Serra G, Traina GC et al: Entrapment of the suprascapular nerve at the spinoglenoid notch. Ann Neurol 12:314, 1982
10. Gardnere E: The innervation of the shoulder joint. Anat Rec 102:1, 1948
11. Matsen FA III, Arntz CT: Rotator cuff tendon failure. p. 648. In Rockwood CA, Matsen FA III (eds): The Shoulder. WB Saunders, Philadelphia, 1990

12. Howell SM, Imobersteg AM, Seger DH et al: Clarification of the role of the supraspinatus muscle in shoulder function. J Bone Joint Surg 68A:398, 1986

13. Strohm BR, Colachis SC Jr: Shoulder joint dysfunction following injury to the suprascapular nerve. Phys Ther 45:106, 1965

14. Ferretti A, Cerullo G, Russo G: Suprascapular neuropathy in volleyball players. J Bone Joint Surg 69A:260, 1987

15. Callahan JD, Scully TB, Shapiro SA et al: Suprascapular nerve entrapment. J Neurosurg 74:893, 1991

16. Zoltan JD: Injury to the suprascapular nerve associated with anterior dislocation of the shoulder: case report and review of the literature. J Trauma 19:203, 1979

17. Garcia G, McQueen D: Bilateral suprascapular nerve entrapment syndrome. J Bone Joint Surg 63A:491, 1981

18. Rengachary SS, Burr D, Lucas S et al: Suprascapular entrapment neuropathy: a clinical, anatomical, and comparative study part 1: clinical study. Neurosurgery 5:441, 1979

19. Ganzhorn RW, Hocker JT, Horowitz M et al: Suprascapular-nerve entrapment: a case report. J Bone Joint Surg 63A:492, 1981

20. Thompson RC, Schneider W, Kennedy T: Entrapment neuropathy of the inferior branch of the suprascapular nerve by ganglia. Clin Orthop 166:185, 1982

21. Fritz RC, Helms CA, Steinbach LS et al: Suprascapular nerve entrapment: evaluation with MR imaging. Radiology 182:437, 1992

22. Edeland HG, Zachrisson B: Fracture of the scapular notch associated with lesion of the suprascapular nerve. Acta Orthop Scand 46:758, 1975

23. Neviaser TJ, Ain BR, Neviaser RJ: Suprascapular nerve denervation secondary to attenuation by a ganglionic cyst. J Bone Joint Surg 68A:627, 1986

24. Wood VE, Marchinski L: Congenital anomalies of the shoulder. p. 135. In Rockwood CA, Matsen FA III (eds): The Shoulder. WB Saunders, Philadelphia, 1990

25. Clein LJ: Suprascapular entrapment neuropathy. J Neurosurg 43:337, 1975

26. Ringel SP, Treihaft M, Carry M et al: Suprascapular neuropathy in pitchers. Am J Sports Med 18:80, 1990

27. Swafford AR, Lichtman DH: Suprascapular nerve entrapment—case report. J Hand Surg 7:57, 1982

28. Glennon TP: Insolated injury of the infraspinatus branch of the suprascapular nerve. Arch Phys Med Rehabil 73:201, 1992

29. Agre JC, Ash N, Cameron MC et al: Suprascapular neuropathy after intensive progressive resistive exercise: case report. Arch Phys Med Rehabil 68:236, 1987

30. Rask MR: Suprascapular nerve entrapment: a report of two cases treated with suprascapular notch resection. Clinical Orthop 123:73, 1977

31. Takagishi K, Maeda K, Ikeda T et al: Ganglion causing paralysis of the suprascapular nerve: diagnosis by MRI and ultrasonography. Acta Orthop Scand 62:391, 1991

32. Wells R: Suprascapular nerve entrapment. p. 173. In Zarins B, Andrews JR, Carson WG (eds): Injuries to the Throwing Arm. WB Saunders, Philadelphia, 1985

33. Butters KP: The scapula. p. 335. In Rockwood CA, Matsen FA III (eds): The Shoulder. WB Saunders, Philadelphia, 1990

# 27

# Acromioclavicular Joint Injuries

*CHRIST J. PAVLATOS*

Injuries to the acromioclavicular joint that result in instability, subluxation of the joint, or dislocation are common. The mechanism of injury is most commonly from direct blows to the point of the shoulder or to its anterior or posterior surfaces. Treatment may range from skillful neglect to the use of slings, braces, harnesses, or different surgical procedures, depending on the severity and one's school of thought.

## ANATOMY

The acromioclavicular joint is classified as a diarthrodal joint, and the articular surfaces are covered with fibrocartilage. There may be two types of fibrocartilaginous interarticular discs—complete and partial (meniscoid). There is great variation in size and shape. DePalma[1] showed that with age, the meniscus undergoes rapid degeneration until it is essentially no longer functional by the fourth decade. Nerve supply is from the branches of the axillary, suprascapular, and lateral pectoral nerves.

The acromioclavicular joint is inherently an unstable joint. It is stabilized by a set of ligaments and two muscles (Fig. 27-1). The first set of ligaments is the acromioclavicular. This ligament envelops the joint. It is thick on the superior aspect and thin on the inferior aspect. Horizontal stability is controlled by the acromioclavicular ligament.[2] At small displacement, the acromioclavicular ligaments are the primary restraints to posterior and superior translation of the clavicle.[3]

The second set of ligaments is the coracoclavicular. This is a very strong and heavy ligament whose fibers run from the outer inferior surface of the clavicle to the base of the coracoid process of the scapula. This ligament is divided into two parts. The conoid ligament[4] is cone-shaped, running from the posterior medial side of the coracoid to the conoid tubercle on the posterior medial side of the clavicle. The trapezoid[4] arises anterior and lateral to the conoid ligament on the coracoid process and extends to the undersurface of the clavicle, anterior and lateral to the conoid tubercle. The coracoclavicular ligaments play an important role in vertical stability. Studies by Fukuda et al[3] showed at large displacement, the conoid ligament provides primary restraint to superior displacement. The trapezoid ligament was primary restraint to acromioclavicular joint compression at small and large displacements.

According to Inman et al,[5] the clavicle rotates as the arm is elevated. There is a total range of motion of the acromioclavicular joint of 20 degrees, which occurs both early (in the first 30 degrees of abduction) and late (after 135 degrees of elevation of the arm). During full elevation of the arm, the clavicle rotates about 40 degrees.

## MECHANISM

Most acromioclavicular injuries are caused by direct fall on the point of the shoulder with the arm at the side in the adducted position (Fig. 27-2). The result of the downward force on the acromion is that a fracture of the clavicle occurs. If no fracture occurs, the acromioclavicular ligaments are first stretched (mild sprain); then as the force continues, the acromioclavicular ligaments tear and the coracoclavicular ligaments are stressed (moderate sprain). As the downward force continues, the coracoclavicular ligaments tear along

291

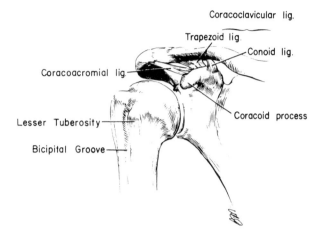

**Fig. 27-1.** Normal anatomy of the acromioclavicular joint. (From Rockwood,[6] with permission.)

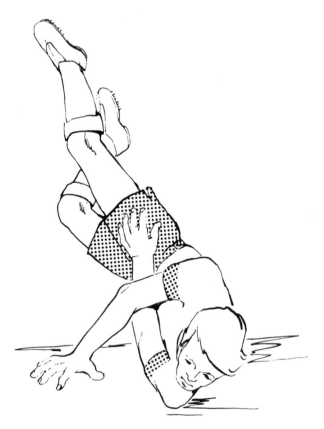

**Fig. 27-2.** The most common mechanism of injury is a direct force that occurs from a fall on the point of the shoulder. (From Rockwood,[6] with permission.)

with the muscle attachments of the deltoid and trapezius muscles, resulting in a severe acromioclavicular sprain (complete dislocation).

## CLASSIFICATION

Injuries to the acromioclavicular joint are best classified according to the amount of damage created by a given force. Classically, Allman classified injuries to the acromioclavicular joint into grade I, II and III.[1] Rockwood[2] identified six types, the first three of which are the same as Allman's grades. Their additional type IV, V, and VI are Allman's grade III injuries, varying only in the degree of direction of displacement of the distal part of the clavicle. The modified classification of Rockwood[6] is as follows (Fig. 27-3):

*Type I*
Sprain of the acromioclavicular ligament
Acromioclavicular ligament intact
Coracoclavicular ligament, deltoid and trapezius muscles intact
*Type II*
Acromioclavicular joint is disrupted with tearing of the acromioclavicular ligament
Coracoclavicular ligament is sprained
Deltoid and trapezius muscles are intact
*Type III*
Acromioclavicular ligament is disrupted
Acromioclavicular joint displaced and the shoulder complex displaced inferiorly
Coracoclavicular ligament disrupted with a coracoclavicular interspace 25 to 100 percent greater than the normal shoulder
Deltoid and trapezius muscles usually detach from distal end of the clavicle
*Type IV*
Acromioclavicular ligaments disrupt with the acromioclavicular joint displaced and the clavicle anatomically displaced posteriorly through the trapezius muscle
Coracoclavicular ligaments disrupted with wider interspace
Deltoid and trapezius muscles detached

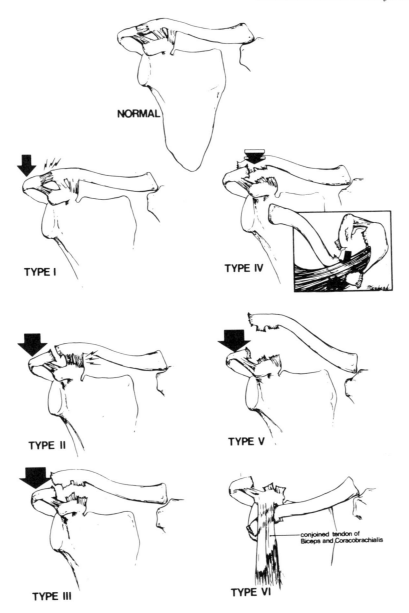

**Fig. 27-3.** Schematic drawings of the classification of ligamentous injuries that can occur to the acromioclavicular ligament. *Type I:* A mild force applied to the point of the shoulder does not disrupt either the acromioclavicular or the coracoclavicular ligaments. *Type II:* A moderate to heavy force applied to the point of the shoulder will disrupt the acromioclavicular ligaments, but the coracoclavicular ligaments remain intact. *Type III:* When a severe force is applied to the point of the shoulder, both the acromioclavicular and coracoclavicular ligaments are disrupted. *Type IV:* In this major injury, not only are the acromioclavicular and coracoclavicular ligaments disrupted, but the distal end of the clavicle is displaced posteriorly into or through the trapezius muscle. *Type V:* A violent force has been applied to the point of the shoulder that not only ruptures the acromioclavicular and coracoclavicular ligments but also disrupts the deltoid and trapezius muscle attachments and creates a major separation between the clavicle and the acromion. *Type VI:* Another major injury is an inferior dislocation of the distal end of the clavicle to the subcoracoid position. The acromioclavicular and coracoclavicular ligaments are disrupted. (From Rockwood,[6] with permission.)

*Type V*
Acromioclavicular and coracoclavicular ligaments disrupted

Acromioclavicular joint is dislocated and gross displacement between the clavicle and the scapula (100 to 300 percent greater than the normal shoulder)

Deltoid and trapezius muscles detached from distal end of the clavicle

*Type VI*
Acromioclavicular and coracoclavicular ligaments disrupted

Distal clavicle is inferior to the acromion or the coracoid process

Deltoid and trapezius muscles detached from distal end of the clavicle

## INCIDENCE

Acromioclavicular dislocations account for 12 percent of all dislocations about the shoulder.[2] Injuries are more common in male patients from 5 to 10:1. Incomplete injuries to the acromioclavicular joint are twice as common as complete dislocations.

## SIGNS AND SYMPTOMS

Pain and swelling are the most common symptoms seen in injuries to the acromioclavicular joints. Mild to moderate pain is noted in type I and II acromioclavicular joint injuries, respectively. Swelling, although minimal in type I acromioclavicular joint sprains, is more prominent in type II acromioclavicular joint injuries, making palpation of the slightly prominent clavicle difficult.

In type III acromioclavicular joint injuries, significant pain and swelling is noted with a prominence of the distal calvicle quite noticeable. Gross displacement of the distal end of the clavicle and tenting of the skin is seen in type V acromioclavicular joint injuries (Fig. 27-4). The patient characteristically presents with the upper extremity adducted close to the body and held upward by the other arm to relieve the discomfort in the acromioclavicular joint. The entire upper extremity is depressed when compared with the normal shoulder.

Patients with type IV dislocations often present with significant pain, with a prominence noted on the posterior aspect of the shoulder. When viewed from above

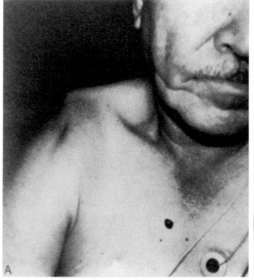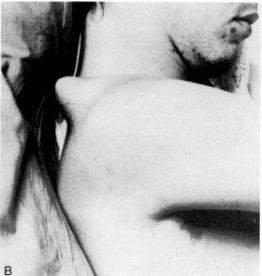

**Fig. 27-4.** Clinical photographs of patients with type V acromioclavicular dislocations. (**A**) The clavicle is quite prominent secondary to the downward displacement of the right upper extremity. (**B**) Severe prominence of the right clavicle. (From Rockwood and Matsen,[69] with permission.)

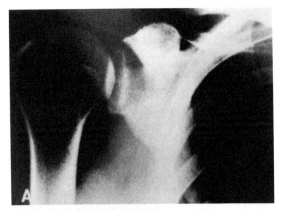

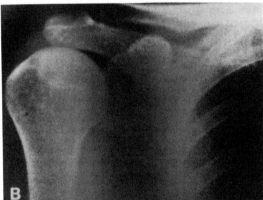

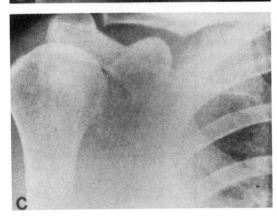

**Fig. 27-5.** Explanation of why the acromioclavicular joint is poorly visualized on routine shoulder radiographs. (**A**) This routine anteroposterior view of the shoulder shows the glenohumeral joint well. However, the acromioclavicular joint is too dark to interpret, because that area of the anatomy has been overpenetrated by the x-ray technique. (**B**) When the exposure usually used to take the shoulder films is decreased by two-thirds, the acromioclavicular joint is well visualized. However, the inferior corner of the acromioclavicular joint is superimposed on the acromion process. (**C**) Tilting the tube 15 degrees upward provides a clear view of the acromioclavicular joint. (From Rockwood,[6] with permission.)

and behind the patient, one may see the distal end of the clavicle displaced through the fibers of the trapezius muscle.

# RADIOGRAPHIC EVALUATION

Radiographic evaluation of the acromioclavicular joint will clearly demonstrate any displacement of the distal clavicle. Standard radiograph should include an anteroposterior view and a lateral view of the acromioclavicular joint.[2] Standard anteroposterior views (Fig. 27-5) are taken with a 10 to 15-degree cephalic tilt (Fig. 27-6) to avoid superimposition of the acromioclavicular joint on the spine of the scapula.[7] Upward displacement of the clavicle as well as increased distance between the undersurface of the clavicle and the coracoid process will confirm acromioclavicular dislocations. Posterior dislocations may be missed on standard anteroposterior views. A scapular lateral view as described by Alexander[8] will help identify posterior dislocations.

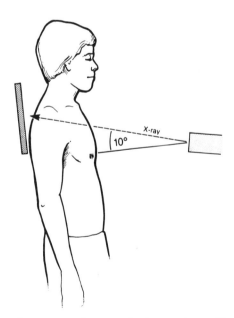

**Fig. 27-6.** Position of patient for Zanca view—10- to 15-degree cephalic tilt of the standard view for the acromioclavicular joint. (From Rockwood and Matsen,[69] with permission.)

Patients in whom it is difficult to differentiate from type II and type III acromioclavicular joint injuries may require stress films of both shoulders. These stress films will test the integrity of the coracoclavicular ligaments and assist in evaluating the degree of displacement of the distal end of the clavicle. These films are taken with the patient sitting or standing and 10 to 15 lb of weights suspended from each wrist. Anteroposterior views of both shoulders are taken. A difference of 25 percent in the distance from the coracoid process to the clavicle in the injured and normal shoulder will confirm a complete acromioclavicular dislocation.

# TREATMENT

The management of injuries to the acromioclavicular joint may range from benign neglect to the use of slings,[9] braces,[10] harnesses,[11] or several surgical procedures described in the literature.[12-20] Most authors agree on conservative or nonoperative management of acute type I and type II acromioclavicular sprains. The treatment of acute type III acromioclavicular joint dislocations is controversial. There are three basic and fundamental different schools of thought in the management of the acute type III acromioclavicular joint dislocations:

1. Those whose approach is nonoperative or conservative
2. Those who recommend surgical repair in all patients
3. Those who recommend surgical repair for selected patients

## Treatment of the Type I Injuries

The type I injury involves a mild sprain of the acromioclavicular ligaments, with the acromioclavicular and coracoclavicular ligaments intact. Treatment consists of application of ice bags to relieve discomfort and a sling to support the extremity for several days. Active assisted range of motion is initiated immediately and then isometric strengthening. Once full motion and strength has returned the patient may return to normal activities.

## Treatment of Type II Injuries

The type II injury involves disruption of the acromioclavicular ligament with the coracoclavicular ligament intact. Most authors agree that nonsurgical measures are indicated to treat this injury. However, there are differences of opinion as to which conservative measure is indicated. Many authors use the sling[9] for 7 to 14 days to rest the shoulder, followed by gradual rehabilitation program. Others recommend the use of adhesive tape strappings,[21] harnesses,[10] and plaster cast.[22] Allman[23] recommended the use of the sling harness immobilizing device—the Kenny Howard sling (Fig. 27-7)—for 3 weeks. Some authors recommend a plaster cast device (Fig. 27-8) as described by Urist,[22] with a strap over the top of the clavicle in an effort to depress the clavicle down to the acromion. However, the problem is a depressed upper extremity and not an elevated clavicle. When used, these harnesses and devices have been used for 3 to 6 weeks to prevent another injury from converting a type II subluxation to a type III dislocation. Heavy lifting and contact sports should be avoided for approximately 8 to 12 weeks until the ligaments have completely healed.

Although conservative management has been recommended for type I and type II injuries, reports from Bergfeld et al[24] and a study by Cox[25] suggested that type I and II injuries may cause more problems than previously recognized. In type I injuries, 36 percent had residual symptoms, with 70 percent disclosing radiographic changes. In type II injuries, 48 to 65 percent have symptoms, with 75 percent disclosing radiographic changes. These injuries may require excision of the outer 2 cm of the clavicle as described by Mumford.[26] This can be performed via an open or arthroscopic technique with gratifying results. In athletes, the Mumford procedure has shown successful results as reported by Cook and Tibone.[27] Twenty-three athletes were followed for an average of 3.7 years after Mumford procedure for type I and II acromioclavicular joint injuries. Most of the athletes achieved preinjury performance levels after the procedure, with little weakness noted on slow-speed and none with high-speed isokinetic testing.

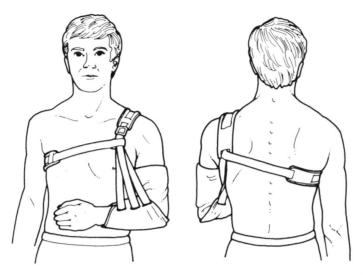

**Fig. 27-7.** Kenny-Howard shoulder halter for acromioclavicular separations. (From Rowe,[70] with permission.)

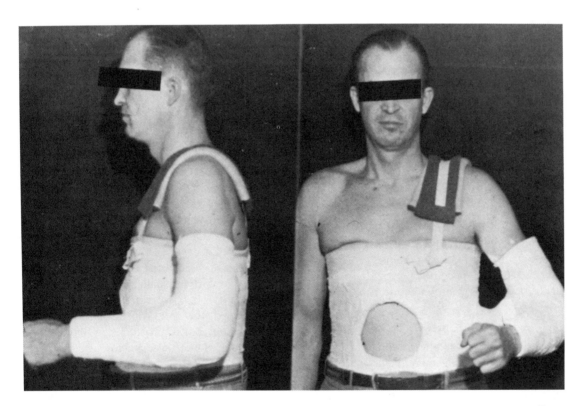

**Fig. 27-8.** Plaster cast device, older method used in 1952, for acromioclavicular separations. (From Rowe,[70] with permission.)

## Treatment for Type III Injuries

The management of type III acromioclavicular injuries has created much controversy in the orthopaedic literature. Many authors have recommended the nonoperative approach.[9,28-36] Most authors agree a simple sling is adequate for rest and comfort. As in type II injuries, a gradual rehabilitation program begins as symptoms subside over a 7 to 14-day period. The use of a harness to reduce the dislocation has not been as rewarding. The harness must be continuously worn for 6 weeks to maintain a reduction. Few patients are able to comply with this form of management.

This conservative approach has become more popular during the past 10 years, as the patient loses little time from work or athletics and does not have to be hospitalized. Cox[25] reported improved results with no support to the arm in 62 percent of his patients, whereas with immobilization and a sling only 25 percent improved at 3 to 6 weeks.

Further reports have also recommended conservative treatment of type III acromioclavicular injuries. Glick and associates[32] reported on 35 unreduced type III acromioclavicular dislocations in athletes. They concluded that a complete reduction is not necessary and that none of the athletes were disabled at follow-up. Bjerneld et al,[29] Dias et al,[30] Sleeswijk et al,[36] and Schwarz and Leixnering[35] also reported on a series of patients with type III acromioclavicular injuries treated nonoperatively, with 90 to 100 percent satisfying results, with follow-up averaging 5 to 7 years.

Studies comparing operative and nonoperative treatment of type III have also supported conservative measures. Bannister,[28] Galpin,[31] Hawkins,[9] Larsen et al,[34] and Imatani et al[33] in their comparative studies concluded that nonoperative treatment yields as good, if not better, results than surgical treatment.

Operative management of complete type III acromioclavicular dislocations is grouped into four basic operations:

1. Primary acromioclavicular joint fixation
2. Primary coracoclavicular ligament fixation
3. Excision of the distal clavicle with or without coracoclavicular ligament repair with ligament transfer or synthetic material
4. Dynamic muscle transfer

Primary stabilizer of the acromioclavicular joint remains popular among some physicians. Most use the small, smooth, or threaded Steinmann pins (Fig. 27-9). The use of the Kirschner wires has been discouraged because of reports of pin breakage and migration.[36-39] Careful technique is necessary to avoid the pins penetrating the medial cortex of the clavicle, as the pins may migrate into the lungs, chest, spinal cord, heart, etc. Along with pin fixation, repair or reconstruction of the acromioclavicular or coracoclavicular ligaments may be performed. With the pin in place most authors recommend motion below 40 degrees of elevation and gentle isometrics. Once the pins are removed at 6 to 8 weeks the rehabilitation may be accelerated.

Primary coracoclavicular ligament fixation was popularized by Bosworth[15] (Fig. 27-10). Bosworth described screw fixation of the clavicle to the coracoid process. More recently, Rockwood and Green[40] devised a clavicular coracoid lag screw that is inserted 1 inch medial to the acromioclavicular joint so it enters the base of the coracoid. Different authors[21,41-44] have reported successful results with this screw fixation. Calcification and ossification may be seen between the clavicle and the coracoid that were found not to interfere with the functional or normal clavicular rotation and produced essentially normal range of motion in the shoulder.

The use of stainless steel wires[14,45] and Dacron grafts[46-48] have also been used to repair dislocations of the acromioclavicular joint. Looping the wire or Dacron grafts around the coracoid process and the clavicle has resulted in successful repairs. However, Dahl[49] reported pressure necrosis with erosion of the Dacron graft through the entire clavicle. The rehabilitation following stainless steel wires or synthetic grafts is much more accelerated. We use a sling for several days to manage postoperative soreness and immediate motion is employed. Usually by 10 to 20 days full motion is accomplished. Isometrics strengthening is employed immediately and progressed to isotonics. Usually the patient can return to heavy lifting or sports approximately 8 to 10 weeks after surgery.

Comparisons of the acromioclavicular and coracoclavicular operative repairs have been published in the literature.[50-53] Lancaster et al[52] compared acromioclavicular and coracoclavicular fixation and found a higher minor complication rate with acromioclavicular fixa-

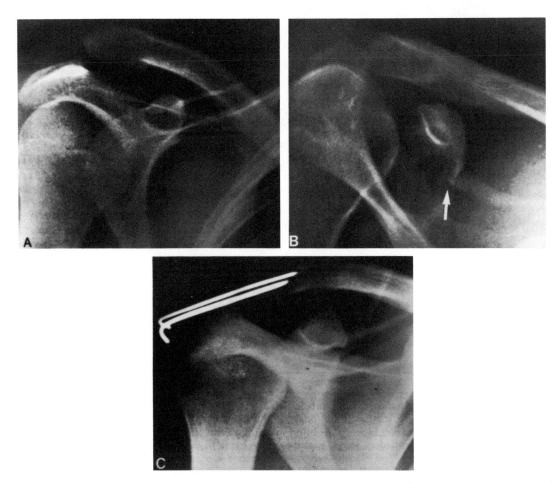

**Fig. 27-9.** Dislocation of the right acromioclavicular joint associated with an avulsion fracture of the base of the coracoid process. (**A**) The distal end of the clavicle is completely dislocated away from the acromion, but the coracoclavicular distance is about the same as in the normal shoulder. (**B**) A cephalic tilt view of the shoulder reveals a fracture at base of coracoid. A Stryket notch view probably would have better defined the fracture of the base of the coracoid. (**C**) Open reduction of the acromioclavicular joint and stabilization of the joint with two pins effectively reduced the fractured coracoid. Note that the distal ends of the pins have been bent to prevent medial migration. (From Rockwood,[6] with permission.)

tion but a higher failure rate with coracoclavicular fixation. However, Bargren et al[50] and Taft et al[53] found superior results with coracoclavicular fixation. Taft et al found that patients with acromioclavicular fixation had a higher incidence of post-traumatic arthritis than those managed with a coracoclavicular screw. They further found a greater incidence of post-traumatic arthritis in those patients who failed to maintain an anatomic reduction.

In 1972, Weaver and Dunn[19] described in 12 patients

a technique that combines an oblique resection of the distal end of the clavicle with intramedullary transfer of the coracoacromial ligament to the clavicle (Fig. 27-11). The distal clavicle resection avoids any post-traumatic changes with transfer of the coracoacromial ligament reconstructing the coracoclavicular ligaments. Successful results have been reported by Rauschning et al[54] in 18 patients.

Smith and Stewart[55,56] compared acomioclavicular fixation and coracoclavicular ligament repairs with and

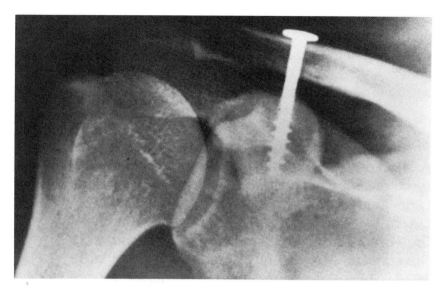

**Fig. 27-10.** Postoperative anteroposterior radiograph of shoulder with Bosworth screw in place. Note that the acromioclavicular joint has been reduced and the coarse lag threads of the screw are well seated into the coracoid process. (From Rockwood,[6] with permission.)

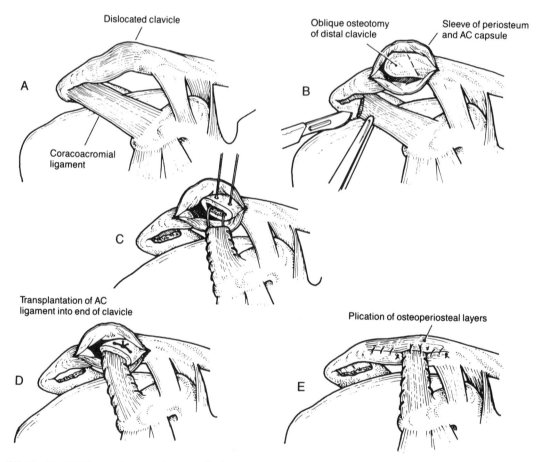

**Fig. 27-11.** (*A–E*) Weaver-Dunn technique of releasing the coracoacromial ligament from the acromion, obliquely osteotomizing the distal clavicle, and transplanting the coracoacromial ligament into the end of the clavicle. Plication of osteoperiosteal flaps gives extra support. (Adapted from Weaver and Dunn,[19] with permission.)

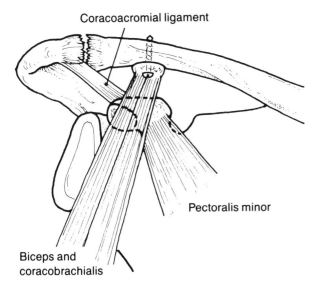

**Fig. 27-12.** Dewar technique: transfer of the coracoid process with the attached muscles by screw fixation to the undersurface of the clavicle—the "dynamic" transfer. (Adapted from E. Hopper Ross by Dewar and Barrington,[17] with permission.)

without distal clavicle excision. They found no difference in symptomatology, range of motion, or strength, although there was a higher incidence of degenerative changes in patients without distal clavicle excision (24.3 percent) compared with those with distal clavicle excision (4.5 percent).

The use of a dynamic muscle transfer[57-59] (Fig. 27-12) has also been reported in treating dislocations of the acromioclavicular joint. Dewar and Barrington[17] recommended transplanting the osteotomized coracoid with its muscular attachments of the short head of the biceps and coracobrachialis to the undersurface of the clavicle by screw fixation. Although no complications were reported in their five patients, Caspi et al[60] warn of injury to the musculocutaneous nerve with this technique.

## Treatment of Type IV, V, and VI Injuries

Because of the severe posterior displacement in type IV injuries and gross displacement in type V injuries, most authors have recommended a surgical repair.[41,61-64] Repairs have been reported with the pre-

viously described operative techniques. Few type VI injuries have been described in the literature[65-68]; all were treated with surgery. Attempts at closed reduction are usually unsuccessful. Gerber and Rockwood[65] reported using the extra-articular technique with a coracoclavicular lag screw, repair of the ligaments, and imbrication of the deltoid trapezius fascia over the top of the clavicle with successful results. The rehabilitation following surgery to correct a type IV, V, and VI sprain tends to be somewhat slower because of the severity of the initial injury. The program is similar to the previously discussed ones and matches the exact surgical procedure and specific patient demands and desires.

## Summary of Treatment

On review of the literature, type I and type II acromioclavicular joint injuries are best treated conservatively, with good results seen in most of the patients. A certain percentage of these patients may have residual pain and stiffness as a result of degenerative changes. This may necessitate excision of the distal clavicle in some patients. In both classes of injury immediate motion and strengthening appears to render better success.

Results of treatment of type III acromioclavicular joint injuries have been successful in both nonoperative and operative groups. Based on these findings, a nonoperative approach to this injury would be appropriate for most patients. If pain is noted on follow-up, an operative approach may be performed using either a Bosworth screw, synthetic graft, or a Weaver-Dunn procedure. Type IV, V, and VI injuries are best treated with open reduction and surgical stabilization of the acromioclavicular joint.

## REFERENCES

1. DePalma AF: The role of the disks of the sternoclavicular and acromioclavicular joints. Clin Orthop 13:7, 1959
2. Rockwood CA, Young DC: Disorders of the acromioclavicular Joint. p. 413. In Rockwood CA, Matsen FA III (eds): The Shoulder. WB Saunders, Philadelphia, 1990
3. Fukuda K, Craig EV, An K-N et al: Biomechanical study of the ligamentous system of the acromioclavicular joint. J Bone Joint Surg 68A:434, 1986
4. Johnston TB, Davies DV, Davies F (eds): Gray's Anatomy. 32nd Ed. Longmans, Green, and Co., London, 1958

5. Inman VT, Saunders JB, Abbott LC: Observations on the function of the shoulder joint. J Bone Joint Surg 26:1, 1944

6. Rockwood CA Jr: Injuries to the acromioclavicular joint. p. 860. In Rockwood CA Jr, Green DP (eds): Fractures in Adults. Vol. 1. 2nd Ed. JB Lippincott, Philadelphia, 1984

7. Zanca P: Shoulder pain: involvement of the acromioclavicular joint: analysis of 1,000 cases. AJR 112:493, 1971

8. Alexander OM: Dislocation of the acromio-clavicular joint. Radiography 15:260, 1949

9. Hawkins RJ: The acromioclavicular joint. Paper prepared for AAOS Summer Institute, Chicago, July 10–11, 1980

10. Giannestras NJ: A method of immobilization of acute acromioclavicular separation. J Bone Joint Surg 26:597, 1944

11. Warner AH: A harness for use in the treatment of acromioclavicular separation. J Bone Joint Surg 19:1132, 1937

12. Augereau B, Robert H, Apoil A: Treatment of severe acromioclavicular dislocation: a coracoclavicular ligamentoplasty technique derived from Cadenat's procedure. Ann Chir 35:720, 1981

13. Bateman JE: Athletic injuries about the shoulder in throwing and body-contact sports. Clin Orthop 23:75, 1962

14. Bearden JM, Hughston JC, Whatley GS: Acromioclavicular dislocation: method of treatment. J Sports Med 1:5, 1973

15. Bosworth BM: Acromioclavicular separation: new method of repair. Surg Gynecol Obstet 73:866, 1941

16. Bundens WD Jr, Cook JI: Repair of acromioclavicular separations by deltoid-trapezius imbrication. Clin Orthop 20:109, 1961

17. Dewar FP, Barrington TW: The treatment of chronic acromioclavicular dislocation. J Bone Joint Surg 47B:32, 1965

18. Sage FP, Salvatore JE: Injuries of acromioclavicular joint: study of results in 96 patients. South Med J 56:486, 1963

19. Weaver JK, Dunn HK: Treatment of acromioclavicular injuries, especially complete acromioclavicular separation. J Bone Joint Surg 54A:1187, 1972

20. Weitzman G: Treatment of acute acromioclavicular joint dislocation by a modified Bosworth method: report on twenty-four cases. J Bone Joint Surg 49A:1167, 1967

21. Rawlings G: Acromioclavicular dislocations and fractures of the clavicle. A simple method of support. Lancet 2:789, 1939

22. Urist MR: Complete dislocation of the acromioclavicular joint: the nature of the traumatic lesion and effective methods of treatment with an analysis of 41 cases. J Bone Joint Surg 28:813, 1946

23. Allman FL Jr: Fractures and ligamentous injuries of the clavicle and its articulation. J Bone Joint Surg 49A:774, 1967

24. Bergfeld JA, Andrish JT, Clancy WG: Evaluation of the acromioclavicular joint following first- and second-degree sprains. Am J Sports Med 6:153, 1978

25. Cox JS: The fate of the acromioclavicular joint in athletic injuries. Am J Sports Med 9:50, 1981

26. Mumford EB: Acromioclavicular dislocation. J Bone Joint Surg 23:799, 1941

27. Cook FF, Tibone JE: The Mumford procedure in athletes: an objective analysis of function. Am J Sports Med 16:97, 1988

28. Bannister GC, Wallace WA, Stableforth PG, Hutson MA: The management of acute acromioclavicular dislocation. J Bone Joint Surg 71B:848, 1989

29. Bjerneld H, Hovelius L, Thorling J: Acromio-clavicular separations treated conservatively: a 5-year follow-up study. Acta Orthop Scan 54:743, 1983

30. Dias JJ, Steingold RA, Richardson RA et al: The conservative treatment of acromioclavicular dislocation: review after five years. J Bone Joint Surg 69B:719, 1987

31. Galpin RD, Hawkins RJ, Grainger RW: A comparative analysis of operative versus nonoperative treatment of grade III acromioclavicular separations. Clin Orthop 193:150, 1985

32. Glick JM, Milburn LJ, Haggerty JF, Nishimoto D: Dislocated acromioclavicular joint: follow-up study of 35 unreduced acromioclavicular dislocations. Am J Sport Med 5:264, 1977

33. Imatani RJ, Hanlon JJ, Cady GW: Acute complete acromioclavicular separation. J Bone Joint Surg 57A:328, 1975

34. Larsen E, Bjerg-Neilsen A, Christensen P: Conservative or surgical treatment of acromioclavicular dislocation: a prospective, controlled, randomized study. J Bone Joint Surg 68A:552, 1986

35. Schwarz N, Leixnering M: [Results of nonreduced acromioclavicular Tossy III separations.] Unfallchirurg 89:248, 1986

36. Sleeswijk Visser SV, Haarsma SM, Speeckaert MTC: Conservative treatment of acromioclavicular dislocation: Jones strap versus mitella (abstr). Acta Orthop Scand 55:483, 1984

37. Grauthoff VH, Klammer HL: [Complications due to migration of a Kirschner wire from the clavicle] Fortschr Rontgenstr 128:1978

38. Mazet RJ: Migration of a Kirschner wire from the shoulder region into the lung: report of two cases. J Bone Joint Surg 25A:477, 1943

39. Norrell H, Llewellyn RC: Migration of a threaded Steinmann pin from an acromioclavicular joint into the spinal canal: a case report. J Bone Joint Surg 47A:1024, 1965

40. Rockwood CA Jr, Green DP (eds): Fractures in Adults. 2nd Ed. JB Lippincott, Philadelphia, 1984

41. Barber FA: Complete posterior acromioclavicular dislocation: a case report. Orthopedics 10:493, 1987

42. Kennedy JC, Cameron H: Complete dislocation of the acromioclavicular joint. J Bone Joint Surg 36B:202, 1954

43. Kennedy JC: Complete dislocation of the acromioclavicular joint: 14 years later. J Trauma 8:311, 1968

44. Lowe GP, Fogarty MJP: Acute acromioclavicular joint dislocation: results of operative treatment with the Bosworth screw. Aust N Z J Surg 47:664, 1977

45. Alldredge RH: Surgical treatment of acromioclavicular dislocation. Clin Orthop 63:262, 1969

46. Kappakas GS, McMaster JH: Repair of acromioclavicular separation using a Dacron prosthesis graft. Clin Orthop 131:247, 1978

47. Park JP, Arnold JA, Coker TP et al: Treatment of acromioclavicular separations: a retrospective study. Am J Sports Med 8:251, 1980

48. Tagliabue D, Riva A: [Current approaches to the treatment of acromioclavicular joint separation in athletes.] Ital J Sports Traumatol 3:15, 1981

49. Dahl E: Velour prosthesis in fractures and dislocations in the clavicular region. Chirurgerie 53:120, 1982

50. Bargren JH, Erlanger S, Dick HM: Biomechanics and comparison of two operative methods of treatment of complete acromioclavicular separation. Clin Orthop 130:267, 1962

51. Kiefer H, Claes L, Burri C, Holzworth J: The stabilizing effect of various implants on the torn acromioclavicular joint: a biomechanical study. Arch Orthop Trauma Surg 106:42, 1986

52. Lancaster S, Horowitz M, Alonso J: Complete acromioclavicular separations: a comparison of operative methods. Clin Orthop 216:80, 1987

53. Taft TN, Wilson FC, Oglesby JW: Dislocation of the acromioclavicular joint: an end-result study. J Bone Joint Surg 69A:1045, 1987

54. Rauschning W, Nordesjo LO, Nordgren B et al: Resection arthroplasty for repair of complete acromioclavicular separations. Arch Orthop Traumatol Surg 97:161, 1980

55. Smith DW: Coracoid fracture associated with acromioclavicular dislocation. Clin Orthop 108:165, 1975

56. Smith MJ, Stewart MJ: Acute acromioclavicular separations. Am J Sport Med 7:62, 1979

57. Bailey RW, O'Connor GA, Tilus PD, Baril JD: A dynamic repair for acute and chronic injuries of the acromioclavicular area (abstr). J Bone Joint Surg 54A:1802, 1972

58. Bailey RW: A dynamic repair for complete acromioclavicular joint dislocation (abstr). J Bone Joint Surg 47A:858, 1965

59. Berson BL, Gilbert MS, Green S: Acromioclavicular dislocations: treatment by transfer of the conjoined tendon and distal end of the coracoid process to the clavicle. Clin Orthop 135:157, 1978

60. Caspi I, Ezra E, Neurbay J, Horoszovski H: Musculocutaneous nerve injury following dynamic fixature of distal clavicle. Clin Orthop 1985

61. Hastings DE, Horne JG: Anterior dislocation of the acromioclavicular joint. Injury 10:285, 1978

62. Malcapi C, Grassi G, Oretti D: Posterior dislocation of the acromioclavicular joint: a rare or an easily overlooked lesion? Ital J Orthop Traumatol 4:79, 1978

63. Nieminen S, Aho AJ: Anterior dislocation of the acromioclavicular joint. Ann Chir Gynaecol 73:21, 1984

64. Sondergard-Petersen P, Mikkelsen P: Posterior acromioclavicular dislocation. J Bone Joint Surg 64B:52, 1982

65. Gerber C, Rockwood CA Jr: Subcoracoid dislocation of the lateral end of the clavicle: a report of three cases. J Bone Joint Surg 69A:924, 1987

66. McPhee IB: Inferior dislocation of the outer end of the clavicle. J Trauma 20:709, 1980

67. Patterson WR: Inferior dislocation of the distal end of the clavicle. J Bone Joint Surg 49A:1184, 1967

68. Sage J: Recurrent inferior dislocation of the clavicle at the acromioclavicular joint. Am J Sports Med 10:145, 1982

69. Rockwood CA, Matsen FA III: The Shoulder. Vol. 1. p. 427. WB Saunders, Philadelphia, 1990

70. Rowe CR: Acromioclavicular and sternoclavicular joints. p. 293. In Rowe CR (ed): The Shoulder. Churchill Livingstone, New York, 1988

# 28

# Scapulothoracic Disorders

*GEORGE M. McCLUSKEY III*
*LOUIS U. BIGLIANI*

Disorders of the scapulothoracic joint are not as common as glenohumeral, acromioclavicular, or subacromial lesions. However, they can be a source of persistent pain and disability and thus limit shoulder function. Any soft tissue or osseous lesion that interrupts the smooth gliding movement of the scapula on the posterior chest wall can result in scapular pain. These lesions are better recognized and appreciated with recent advances in imaging modalities including magnetic resonance imaging and computed tomography. Electromyographic analysis has proven valuable in verifying the presence of a suspected neurologic lesion.

Some of the more common scapulothoracic joint disorders seen in the athletic population include the snapping scapula syndrome, scapulothoracic bursitis, and paralysis of the trapezius or serratus anterior muscles. This chapter discusses these different lesions including diagnosis and common methods of treatment.

## FUNCTIONAL ANATOMY

The scapula is a thin triangular bone that serves as an attachment site for most of the extrinsic and intrinsic muscles that provide stability and movement of the glenohumeral and scapulothoracic joints. The muscles responsible for movement of the scapula are divided into groups including elevators, depressors, protractors, retractors, and rotators. Protraction refers to the lateral and forward movement of the scapula on the thorax. Retraction refers to medial scapula movement toward the vertebral column. During upward rotation, the inferior angle of the scapula moves lateral and

forward, thus orienting the glenoid articular surface upward. The glenoid surface moves downward during downward rotation of the inferior angle of the scapula.[1]

Elevation of the scapula is primarily achieved by the actions of the upper portion of the trapezius that inserts into the distal clavicle, acromion, and lateral spine of the scapula, the levator scapulae, and the rhomboideus minor and major. Depression of the scapula occurs with gravity, especially the lateral angle. The primary active depressor of the scapula is the latissimus dorsi. However, several muscles serve as accessory depressors including the lower portion of the serratus anterior, pectoralis minor, and lower portion of the trapezius.[1]

The primary upward rotators of the scapula are the serratus anterior and trapezius (Fig. 28-1). The middle portion of the trapezius initiates upward rotation, and at 45 degrees of scapular abduction, the serratus anterior contracts and pulls the inferior angle forward. The upper trapezius assists in this movement by elevating the lateral angle of the scapula while the lower part of the trapezius pulls down on the base of the scapular spine. The upper portion of the trapezius is the only muscle that elevates the lateral border of the scapula. Downward rotation of the scapula is assisted by several muscles including the levator scapulae and rhomboideus minor and major that insert on the medial scapula and elevate the scapula, as well as the pectoralis minor, lower portion of the pectoralis major, and the latissimus dorsi that insert laterally and depress the scapula (Fig. 28-2).

Protractors or abductors of the scapula include the serratus anterior and the pectoralis minor and major. Together these muscles provide lateral and forward

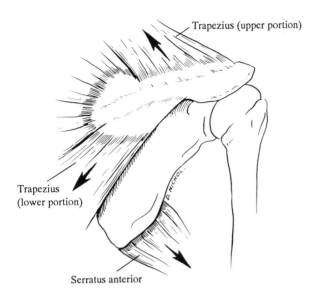

**Fig. 28-1.** Upward scapular rotators include serratus anterior and trapezius.

movement of the scapula. The trapezius, especially the middle portion, and the rhomboideus major and minor serve as primary retractors or adductors of the scapula (Fig. 28-3). They are important muscles, creating medial scapular stability.

Investigators have demonstrated that the posterior scapular muscles control forces at the glenohumeral joint and stabilize this joint with a graded coordinated firing pattern during shoulder motion.[2–4] During the windup and cocking phases of throwing, the trapezius, rhomboid major, and rhomboid minor act to maximally retract the scapula.

With the acceleration and follow-through phases, protraction of the scapula by the serratus anterior and pectoralis major and minor allows for appropriate positioning of the scapula to enhance the dissipation of forces generated with throwing. Normal protraction allows the scapula to follow the humeral head and shaft during acceleration and follow-through, thus providing a stable glenohumeral joint that protects the capsular ligaments from tensile overload injury.[2] Kibler[2] and others[4] have emphasized the importance of the scapular stabilizing muscles in decelerating the arm by dissipating acceleration forces during the follow-through phase of throwing using electromyelo-

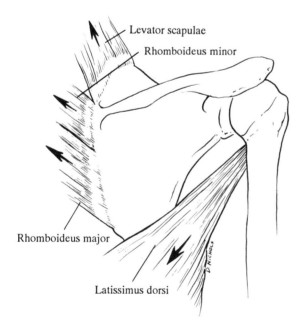

**Fig. 28-2.** Downward scapular rotators include levator scapulae, rhomboideus major and minor, and latissimus dorsi.

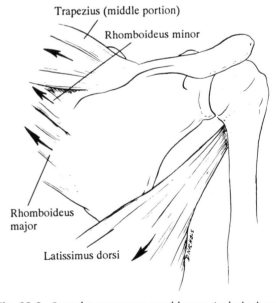

**Fig. 28-3.** Scapular retractors or adductors include the trapezius, rhomboid major, and rhomboid minor.

graphic studies. Force couples must act efficiently to provide smooth scapulohumeral motion during throwing to minimize the risk of injury and maximize performance.

# SNAPPING SCAPULA

The term *snapping scapula* was initially used by Boinet[5] in 1867 to describe crepitation caused by movement of the scapula on the posterior thorax. Milch[6] subsequently differentiated between scapular snapping and scapular crepitus based on the quality and etiology of the sounds caused by osseous and soft tissue lesions involving the scapulothoracic interval.

Scapular snapping refers to the sound that occurs when an osseous or osteocartilaginous lesion, arising from either the anterior scapula or the posterior thorax, moves against the opposite surface. This interruption of the normal smooth gliding scapulothoracic mechanism causes snapping and pain in the periscapular region. Although scapular noises are not uncommon in the normal population, this loud grating and snapping sound is distinctive and easily felt with the examiner's hand.

In many cases, an anatomic lesion cannot be identified with routine x-ray views of the scapula and shoulder. Tangential views of the lateral scapula, computed tomography scans, or magnetic resonance imaging are often necessary to localize the lesion correctly.

Clinically, most patients present with pain in the periscapular region associated with an audible and palpable snapping sound as the scapula moves on the posterior thorax. Fullness in the posterior shoulder girdle or winging of the scapula may indicate a space-occupying osseous lesion in the scapulothoracic interval. Neurovascular examination is usually negative.

Some of the offending osseous or osteocartilaginous lesions causing scapular snapping include the osteochondroma, Luschka's tubercle, an excessively long or curved superior angle of the scapula with a protruding scapular hook, and malunion of either scapular or rib fractures.[6] Bateman[7] attributed scapular snapping and crepitus to repetitive episodes of trauma to the periscapular region that produce periosteal microtears along the medial border of the scapula, eventually producing a reactive bone spur at the avulsed muscle attachment site on the scapula.

The osteochondroma or exostosis is a common benign osteocartilaginous skeletal growth. Most of these exostoses occur as single isolated lesions, but they may be multiple in patients with a hereditary predisposition. In the periscapular region, they project from the anterior scapula and the posterior thorax and commonly assume a mushroom-shaped appearance (Fig. 28-4). "Pseudo-winging" of the scapula has been described in cases in which a large osteochrondroma forces the scapula and posterior thorax apart. A specific lesion called Luschka's tubercle is an osteochondroma that occurs at the superomedial angle of the scapula and produces scapular snapping.[6] It varies in size and is often associated with a large bursa.

Occasionally, the superior angle of the scapula is excessively long and curved. This may cause scapular snapping when the arm is abducted and the scapula rotated. Sprengel's deformity with its associated omo-vertebral bone, as well as a malunion of a scapula or rib fracture, may also produce periscapular symptoms of pain and snapping with motion of the shoulder girdle.

Treatment of the snapping scapula is generally conservative. Strengthening exercises for the scapular retractors, protractors, and rotators, along with heat, non-steroidal anti-inflammatory medication, and occasional local steroid injections provide relief of symptoms in most cases. Scapular noises and sounds may not be associated with symptoms and therefore do not always require treatment. Osteochondromas or other osseous lesions that protrude into the scapulothoracic interval and cause symptoms that prove to be refractory to conservative therapy should be excised. Partial scapulectomy or removal of the superomedial angle of the scapula has been advocated by many authors when crepitation and pain are localized to this region.[6,8–10]

The surgical technique of excision of the osteochondroma or other bony protuberance in the scapulothoracic interval is similar to that described for scapulothoracic bursitis. Care must be taken during this approach to search for all potential bone and soft tissue lesions that may be present, as sometimes these are undetected preoperatively.

Often, an osteochondroma or bone protuberance can be associated with an overlying bursa or soft tissue lesion that should be excised in conjunction with the bone lesion. Removal of too much bone may weaken the important intrinsic and extrinsic muscles with scap-

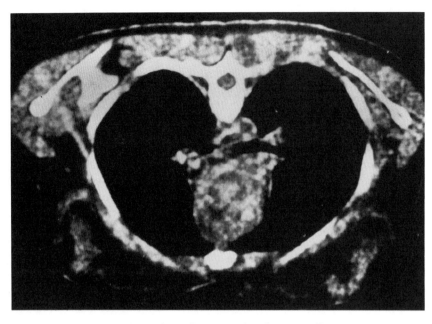

**Fig. 28-4.** This computed tomography scan showed an osteochondroma on the anterior aspect of the scapula in a patient with "pseudo-winging" of the scapula, with scapular snapping and pain.

ular attachments and can lead to instability and dysfunction with respect to scapulohumeral rhythm.

## SCAPULOTHORACIC BURSITIS

Milch[6] differentiated between patients with true scapular snapping and those with scapular crepitus. Scapular snapping is the result of an osseous or osteocartilaginous lesion involving the scapulothoracic interval. Scapular crepitus, however, occurs as the result of inflammation involving periscapular bursae and soft tissues that result from overuse activity or local trauma. Three bursae, located in the periscapular region, have clinical significance.[11] These bursae normally reduce friction between the scapula and the posterior thorax, thus providing for smooth gliding scapulothoracic motion. One bursa, called the bursa mucosa angulae superioris scapulae, is located at the upper angle of the scapula between the serratus anterior and the subscapularis. A second bursa is found between the serratus anterior and the lateral chest wall, called the bursa mucosa serrata. A third bursa is situated at the inferior angle of the scapula.

Scapulothoracic bursitis is primarily a clinical diagnosis and is based on characteristic periscapular pain associated with audible and palpable crepitus with scapulothoracic motion. The crepitus is usually located at the superomedial border of the scapula. Local injections of 1 percent Xylocaine are helpful in establishing the diagnosis and affording relief of symptoms in most cases.

Trauma to the periscapular region is responsible for the onset of symptoms in most cases. This trauma may be direct as in injury from a motor vehicle accident or a direct blow to the periscapular region. Indirect trauma may occur as the result of a fall on an extended extremity that indirectly injures soft tissues in the scapulothoracic interval. In a series reported by Arntz and Matsen,[9] 10 of 12 patients (88 percent) attributed the onset of their symptoms to some kind of traumatic event. Richards and McKee[10] presented three healthy young male laborers that developed unilateral scapulothoracic crepitus with a history of direct trauma to the involved shoulder in two patients. They believed that trauma to the scapula initiated an inflammatory process in the scapulothoracic bursa, which together with a "prominent" superomedial scapular angle created the syndrome of scapulothoracic impingement. Recently, we reported on a series of nine patients with refractory scapulothoracic bursitis of which a traumatic episode was noted in six patients.[12] Three patients had direct trauma to the periscapular region (i.e., motor vehicle accident) whereas three had indirect trauma. A professional baseball player fell backward onto his extended arm and indirectly injured the muscles and soft tissue structures in the scapulothoracic interval.

Many patients with this disorder have no history of trauma to the shoulder or periscapular region. Overuse type syndromes, including overhead sports such as throwing, swimming, and tennis, or any type of work that requires repetitive or constant movement of the scapula on the posterior thorax may irritate the soft tissue located in the scapulothoracic interval. This repetitive irritation continues until a chronic bursitis and inflammation of the surrounding soft tissue evolves, resulting in scarring and fibrosis of the involved tissues with eventual crepitus and pain. Sisto and Jobe[13] attributed symptoms in their group of professional pitchers to a flaw in delivery style and to repetitive irritation and pressure between the scapula and posterior thorax secondary to alternate firing times in the pitching cycle in the two main muscle groups involved in the throwing motion. In our recent report, [12] three of nine patients had overuse syndromes that resulted in scapulothoracic bursitis that was surgically treated.

Scapulothoracic bursitis rarely requires surgical intervention, as it generally responds favorably to conservative management. Rest, analgesics, nonsteroidal anti-inflammatory medication, physical therapy, heat, and local steroid injections usually provide adequate relief of symptoms. Specific exercises designed to strengthen the scapular stabilizers and the internal and external rotators have proved extremely beneficial. However, occasionally patients may prove to be refractory to conservative therapy.

In the literature, it seems that most authors recommended partial scapulectomy in patients with scapular crepitus and pain that have failed conservative treatment, even when no osseous lesion is present.[6,8–10] The question arises as to whether partial scapulectomy is necessary in situations in which no bony abnormality can be identified, either preoperatively or intraoperatively. Sisto and Jobe[13] reported on four professional baseball pitchers with scapulothoracic bursitis at the inferomedial angle of the scapula that became refrac-

tory to conservative therapy. No bone abnormalities were found in any of their patients. Excision of the offending bursa, without resection of bone, allowed all four players to return to professional baseball at their former level of pitching within 1 year. In our series,[12] 88 percent satisfactory results were reported after bursal excision alone in a group of patients with refractory scapulothoracic bursitis in which no bone abnormality was found. The operative findings included a thickened, fibrotic bursa located between the serratus anterior and the posterior thorax in all cases. Strict adherence to proper surgical technique with adequate repair of the medial scapular stabilizing muscles can lead to a satisfactory result in most cases.

The surgical technique involves making a vertical incision just medial to the vertebral border of the scapula (Fig. 28-5). The trapezius is dissected free. Using subperiosteal dissection, the rhomboid minor and the rhomboid major are elevated from the medial scapular border and retracted medially. A plant is developed between the deep surface of the serratus anterior and the posterior thorax. The anterior surface of the scapula

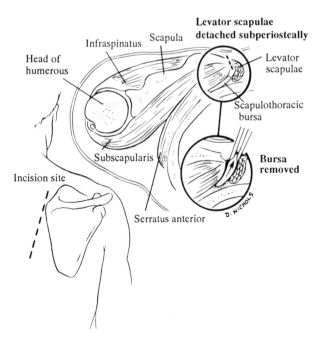

**Fig. 28-5.** A vertical incision is made medial to the vertebral scapular border. The trapezius and rhomboid muscles are retracted medially. The bursa is typically found in the interval between the serratus anterior and the posterior thorax.

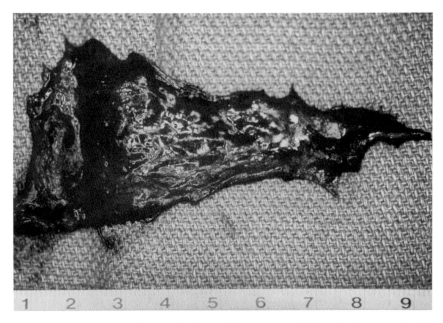

**Fig. 28-6.** Typical surgical specimen shows a thickened fibrotic scapulothoracic bursa excised from a patient with scapular crepitus and pain located at the superomedial angle of the scapula.

and the posterior ribs are carefully palpated for any evidence of bony projections or osteophytes. The thickened bursa is excised in its entirety (Fig. 28-6). The rhomboids are sutured back to the medial scapular border, and the trapezius is repaired. The wound is closed in layers.

Postoperatively, the patient is placed in a sling for comfort. Pendulum and early passive motion exercises are started immediately. Active motion is begun at 3 weeks, and strengthening exercises for the scapular stabilizers and external rotators are started at 6 weeks. Throwing is begun at 12 weeks with short gentle tossing and is progressed to full-speed throwing as tolerated.

## SERRATUS ANTERIOR PARALYSIS

The serratus anterior is a large muscle that originates from the anterior thorax along the upper eight or nine ribs, covers the lateral aspect of the thorax, and inserts along the costal surface of the medial scapula.[1] Its chief function is to protract the scapula or draw it forward onto the posterior thorax while allowing the scapula to rotate upward. This movement allows abduction and flexion of the shoulder to occur.

The long thoracic nerve innervates the serratus anterior.[1] It is composed of the anterior rami of the C5, C6, and C7 cervical nerves as they exit their respective intervertebral foramina. The nerve passes posterior to the remaining brachial plexus and axillary vessels to the superficial surface of the serratus anterior along the lateral thorax.

Injury to the long thoracic nerve generally occurs as the result of trauma, although viral illness, some inoculations, prolonged bed rest, and general anesthesia have been reported to cause paralysis of the serratus anterior.[14–16]

Trauma to the long thoracic nerve may result from repetitive use of the shoulder and upper extremity either from a work-related activity or from sports (including overhead sports and gymnastics in particular). Traction injuries involving the neck or the arm, when in the abducted position, can injure the long thoracic nerve. Surgical procedures such as radical mastectomy, rib resection, or any operation in the region of the axilla may result in nerve injury and serratus anterior paralysis. Often the cause for paralysis is idiopathic.

As the serratus anterior serves as a primary scapular stabilizer in pushing and elevating movements, paralysis of this muscle causes the scapula to move medially toward the vertebral column and to rotate downward and inward. This posture is commonly referred to as scapular winging. Normal flexion and abduction of the arm above the horizontal is usually not possible as the upward rotation function of the scapula is lost. Scapular winging is easily demonstrated clinically by having the patient push against a wall using both hands (Fig. 28-7). This winging posture of the scapula may not be obvious with the patient in a resting and sitting position. Pain with attempted elevation of the arm and with functional activities such as lifting and pushing is commonly experienced by the patient because of the loss of scapular stabilization normally provided by the serratus anterior and also because of the poor success of adjacent muscles to compensate for the ineffective serratus anterior.

Conservative therapy is the mainstay of treatment in early closed injuries involving the long thoracic nerve. Passive range of motion exercises to avoid stiffness and contracture, as well as strengthening exercises for the deltoid and other scapular stabilizers, should be used during the waiting period for recovery. This nonoperative regimen may halp reduce pain and improve shoulder function. Braces and orthotics have not been successful and are not advised.[15]

Serratus anterior paralysis usually disappears spontaneously, especially in idiopathic cases. Electromyographic studies are recommended at 3-month intervals, along with repeated clinical examinations to monitor recovery.[15] Although recovery of serratus function after 2 or 3 years has recently been reported,[14] patients with symptomatic scapular winging or dysfunction caused by serratus palsy of 1 year or more in duration may be candidates for surgical intervention. Not all patients with permanent serratus anterior paralysis desire surgery, as they learn to de-emphasize their disability by altering their work and sports-related activities.

Several surgical options exist for serratus anterior paralysis. Scapulothoracic fusion is not recommended as a primary surgical alternative.[15] Several types of tendon transfers have been described in the literature. These include transfer of the pectoralis minor, transfer of the pectoralis major,[17] and transfer of the teres major and rhomboids. Our procedure of choice involves transfer of the sternal head of the pectoralis major using a fascial extension through the inferior angle of the scapula as described by Marmor and Bechtol in 1983.[17] Transplanting only the costosternal portion of the pectoralis major preserves the function of

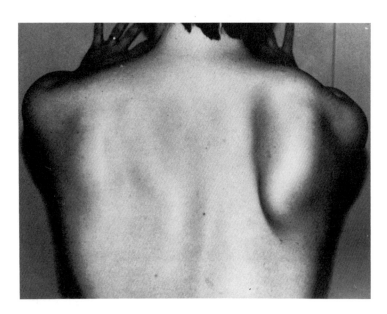

**Fig. 28-7.** Scapular winging in patient with serratus anterior paralysis secondary to long thoracic nerve palsy.

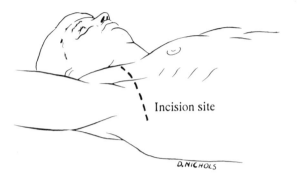

**Fig. 28-8.** Skin incision is made from the pectoralis major muscle anteriorly to the inferior tip of the scapula.

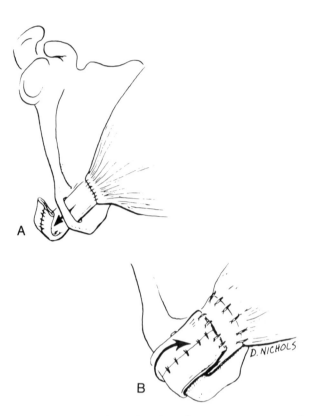

**Fig. 28-10.** Pectoralis tendon, fascia lata composite is passed through the inferior tip of the scapulae **(A)** and sutured to itself **(B).** The wound is closed in layers.

the clavicular portion of the pectoralis major, which is important in normal shoulder function.

The surgical procedure requires a skin incision from the middle of the pectoralis major muscle to the tip of the scapula through the axilla (Fig. 28.8). The sternal head of the pectoralis major tendon is released from its insertion into the bicipital ridge. A fascia lata graft is harvested from the lateral thigh and sutured into the distal portion of the freed pectoralis tendon to form a tube (Fig. 28-9). This tube is passed through a hole

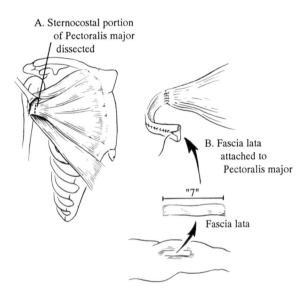

**Fig. 28-9. (A&B)** Sternal head of the pectoralis major tendon is released from its humeral head insertion. A fascia lata graft, harvested from the lateral thigh, is sutured into this freed sternal head of the pectoralis major.

made in the inferior tip of the scapula and secured (Fig. 28-10). The incision is closed in layers.

Postoperatively, the arm is placed in a sling for comfort. Early passive motion exercises are started immediately and progressed to active assisted exercises in 10 days. Strengthening exercises and active motion are begun at 6 weeks.

## TRAPEZIUS PARALYSIS

Paralysis of the trapezius muscle, caused by injury to the spinal accessory nerve (11th cranial nerve), is a painful and disabling problem. Blunt trauma to the posteromedial shoulder girdle or posterior cervical triangle region, from either a direct blow or stretching of the nerve, results in drooping of the shoulder, asymmetry of the neck line, winging of the scapula, and weakness of forward elevation in abduction. Penetrating injuries from a stab wound, gunshot, or inadvertent injury during a surgical procedure such as cervical node biopsy, may also damage the spinal accessory nerve.[18–21] The smooth scapulohumeral rhythm is lost as the intricate balance of muscle forces about the scapula is disrupted. Muscle spasm, frozen shoulder, subacromial impingement, and radiculitis from traction on the brachial plexus may cause severe pain and disability in the shoulder girdle.

The trapezius muscle is the largest and most superficial of the scapulothoracic muscles (Fig. 28-11). This muscle originates from the spinous processes of the

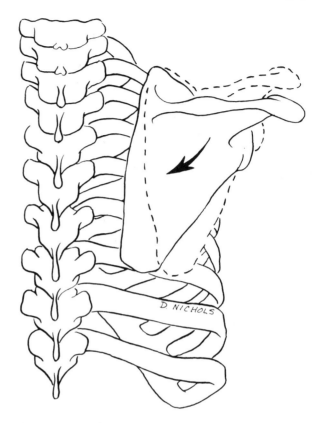

**Fig. 28-12.** Paralysis of the trapezius muscle causes drooping of entire extremity.

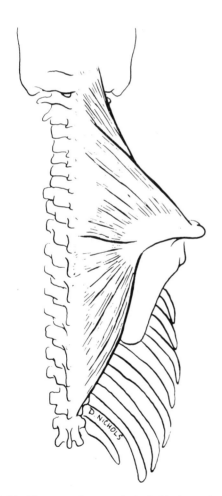

**Fig. 28-11.** The trapezius muscle is divided into three components. The upper portion elevates and rotates the scapula upward. The middle portion adducts the scapula, and the lower portion depresses and rotates the scapula downward.

C7 through the T12 vertebrae. The trapezius is divided into distinct upper, middle, and lower components that work as a unit but with individual functions.[1] The upper portion inserts over the distal one-third of the clavicle and functions to rotate and elevate the scapula upwardly. The middle portion inserts over the acromion and the spine of the scapula and functions to stabilize and adduct the scapula. The lower portion inserts along the base of the scapular spine and downwardly rotates and depresses the scapula. The most important function of the trapezius is to elevate the lateral tip of the scapula. It also abducts the arm and facilitates overhead activities. The spinal accessory nerve is the sole motor innervation to the trapezius.[1,20] The nerve lies superficial in subcutaneous tissue on the floor of the posterior cervical triangle, on its course to innervating the trapezius, and is thus vulnerable to injury. Paralysis of the trapezius causes drooping of the entire upper extremity (Fig. 28-12).

Conservative treatment of trapezius paralysis is not that effective, as resistance exercises will not strengthen the adjacent scapular muscles adequately to substitute for the trapezius.[19] These muscles are unable to prevent scapular winging because their medial insertion places them at a biomechanical disadvantage.

Initial operative treatment of a traumatized spinal accessory nerve within 1 year after injury involves lysis of the nerve or nerve repair, or both. However, if this is unsuccessful or if the diagnosis is made more than 1 year after injury, muscle transfers should be performed. Most commonly, the levator scapulae, rhomboideus major, and rhomboideus minor muscles are transferred.[23] Other procedures including scapular suspension, static scapular stabilization, and scapulothoracic fusion have significant disadvantages and are considered only in patients with neuromuscular disorders or as salvage-type procedures.[20,23–29]

In 1985, Bigliani et al[22] reported on a series of 10 patients with trapezius paralysis who underwent operative reconstruction using the Eden-Lange transfers. The Eden-Lange procedure involves transfer of the levator scapulae and rhomboid major and minor to substitute for the complex functions of the three portions of the trapezius. Lateral transfer of each of these muscles to the spine and body of the scapula allows them to stabilize the scapula and correct the laterally displaced and winging posture of the scapula. The levator scapulae substitutes for the upper portion of the trapezius, the rhomboideus minor replaces the middle portion of the trapezius, and the rhomboideus major replaces the middle and lower portions. Seven patients had greater than 2 years of follow-up with five excellent, one satisfactory, and one unsatisfactory results. All patients had improved function and correction of scapular deformity, and six had good pain relief. This series has enlarged to more than 20 patients, and the results continue to be satisfactory. Of importance is that nine patients had a misdiagnosis before evaluation at the author's institution. The most common misdiagnosed lesions included herniated nucleus pulposus and serratus anterior paralysis. In most misdiagnosed cases that had electromyographic studies performed initially, the trapezius was not tested, and thus the trapezius paralysis was missed. This emphasizes the need for a thorough physical examination of the back, neck, and chest, in addition to an electromyographic examination to confirm the diagnosis. Without specific information provided by appropriate electromyography, it is not possible to assess thoroughly which muscles are involved or the extent of their involvement.

The surgical technique involves two incisions with the patient in a lateral, slightly tilted position (Fig. 28-13A). The first incision is made along the medial scapular border. The levator scapulae, rhomboideus minor, and rhomboideus major are detached from the medial scapula border with a thin portion of insertional bone. The infraspinatus is carefully elevated from its fossa on the posterior scapula to allow drill holes to be placed 5 cm lateral to the medial border of the

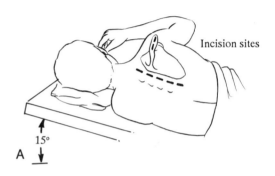

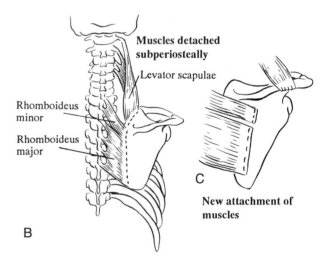

**Fig. 28-13.** **(A)** Patient is placed in the lateral position with the head of the table tilted 15 degrees. Two incisions are used. **(B)** Levator scapulae, rhomboideus minor, and rhomboideus major normally insert along the medial border of the scapula. **(C)** Levator scapulae is transferred to the scapular spine, and the rhomboid muscles are transferred to the body of the scapula.

scapula and 1 cm below the scapular spine. The rhomboideus minor and rhomboideus major are transferred laterally and sutured to the scapula through these drill holes (Fig. 28-13B and C). The scapula should be reduced with the arm abducted 90 degrees. A second incision is made over the spine of the scapula, and a tunnel is created that connects both incisions. The levator scapulae is passed through this tunnel and sutured to the spine of the scapula through the drill holes. Both incisions are then closed in layers.

Postoperatively, an abduction brace is worn for 6 weeks. Passive assistive exercises are performed to maintain forward flexion and external rotation. At 6 weeks, the patient is begun on a strengthening program concentrating on the posterior scapular stabilizers, deltoid, and rotator cuff. Gentle throwing is started at 9 weeks and is progressed as tolerated to full-speed throwing.

## DIFFERENTIAL DIAGNOSIS

Several other shoulder conditions must be considered in the differential diagnosis of scapulothoracic disorders, all of which may present with scapular pain. Referred pain to the scapula may originate from inflammation of the cervical nerve roots. Any pathologic condition, primarily affecting the glenohumeral joint (e.g., arthritis, adhesive capsulitis, rotator cuff tears) or the subacromial space (e.g., impingement syndrome, bursitis) may secondarily cause pain in the periscapular region. After severe injury to the coracoclavicular ligaments, drooping of the shoulder may occur, causing scraping of the scapula against the posterior chest wall, thus irritating sift tissue on the medial border of the scapula. This irritation may induce muscle spasm in the periscapular region, which may potentiate the muscle weakness and sagging posture of the scapula. Shoulder instability, especially posterior recurrent subluxations and dislocations, may present clinically with scapular pain and winging posture of the scapula. Electromyograms, in these cases, are generally negative for any neurologic lesion of the spinal accessory nerve or long thoracic nerve, and careful clinical scrutiny will reveal the instability. Lesions of the suprascapular nerve, which are covered in another chapter, also lead to periscapular symptoms of pain, muscle atrophy, and occasional crepitus.

## REFERENCES

1. Hollinshead WH: Anatomy for Surgeons. Vol. 3. The Back and Limbs. 3rd Ed. Harper and Row, Philadelphia, 1982
2. Kibler WB: Role of the scapula in the overhead throwing motion. Contemp Orthop 22:525, 1991
3. Kibler WB, Shapiro RL, Chandler TJ et al: Posterior Shoulder Muscle Firing Patterns in Tennis Players. AOSSM Interim Meeting, New Orleans, 1990
4. Glousman RE, Jobe FW, Tibone JE et al: Dynamic electromyographic analysis of the throwing shoulder with glenohumeral instability. J Bone Joine Surg 70:220, 1988
5. Boinet M: BWW. Soc Imperalede Chir 8:458, 1867
6. Milch H: Snapping scapula. Clin Orthop 20:139, 1961
7. Bateman JE: The Shoulder and Neck. 2nd Ed. WB Saunders, Philadelphia, 1978
8. Cameron H: Snapping scapulae: a report of three cases. Eur J Rheumatol Inflamm 7:66, 1984
9. Arntz CT, Matsen FA: Partial scapulectomy for disabling scapulothoracic snapping. ASES Annual Meeting, New Orleans, LA, February 1990
10. Richards RR, McKee MD: Treatment of painful scapulothoracic crepitus by resection of the superomedial angle of the scapula: a report of three cases. Clin Orthop 247:111, 1989
11. Von Gruber W: Die bursae mucosa der inneren Achselwand, Arch fuer Anatomie. Physiol Wissenschaftliche Med 358: 1984
12. McCluskey GM, Bigliani LB: Surgical Management of Refractory Scapulothoracic Bursitis. AAOS, 58th Annual Meeting, Anaheim, CA, March 1991
13. Sisto DJ, Jobe FW: The operative treatment of scapulothoracic bursitis in professional pitchers. Am J Sports Med 14:192, 1986
14. Leffart RD: Neurological problems. p. 768. In Rockwood CA, Matsen FA eds: The Shoulder. Vol. 2. 1st Ed. WB Saunders, Philadelphia, 1990
15. Horowitz MT, Tocantins LM: An anatomic study of the role of the long thoracic nerve and the related scapular bursae in the pathogenesis of local paralysis in the serratus anterior muscle. Anat Rec 71:375, 1938
16. Chavez JP: Pectoralis minor transplanted for paralysis of the serratus anterior. J Bone Joint Surg 33B:2128, 1985
17. Marmor L, Bechtol CO: Paralysis of the serratus anterior due to electric shock relieved by transplantation of the pectoralis major muscle. A case report. J Bone Joint Surg 45A:156, 1983
18. Dunn AW: Trapezius paralysis after minor surgical procedures in the posterior cervical triangle. South Med J 67:312, 1974

19. Sunderland S: Nerves and Nerve Injuries. 2nd Ed. Churchill Livingstone, Edinburgh, 1978

20. Wright PE, Simmons JCH: Peripheral nerve injuries. p. 1642. In Edmonston AS, Crenshaw AH (eds): Campbell's Operative Orthopaedics. Vol. 2. 6th Ed. CV Mosby, St. Louis, 1980

21. Woodhall B: Trapezius paralysis following minor surgical procedures in the posterior surgical triangle. Ann Surg 136:375, 1952

22. Bigliani LU, Perez-Sanz JR, Wolfe IN: Treatment of trapezius paralysis. J Bone Joint Surg 67A:871, 1985

23. Henry AK: An operation for slinging a dropped shoulder. Br J Surg 15:95, 1927

24. Whitman A: Congenital elevation of scapula and paralysis of serratus magnus muscle. JAMA 99:1332, 1932

25. Ketenjiaw AY: Scapulocostal stabilization for scapular winging in fascioscapulohumeral muscular dystrophy. J Bone Joint Surg 60A:476, 1978

26. Dewar FP, Harris RI: Restoration and function of the shoulder following paralysis of the trapezius by fascial sling fixation and transplantation of the levator scapulae. Ann Surg 132:1111, 1950

27. Lange M: Die Behandlung der irreparablem Trapeziuslaehmung. Langebecks Arch Klin Chir 270:437, 1951

28. Lange M: Die Operative Behandlung der irreparablem Trapeziuslaehmung. TIP Fakuelt Mecmuasi 22:137, 1959

29. Foo CL, Swann M: Isolated paralysis of the serratus anterior. A report of 20 cases. J Bone Joint Surg 65B:552, 1983

# 29

# Total Shoulder Arthroplasty

*FRED J. McGLYNN*

Total hip and total knee replacements are commonly performed for primary and secondary arthritis, avascular necrosis, and rheumatoid arthritis of the hip and knee. Hungerford stated that total hip replacement may be the "single most predictable surgery of the century." (American Academy of Orthopaedic Surgeons meeting, San Francisco, 1993) The successful results (greater than 95 percent) have made arthrodesis, osteotomy, resection, and debridement less acceptable treatment methods for severe joint afflictions. Joint implant innovations have made arthroplasty more predictable and have expanded indications to include younger, more active individuals. Some of the main improvements include

1. Better materials (metals, plastics, ceramics)
2. Precise instrumentation systems
3. Modularity of components
4. Application of biologic ingrowth
5. Improvements in cement fixation techniques

The evolution of hip and knee arthroplasty has directly affected the advances seen in total shoulder replacement (Fig. 29-1). The factors that make total shoulder arthroplasty different are

1. Goals and results depend on specific disease states
2. Total shoulder replacement depends on the integrity of the soft tissues for stability, strength, and ultimate function
3. Optimal function requires coordinated involvement of the patient, surgeon, and physical therapist in the rehabilitation process

This chapter gives an overview and hopefully promotes better understanding of the most challenging and least forgiving of joint arthroplasties—total shoulder replacement.

## HISTORICAL BACKGROUND

The first total shoulder replacement is credited to French surgeon Péan.[1] In 1893, he inserted a platinum shaft attached to a rubber ball to replace a glenohumeral joint that had been destroyed by tuberculous arthritis (Fig. 29-2). It functioned for approximately 2 years until overwhelming infection ensued. This was one of the first arthroplasties to be attempted in any joint in the human body.

The modern era of total shoulder replacement began in the 1950s. Charles Neer is credited with stimulating and advancing interest in total shoulder replacement.[2-13] His early experience was with proximal humeral prosthetic replacement (hemiarthroplasty) for complex fractures. In the early 1970s, Neer developed a polyethylene glenoid and expanded the indications for arthroplasty to include patients with rheumatoid arthritis, old trauma, and primary and secondary osteoarthritis. In 1972, he developed design criteria for successful total shoulder replacement:

1. Anatomic shape for maximum range of motion
2. Minimum bone removal at insertion
3. Avoidance of mechanical locking
4. Repair and rehabilitation of soft tissues

Neer stressed the importance of monitored rehabilitation, and he kept his patients in the hospital for many weeks. There have been modifications and improvements in the surgical technique, implants, and rehabilitation programs, but little has changed from the basic concepts espoused in the Neer system.

317

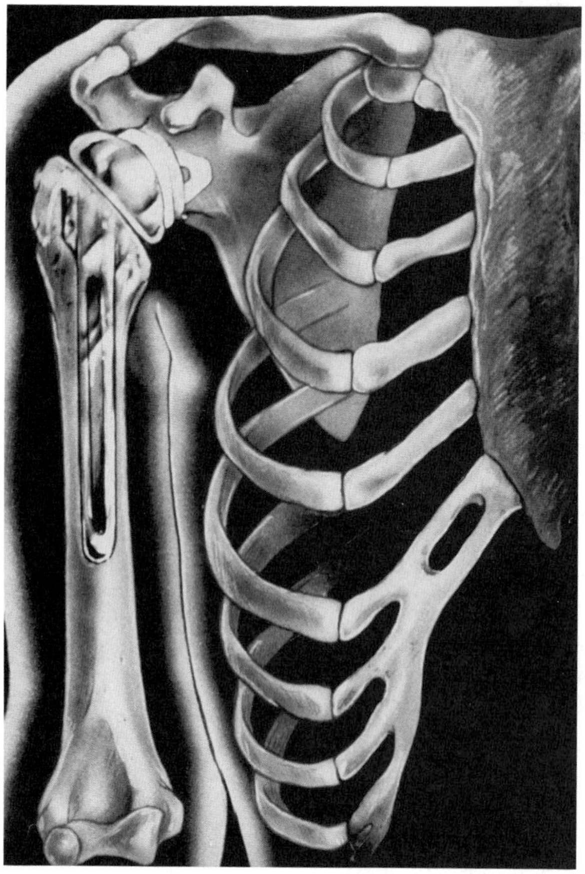

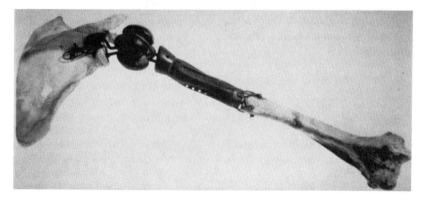

**Fig. 29-1.** Unconstrained total shoulder replacement.

## FUNCTIONAL ANATOMY

The glenohumeral articulation is the most mobile joint in the body. There is minimal static (bony) stability. The humeral head articulates with the glenoid very much like a "golf ball sits on a tee" (Fig. 29-3). The soft tissues play an integral role in the stability and strength of the shoulder. The rotator cuff muscles are the subscapularis, supraspinatus, infraspinatus, and teres minor. They serve at least three main functions:

1. Dynamic stability of the humeral head within the glenoid fossa
2. Compressive force of the humeral head within the glenoid fossa to work in concert with function of the deltoid
3. Rotation of the humeral head

The supraspinatus and long head of the biceps are important depressors of the humeral head. If there is deficiency of the rotator cuff, superior migration, pain, and subsequent atrophy and stiffness become clinically apparent (Fig. 29-4). An intact rotator cuff, or the ability to reconstruct a functioning rotator cuff, is thus extremely important with respect to the final functional result of the total shoulder replacement.

Inferiorly, there is a redundancy of the glenohumeral joint capsule. This must be present to allow for overhead activity and the necessary concomitant

**Fig. 29-2.** Original prosthesis inserted by Jules Emile Péan. (Courtesy of The National Museum of American History, Smithsonian Institute.)

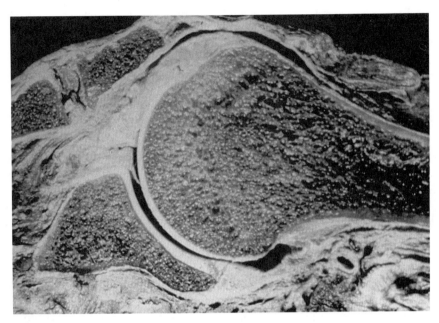

**Fig. 29-3.** Anatomic cross section showing shallow glenoid and limited bony contact between humeral head and glenoid.

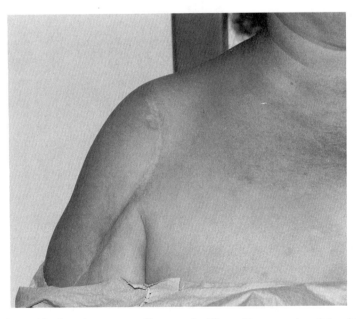

**Fig. 29-4.** Patient with chronic rotator cuff tear and stiffness. Note atrophy of shoulder muscles.

external rotation. With the hand overhead, the inferior glenohumeral ligament prevents anterior translation of the humeral head. The coracoacromial arch is made up of the acromion, coracoacromial ligament, and acromioclavicular joint. The rotator cuff must have adequate clearance under this roof or symptoms of impingement will occur. Anterior acromioplasty, excision of the coracoacromial ligament, and partial excision of the acromioclavicular joint are commonly performed in total shoulder replacement to avoid impingement.

Scapulothoracic motion plays an important role in normal shoulder function. Approximately 60 degrees of motion usually occur between the scapula and the thorax. Maintaining full excursion of the scapula increases total range of motion, increases stability of the shoulder joint, prevents impingement, and allows better mechanical advantage of the deltoid muscle.

Finally, approximately 20 degrees of external rotation are needed for full overhead motion. Without external rotation, the greater tuberosity of the humerus abuts against the acromion, limiting full flexion and causing discomfort due to impingement.

When considering total shoulder replacement, soft tissue involvement is critical in operative planning and postoperative rehabilitation.

## PROSTHETIC DESIGN

Prostheses are classified into constrained (ball-and-socket), semiconstrained (hooded), and nonconstrained (anatomic) devices (Fig. 29-5). The constrained prosthesis has a linked ball-and-socket joint that allows rotation but prevents translation. The constrained prosthesis is rarely used because of the high failure rate caused by increased stresses at the bone cement interface.[14–22] A constrained-type prosthesis may rarely be indicated in tumor resection surgery.

A semiconstrained prosthesis provides added stability by adding a superior hood to the glenoid component.[13,14] In deficient rotator cuff situations, the hood helps to prevent superior migration of the humeral prosthesis.

The most commonly used prosthesis is the nonconstrained variety (Fig. 29-6). The prosthesis has similar

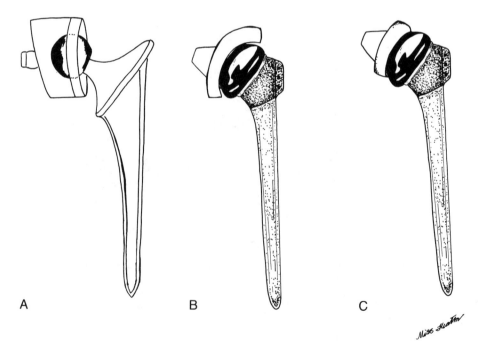

**Fig. 29-5.** Total shoulder replacement has a variable amount of built-in constraint dependent on the particular design. Components may be **(A)** constrained, **(B)** semiconstrained, or **(C)** nonconstrained.

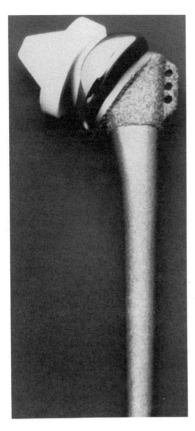

**Fig. 29-6.** Nonconstrained prosthesis with similar radius of curvature of humeral and glenoid components allowing full range of motion. (Courtesy of Biomet.)

geometry to the anatomic humeral head and glenoid. The humeral head component is usually made from cobalt chrome or titanium and has a rough proximal surface to allow biologic ingrowth or better interlock with cement. The stems have different lengths and widths to allow better filling of the humeral shaft, and proximally there are holes to help anchor the greater and lesser tuberosities in complex fracture situations (Fig. 29-7). The humeral heads are modular. They come in different sizes and widths and can be interchanged on the fixed humeral stem (Fig. 29-8). This allows "fine tuning" of the rotator cuff to allow optimum range of motion and stability.

The glenoid component is made of polyethylene and also comes in different sizes. The glenoid component comes with the option of metal backing (Fig. 29-9), which has the theoretic advantages of better distribu-

tion of stresses, improved fixation, and decreased polyethylene deformation.

The humeral and glenoid components have a matched radius of curvature (Fig. 29-10). Because little restraint is built into the prosthesis, the soft tissue complex (capsule, rotator cuff, and deltoid) must be reconstructed and rehabilitated to provide stability and achieve maximum function.

## PATIENT SELECTION AND SPECIFIC PATHOLOGIC ENTITIES

Pain, loss of function, and destruction of the glenohumeral joint cartilage can occur from many diseases. Osteoarthritis, rheumatoid arthritis, and arthritis associated with past trauma account for most patients indicated for total shoulder replacement. Avascular necrosis, rotator cuff arthropathy, and previous failed surgery account for a small percentage of patients undergoing total shoulder replacement. It is useful to understand the characteristics of these diseases to better comprehend the selection of a prosthesis and the surgical nuances in reconstructing the rotator cuff. The status of the rotator cuff will be the prime determinant in passive and active range of motion allowed in the immediate postoperative period.

### Osteoarthritis

Patients with osteoarthritis usually have an enlarged and deformed humeral head. The glenoid is flattened and often eroded (deficient) posteriorly. Inferior osteophytes are often prominent (Fig. 29-11). The rotator cuff is usually intact (95 percent). The subscapularis is sometimes contracted, limiting external rotation, and needs to be lengthened at surgery approximately 10 to 15 percent of the time. Concomitant acromioclavicular joint arthritis is often present, and excision of the distal clavicle may be performed at surgery.

In summary, with regard to postoperative rehabilitation, the rotator cuff must be appropriately strengthened, and the communication between physical therapist and surgeon is mandatory to determine the appropriate amount of external rotation depending on whether the subscapularis was lengthened and the amount of external rotation noted at the time of surgery.

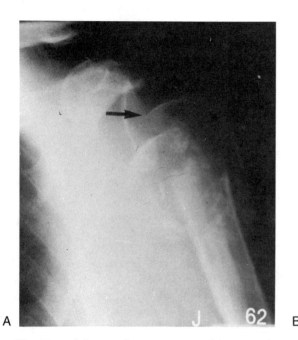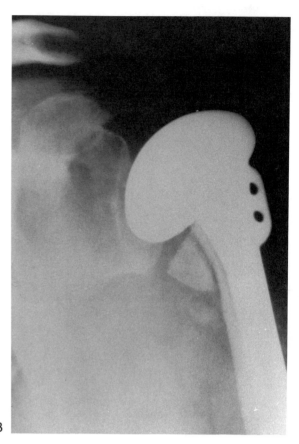

**Fig. 29-7.** **(A)** Acute four-part proximal humerus fracture; **(B)** hemiarthroplasty for immediate management of four-part fracture.

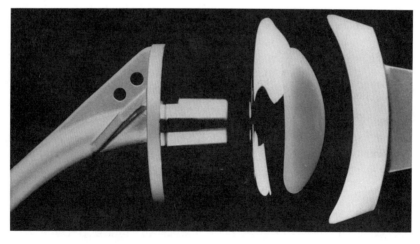

**Fig. 29-8.** Modular humeral component. (Courtesy of Zimmer.)

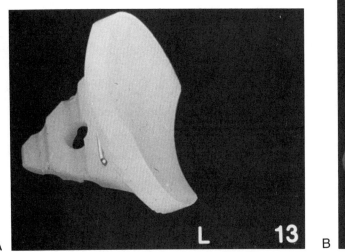

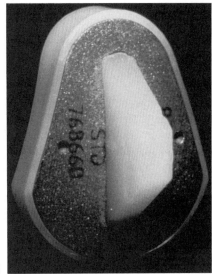

**Fig. 29-9.** **(A)** Polyethylene glenoid component. (Courtesy of 3M.) **(B)** metal-backed polyethylene glenoid component. (Courtesy of Biomet.)

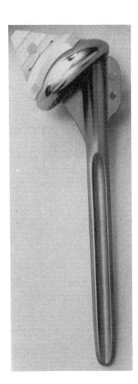

**Fig. 29-10.** Neer II prosthesis. (Courtesy of 3M.)

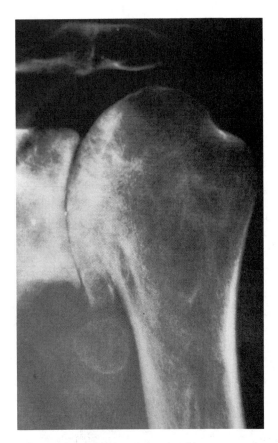

**Fig. 29-11.** Osteoarthritis of the shoulder. Note enlarged, flattened, and deformed humeral head and osteoarthritis of acromioclavicular joint.

## Rheumatoid Arthritis

All tissues, including the rotator cuff, are involved in rheumatoid arthritis. The rotator cuff is often deficient or torn (40 to 50 percent), and rotator cuff involvement often parallels the extent of joint destruction. The bone is soft (osteopenic) with erosion and cysts, and marked resorption is sometimes present (Fig. 29-12). Rarely, severe glenoid bone loss in the rheumatoid patient may preclude use of a glenoid component, and a humeral head component with rotator cuff reconstruction around the implant may be considered in these patients. The physical therapist must be aware of the status of the reconstructed rotator cuff and often needs to delay active range of motion against gravity, which would unduly stress the repaired tissue for up to 6 to 8 weeks.

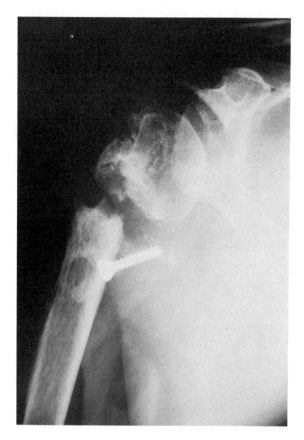

**Fig. 29-13.** Traumatic arthritis with nonunion, deformity, and scarring.

## Post-traumatic Degenerative Disease

Operations performed after old trauma are especially difficult, and peculiar situations are encountered that result in higher complication rates and special rehabilitation concerns. Several factors are responsible, including scarring of the rotator cuff and capsule from previous surgery and bony deformity or erosion from trauma (Fig. 29-13). Associated nerve deficits, muscle contractures, and atrophy are usually present. Capsular releases, tendon lengthening, rotator cuff reconstruction, and bone grafting may make rehabilitation a unique challenge.

## Avascular Necrosis

The results of total shoulder replacement in patients with significant deformity and persistent severe pain

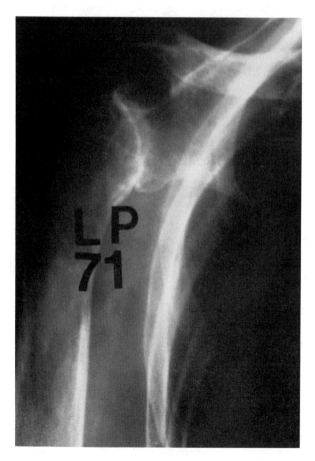

**Fig. 29-12.** Rheumatoid arthritis of the shoulder.

from avascular necrosis are particularly gratifying. This is because the pathology usually involves only the humeral head (Fig. 29-14). The rotator cuff and capsule are usually intact, with a normal amount of excursion. The glenoid is usually spared unless long-standing osteonecrosis has been present. Hemiarthroplasty (replacement of the humeral head) is usually the treatment of choice (Fig. 29-15). Immediate passive range of motion can proceed quickly, and active exercises against gravity may begin 2 to 4 days postoperatively.

## Rotator Cuff Tear Arthropathy

Rotator cuff tear arthropathy is defined as severe rotator cuff deficiency with associated shoulder arthritis. These patients fit into a "limited goals" category for rehabilitation. The massive rotator cuff tearing limits the reconstruction of the soft tissues and therefore limits total shoulder replacement. Resurfacing of the joint gives predictably good pain relief, and the focus of therapy should be on obtaining improved rotation and limited (80 to 90 degrees) forward flexion.

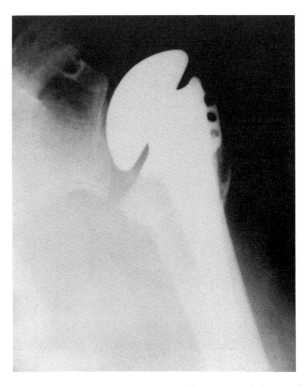

**Fig. 29-15.** Hemiarthroplasty (replacement of humeral head to articulate with nonreplaced glenoid hyaline cartilage).

## SURGICAL TECHNIQUE

The patient's head is stabilized on a special neurosurgical head rest, and the endotracheal tube is protected. The patient is placed in a beach chair (semireclined) position with the affected arm on an armboard. A pad is placed behind the scapula, and the entire arm and shoulder girdle are prepared and draped (Fig. 29-16). This allows free motion of the arm and shoulder throughout the procedure.

An incision is made starting just medial to the acromioclavicular joint, passing over the coracoid and continuing in a straight line toward the insertion of the deltoid (Fig. 29-17). The deltopectoral interval is identified, and then blunt dissection is used to retract the deltoid laterally. The cephalic vein and pectoralis muscle are retracted medially. This exposure allows retraction of the deltoid without removing the clavicular

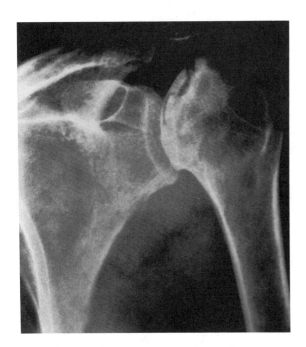

**Fig. 29-14.** Avascular necrosis associated with steroid use.

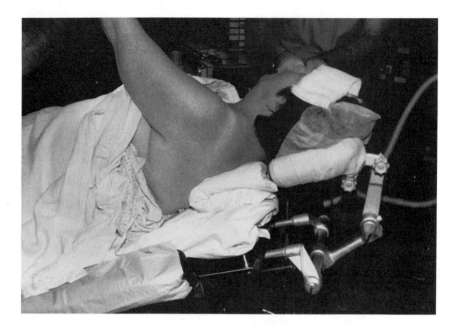

**Fig. 29-16.** Preparation for total shoulder arthroplasty.

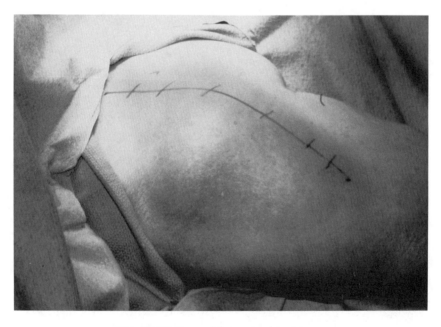

**Fig. 29-17.** Long deltopectoral incision.

attachment and expedites postoperative recovery because flexion and extension can begin without fear of pulling off the repaired anterior deltoid from the clavicle.

The subdeltoid bursa is bluntly exposed, and the coracoacromial ligament is excised. An anterior acromioplasty is performed removing the anteroinferior one-third of the acromion. Palpation of the acromioclavicular joint determines whether excision of the distal clavicle is warranted.

The rotator cuff is then carefully inspected. If the rotator cuff is intact (i.e., osteoarthritis, avascular necrosis), the amount of external rotation is noted. If greater than 20 degrees of external rotation is present, the subscapularis is vertically divided 1 to 2 cm medial to the tendinous insertion on the lesser tuberosity (Fig. 29-18). If there is an internal rotation contracture, as in osteoarthritis, the subscapularis is lengthened by performing a Z-plasty.

The arm is extended and externally rotated, exposing the proximal humerus (Fig. 29-19). The osteophytes are removed, and a small (10 to 12 mm) amount of humeral head is excised. The humerus is resected so that the humeral component is placed in

the normal amount of retroversion (30 to 45 degrees). The humeral canal is opened with a hand awl, and then rasps corresponding to the diameters of the different humeral components are used. The humeral component trial is then placed, and appropriate depth of insertion of the prosthesis into the shaft of the humerus is noted relative to the glenoid and the greater tuberosity. Trial reduction is accomplished, and soft tissues are carefully assessed. Modular heads allow "finetuning" of the rotator cuff tension by increasing or decreasing the size and width of the head to obtain optimum stability and range of motion. The trail component is removed, and the glenoid is exposed.

There is a trend toward not replacing the glenoid if normal articular cartilage is present, as is often seen in early avascular necrosis and osteoarthritis or acute fractures. If eburnated bone, cysts, or bony deformity are noted, the glenoid is carefully exposed with retractors. A burr is used to remove any remaining cartilage, and a keel slot is made into the neck of the scapula to allow complete seating of the glenoid component. The glenoid vault is then thoroughly irrigated with pulsatile lavage, and methyl methacrylate is placed in the slot and along the surface of the glenoid. The glenoid com-

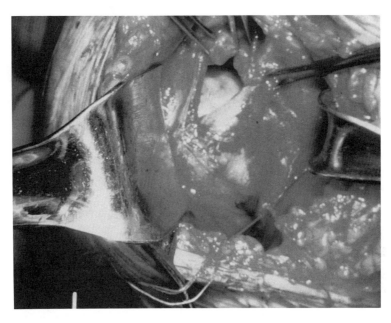

**Fig. 29-18.** Subscapularis is divided for entry into the joint. In most cases, subscapularis is the only tendon divided during the procedure.

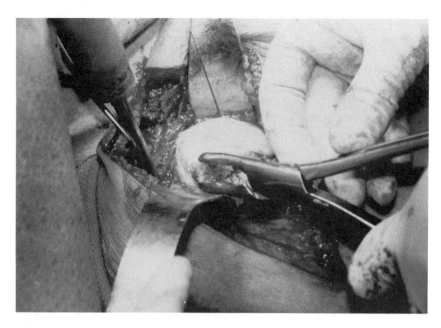

**Fig. 29-19.** Humeral head is exposed while protecting surrounding rotator cuff.

ponent is then cemented in place. The humeral component can then be either press-fitted or cemented in place. Once the humeral stem is in place, the modular heads are again used to determine appropriate size for motion and stability (Fig. 29-20). If the prosthesis is acceptable, the subscapularis is repaired and external

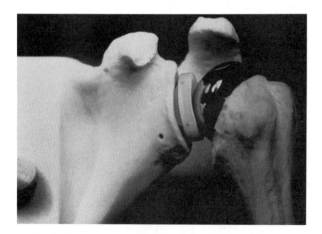

**Fig. 29-20.** Trial components in place. "Fine-tuning" of stability accomplished with interchangeable modular humeral heads.

rotation is assessed and *documented*. A Hemovac drain is placed deep to the deltopectoral fascia, and then the fascia is loosely closed. The subcutaneous tissue is approximated and the skin closed with staples or preferably by subcuticular stitches. A dressing and shoulder immobilizer are applied and an abdominal bandage dressing with baby powder is placed in the axilla.

The postoperative note should carefully document the amount of external rotation that could be obtained intraoperatively without stress on the closure. Also, the status of the rotator cuff and whether any special protection for the repaired rotator cuff or anterior deltoid if required should be documented and communicated to the physical therapist.

## POSTOPERATIVE REHABILITATION

A brief review from a surgeon's perspective of the critical aspects of postoperative rehabilitation is outlined in Table 29-1. The surgeon, patient, and physical therapist must be a coordinated team in communicating and giving feedback to each other to gain optimum success. The surgeon must document reconstruction

**Table 29-1. Postoperative Total Shoulder Rehabilitation**

| Postoperative Period | Exercises | Function |
| --- | --- | --- |
| Day 1 | Pendulum exercises<br>Isometric exercises<br>  Hand<br>  Wrist<br>  Elbow | Sling × 24 h after surgery<br>Ambulate with assistance |
| Day 2 | Gravity-assisted free-swing<br>  exercises<br>Active assisted forward flexion<br>Assisted external rotation[a] | Remove drains, intravenous lines<br>Change dressing to Bandaid<br>Independent ambulation and<br>  transfer<br>Sling while asleep |
| Days 3 to 10 | Supine to sitting exercises<br>Active assisted forward flexion,<br>  internal rotation, external<br>  rotation[a]<br>Pulley exercises<br>Active exercises[b] | No sling during awake hours<br>Sling at night and for naps<br><br><br>Independent transfer<br>Occupational therapy–activities<br>  of daily living training<br>Active patient participation<br>Discharge home |
| Discharge home to 6 wk | Continue above | Continue outpatient physical<br>  therapy<br>Sling at night |
| 6 Wk to 3 mo | Strengthening exercises<br>  Rotator cuff and deltoid<br>Stretching—pulley, etc. | Discontinue sling<br>Accomplish normal activities of<br>  daily living<br>Monitor progress |

[a] External rotation by status of subscapularis repair noted at time of surgery.
[b] Forward flexion and external rotation delayed 6 wk with rotator cuff repair or if deltoid taken off clavicle.

of the soft tissues to guide the therapist in limiting the postoperative arcs of motion. The therapist must be aware of any deviations from the normal postoperative progression, such as changes in pain, range of motion, or expected strength. The patient must understand his or her expected active role in the rehabilitation process. This is true both in the immediate supervised hospital setting and over the long term at home and in an outpatient monitored physical therapy program.

The patient usually remains in the hospital about 1 week (5 to 10 days). The physical therapist should be very familiar with the specific needs of the patient and the limitations described by the operating surgeon. Even though the hospitalization is quite brief, the initial phase of mobilization and education is key for a smooth postoperative transition to the home setting.

The patient is placed in a sling or shoulder immobilizer with a pillow placed behind the ipsilateral elbow. On the first postoperative day, the patient is educated in range of motion and isometric exercises for the nonoperated joints—elbow, wrist, and hand. On the

second postoperative day, the bulky dressing, drains, and intravenous lines are removed, making ambulation easier. The patient is usually more comfortable with beginning pendulum and gravity assisted free-swing exercises. Active assisted forward flexion can begin on the second postoperative day. Also on the second day, active assisted external rotation is begun, limited by the intraoperative range determined after closure of the subscapularis tendon. The patient is gradually taught to do active assisted forward flexion and external rotation exercises using the opposite hand, first in the supine position and then against gravity. If the anterior deltoid has not been taken off the clavicle, active exercises can begin immediately. Pulleys are added on the third or fourth postoperative day to help with passive range of motion and to encourage patient involvement. Patient participation and cooperation is vital.

The patient is usually transferred from the hospital to a home monitored outpatient physical therapy program when forward flexion approaches 100 to 120 degrees and external rotation reaches 10 to 20 degrees.

At discharge, the patient should understand the early rehabilitation goals:

1. Prevent adhesions, regain passive range of motion
2. Protect the repair (rotator cuff)
3. Strengthening through active exercises of the non-repaired rotator cuff and deltoid

As a general rule, patients with osteoarthritis and avascular necrosis can progress with a vigorous early active range of motion program. Those patients with old trauma, rheumatoid arthritis, and cuff arthropathy have to focus on a passive range of motion program and delay active range of motion for 6 to 8 weeks, depending on the status of the reconstructed rotator cuff.

Most patients may wear a sling during the day but should wear a shoulder immobilizer at night for protection and comfort. If available, the patient's spouse, companion, or relative should be included in the therapy program to act as a motivator and supervisor.

A supervised outpatient program should continue at least biweekly with advancement of active and passive range of motion and monitoring progress. The physician should be alerted to any setbacks in recovery. Patients are encouraged to perform a home therapy program on their own at least three times per day. Patients are given goals to strive toward, such as 130 degrees of forward flexion and 20 degrees of external rotation by 4 weeks.

At 4 to 6 weeks, gentle stretching in all planes and active range of motion begins. Progressive resistance, working on both external rotation and internal rotation, is begun approximately 2 to 3 months postoperatively. Surgical tubing and light weights (soup cans, etc.) are added. Patients must understand that the rehabilitation process is a continuous one and that there cannot be any absences from the daily program. The patient should be informed that motion, strength, and function will improve well after 1 year and that patience and persistence are important virtues. Because each patient's motivation and pain threshold is different, the degree of supervision and coaxing varies. The patient should be given positive reinforcement for efforts and gains. Steady improvements with decreased discomfort should be the rule.

Continuous passive range of motion machines may be an adjunct in the early phases of total shoulder

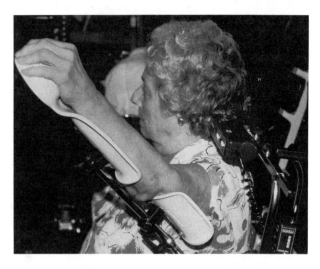

**Fig. 29-21.** Continuous passive motion machine (sitting position).

replacement rehabilitation (Fig. 29-21). Craig[23] noted earlier range of motion, earlier discharge from the hospital, and less need for postoperative narcotics. Our experience has been positive, but careful monitoring in the hospital or at home must be performed by the physical therapist or physician.

In summary, the rehabilitation program must be suited and adapted to the particular patient and to his or her distinct disease entity. Total shoulder replacement rehabilitation does not fit into a "cookbook" approach, but the above guidelines should help in the timing of the range of motion and strengthening activities for each patient.

## RESULTS

As expected, the results of total shoulder replacement are dependent on the underlying disease entity. In particular, with those diseases in which the rotator cuff is usually intact (osteoarthritis, avascular necrosis), pain relief and range of motion are excellent. Nearly all series report that greater than 90 percent of patients are pain-free, and range of motion approaches normal.[3,6,10,24–27]

Those diseases that usually require rotator cuff reconstruction (rheumatoid arthritis, old trauma) achieve pain relief greater than 80 percent of the time, but gains in range of motion are more modest.[5,28–40] Range of motion in these patients varies among series but seems to be in the range of one-half to three-quarters normal arc of motion.

Neer et al[11,13] suggested that a separate class of patients should be regarded as a "limited goals" category. These cuff tear arthropathy patients have massive rotator cuff defects for which reconstruction is impossible. These patients have "satisfactory" results greater than 90 percent of the time, meaning good pain relief but forward elevation of only about 90 degrees.

Therefore, as a rule, patients having total shoulder replacement achieve satisfactory pain relief predictably (greater than 90 percent of the time), but the amount of motion regained is variable and is dependent on diagnostic category.

The early results with constrained prostheses were poor.[41–45] Revision surgery was required in 40 to 50 percent of the cases because of loosening. The indication for a constrained prosthesis is extremely rare (i.e., tumor).

Biologic ingrowth in total shoulder replacement may be appropriate in the younger, more active individual. Clinical results on the humeral side have been good. Glenoid fixation is more difficult, and clinical enthusiasm is more guarded (perhaps because of the problem in obtaining bony ingrowth into the tibia seen in total knee replacement). "Hybrid" implantation—biologic ingrowth humerus and cemented glenoid—seems to be the most common fixation choice of shoulder surgeons. Patients with osteopenic bone (rheumatoid arthritis) should have cement fixation of both humeral and glenoid components. In acute fractures, bony stability of the proximal humerus is usually compromised, and cement is required in most cases.

## COMPLICATIONS

The complications for total shoulder replacement are listed in Table 29-2. Patients who have scar tissue from previous surgery or old trauma have the highest rate of complications. Overall, the complication rate is less than 5 percent when reviewing all major series using the nonconstrained (Neer-type) total shoulder replacement.

**Table 29-2. Complications of Total Shoulder Replacement**

| Complication | Incidence (%) |
|---|---|
| Rotator cuff tear | 3–5 |
| Impingement | 1–2 |
| Infection | <1 |
| Nerve injury | |
| Primary | <1 |
| Revision | 5–6 |
| Intraoperative fracture | 1–2 |
| Postoperative instability | 2–3 |
| Loosening | |
| Glenoid | 2–3 |
| Humerus | <1 |

The most common complication after total shoulder replacement is with the rotator cuff.[10,33,46–49] Subsequent rotator cuff tears (about 10 percent in rheumatoid arthritis) or impingement problems (2 percent) may develop. Therefore, if there is a noticeable loss of strength associated with increasing pain 3 to 4 or more months after surgery, the physical therapist should alert the surgeon of the condition.

Infection is uncommon (less than 1 percent). Nerve injuries are rare (less than .1 percent) except in old trauma cases (5 percent). Temporary paresthesias or numbness do occur, but fortunately they typically resolve. Fractures, intraoperatively or with vigorous postoperative activities, sometimes occur in patients with rheumatoid arthritis who have marked osteopenia (1 percent). Instability used to be a concern in total shoulder replacement. With the newer prosthetic systems, the modular heads allow the soft tissues to be "fine-tuned," and instability should be a rare concern.

A major concern is glenoid loosening.[46,48–52] To date this has been more of a theoretic and radiographic concern than a clinical problem. Radiographic radiolucent lines about the glenoid component are seen in one-third to two-thirds of the patients in most series. This x-ray finding is bothersome, but rarely has revision surgery been indicated. Only longer follow-ups will give us the survival data in total shoulder replacement. The new metal-backed glenoid component has been developed theoretically to distribute stress to the glenoid more evenly.

## SUMMARY

Total shoulder arthroplasty has been successful in relieving pain and improving function and quality of life for many patients with disabling shoulder problems (Fig. 29-22). When used in the acute complex fracture situation, management is greatly simplified. For disabling glenohumeral arthritis, pain relief is predictable, and expected improvement in arcs of motion is dependent on the specific disease entity. With meticulous attention to patient selection, proper surgical technique, and postoperative rehabilitation, end results can be maximized. Soft tissue repair, balance, and proper postoperative protection (with appropriate progression in passive and active range of motion) are the limiting factors in predicting return to full activity.

Rehabilitation after shoulder arthroplasty is critical for optimum success. Unless the motion obtained in surgery is maintained in the early postoperative period, adhesions, stiffness, and subsequent atrophy will occur. Early motion should focus on elevation of the scapula, internal rotation, external rotation, and forward flexion. The specific type, speed, and extent of postoperative exercises must be adapted to the individual patient and his or her specific disease process. The goals and aims of the patient must be in line with the environment of the repaired rotator cuff. The rehabilitation of each patient should be individualized according to the quality of bone and soft tissue, as well as specific needs and desires of the patient.

Refinements in implant design, modifications in surgical technique dependent on the disease process, bet-

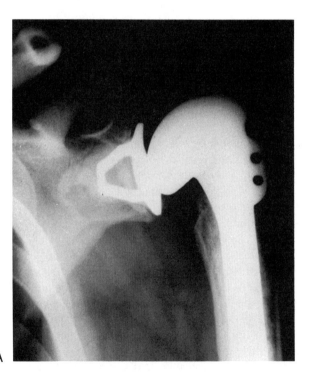
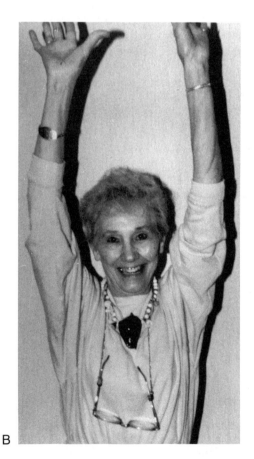

**Fig. 29-22. (A)** Radiograph of total shoulder arthroplasty of patient shown in B; **(B)** rheumatoid patient with total shoulder replacement.

ter patient selection, and recognition of the critical nature of short-term and long-term rehabilitation have made total shoulder replacement results predictable. Total shoulder replacement has taken its place as being on the same plane as total hip replacement and total knee replacement in relieving pain and improving quality of function.

# REFERENCES

1. Lugli T: Artificial shoulder joint by Péan (1893). The facts of an exceptional intervention and the prosthetic method. Clin Orthop 133:215, 1978

2. Neer CS, Brown TH Jr, McLaughlin HL: Fracture of the neck of the humerus with dislocation of the head fragment. Am J Surg 85:252, 1953

3. Neer CS II: Articular replacement for the humeral head. J Bone Joint Surg 37A:215, 1955

4. Neer CS II: Follow-up notes on articles previously published in the journal. Articular replacement for the humeral head. J Bone Joint Surg 46A:1607, 1964

5. Neer CS II: The rheumatoid shoulder. p. 117. In Cruess RR, Mitchell NS (eds): Surgery of Rheumatoid Arthritis. JB Lippincott, Philadelphia, 1971

6. Neer CS II: Replacement arthroplasty for glenohumeral osteoarthritis. J Bone Joint Surg 56A:1, 1974

7. Neer CS II: Reconstructive surgery and rehabilitation of the shoulder. p. 1944. In Kelley WN, Harris ED Jr, Ruddy S, Sledge CS (eds): Textbook of Rheumatology. WB Saunders, Philadelphia, 1981

8. Neer CS II: Surgical Protocol. Neer II Proximal Humerus. Arthroplasty of the Shoulder: Neer Technique. Minnesota Mining and Manufacturing Company, St Paul, MN, 1982

9. Neer CS II, Kirby RM: Revision of the humeral head and total shoulder arthroplasties. Clin Orthop 170:189, 1982

10. Neer CS II, Watson KC, Stanton FJ: Recent experience in total shoulder replacement. J Bone Joint Surg 64A:319, 1982

11. Neer CS II, Craig EV, Fukuda H: Cuff-tear arthropathy. J Bone Joint Surg 65A: 1232, 1983

12. Neer CS II, McCann PD, Macfarlane EA, Padilla N: Earlier passive motion following shoulder arthroplasty and rotator cuff repair. A prospective study. Orthop Trans 2:231, 1987

13. Neer CS, Morrison DS: Glenoid bone-grafting in total shoulder arthroplasty. J Bone Joint Surg 70A:1154, 1988

14. Coughlin MJ, Morris JM, West WF: The semiconstrained total shoulder arthroplasty. J Bone Joint Surg 61A:574, 1979

15. Engelbrecht E, Stelbrink G: Totale Schulterendoprosthese Modell "St. Georg." Chirurg 47:525, 1976

16. Fenlin JM Jr: Total glenohumeral joint replacement. Orthop Clin North Am 6:565, 1975

17. Gristina AG, Webb LX: The monospherical shoulder prosthesis (abstr). Orthop Trans 8:88, 1984

18. Gristina AG, Forte MR, Rovere GD et al: The trispherical total shoulder prosthesis—biomechanical, anatomical, and surgical considerations. Trans Orthop Res Soc 3:302, 1978

19. Kessel L, Bayley I: The Kessel total shoulder replacement. In Bayley I, Kessel L (eds): Shoulder Surgery. Springer-Verlag, New York, 1982

20. Kölbel R, Rohlmann A, Bergmann G et al: Schultergelenkersatz nach Kolbel-Friedebold. Aktuel Probl Chir Orthop 1:50, 1977

21. Kölbel R, Friedebold G: Schultergelenkersatz. Z Orthop 113:452, 1975

22. Lettin AWF, Copeland SA, Scales JT: The Stanmore shoulder replacement. J Bone Joint Surg 64B:47, 1982

23. Craig EV: Continuous passive motion in the rehabilitation of the surgically reconstructed shoulder. A preliminary report. Orthop Trans 10:233, 1986

24. Cruess RL: Steroid-induced avascular necrosis of the head of the humerus. J Bone Joint Surg 58B:313, 1976

25. Cruess RL: Corticosteroid-induced osteonecrosis of the humeral head. Orthop Clin North Am 16:789, 1985

26. Rutherford CS, Cofield RH: Osteonecrosis of the shoulder. Orthop Trans 11:239, 1987

27. Zuckerman JD, Cofield RH: Proximal humeral prosthetic replacement in glenohumeral arthritis. Orthop Trans 10:231, 1986

28. Barrett WP, Thornhill TS, Thomas WH et al: Nonconstrained total shoulder arthroplasty in patients with polyarticular rheumatoid arthritis. J Arthroplasty 4:91, 1989

29. Brenner BC, Ferlic DC, Clayton ML, Dennis DA: Survivorship of unconstrained total shoulder arthroplasty. J Bone Joint Surg 71A:1289, 1989

30. Hawkins RJ, Bell RH, Jallay B: Total shoulder arthroplasty. Clin Orthop 242:188, 1989

31. Hawkins RJ, Neer CS II, Pianta RM, Mendoza FX: Locked posterior dislocation of the shoulder. J Bone Joint Surg 69A:9, 1987

32. Huten D, Duparc J: L'arthroplastic prothétique dans les traumatismes complexes récents et anciens de l'épaule. Rev Chir Orthop 72:517, 1986

33. Kelly IG, Foster RS, Fisher WD: Neer total shoulder replacement in rheumatoid arthritis. J Bone Joint Surg 69B:723, 1987

34. McCoy SR, Warren RF, Bade HA III et al: Total shoulder arthroplasty in rheumatoid arthritis. J Arthroplasty 4:105, 1989

35. Petersson CJ: Painful shoulders in patients with rheumatoid arthritis. Scand J Rheum 15:375, 1986

36. Petersson CJ: Shoulder surgery in rheumatoid arthritis. Acta Orthop Scand 57:222, 1986

37. Pritchett JW, Clark JM: Prosthetic replacement for chronic unreduced dislocations of the shoulder. Clin Orthop 216:89, 1987

38. Rowe CR, Zarins B: Chronic unreduced dislocations of the shoulder. J Bone Joint Surg 64A:494, 1982

39. Tanner MW, Cofield RH: Prosthetic arthroplasty for fractures and fracture-dislocations of the proximal humerus. Clin Orthop 179:116, 1983

40. Vahavanen V, Hamalainen M, Paavolainen P: The Neer II replacement for rheumatoid arthritis of the shoulder. Int Orthop 13:57, 1989

41. Coughlin MJ, Morris JM, West WF: The semiconstrained total shoulder arthroplasty. J Bone Joint Surg 61A:574, 1979

42. Gristina AG, Webb LX: The trispherical total shoulder replacement. p. 153. In Bayley I, Kessel L (eds): Shoulder Surgery. Springer-Verlag, Berlin, 1982

43. Kessel L, Bayley I: The Kessel total shoulder replacement. p. 160. In: Shoulder Surgery. Springer-Verlag, New York, 1982

44. Lettin AWF, Copeland SA, Scales JT: The Stanmore total shoulder replacement. J Bone Joint Surg 64B:47, 1982

45. Post M, Haskell SS, Jablon M: Total shoulder replacement with a constrained prosthesis. J Bone Joint Surg 62A:327, 1980

46. Bade HA III, Warren RF, Ranawat C, Inglis AE: Long term results of Neer total shoulder replacement. p. 294. In Bateman JE, Welsh RP (eds): Surgery of the Shoulder. CV Mosby, St. Louis, 1984

47. Barrett WP, Franklin JL, Jackins SE et al: Total shoulder arthroplasty. J Bone Joint Surg 69A:865, 1987

48. Cofield RH: Total shoulder arthroplasty with the Neer prosthesis. J Bone Joint Surg 66A:899, 1984

49. Wilde AH, Borden LS, Brems JJ: Experience with the Neer total shoulder replacement. p. 224. In Bateman JE, Welsh RP (eds): Surgery of the Shoulder. CV Mosby, St. Louis, 1984

50. Amstutz HC, Sew Hoy AL, Clarke IC: UCLA anatomic total shoulder arthroplasty. Clin Orthop 155:7, 1981

51. Neer CS, Watson KC, Stanton FJ: Recent experience in total shoulder replacement. J Bone Joint Surg 64A:319, 1982

52. Thornhill TS, Karr MJ, Averill RM et al: Total shoulder arthroplasty: the Brigham experience. Orthop Trans 7:497, 1983

# 30

# Current Concepts in the Rehabilitation of Athletic Shoulder Injuries

*KEVIN E. WILK*

In the past several years, there has been an influx of information pertaining to the evaluation and treatment of the shoulder joint complex and, in particular, the athletic shoulder. This increased interest has stemmed from a general population that has become more health conscious and, consequently, more active in weight training and sporting activities. As a result of this increased activity, shoulder injuries now appear more frequently. With the number of these injuries increasing, the members of the basic and clinical science community have begun to focus increased attention on advancing techniques to properly identify and manage injuries of the shoulder complex.

In the past, after shoulder surgery or injury, the active rehabilitation process was frequently delayed for several weeks to allow the patient to become more comfortable and the pain and inflammation to subside. Often, after rotator cuff surgery or open anterior acromioplasty, the postoperative management consisted of 4 to 6 weeks of immobilization, progressing to passive range of motion and finally active motion at approximately 8 weeks. This type of treatment approach resulted in significant atrophy of the glenohumeral joint musculature and motion compensation by the scapular muscles during arm elevation. Currently, the trend in rehabilitation is toward earlier motion, early strengthening activities, and stabilizing exercises for the rotator cuff muscles to re-establish voluntary control of the humeral head. This trend toward earlier aggressive rehabilitative exercises has occurred be-

cause of improved surgical techniques,[1,2] advances in arthroscopic procedures,[3-8] and improved soft tissue fixation techniques and devices.[9,10] These improved techniques have lessened the tissue morbidity of the deltoid and surrounding shoulder musculature, allowing an earlier functional return to activities after rotator cuff repairs and capsular stabilization procedures.

The athletic shoulder presents unique challenges to the rehabilitative team. The athlete is usually a highly motivated, overly compliant, energetic patient. Each athletic patient presents with a specific and unique musculoskeletal profile, which the rehabilitation specialist should first recognize and identify. An ectomorphic baseball pitcher presents the clinician with a much different set of challenges than does the mesomorphic football linebacker. In this example, the baseball player may require a treatment program that focuses on improving dynamic glenohumeral joint stability and thus emphasize strengthening exercises to control the excessive shoulder motion necessary to throw a baseball. In contrast, the football linebacker is more likely to exhibit hypomobility of the shoulder, and mobility exercises, such as stretching, may be more appropriate.

The overhead athlete (tennis player, thrower, swimmer) presents the most significant challenge to the clinician. Often these athletes present with glenohumeral joint hypermobility resulting from significant laxity of the shoulder capsule. This increased shoulder laxity is necessary to allow the athlete the excessive motion required to cock the arm during the throwing motion and tennis serve, as well as to perform several swimming strokes. Because of this glenohumeral joint capsular laxity, the rotator cuff muscles must contract forcefully to maintain compression of the humeral head into the glenoid fossa. The rotator cuff muscles serve to prevent excessive humeral head displacements during various motions of the arm. The role of the rotator cuff is one of dynamic stability: to steer and control the humeral head within the glenoid fossa. In the overhead athlete, the stresses imparted on the shoulder are repetitive in nature. Therefore, with these repetitively high stresses placed on the shoulder, inflammation of the rotator cuff muscles may ensue. This prolonged inflammatory process will eventually result in decreased muscular efficiency, poor dynamic stability, increased humeral head displacement, and possibly functional instability. The difference between functional instability and stability is the ability of the athlete to dynamically stabilize the humeral head. Thus, in the athletic shoulder there exists a continuous interplay between (1) functional stability and functional instability, (2) instability and laxity, and (3) too loose versus too tight of a shoulder capsule. The shoulder capsule must be loose enough to allow the extreme motions for sport; however, the capsule must be able to be tight enough to provide stability.

Six basic principles of rehabilitation serve as the foundation for the philosophy and clinical approach to shoulder rehabilitation presented in this chapter. This philosophy has been developed to compliment the current surgical techniques and functional biomechanics of the shoulder complex. These basic principles of rehabilitation are

1. The effects of immobility must be minimized.
2. Healing tissue should never be overstressed.
3. The patient must fulfill specific criteria to progress from one stage of rehabilitation to another.
4. The rehabilitation program must be based on current clinical and basic science research.
5. The rehabilitation program must be adaptable to each patient, allowing for the desired goals of each individual patient.
6. The rehabilitation process is a team effort with the physician, therapist, trainer, patient, coach, and family all working together toward a common goal.

**Table 30-1. Shoulder Rehabilitation Clichés**

1. Structure governs function
2. More to the shoulder complex than the shoulder
3. Proximal stability for distal mobility
4. Normalize arthrokinematics for normal motion
5. Circle stability concept
6. Classification of shoulder instability
7. The key to the shoulder is the rotator cuff
8. More to the shoulder than the rotator cuff
9. More to strength training than dumbbells
10. Treat the shoulder joint as one part of the kinetic chain
11. Functional stability results in successful outcome
12. Isolated movement patterns strengthen weak muscles—combined movement patterns re-establish functional activities

Besides these six basic principles of rehabilitation, I have also developed a list of rehabilitative clichés that need to be considered before rehabilitating an athletic shoulder injury. These clichés are listed in Table 30-1.

"The structure of the glenohumeral joint governs its function." This statement is true of any synovial joint but is of particular importance when considering the shoulder joint. The glenohumeral joint is a ball-and-socket-type joint, with a large humeral head articulating with a relatively small glenoid fossa (Fig. 30-1). At any

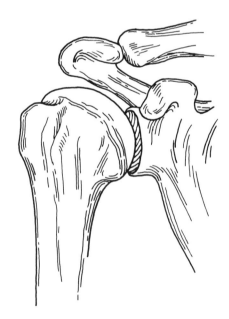

**Fig. 30-1.** Osseous structures of glenohumeral joint. Large oval humeral head articulates with small concave glenoid fossa.

given time during shoulder motion, only 25 to 30 percent of the humeral head is in contact with the glenoid fossa.[11-14] This type of joint geometry inherently affords tremendous amounts of mobility; however, it renders minimal static joint stability. Although the glenohumeral joint exhibits inherent laxity, during normal shoulder motion the humeral head translates only a few millimeters on the glenoid fossa.[15-19] It is the role of the rotator cuff and the deltoid to stabilize the humeral head within the glenoid. Glenohumeral joint stability is accomplished through static (passive) and dynamic (active) mechanisms that interact with each other (Table 30-2).

"There is more to the shoulder complex than merely the shoulder joint." Often clinicians will isolate their attention entirely on the glenohumeral joint, especially when motion is restricted. Arm elevation requires the interplay of the sternoclavicular, acromioclavicular, and scapulothoracic joints.[20-27] During arm elevation, the lateral segment of the clavicle must elevate 30 to 40 degrees to allow the scapulae to rotate upwardly.[20,22] Inman et al[27] reported 4 degrees of clavicular elevation for every 10 degrees of humeral elevation. The scapulae must be able to rotate upwardly approximately 45 to 60 degrees to enable the glenoid fossa to follow the humeral head as the arm elevates to 180 degrees.[20,22] Thus, when arm motion is restricted, the entire kinematic chain must be evaluated and treated to restore normal functioning of the arm and shoulder. The sternoclavicular, acromioclavicular, scapulothoracic, and glenohumeral joints should all receive equal attention.

"The scapulae is an important component of the kinematic chain." One of its main roles is in providing proximal stability enabling the distal segment (the arm) to move through space. The scapula acts as a stable base of support and provides an anchor to which 17 different muscles firmly attach.[23] Another role of the scapula is to follow the proximal humeral head during motion to maintain a normal relationship between the glenohumeral and scapulothoracic joints. This relationship will allow a consistent length tension balance among the muscles of the glenohumeral joint and additionally may prevent structural impingement. The scapula must be free to move and to follow the head of the humerus. The movement of the scapula can be described in relation to the degree of arm elevation. During the first 30 degrees of arm elevation, the scapula is setting itself on the thoracic wall; thus little movement can be observed.[24-26] During 30 to 90 degrees of arm elevation, the scapula is moving approximately 1 degree to every 2 degrees of glenohumeral elevation, and finally from 90 degrees to full elevation (160 to 180 degrees), the ratio is increased to 1 degree of scapula motion to every degree of humeral motion. The overall glenohumeral-to-scapulothoracic joint movement ratio can be expressed in a range from 1.5 to 2.2 to 1.[12,24-27] It is not only the movement of the scapulae that is important but also the ability of the individual to stabilize the scapulae at any point in the range of motion.

"Normalization of joint arthrokinematics will reestablish normal shoulder motion." Arthrokinematics is described as the study of articular movements between two adjacent joint surfaces.[28-30] During arm elevation, the convex humeral head moves on the concave glenoid fossa in a somethat predictable fashion. During the first 90 degrees of elevation, the humeral head glides inferiorly and posteriorly, whereas the last 90 degrees of arm elevation is characterized by an inferior and anterior humeral glide. Based on the clinical assessment of range limitations, specific mobilization techniques can be used at that point in the range to stretch the capsule and restore normal motion. The specific mobilization techniques have been thoroughly described by numerous authors including Maitland,[30] Kaltenborn,[31] Paris,[32] and Donatelli.[33]

The fifth cliché attempts to address the concept of humeral head translation on the glenoid fossa, referred to as the "circle stability concept."[34-38] This concept, best explained as excessive translation in one direction, is probably related to the integrity of capsular structures on both sides of the joint.[37] Thus, for a shoulder to dislocate anteriorly, both the anterior and posterior structures must be insufficient. This can further be explained through primary, secondary, and dynamic restraints.

**Table 30-2. Glenohumeral Joint Stability**

| Passive Mechanisms | Active Mechanisms |
| --- | --- |
| Joint geometry | Compression of joint |
| Limited joint volume |   surfaces |
| Adhesion/cohesion of joint | Dynamic ligament tension |
|   surfaces | Neuromuscular control |
| Ligamentous restraints | |
| Soft tissue barrier | |
| Glenoid labrum | |

*Primary restraint* is located on the side or direction the humeral head is translating toward

*Secondary restraint* is located on the opposite side of the joint of humeral head translation

*Dynamic restraint* is located on both sides of the joint and all around the joint

For significant humeral head translation to occur (i.e., dislocation), injury must occur on both sides of the joint (Fig. 30-2). In the example of an anterior dislocation, the primary restraint is the anterior glenohumeral ligament; however, the secondary restraint is the posterior glenohumeral ligament.[39,40] Warren et al[36] studied posterior instability in the cadaveric shoulder. They reported that incising only the posterior capsule will cause increased posterior humeral translation but will not cause the glenohumeral joint to dislocate posteriorly. For this to occur, the anterior superior capsule had to be incised as well. Also, the rotator cuff muscles around the joint provide stability through a combined contraction that will compress the humeral head into the glenoid fossa and thus minimize humeral head translation.[41–44] Shoulder stability and instability should be thought of in a "circle stability concept," with structures on both sides of the joint providing stability. We refer to this as the "circle dynamic stability concept."

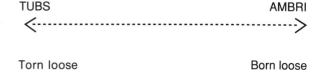

TUBS                  AMBRI

Torn loose             Born loose

**Fig. 30-3.** Shoulder instability spectrum.

The degree, direction, and associated findings in glenohumeral instability testing is difficult to determine on clinical examination. Excessive humeral head translation does not warrant the diagnosis of shoulder instability. Shoulder instability is based on the clinical history and the examination process.[45] In an attempt to help the clinician understand shoulder instability syndromes, Matsen et al[44] introduced two acronyms, TUBS and AMBRI, to classify shoulder instability syndromes. These two instability syndromes represent the two ends of the instability spectrum (Fig. 30-3).

TUBS represents a patient with a traumatic, unidirectional instability pattern, with a Bankart lesion that usually requires surgery to correct. This may be a ball player whose arm was forcefully abducted and externally rotated, thus causing injury to the anterior capsulolabral complex, and instability may ensue.

On the other end of the spectrum is the AMBRI type of instability, which illustrates the patient with an atraumatic etiology in which the instability is multidirectional in nature is usually present in both shoulders, and responds well (usually) to aggressive rehabilitation; and if surgery is necessary, an inferior capsular shift is usually the surgical procedure of choice. This type of patient is the congenitally ligamentously lax individual who exhibits increased hypermobility at several other joints as well. The TUBS variety of injury in the athlete usually requires surgery if overhead motions are necessary to sporting activities. The reader is encouraged to appreciate that most athletes involved in repetitive overhead activities fall somewhere on the right side of the shoulder instability spectrum seen in Fig 30-3. However, as repetitive overhead motions continue, glenohumeral ligamentous capsular laxity often increases, and this is referred to as acquired laxity. The inferior glenohumeral ligament complex is prone to considerable plastic deformation before ultimate failure.[46]

The next cliché is "the key to the shoulder is the rotator cuff." The primary role of the rotator cuff is dynamic stability of the humeral head during arm

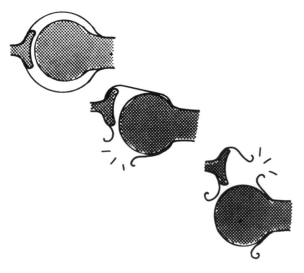

**Fig. 30-2.** "Circle stability concept" describes injury to glenohumeral ligamentous capsule. Translation of humeral head is increased in one direction when injury to one side of the capsule exists. Dislocation requires injury on both sides of joint. (From Bowen and Warren,[38] with permission.)

movements. The function of the rotator cuff is isometric control of the humeral head. The muscles responsible for this act are several force couples; the subscapularis counterbalanced by the infraspinatus and teres minor muscles form one very important force couple.[47] Another critical force couple is formed by the anterior deltoid opposed by the infraspinatus/teres minor muscles. Basmajian and DeLuca[48] stated that the primary depressors and stabilizers of the humeral head are the force couples of the infraspinatus, teres minor, and subscapularis. These muscles act together as force couples to compress the humeral head into the glenoid fossa and to minimize humeral head translation. Also, the musculotendinous unit of the rotator cuff may act as a static restraint or barrier to humeral head movement.[38] The prime movers of the shoulder are the latissimus dorsi, pectoralis major, and the deltoid muscles.[27,49] With this classification of shoulder muscles in place, the rotator cuff musculature is considered the "fine tuner" of the glenohumeral joint. Often, when a tear in the rotator cuff is present, functional activities requiring dynamic shoulder stability are extremely difficult if possible at all. Often high-level functional activities require that the rotator cuff defect be repaired. This may occur because of a decrease in the dynamic stabilizing forces of the musculature and changes in the intra-articular pressure.[50–53] The normal intact glenohumeral joint capsule is an air-tight, sealed structure with limited volume. During shoulder movements, the capsule expands, causing an increase in the negative intra-articular pressure. This increase in the negative intra-articular pressure may limit glenohumeral translation. Clinically, a redundant capsule (greater capsular volume) or a capsule that is torn will result in smaller pressures occurring during movement and an increase in glenohumeral translation.[51,53]

Also, the rotator cuff muscles should be thought of as a dynamic musculoligamentous stabilizing system. When the muscles of the rotator cuff contract, the ligamentous capsule becomes taut and contributes additional static stability. In contrast, when the capsule is excessively stretched, the muscles about the shoulder should contract to provide dynamic stability. We have developed a specific program to enhance humeral head stability in the early phases of the rehabilitation process either immediately postsurgery or after an injury. These are referred to as "humeral head stabilizing exercises" (Table 30-3). If a patient is unable to elevate his or her arm without substitution of the scapular

**Table 30-3. Humeral Head Stabilizing Exercises**

Phase 1—Submaximal Isometrics
    Abductive at 30° and 60°
    Supraspinatus at 30° and 60°
    External rotation arm at side
    Internal rotation arm at side
    Elbow flexion

Phase 2—Short Arc Isotonics
    Abduction (45°–90°)
    Supraspinatus (45°–90°)
    Shoulder flexion (45°–90°)
    Internal rotation/External rotation with exercise tubing (towel under arm)
    Proprioceptive neuromuscular facilitation D2 flexion rhythmic stabilization holds at 30°, 60°, 90°

Phase 3—Dynamic Stabilizing Exercises
    Shoulder flexion (0°–60°) isometric hold at end ranges
    Shoulder flexion (60°–120°) isometric hold at end ranges
    Supraspinatus (0°–60°) isometric hold at end ranges
    Supraspinatus (45°–90°) isometric hold at end ranges
    D2 flexion Proprioceptive neuromuscular facilitation with exercise tubing

musculature, he or she will immediately be placed on specific exercises to enhance voluntary control of the humeral head and prevent excessive humeral head migration.

The rotator cuff is the key to the shoulder, but "there is more to the shoulder than just the rotator cuff." The scapular muscles play a vital role in normal shoulder function. If the scapulothoracic rhythm is impaired during normal arm movements, the glenohumeral joint is at greater risk of injury. Clinically, patients who exhibit significant glenohumeral laxity often exhibit weakness and excessive scapulothoracic motion. As previously stated, the prime movers of the shoulder are the pectoralis major, deltoid, and latissimus dorsi muscles. These muscles are primarily responsible for acceleration of the arm in space, such as during the acceleration phase in throwing or with a tennis serve. The deltoid and the inferior rotator cuff muscles form a critical force couple for shoulder elevation and assist in stabilizing the humeral head in the glenoid fossa.[47]

The next cliché states that "there is more to strength training than just dumbbells." The muscles of the shoulder have already been classified into stabilizers and prime movers. This classification can be further subdivided into accelerators and decelerators. The accelerators are the pectoralis major, latissimus dorsi, teres major, and long head of the triceps. These muscles are two joint muscles and generally function to extend, adduct, and internally rotate the shoulder.

These muscles should be trained primarily with concentric exercise. In contrast, the decelerators of the shoulder are the infraspinatus, teres minor, and the posterior fibers of the deltoid. These muscles should be trained eccentrically with elastic tubing exercises to control and limit joint motion. The use of exercise tubing allows the patient to perform a concentric/eccentric muscle contraction and allows constant loading on the musculotendinous unit throughout the entire range of motion[54] (Fig. 30-4). Other ways of accomplishing concentric/eccentric muscular loading include manual resistance, isokinetic exercise, and plyometric exercise training.[55]

The tenth cliché is "treat the shoulder joint as only one part of the kinetic chain." As stated earlier, the scapulae, the clavicle, and the trunk all play a significant role in normal shoulder function. The clinician should always consider the glenohumeral joint as merely one part of a closed-link system and should routinely evaluate and treat the joints and muscles distal and proximal to the shoulder joint. This type of closed-link system treatment approach should be routinely used when the shoulder joint is involved.

The next cliché is "functional stability results in a successful outcome." This cliché addresses the phenomenon frequently seen on clinical examination. Some patients with a very loose shoulder joint never complain of instability, whereas another patient who appears relatively stable on clinical examination reports frequent episodes of glenohumeral subluxations. Possibly the best explanation available is from Matsen et al.[44] They stated that shoulder laxity is the ability to translate passively the humeral head on the glenoid fossa. Whereas, instability is a clinical condition in which unwanted humeral head translation compromises the comfort and function of the shoulder. Thus, instability is the inability of the patient to control the translation of the humeral head in a dynamic situation. The ultimate key to sporting activities is functional stability. Functional stability occurs through the interaction of the dynamic and static stabilizers and, specifically, the patient's proprioceptive ability.

The last cliché is "isolated movement patterns strengthen weak muscles, and combined movement patterns re-establish functional activities." Isolated movement patterns such as shoulder abduction or external rotation are used to strengthen a muscle that has been identified as weak. By exercising this muscle in an isolated pattern, the compensation by strong mus-

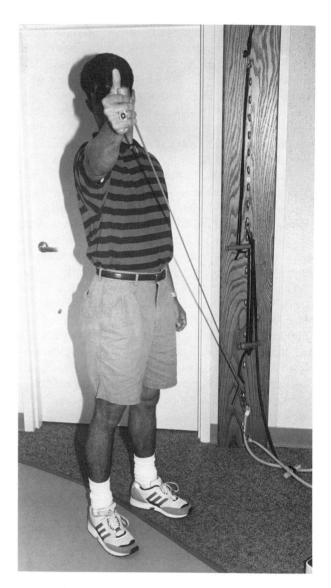

**Fig. 30-4.** Diagonal pattern consisting of shoulder abduction, external rotation, and flexion using exercise tubing (Berg Corp., Vista, CA). Exercise tubing allows constant loading of muscle while performing concentric and eccentric muscular contractions.

cles is not allowed. Combined movement patterns, such as proprioceptive neuromuscular facilitation D2 flexion pattern for the upper extremities, which uses abduction, flexion, and external rotation, is used to re-establish and encourage a specific functional movement (Fig. 30-4). In a combined movement pattern, the quality of motion is emphasized, and strong muscles may compensate for weak muscles. Both movement patterns and exercises are important in the rehabilitation process and should be incorporated at appropriate intervals.

Many concepts and principles are currently used in the rehabilitation of the shoulder complex. Several of these concepts are briefly discussed in hopes of providing the scientific rationale for some of these treatment principles. The concepts to be discussed are listed in Table 30-4.

Immediately after a shoulder injury or surgery, motion exercises are allowed in a protected, minimally painful arc of motion. By allowing immediate motion, the deleterious effects of immobilization, such as adverse collagen alignment, articular cartilage degeneration, and muscular atrophy, may be minimized.[56–61] Also, early motion may also assist in aligning collagen fibers to appropriate stress patterns.[56,61] Last, early motion for the glenohumeral joint may assist in the prevention of glenohumeral musculature disassociation and the substitution of scapular muscles to elevate the arm.[21] These early motion exercises can be performed passively, actively, or with active assisted movements. Passive movement may use a continuous passive motion device (Fig. 30-5) or a therapist moving the limb through a prescribed arc of motion. Active assisted movements can be performed using an L- bar (Fig. 30-6), cane, and/or rope and pulley. Active movements are usually used slightly later in the rehabilitation process, once passive motion has increased and healing constraints allow this type of activity to occur.

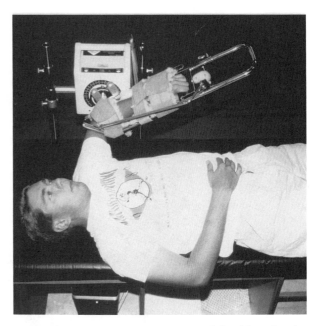

**Fig. 30-5.** Continuous passive motion of shoulder. Therakinetics.

Another form of passive motion is joint mobilization. This is a passive technique to assess and restore normal joint mobility through the movement of one joint surface on another.[30–32] In using these tehcniques, the therapist manually glides the humeral head in an appropriate direction to stretch the capsule and restore a normal movement pattern. The direction of the glide is determined by the restriction in movement evaluated and the desired outcome (Table 30-5). The magnitude of the glide is determined by the amount of stretch desired on the capsule and is referred to in grades. These grades range from I to IV, with grade IV glides using a vigorous stretch on the joint capsule.[30] Grade I and II oscillations are used to decrease the patient's pain, whereas grades III and IV glides are used to stretch the joint capsule.[30]

**Table 30-4. Current Concepts in Shoulder Rehabilitation**

Immediate Motion
    Continuous passive motion
    Active assisted motion
    Passive motion
    Joint mobilization techniques
Early Strengthening Exercises
    Isometrics
    Isotonics
Proprioceptive Neuromuscular Facilitation
    Combined movement patterns
Proprioception/Kinesthesia
    Movement awareness drills
Neuromuscular Control Exercises
    Quality movement drills
Closed Chain Rehabilitative Exercises
Eccentric Muscular Contraction
Plyometric Muscular Training
Isokinetic Exercise and Testing
Soft Tissue Mobilization

**Table 30-5. Arthrokinematics of the Glenohumeral Joint**

| Osteokinematic Motion | | Arthrokinematics |
|---|---|---|
| Flexion | 0–90° | Posterior-inferior glide/anterior-superior roll |
| | 90–180° | Anterior-inferior glide/posterior-superior roll |
| External rotation | | Anterior glide/posterior roll |
| Internal rotation | | Posterior glide/anterior roll |

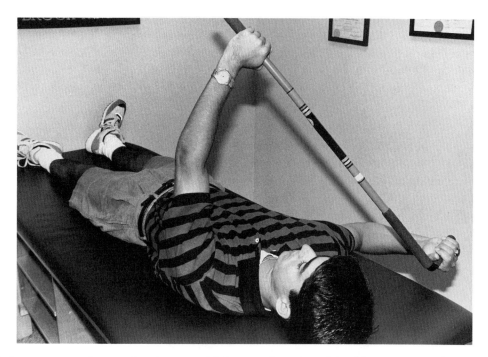

**Fig. 30-6.** Active assisted range of motion to establish external rotation of shoulder joint using L bar (Berg Corp., Vista, CA).

Also, motion exercises are useful in decreasing the patient's perception of pain. By allowing controlled movement, the type I and II mechanoreceptors of the joint are stimulated, which presynaptically inhibits pain fiber transmission at the spinal cord level.[62,63] Thus, by allowing immediate motion, patients feel better and achieve humeral head control much faster. Also, the need for prolonged pain medication is minimized.

Another method of obtaining control of the humeral head is through early strengthening exercises. Immediately after a shoulder injury or surgery, it is common to observe a functional decrease in strength of the rotator cuff musculature secondary to pain, swelling, and injury. The function of the rotator cuff is to stabilize and steer the humeral head dynamically during arm movements.[49] Therefore, it is critical to initiate voluntary control and function of the rotator cuff as quickly as possible after trauma. This is imperative to prevent excessive uncontrollable humeral head migration.[64] Isometrics are a useful form of strengthening exercise to re-establish this humeral head control. Isometric contractions are performed submaximally and in a pain-free fashion at different points in the range of motion. An exercise progression has been established

for the patient with poor humeral head control. This program is referred to as humeral head stabilizing exercises (see Table 30-3).

Proprioceptive neuromuscular facilitation exercises were first developed by Kabat in 1965[65] and later by Knott and Voss in 1968.[66] This form of exercise uses specific skilled sensory input from the clinician to bring about or facilitate a specific activity or movement pattern. A commonly used movement for the shoulder is referred to as a D2 flexion pattern. This movement pattern uses shoulder flexion, abduction, and external rotation (Fig. 30-7). The reverse of this movement pattern is a D2 extension pattern, in which shoulder extension, adduction, and internal rotation are facilitated (Fig. 30-8). The advantage of this form of exercise is that it allows the clinicain to provide a hands-on treatment technique. This treatment technique allows the clinician to increase the awareness of specific movement patterns and reinforce or facilitate weak patterns through irradiation from strong patterns of motion. The clinician uses specific techniques (slow reversal, rhythmic stabilization, contact relax, timing for emphasis, etc.) and different elements (quick stretch, traction, brushing, manual contacts, etc.) to

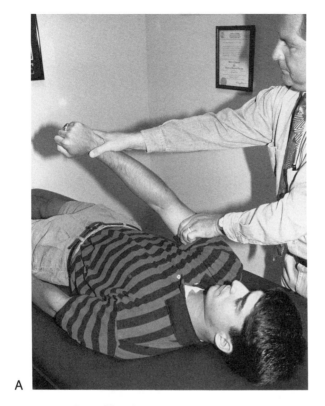

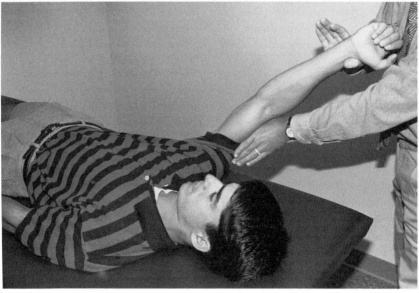

**Fig. 30-7.** (**A,B**) Manual resistance applied during a $D_2$ flexion proprioceptive neuromuscular facilitation exercise. Rhythmic stabilization (RS) technique is employed at various points in the plane of motion; patients are instructed to lead the motion with their thumb, and when the RS is applied to rotation the arm in the direction of the resistance.

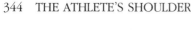

**Fig. 30-8.** D$_2$ extension pattern for shoulder musculature.

facilitate a desired functional movement pattern.[66–69] The author routinely uses the rhythmic stabilization technique at various points of the range of motion of the D$_2$ extension flexion pattern. Rhythmic stabilization is most commonly performed at 30, 60, 90, 120 and 150 degrees of elevation. I believe this specific technique enhances dynamic humeral head control and maximally challenges the glenohumeral force couples.

The awareness of the glenohumeral or scapulothoracic joint posture, movements, and positional changes is referred to as *proprioception*.[70] The ability to perceive the extent and direction of specific movements is defined as *kinesthesia*.[70] Smith and Brunolti[71] documented that after anterior glenohumeral joint dislocation, there is a significant deficit in joint proprioception when compared with the contralateral uninvolved side. The patient's ability to recognize the posture and position of the glenohumeral and scapulothoracic joint is most likely an important factor in preventing shoulder injuries.[72] This type of rehabilitation component should use specific drills and procedures to challenge and, thus, improve the proprioception and kinesthesia of the upper extremity. The author has incorporated specific proprioceptive drills for the glenohumeral joint after anterior shoulder instability. These drills are designed to provide static and dynamic stress to the

anterior shoulder capsule as the arm is positioned into the frequent position of dislocation, shoulder abduction, and external rotation. These drills begin by positioning the arm in the most tolerable degree of abduction and external rotation. Then the patient is asked to hold that position isometrically as rhythmic stabilization techniques are applied in an attempt to rotate the arm externally and internally. The patient must maintain this static position for successful completion of the activity (Fig. 30-9). As the patient improves, the arm is taken further into an apprehensive posture (abduction and external rotation). More advanced drills involve the use of a ball (either weighted or nonweighted). With the arm positioned in different degrees of abduction, the ball is thrown to overload the arm into external rotation. The patient must recognize the degree of external rotation and prevent excessive glenohumeral joint motion from occurring. These drills can be performed with the patient supine or standing against a wall. The wall or floor will provide a static barrier and assists in preventing excessive motion (Fig. 30-10). As the patient progresses, these drills can be performed without the external support of the wall or floor[72] (Fig. 30-11). Table 30-6 illustrates the progression of this program. Additionally, PNF diagonal patterns such as D$_2$ flexion/extension can be per-

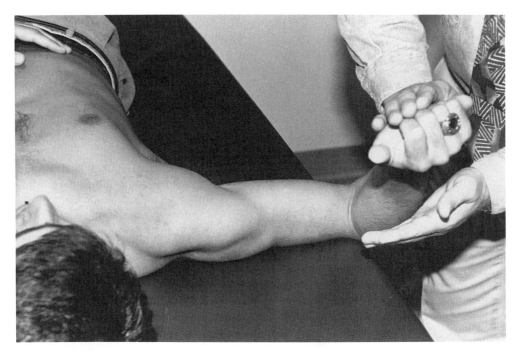

**Fig. 30-9.** Rhythmic stabilization exercises and drills for unstable shoulder patient. Arm is abducted and externally rotated, and patient is instructed to maintain that position as force is applied.

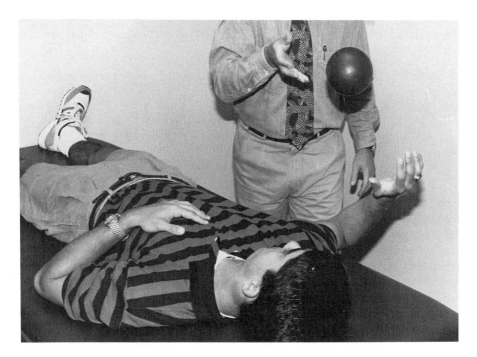

**Fig. 30-10.** Unstable shoulder patient's arm is abducted and externally rotated to maximal tolerance in supine position. Weighted ball is thrown to create an overload into further external rotation; patient must dynamically stabilize arm in that position.

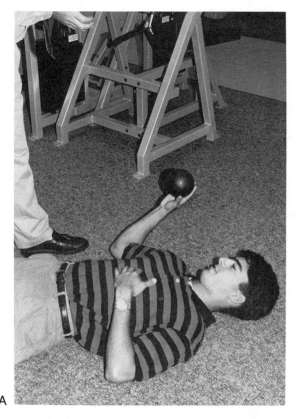
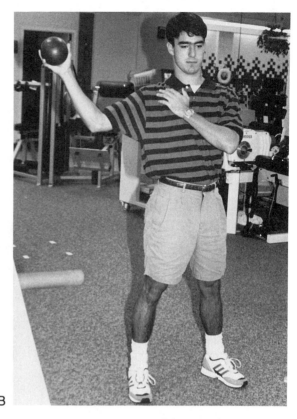

**Fig. 30-11.** Same exercise drill as described in Fig. 30-10 is used with **(A)** and without **(B)** external support of the floor.

formed with exercise tubing and manual resistance applied either through a movement plane or at a particular point in the movement plane (rhythmic stabilization) (Fig. 30-12).

The ability to perceive joint position is an important component to the rehabilitation process, but the ability to make a postural change based on proprioceptive input is vital to the successful rehabilitation of the active individual. This process is referred to as neuromuscular control. It is the ability to couple afferent sensory input and use the muscular system to make a positional change that is advantageous to increase performance (efferent output). Neuromuscular control exercises are commonly used for the scapulothoracic joint. The scapula must be able to move (upward rotation and abduction) to allow full arm elevation.[18,20,27] Also, the scapulothoracic musculature plays a significant role in providing adequate scapular mobility and, more importantly, a stable base for the glenohumeral musculature. This stable base allows a consistent length–tension relationship of the rotator cuff musculature.

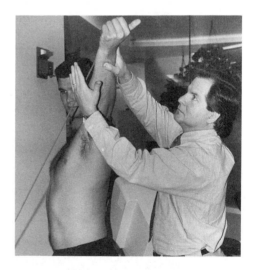

**Fig. 30-12.** Proproceptive neuromuscular facilitation drills utilizing exercise tubing and manual resistance concomitantly. Rhythmic stabilization can be performed as the patient holds a static point in the range with the tubing and force is applied by the clinician.

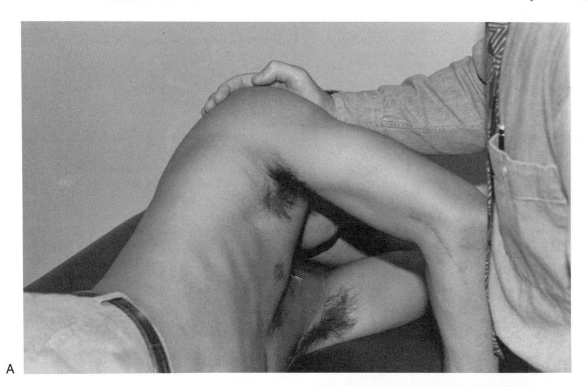

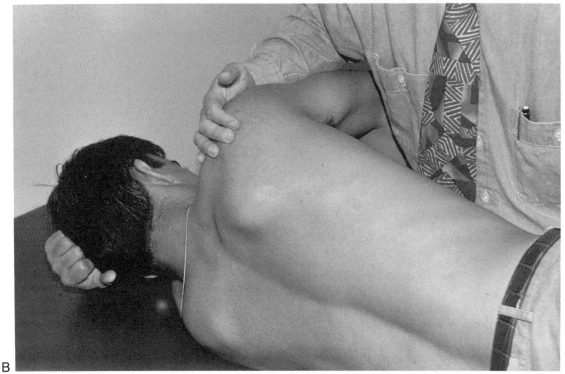

**Fig. 30-13.  (A & B)** Neuromuscular control exercises for scapular musculature. Note, the patient's hand is placed on the table to close the kinetic chain and better isolate the proximal scapular muscles.

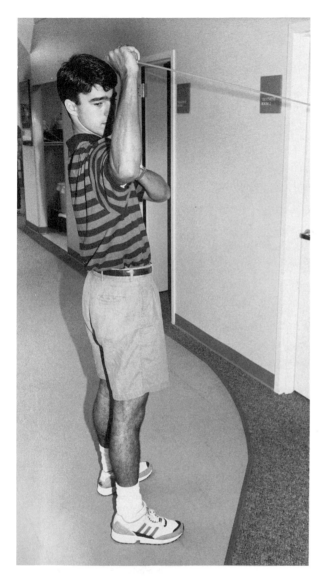

**Fig. 30-14.** Eccentric muscular strengthening exercises for shoulder's external rotators.

Neuromuscular control exercises and drills are routinely instituted for the shoulder patient to ensure improvement in the volitional motor control and movement of the scapulae. These exercises originally described by Feldenkrais[73-75] have been modified by the author for the orthopaedic and sports medicine patient.[21] The exercises are performed with the patient lying on the contralateral side. The involved shoulder is free to move while the hand is placed on the table with the shoulder abducted to 90 degrees and inter-

nally rotated (this position of abduction can be modified, if necessary). The neuromuscular drill is performed with the patient slowly elevating and depressing the scapula and then slowly retracting and protracting the scapula. The goal of this drill is quality-controlled movements that can isolate specific scapular muscles. Manual resistance can be used to assist in the motor learning process of these drills (Fig. 30-13). The scapular neuromuscular control drills progress from straight planes to diagonal planes to circles, etc. The manual resistance may progress to rhythmic stabilization at various positions to slow reversal holds, etc. Also, scapular stabilizing exercises can be performed in the quaduped position and in the triped and biped positions (Fig. 30-14). The patient is asked to stabilize the scapula and humerus proximally as the therapist applies rhythmic stabilization forces at the glenohumeral joint. A physioball or swiss ball can also be used to incorporate the posterior scapular muscles (Fig. 30-15).

The concept of closed chain exercise has been popularized for the lower extremity.[76-79] However, this concept is often used for the upper extremity. The concept of closed kinetic chain exercise is defined as the distal segment being fixed to an immovable object. Examples of closed kinetic chain exercises or drills include push-ups, hand stands, and dips. Closed chain exercise is useful in providing joint approximation forces that promote a co-contraction about the joint and provides joint stability. This form of exercise is useful for the athlete who must spend time on his or her hands such as a gymnast, a wrestler, or any athlete who may fall onto his or her hands repetitively (football, hockey, etc.). Many drills are routinely used to promote joint stability through closed kinetic chain exercises. These exercises include weight shifts with resistance, push-ups with rhythmic stabilization, push-ups on a ball, and press-ups (Fig. 30-15). These drills are especially beneficial during the early stages of the rehabilitation program to initiate a muscular contraction.

The ability of the athlete to decelerate the arm after ball release in throwing or after hitting a tennis or golf ball is an important component to injury-free sports participation. The posterior shoulder musculature (infraspinatus, teres minor, and posterior deltoid), as well as the elbow flexors (biceps, brachialis), is responsible for this through an eccentric muscular contaction. These muscles must have the ability to elongate while resisting a load and thus slow functional arm move-

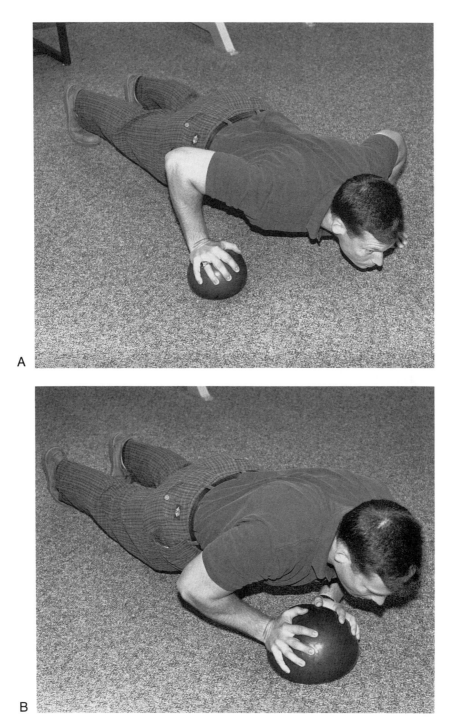

**Fig. 30-15.** Closed chain exercises for the upper quarter. **(A)** Single balance push-ups on a ball and **(B)** two-arm push-ups into a ball. (*Figure continues.*)

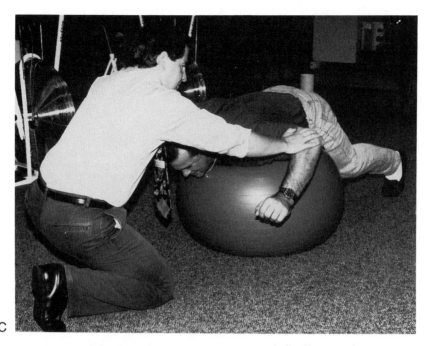

**Fig. 30-15** (*Continued*). **(C)** Prone scapular retraction over a swiss ball. All are used to improve upper extremity proprioception and kinesthesia.

ments and prevent shoulder and/or elbow injury. This form of contraction allows the arm to decelerate and absorb much of the stress during the ball release and follow-through phases of throwing. Specific rehabilitative exercises must be used to create an eccentric overload on the posterior shoulder muscles to replicate these forces. Frequently, eccentric exercises are used with exercise tubing during internal and external rotation of the arm at 90 degrees of abduction, as well as the D2 flexion pattern, to accomplish this activity (Fig. 30-16).

**Table 30-6. Drills to Challenge and Improve Proprioception and Kinesthesia of the Upper Extremity**

| Abduction | Movement Awareness Drills |
|---|---|
| 0° | supine table (arm support) |
| ⇓ | ⇑ |
| 45° | standing wall (arm support) |
| ⇓ | ⇑ |
| 90° | slightly away from wall (minimal support) |
| ⇓ | ⇑ |
| >90° | standing without support |

Plyometric drills have become increasingly popular for the overhead athlete, particularly the baseball thrower, in the past several years. These drills refer to a quick, powerful movement involving a prestretch of the muscle, thereby activating its stretch–shortening cycle (see Ch. 44)[80-82] Plyometrics are designed to increase the excitability of the neurologic receptors for improved reactivity of the neuromuscular system. All movements in competitive athletics involve a repeated series of stretch–shortening cycles. This is especially true for the throwing athlete who relies on the prestretch of the internal rotators and adductors during the cocking phase to facilitate a concentric muscular contraction during the acceleration phase of throwing. This also applies to other athletes such as tennis players, swimmers, and even golfers, all of whom rely on the stretch–shortening cycle for arm speed and power movements during activity.

Plyometric exercises use three phases, all intended to use the elastic and reative properties of the muscle to generate maximal force production. The setting phase or eccentric period is the phase in which the prestretch is applied to the muscle stimulating the mus-

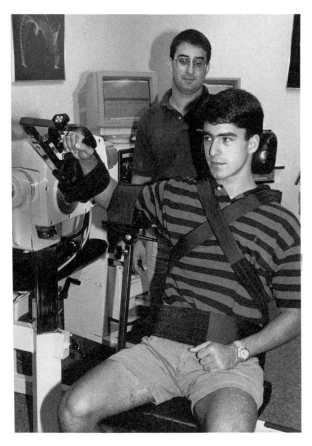

**Fig. 30-16.** Isokinetic exercise for shoulder's internal and external rotators performed in 90 degree abducted position.

ing throughout the entire arc of motion. Thus, theoretically, with maximal patient intensity, the patient should be receiving maximal muscle loading throughout the range of motion. Isokinetic testing is commonly used to document the patient's muscular performance in an objective reproducible method.[83] The clinician can document the strength, power, work, and endurance variables of the injured shoulder. Several authors have documented the muscular performance characteristics of the throwing athlete,[84–89] tennis player,[90] and the swimmer (Murphy, unpublished data). Shoulder internal/external rotation is a commonly performed isokinetic exercise movement (Fig. 30-16). Several authors have shown significant torque value variations by altering the shoulder position.[91–96] Soderberg and Blaschek[91] tested (IR/ER) in six different test positions and concluded IR torque was highest in the neutral position (arm at side) and that ER was highest with the arm in neutral or at 90 degrees of abduction. Greenfield et al[93] reported ER values being higher in the scapular plane versus the frontal plane. Ellenbecker et al [95] found no difference in ER/IR torque values in the frontal plane versus the scapular plane. Therefore, there appears to be no clear conclusion as to the plane of the scapula enhancing ER torque. Thus, the clinician must be aware that significant variation in torque production may occur when the arm position is changed during isokinetic exercise. A thorough discussion of the advantages of exercise in the scapular plane can be found in Chapter 42 and of isokinetic testing/exercise in Chapter 43.

The human body is composed of different soft tissue layers consisting of connective tissue. Two of these soft tissue layers are referred to as a superficial and deep fascia layer.[97–99] The superficial fascial plane is composed of loose connective tissue and adipose tissue. This superficial layer is connected to the underlying deeper fascia consisting of periosteum or aponeurosis. Soft tissue mobilization techniques attempt to free these fascia planes so that they glide freely and may move in all directions. A common region for soft tissue adhesions is over the upper trapezius and middle rhomboideus muscles. These fascia layers are continuous soft tissue planes throughout the entire body. Several therapeutic techniques may benefit the patient in pain relief and assist in motion restoration.[97–99] These techniques attempt to restore the freedom of movement between these fascial planes.[97]

cle spindle. The second phase is referred to as the amortization phase and represents the time between the eccentric and concentric phase. The final plyometric phase is the resultant concentric phase. This is the resultant facilitated contraction from the prestretch stimulus. The author has found stretch shortening exercise drills beneficial for sports performance training and enhancement. These drills appear to enhance the neuromuscular coordination, neural adaption and muscular recruitment rather than morphologic changes of the muscles. A description of different exercises can be found in Chapter 44.

Isokinetic exercise and testing is commonly used for the athletic shoulder. Isokinetic muscular contractions are accomplished through the use of an isokinetic dynamometer. This form of exercise uses a pre-set speed (0 to 450 degrees) and resistance that is accommodat-

# CONCLUSION

Treatment of the athletic shoulder has changed dramatically in the past several years. Currently, rehabilitation plays a vital role in the successful outcome after shoulder injuries or surgeries. The rehabilitation of the shoulder should include the evaluation and treatment of the sternoclavicular, acromioclavicular, and scapulothoracic joints as well as an eclectic approach to the treatment plan. The rehabilitation techniques used must have basic and clinical science basis for their application.

# REFERENCES

1. Hawkins RJ, Misamore GW, Hobecka PE: Surgery for full thickness rotator cuff tears. J Bone Joint Surg 67A:1349, 1985
2. Jobe FW, Glousman RE: Anterior capsulolabral reconstruction. Techniques Orthop Shoulder 3:29, 1985
3. Andrews JR, Angelo RL: Shoulder arthroscopy for the throwing athlete. p. 79. In Paulos LE, Tibone JE (eds): Operative Techniques in Shoulder Surgery. Aspen Publishers, Rockville, MD, 1991
4. Andrews JR, Carson WG: The arthroscopic treatment of glenoid labrum tears in the throwing athlete. Orthop Trans 8:44, 1984
5. Andrews JR, Broussard TS, Carson WG: Arthroscopy of the shoulder in the management of partial tears of the rotator cuff; a preliminary report. Arthroscopy 1:117, 1985
6. Ellman H: Shoulder arthroscopy: current indications and techniques. Orthopedics 11:45, 1988
7. Johnson LL: Shoulder arthroscopy. In Johnson LL (ed): Arthroscopic Surgery, Principles and Practice. CV Mosby, St Louis, 1986
8. Morgan CD, Bodenstab AB: Arthroscopic Bankart suture repair. Technique and early results. Arthroscopy 3:111, 1987
9. Feldman A, Harner C, Fu FH: Arthroscopic repair of glenoid capsular labral tears using the Mitek anchor. Presented at the American Academy of Orthopaedic Surgeons Annual Meeting, New Orleans, 1990
10. Warren RF: Anterior shoulder instability: arthroscopic capsular repair. Presented at Controversies in Arthroscopy and Sports Medicine, American Sports Medicine Institute Course, Bermuda, August 1990
11. Bost FC, Inman VTG: The pathological changes in recurrent dislocations of the shoulder. J Bone Joint Surg 24:595, 1942
12. Codman EA: The Shoulder. Thomas Todd, Boston, 1934
13. Saha AK: Dynamic stability of the glenohumeral joint. Acta Orthop Scand 42:491, 1971
14. Steindler A: Kinesiology of the human body under normal and pathological conditions. Charles C Thomas, Springfield, IL, 1955
15. Altchek DW, Schwartz E, Warren RF: Radiologic measurement of superior migration of the humeral head in impingement syndrome. Presented at the Annual Meeting American Shoulder and Elbow Surgeons, New Orleans, 1990
16. Harryman DTI, Sidles JA, Clark JM et al: Translation of the humeral head on the glenoid with passive glenohumeral motion. J Bone Joint Surg 72A:1334, 1990
17. Howell SM, Galinat BJ, Renzi AJ et al: Normal and abnormal mechanics of the glenohumeral joint in the horizontal plane. J Bone Joint Surg 68A:398, 1986
18. Poppen NK, Walker PS: Normal and abnormal motions of the shoulder. J Bone Joint Surg 58A:195, 1976
19. Poppen NK, Walker PS: Forces at the glenohumeral joint in abduction. Clin Orthop 58:165, 1978
20. Kapandji I: The Physiology of Joints. Vol. 1. Williams & Wilkins, Baltimore, 1970
21. Wilk KE, Arrigo CA: An integrated approach to upper extremity exercises. In Timm KE (ed): Exercise Principles. Orthop Phys Ther Clin North Am 9:337, 1992
22. Schenkmann M, Rugo de Cartaya V: Kinesiology of the shoulder complex. J Orthop Sports Phys Ther 8:438, 1987
23. Butters KP: The scapula. p. 335. In Rockwood CA, Matsen FA (eds): The Shoulder. WB Saunders, Philadelphia, 1990
24. Doody SG, Freedman L, Waterland JC: Shoulder movements during abduction in the scapular plane. Arch Phys Med Rehabil 51:595, 1970
25. Freedman L, Munro RR: Abduction of the arm in the scapular plane: scapular and glenohumeral movements. A roentgenographic study. J Bone Joint Surg 48A:1503, 1966
26. Saha AK: Mechanics of elevation of glenohumeral joint. Its application in rehabilitation of flail shoulder in upper brachial plexus injuries and poliomyelitis and in replacement of the upper humerus by prosthesis. Acta Orthop Scand 44:668, 1973
27. Inman VT, Saunders M, Abbott LC: Observations on the function of the shoulder joints. J Bone Joint Surg 26:1, 1944
28. Basmajian JV, MacConail C: In Warwick R, Williams P (eds): Gray's Anatomy. 35th Ed (British). WB Saunders, Philadelphia, 1973
29. Mennell JM: Joint pain: diagnosis and treatment using manipulative techniques. Little, Brown, Boston, 1964
30. Maitland G: Peripheral Manipulation. 2nd Ed. Butterworth, London, 1978

31. Kaltenborn F: Manual Therapy of the Extremity Joints. Olaf Noris Borkhandel, Oslo, 1973
32. Paris SV: Extremity Dysfunction and Mobilization. Institute Press, Atlanta, 1980
33. Donatelli RA, Wooden MJ: Mobilization of the shoulder. p. 271. In Donatelli RA (ed): Physical Therapy of the Shoulder. 2nd Ed. Churchill Livingstone, New York, 1991
34. Hawkins RJ: Basic science and clinical application in the athlete's shoulder. Clin Sports Med 10:4, 1991
35. Schwartz RE, O'Brien SJ, Warren RF et al: Capsular restraints to anterior-posterior motion of the abducted shoulder. A biomechanical study. Orthop Trans 17:727, 1988
36. Warren RF, Kornblatt IB, Marchand R: Static factors affecting posterior shoulder stability. Orthop Trans 8:89, 1984
37. Hawkins RJ, Schutte JP, Huckell GJ et al: The assessment of glenohumeral translation using manual and fluoroscopic techniques. Orthop Trans 12:727, 1988
38. Bowen MK, Warren RF: Ligamentous control of shoulder stability based on selective cutting and static translation experiments. Clin Sports Med 10:757, 1991
39. O'Brien SJ, Neves CM, Arnoczky SJ et al: The anatomy and histology of the inferior glenohumeral ligament complex of the shoulder. Am J Sports Med 18:449, 1990
40. Warner JP, Deng X, Warren RF et al: Static capsuloligamentous restraints to superior-inferior translation of the glenohumeral joint. Presented at the Annual Meeting of the Orthopaedic Research Society, Anaheim, CA, 1991
41. Cain PR, Mutschler TA, Fu FH: Anterior stability of the glenohumeral joint: a dynamic model. Am J Sports Med 15:144, 1987
42. Howell SM, Galinet BJ: The glenoid-labral socket: a constrained articular surface. Clin Orthop 243:122, 1989
43. Howell SM, Inobersteg AM, Seger OH et al: Clarification of the role of the supraspinatus muscle in shoulder function. J Bone Joint Surg 68A:398, 1986
44. Matsen FA, Harryman DT, Sidles JA: Mechanics of glenohumeral instability. Clin Sports Med 10:783, 1991
45. Hawkins RJ: Clinical examination of shoulder problems. In Rockwood CA, Matsen FA (eds): The Shoulder. WB Saunders, Philadelphia, 1990
46. Pollack RG, Bigliani LU, Flatow EL et al: The mechanical properties of the inferior glenohumeral ligament. Presented at the Annual Meeting of the American Shoulder and Elbow Surgeons, New Orleans, 1990
47. Burkhart SS: Arthroscopic treatment of massive rotator cuff tears. Clin Orthop 267:45, 1991
48. Basmajian JV, DeLuca CJ: Muscles Alive. 5th Ed. Williams & Wilkins, Baltimore, 1985
49. Saha AK: Theory of Shoulder Mechanism. Charles C Thomas, Springfield, IL, 1966
50. Harryman DT, Sidles JA, Clark JM et al: Translation of the humeral head on the glenoid with passive glenohumeral motion. J Bone Joint Surg 72:1334, 1990
51. Browne AO, Hoffmeyer P, An KN et al: The influence of atmospheric pressure on shoulder stability. Presented at the Annual Meeting of American Shoulder and Elbow Surgeons, New Orleans, 1990
52. Kumar VP, Balasubraamanian P: The role of atmospheric pressure in stabilizing the shoulder. An experimental study. J Bone Joint Surg 67B:719, 1985
53. Warner JP, Deng X, Warren RF et al: Superior-inferior translation in the intact and vented glenohumeral joint. Presented at the Annual Meeting of the American Shoulder and Elbow Surgeons, Anaheim, CA, 1991
54. Anderson L, Rush R, Shearer L, Hughes CJ: The effects of a Theraband exercise program on shoulder internal rotational strength. Presented at the Annual Meeting of the American Physical Therapy Association, Denver, CO, June 1992
55. Wilk KE, Voight ML, Keirns MA et al: Plyometrics for the upper extremities; theory and clinical application. J Orthop Sports Phys Ther, May 1993
56. Akeson WH, Woo SLY, Amiel D: The connective tissue response to immobility: biomechanical changes in periarticular connective tissue of the immobilized rabbit knee. Clin Orthop 93:356, 1973
57. Dehne E, Tory R: Treatment of joint injuries by immediate mobilization, based upon the spinal adaption concept. Clin Orthop 77:281, 1971
58. Noyes FR, Mangine RE, Barber S: Early knee motion after open and arthroscopic ACL reconstruction. Am J Sports Med 15:149, 1981
59. Perkins G: Rest and motion. J Bone Joint Surg 45B:521, 1954
60. Ericksson E: Rehabilitation of muscle function after sport injury—a major problem in sports medicine. Int J Sports Med 2:1, 1981
61. Woo SLY, Matthews SU, Akeson WH: Connective tissue response to immobility. Arthritis Rheum 18:257, 1975
62. Wyke B: Articular neurology—a review. Physiotherapy 58:94, 1972
63. Melzack R, Torgerson WS: On the language of pain. Anesthesiology 34:50, 1971
64. Wilk KE, Andrews JR: Rehabilitation following arthroscopic subacromial decompression. Orthopedics (accepted for publication, 1993)
65. Kabat H: Proprioceptive facilitation in therapeutic exercises. p. 327. In Licht S (ed): Therapeutic Exercises. Waverly Press, Baltimore, 1965
66. Knott M, Voss D: Proprioceptive Neuromuscular Facilitation. Harper & Row, New York, 1968
67. Sullivan PE, Markos PD, Minor MD: An Integrated Ap-

proach to Therapeutic Exercise: Theory and Clinical Application. Reston Publications, Reston, VA, 1982

68. Harris FA: Facilitation techniques in therapeutic exercise. In Basmajian JU (ed): Therapeutic Exercise. 3rd Ed. Williams & Wilkins, Baltimore, 1978.

69. Voss DE, Knott M, Kabat M: Application of neuromuscular facilitation in the treatment of shoulder disabilities. Phys Ther Rev 33:536, 1953

70. Taber's Cyclopedic Medical Dictionary. FA Davis, Philadelphia, 1977

71. Smith RH, Brunolti J: Shoulder kinesthia after anterior glenohumeral joint dislocation. Phys Ther 69:106, 1989

72. Wilk KE: Current concepts in the evaluation and treatment of shoulder pathologies. Presented in Kansas City, MO, June 1992

73. Feldenkrais M: Awareness Through Movement. Harper & Row, New York, 1972

74. Rywerant Y: Improving the ability to perform: an instance of the Feldenkrais method of functional integration. Somatics 37, 1977

75. Wildman G: Awareness in movement. Presented in Milwaukee, WI, March 1989

76. Gray GW: Rehabilitation of running injuries: biomechanical and proprioceptive considerations. Top Acute Care Trauma Rehabil 1:67, 1986

77. Palmittier RA, An KN, Scott SG et al: Kinetic chain exercise in knee rehabilitation. Sports Med 11:402, 1991

78. Shelbourne DK, Nitz PA: Accelerated rehabilitation after anterior cruciate ligament reconstruction. Am J Sports Med 18:292, 1990

79. Wilk KE, Andrews JR: Current concepts in the treatment of anterior cruciate ligament disruption. J Orthop Sports Phys Ther 15:279, 1992

80. Assmussen E, Bonde-Peterson F: Storage of elastic energy in skeletal muscle in man. Acta Physiol Scand 91:385, 1974

81. Chu D: Plyometric exercise. Natl Strength Cond Assoc J 6:56, 1984

82. Bosco C, Komi P: Potentiation of the mechanical behavior of the human skeletal muscle through pre-stretching. Acta Physiol Scand 106:467, 1979

83. Wilk KE: Dynamic muscle strength testing. p. 123. In Amundsen LR (ed): Muscle Strength Testing; Instrumental and Non-instrument Systems. Churchill Livingstone, New York, 1990

84. Cook EE, Gray VL, Savinor-Nogue E et al: Shoulder antagonistic–agonist strength ratios: a comparison between college level baseball pitchers. J Orthop Sports Phys Ther 8:451, 1987

85. Alderink GJ, Kuck DJ: Isokinetic shoulder strength of high school and college aged pitchers. J Orthop Sports Phys Ther 7:163, 1986

86. Brown LP, Nichues SL, Harrah A et al: Upper extremity range of motion and isokinetic strength of the internal and external rotators in major league baseball players. Am J Sports Med 16:577, 1988

87. Wilk KE, Andrews JR, Arrigo CA et al: The internal and external rotator strength characteristics of professional baseball pitchers. Am J Sports Med 21:61, 1993

88. Wilk KE, Andrews JR, Arrigo CA et al: The isokinetic abductor and adductor strength characteristics of professional baseball pitchers. Am J Sports Med (submitted for publication)

89. Wilk KE, Arrigo CA, Andrews JR: Standardized isokinetic testing protocol for the throwing shoulder. The thrower's series. Isokin Exerc Sci 1:63, 1991

90. Ellenbecker TS: A total arm strength profile of highly skilled tennis players. Isokin Exerc Sci 1:9, 1991

91. Soderberg GJ, Blaschek MJ: Shoulder internal and external rotation peak torque production through a velocity spectrum in differing positions. J Orthop Sports Phys Ther 8:518, 1987

92. Hagemann PA, Mason DK, Rydlund KW et al: Effects of positions and speed on eccentric and concentric isokinetic testing of the shoulder rotators. J Orthop Sports Phys Ther 11:64, 1989

93. Greenfield BH, Donatelli R, Wooden MJ, Wilkens J: Isokinetic evaluation of shoulder rotational strength between plane of scapula and functional place. Am J Sports Med 18:124, 1990

94. Walmsley RP, Szybbo C: A comparative study of the torque generated by the shoulder internal and external rotators in different positions and at varying speeds. J Orthop Sports Phys Ther 9:217, 1987

95. Ellenbecker TS, Feiring DC, DeHart RL, Rich M: Isokinetic shoulder strength: coronal versus scapular plane testing in upper extremity unilaterally dominant athletes. Phys Ther, suppl 72:580, 1992

96. Hellwig EV, Perrin DH: A comparison of two positions for assessing shoulder rotator peak torque: the traditional frontal plane versus the plane of the scapula. Isokin Exerc Sci 1:202, 1991

97. Johnson G, Saliba V: Functional Orthopaedics. Institute of Physical Art, San Anselmo, CA, 1990

98. Gallaudet B: The Planes of Fascia. Columbia University Press, New York, 1931

99. Fung YC: Elasticity of soft tissue in simple elongation. Am J Physiol 213:1532, 1967

# 31

# Biomechanics of the Shoulder During Throwing

GLENN S. FLEISIG
CHARLES J. DILLMAN
JAMES R. ANDREWS

Knowledge of proper biomechanics can help in the development of rehabilitation. In particular, with an understanding of the motions and loads involved in throwing, we can determine the usefulness of different rehabilitation exercises for a throwing injury. Also, an understanding of proper mechanics can help throwers become more efficient. By becoming more efficient, the athlete should be able to minimize the chance of injury and to improve performance.

## DESCRIPTION OF THROWING MOTION

A throw is a complex and highly dynamic athletic motion. Although the exact range of motion and body segment speeds vary from athlete to athlete as well as from sport to sport, there seems to be an optimal pattern. The proper ranges of motion and timing between the different motions will lead to the most efficient throw. Although the specific kinematic parameters must be determined for each sport, this section provides a generalized description of proper throwing mechanics.

A throw can be divided into different phases[1,2] to help understand the mechanics involved, but, in fact, a throw is actually one continuous motion. Here, a throw is broken into five phases:

1. windup (or balance)
2. arm cocking
3. arm acceleration
4. arm deceleration
5. follow-through

### Windup (or Balance)

Windup is the phase with the most variability from sport to sport, because of the rules of different games. The purpose of the windup phase is to put the athlete in a good starting position to throw. The thrower, whom we assume here is right-handed, plants the back foot (right foot) on the ground and places the body perpendicular to the direction of the target so that the left side is closest to the target. In baseball, a pitcher has enough time to lift the left leg high, whereas in other sports such as football, the thrower has limited time, and the lead foot is not lifted high off the ground. Regardless of whether the leg is lifted high, the thrower should reach a balanced position (Fig. 31-1). At the balance point, the athlete has both hands together, anterior to the chest. The thrower then starts to step toward the target with the left foot and at the same time moves the arms away from each other. Except for the potential energy from lifting the lead leg, very little energy is generated in the windup phase.

355

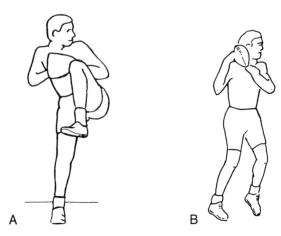

**Fig. 31-1.** Balanced body position: (**A**) for a baseball pitcher; (**B**) for an American football quarterback. (Fig. A from Dillman,[1] with permission.)

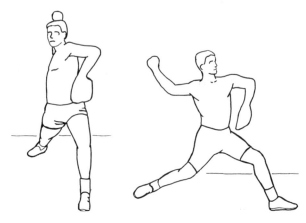

**Fig. 31-3.** Body position at foot contact for a baseball pitcher. (From Dillman,[1] with permission.)

## Arm Cocking

Arm cocking and acceleration are highly dynamic phases of throwing. The athlete generates energy in the different segments of the body and then quickly and systematically passes this energy to the ball. The proper timing and sequence of the motions involved is known as the principle of "kinetic links" to biomechanists and "coordination" to athletes and coaches.

As the arms swing apart, the front leg strides toward the target (Fig.31-2). These motions cause the upper and lower body to stretch out, creating elastic energy to drive the upper body forward in the delivery phase. To maximize the elastic energy available, the upper body should be held back as long as possible. The

stride foot lands almost directly in front of the back foot, with the lead knee flexed 45 degrees.

At foot contact, both arms should be abducted approximately 90 degrees so that both elbows are almost on a line passing through the two shoulders. The throwing arm should be flexed at the elbow and externally rotated at the shoulder (Fig. 31-3). After foot contact, the hips and then the shoulders rotate to face the target. While the hips and shoulders rotate forward, the throwing arm continues to rotate back to a position of maximum external rotation, as shown in Figure 31-4.

At the point of maximum external rotation, a great amount of energy is available to accelerate the arm forward. The energy was generated by, in order, the

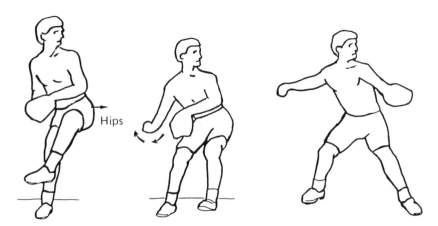

**Fig. 31-2.** Sequence of motion during stride for a baseball pitcher. (From Dillman,[1] with permission.)

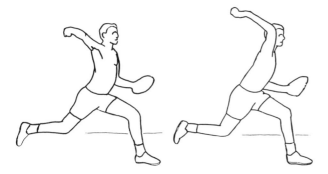

**Fig. 31-4.** Sequence of motion during arm cocking. (From Dillman,[1] with permission.)

legs, the hips, and the trunk. As the arm approaches this position of maximum external rotation, the internal rotator muscles are eccentrically loaded and also elastically stretched.

It is better to refer to this phase as the "arm cocking" rather than simply "cocking." Clearly, only the arm is "cocked" by the end of this phase; the thrower's legs, hips, and trunk have already accelerated.

## Arm Acceleration

As the arm reaches the point of maximum external rotation, the elbow begins to extend. While the arm extends at the elbow, it begins to internally rotate at the shoulder. The arm acceleration phase ends with the release of the ball (Fig 31-5). At release, the throwing shoulder should be abducted about 90 or 100 degrees, regardless of what type of ball is being thrown and the style of the individual thrower. The difference between an "overhand" and a "sidearm" baseball pitcher, for

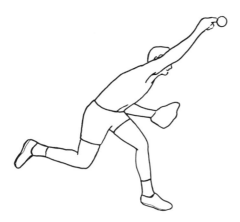

**Fig. 31-5.** Ball release. (From Dillman,[1] with permission.)

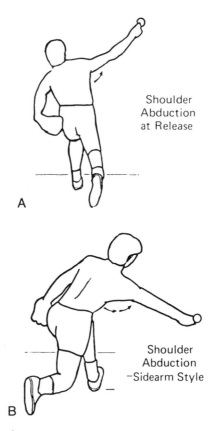

Shoulder Abduction at Release

A

Shoulder Abduction –Sidearm Style

B

**Fig. 31-6.** Comparison of pitching styles at the time of ball release. Shoulder abduction at release for (**A**) an overhand baseball pitcher and (**B**) a sidearm baseball pitcher. (From Dillman,[1] with permission.)

instance, is not the abduction at the shoulder but rather the lateral tilt of the trunk (Fig. 31-6). The biomechanics of throwing seem to indicate that approximately 90 degrees of abduction is the strongest angle for the shoulder during a throw, as well as the angle with minimal chance of impingement or other shoulder injury.

## Arm Deceleration

After ball release, the arm continues to extend at the elbow and to internally rotate at the shoulder. Because of this internal rotation, the hand appears to pronate (Fig. 31-7). During this phase, the external rotator muscles at the shoulder must decelerate the internal rotation and also prevent distraction at the glenohumeral joint. Similarly, the elbow must be decelerated before

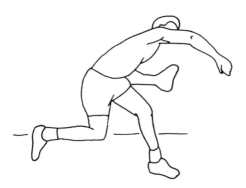

**Fig. 31-7.** Baseball pitcher during deceleration. (From Dillman,[1] with permission.)

it reaches complete extension, and distraction must also be prevented at the elbow.

## Follow-through

The importance of a good follow-through is often overlooked. Although a good follow-through cannot directly improve the throw, it is critical in minimizing the risk of injury. Most overuse injuries to the posterior side of the arm or trunk (such as supraspinatus injuries) occur during deceleration and follow-through.

All the energy generated in the body to accelerate the ball forward must be dissipated after ball release. The key to a good follow-through is to let the larger body parts help dissipate the energy in the throwing arm. This can be accomplished by flexing the trunk forward after ball release. Extension of the left knee can lead to energy absorption by the left leg (Fig. 31-8).

To reduce the deceleration force required, the throwing arm should have a long follow-through path,

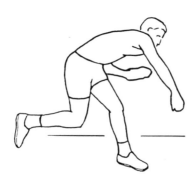

**Fig. 31-8.** Baseball pitcher during follow-through. (From Dillman,[1] with permission.)

allowing the energy to be dissipated over a longer time. With a correct follow-through, a pitcher's right hand will end up near the left leg. (An overhand pitcher's right hand should end up near the left ankle, whereas a three-quarter overhand pitcher's hand should end up near the knee. For a sidearm pitcher, the hand ends up near the left hip.) A pitcher who ends up with the hand toward the target will most likely place excessive distraction loads on the shoulder.

## QUANTITATIVE DESCRIPTION OF ARM MOTION

As mentioned in the preceding section, the throwing motion patterns are similar from one sport to another. In this section, a quantitative description of a baseball pitch is given. The data shown are based on a computer analysis of 17 healthy, successful college and professional pitchers with no history of serious arm injury, seen at the American Sports Medicine Institute. A Motion Analysis Corporation three-dimensional automatic digitizing system was used, as previously described by Wisleder et al[3] and Wick et al[4].

Pitching is one of the fastest throws known; also, it has one of the highest overuse injury rates. An understanding of proper pitching mechanics can therefore be useful not only in learning about pitching but also in learning about proper throwing in general. Because very little energy is generated in the balance phase, the graphs presented do not start until foot contact.

## Shoulder Abduction

Figure 31-9 shows the shoulder abduction during a pitch. For this and all following graphs, the horizontal scale represents time during the pitch. Data from the different pitchers are time-matched where foot contact (FC) is defined as time equal to 0 percent and ball release (REL) occurs at time equal to 100 percent. The time of maximum external rotation (MER) is also shown. The solid line represents the average value for the 17 pitchers, and the vertical bars represent the standard deviation.

From front foot contact to ball release, abduction does not vary greatly from 90 degrees. As mentioned before, this is true for pitchers of different styles, as well as for throwers of different sports.

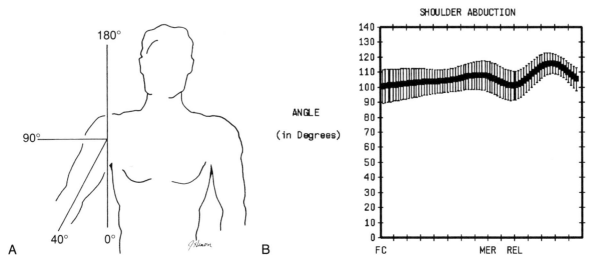

**Fig. 31-9.** Shoulder abduction: (**A**) definition of shoulder abduction; (**B**) shoulder abduction during the pitch. (Fig. A from Dillman et al.,[6] with permission.)

## Horizontal Adduction

Figure 31-10, a graph of horizontal adduction, shows that the arm stays to the side of the trunk throughout most of the pitch (i.e., horizontal adduction stays near 0 degrees). A maximum positive value of about 15 degrees is reached at the time corresponding to maximum external rotation, which is shortly before release. In other words, when the arm is externally rotated,

the elbow is slightly in front of the trunk. As the arm internally rotates, the wrist moves forward and the elbow moves backward.

## Internal/External Rotation

The largest range of motion of the shoulder is external/internal rotation. In Figure 31-11, the arm externally rotates about 180 degrees. This extreme range of mo-

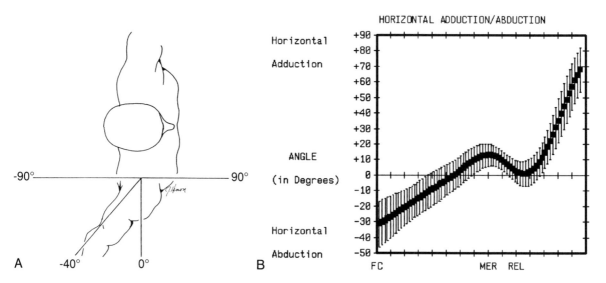

**Fig. 31-10.** Horizontal adduction: (**A**) definition of horizontal adduction; (**B**) horizontal adduction during the pitch. (Fig. A from Dillman et al.,[6] with permission.)

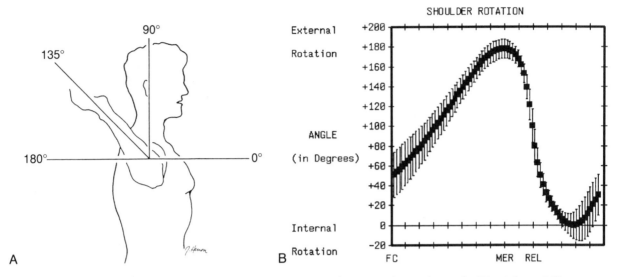

**Fig. 31-11.** (**A**) Definition of external rotation; (**B**) external rotation during the pitch. (Fig. A from Dillman et al.,[6] with permission.)

tion is partially because of the way external rotation was measured. As shown in Figure 31-11A, external rotation is defined here as the angle the forearm makes relative to the trunk. Because of this, the measured angle is the summation of many motions, including extension of the spine, scapulothoracic motion, and true external rotation (glenohumeral motion). From the position of maximum external rotation, the arm is rapidly internally rotated. The maximum internal rotation velocity, measured as the slope of the line in Figure 31-11B, is typically 7,000 degrees/s, making it one of the fastest known human motions in sports.

## Elbow Flexion/Extension

To understand the biomechanics of the shoulder, one must also look at the elbow. Figure 31-12 shows elbow flexion and extension. Notice that in this study the

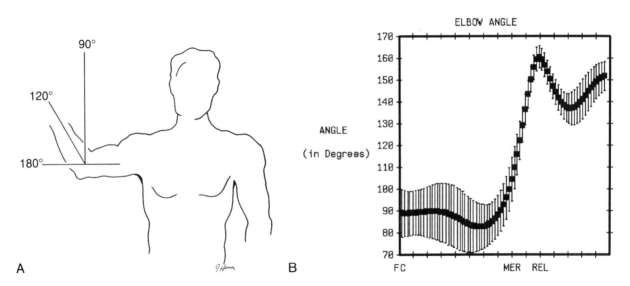

**Fig. 31-12.** (**A**) Definition of elbow angle; (**B**) elbow angle during the pitch.

elbow angle is defined as the angle between the forearm and upper arm, as shown in Figure 31-12A. The elbow should be flexed about 90 degrees from the time of foot contact to maximum external rotation. Rapid elbow extension then occurs, stopping about 20 degrees short of full extension. The maximum elbow extension velocity, measured as the slope of the line in Figure 31-12B, is typically 2,500 degrees/s.

## Kinematics for Baseball Pitchers and Football Quarterbacks

Table 31-1 shows some of the key parameters for proper pitching mechanics. It also shows the same parameters calculated for football throwing. Some variables, such as maximum internal rotation angular velocity, depend on the weight and type of ball being thrown, whereas others, such as abduction at foot contact, do not.

# QUANTITATIVE DESCRIPTION OF SHOULDER KINETICS

Besides kinematics, joint kinetics are also needed for a total understanding of the shoulder's involvement in throwing. From high-speed video data, an estimation of joint forces and torques can be calculated.[5,6] To keep the joint stable and achieve equilibrium, equal and opposite reaction forces and torques must be generated by the joint structure. If the muscles, ligaments, and tendons about the joint cannot generate the necessary forces and torques, instability or injury will occur.

## Torques at the Shoulder Joint

For the shoulder joint, the forces and torques were calculated about the three axes shown in Figure 31-13. All the kinetic graphs show the force or torque applied by the proximal body to the distal segment. Figure 31-14 shows abduction/adduction torque applied by the trunk onto the arm at the shoulder. Because there is not much movement in this direction,

**Table 31-1. Mean Values of Baseball Pitching and Football Passing Kinematic Parameters**

|  | Baseball (n = 23) | Football (n = 14) |
|---|---|---|
| Foot contact parameters (degrees) | | |
| Elbow angle[a] | 100 ± 21 | 75 ± 13 |
| Shoulder external rotation[a] | 65 ± 29 | 88 ± 36 |
| Shoulder abduction | 103 ± 13 | 105 ± 17 |
| Shoulder horizontal adduction | −11 ± 24 | −2 ± 17 |
| Lead knee angle | 132 ± 11 | 137 ± 11 |
| Delivery parameters | | |
| Angular variables (degrees) | | |
| Elbow angle at initial extension[a] | 84 ± 12 | 65 ± 9 |
| Maximum external rotation | 175 ± 12 | 168 ± 12 |
| Angular velocity parameters (degrees) | | |
| Maximum elbow extension[a] | 2,340 ± 351 | 1,716 ± 193 |
| Maximum internal rotation[a] | 7,365 ± 1,503 | 4,586 ± 843 |
| Maximum shoulder horizontal adduction | 657 ± 266 | 519 ± 165 |
| Maximum shoulder[a] | 1,180 ± 294 | 1,017 ± 177 |
| Maximum hip[a] | 662 ± 148 | 518 ± 97 |
| Trunk tilt[a] | 377 ± 76 | 260 ± 71 |
| Release parameters (degrees) | | |
| Elbow angle[a] | 156 ± 6 | 124 ± 28 |
| Shoulder external rotation[a] | 124 ± 22 | 145 ± 25 |
| Shoulder abduction[a] | 99 ± 8 | 114 ± 15 |
| Shoulder horizontal adduction[a] | 10 ± 8 | 21 ± 10 |
| Lead knee angle[a] | 138 ± 17 | 148 ± 6 |
| Trunk tilt forward[a] | 57 ± 9 | 72 ± 9 |
| Trunk tilt lateral | 117 ± 17 | 113 ± 6 |
| Ball velocity (m/s)[a] | 74 ± 5 | 446 ± 4 |
| Duration of throw (s)[a] | 0.15 ± 0.03 | 0.20 ± 0.03 |

[a] Significant difference $P \leq .05$.
(From Wick et al,[4] with permission.)

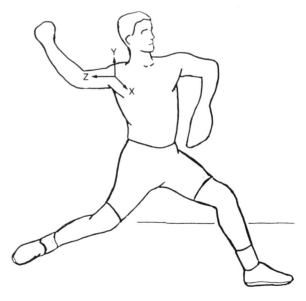

**Fig. 31-13.** Reference frame for shoulder forces and torques.

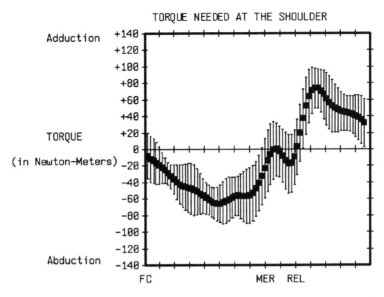

**Fig. 31-14.** Adduction/abduction torque applied onto arm by the trunk at the shoulder.

most of the abduction torque is required simply to resist gravity and keep the arm abducted. After release, an adduction torque is needed. Remember that after release the pitcher's trunk is leaning forward, as was shown in Figure 31-7. The purpose of this adduction torque, therefore, is to stop the arm from passing the flexed body and moving toward the target with excessive abduction.

Figure 31-15 shows horizontal adduction/abduction torque. A horizontal adduction torque is applied to the arm to keep it aside the trunk as the trunk rotates to face the target between the time of foot contact and

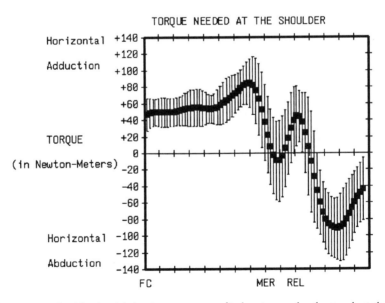

**Fig. 31-15.** Horizontal adduction/abduction torque applied onto arm by the trunk at the shoulder.

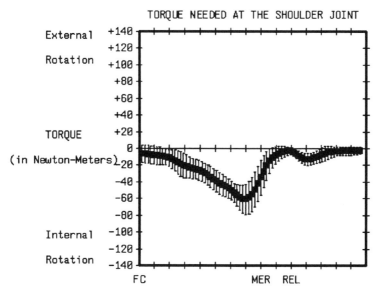

**Fig. 31-16.** Internal/external rotation torque applied onto arm by the trunk at the shoulder.

ball release. After release, the fast-moving throwing arm has a tendency to pass in front of the trunk, and an eccentric horizontal abduction torque is needed to prevent excessive horizontal adduction.

Figure 31-16 shows internal/external rotation torque. As expected, an internal rotation torque is needed to rotate the arm forward. This torque starts at about the time of foot contact and goes until the time of ball release, reaching a maximum value of 60 Nm when the arm is in maximum external rotation. Surprisingly, this graph shows no external rotation torque generated to stop the rapid internal rotation.

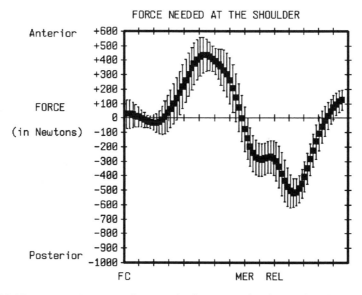

**Fig. 31-17.** Anterior/posterior force applied onto arm by the trunk at the shoulder.

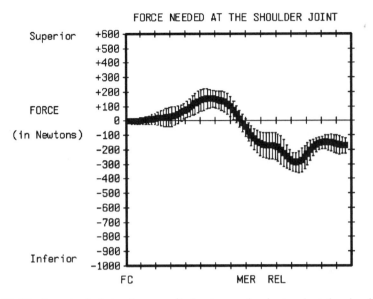

**Fig. 31-18.** Superior/inferior force applied onto arm by the trunk at the shoulder.

This is because after release the arm is nearly fully extended, as was shown in Figure 31-12. Therefore, instead of an external rotation torque, the arm is decelerated at the shoulder with a compression force, as explained in the next section.

## Forces at the Shoulder Joint

The anterior/posterior force applied by the trunk and musculature to the arm at the shoulder is shown in Figure 31-17. This graph is similar to the horizontal

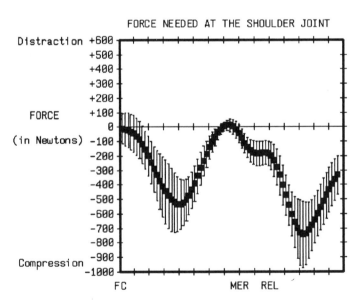

**Fig. 31-19.** Distraction/compression force applied onto arm by the trunk at the shoulder.

adduction/abduction torque curve shown in Figure 31-15. Between the time of foot contact and maximum external rotation, an anterior force is applied to the arm to move it forward with the trunk. After ball release, the arm moves in front of the trunk and a 500-N posterior force must be applied to prevent anterior subluxation at the shoulder.

Figure 31-18 shows the force applied by the trunk and shoulder musculature to the arm in the superior and inferior direction. Until the time of maximum external rotation, an upward force is needed to counterbalance the weight of the arm. After the time of maximum external rotation, the trunk is tilted forward and a force is needed in the inferior direction to resist subluxation at the shoulder joint in the superior direction.

As the body rotates between the time of foot contact and maximum external rotation, the arm has a tendency to swing to the side of the body. To prevent distraction during this time, a 500-N compressive force is applied to the arm at the shoulder, as seen in Figure 31-19. As mentioned above, the fast-moving arm moves ahead of the body after release and a large compression force, as shown in Figure 31-19, must be applied to the arm to prevent distraction. This large compression force is typically about 750 N—roughly 80 percent of the pitcher's body weight.

## IMPLICATIONS FOR THE REHABILITATION OF THE THROWER'S SHOULDER

It would be easy and convenient to look at all the loads and motions separately. Unfortunately, this does not give a realistic description of the dynamics involved at the joint. By looking at some of the more important interactions, a more practical and useful understanding of the shoulder joint can be achieved.

### Angle–Angle Interactions

Recently, many people have come to the realization that the standard isokinetic devices currently being used may not be ideal for the rehabilitation of throwers. This is due to the substantial difference between the speed and motions performed on these devices and those performed during actual throwing. With a better understanding of the kinematics of throwing, medical professionals should be able to design rehabilitative equipment more specific to throwing.

Figures 31-11 and 31-12 showed the two principal motions of the arm—internal/external rotation at the shoulder and elbow flexion/extension. Figure 31-20 shows the angle–angle interaction of these two motions. The figure shows that between the time of foot contact and maximum external rotation, the arm is externally rotated. After maximum external rotation, the arm begins to extend at the elbow, immediately followed by internal rotation at the shoulder.[5] With the arm almost fully extended at the time of release, the arm continues rapidly to internally rotate. One of the biggest problems with most current rehabilitative machines is that during internal/external rotation motion, the arm is not allowed to extend at the elbow. For the muscles and ligaments of the shoulder to be loaded correctly, the arm should move through a pattern similar to that shown in Figure 31-20.

The other main problem with current machines is their inability to approach speeds the body segments actually undergo during throwing. Figures 31-21 and 31-22 show that the maximum angular velocities for shoulder internal rotation and elbow extension are approximately 7,000 and 2,500 degrees/s, respectively. These speeds are significantly greater than those seen on conventional rehabilitative machines. Figure 31-23 shows a cross-plot of these two angular velocities during a pitch. From foot contact to maximum external rotation, minimal arm velocities are present. From maximum external rotation, the arm rapidly extends at the elbow, followed by rapid internal rotation at the shoulder. The closer a rehabilitation exercise can come to the movement patterns shown in Figures 31-20 and 31-23, the more appropriate it is for a thrower.

### Torque–Angle Interactions

Besides the magnitude, the type of joint force or torque is also of importance. Rehabilitative procedures often incorporate a combination of concentric, eccentric, and isometric exercises. Together, the graphs for shoulder rotation motion and torque (see Figures 31-11 and 31-16, respectively) show the magnitude and types of shoulder rotation torque. While the arm is

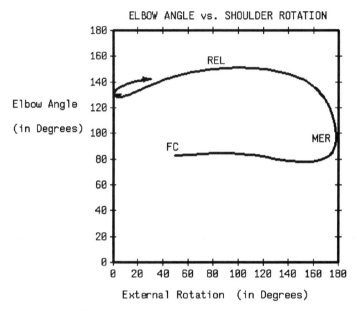

**Fig. 31-20.** Cross-plot of elbow angle versus shoulder rotation. *Arrowhead* indicates temporal direction, starting with time of foot contact.

externally rotated toward maximum external rotation, the internal rotators are eccentrically loaded. From the time of maximum external rotation to release, the arm internally rotates while the internal rotators are concentrically loaded. After release, the arm continues to rotate internally while no significant rotation torque is present; the deceleration is in the form of a compression force instead, as was shown in Figure 31-19. These torque–angle interactions should serve as a model for rehabilitative exercises.

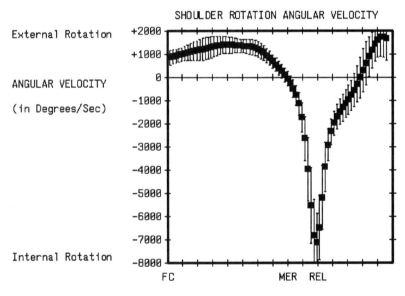

**Fig. 31-21.** Shoulder rotation angular velocity during the pitch.

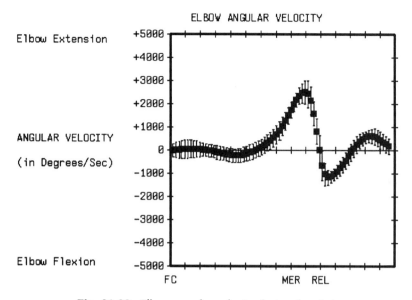

**Fig. 31-22.** Elbow angular velocity during the pitch.

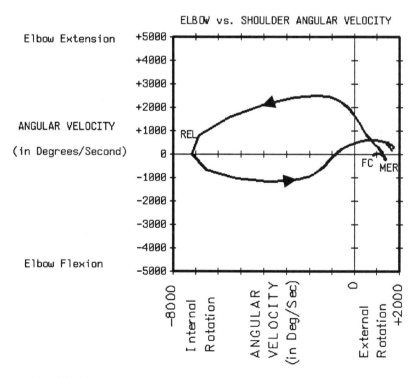

**Fig. 31-23.** Cross-plot of shoulder rotation angular velocity versus elbow angular velocity. *Arrowhead* indicates temporal direction, starting with time of foot contact (*FC*). *MER*, maximum external rotation; *REL*, ball release.

## CONCLUSIONS

Figure 31-11 shows that the arm undergoes a rapid internal rotation, followed by a rapid deceleration at the shoulder. Looking at this as an isolated motion may, however, lead to false conclusions.

A better description is the following:

1. The arm externally rotates. During this motion, the internal rotator muscles are eccentrically loaded. Also, the trunk rotates, inducing the need for more internal rotation torque at the shoulder. While the trunk rotates, a horizontal adduction torque is needed to keep the arm moving with the trunk and a compression force is needed to prevent the swinging arm from distracting at the shoulder.
2. The arm begins to extend at the elbow, immediately followed by internal rotation at the shoulder. During this time, the internal rotators continue to fire concentrically.
3. After ball release, the arm continues to internally rotate as the trunk continues to rotate. Force in the inferior, posterior, and especially compressive directions is applied to the arm to prevent distraction at the shoulder. Adduction and horizontal abduction torques are applied to the arm at the shoulder to stabilize the arm's position relative to the trunk.

For the optimum rehabilitation of a thrower, some exercises specific for throwing should be used. Before exercises can be defined, an understanding of throwing itself must be achieved. In this chapter, a general description of the throwing motion has been presented for this purpose. To design rehabilitation for a particular type of throw, a quantitative description of that throw is needed. Exercises for the rehabilitation for a baseball pitcher's shoulder, for example, should simulate motion patterns and joint loads similar to those shown in this chapter. The rehabilitation and conditioning of the throwing shoulder is dealt with more completely in the final chapters of this book.

## REFERENCES

1. Dillman CJ: Proper mechanics of pitching. Sports Med Update 5:15, 1990
2. Fleisig GS, Dillman CJ, Andrews JR: Proper mechanics for baseball pitching. Clin Sports Med 1:151, 1989
3. Wisleder D, Fleisig GS, Dillman CJ et al: Development of a biomechanical analysis of throwing with clinical applications for pitchers. Sports Med Update 4:28, 1989
4. Wick HJ, Dillman CJ, Wisleder D et al: A kinematic comparison between baseball pitching and football passing. Sports Med Update 6:13, 1991
5. Feltner M, Dapena J: Dynamics of the shoulder and elbow joints of the throwing arm during the baseball pitch. Int J Sport Biomechanics 2:235, 1986
6. Dillman CJ, Fleisig GS, Werner SL, Andrews JR: Biomechanics of the shoulder in sports: Throwing activities. Postgrad Adv Sports Med. Forum Medicum, Inc, Berryville, VA, 1991

# Injuries in Baseball

√DREWS
ILK

,or part of injuries.
Yogi Berra

.tremendous demands placed on the shoul-
.nplex during the throwing motion. Throwing
is a skilled movement that requires excessive motion,
precise coordinated movement, and a synchronized
muscle firing pattern, all of which must occur at a
velocity faster than that of any other movement.[1,2] To
accomplish this difficult task, the shoulder must have
a tremendous amount of passive and dynamic motion
(Fig. 32-1). Although excessive motion is required for
throwing, the shoulder complex must still maintain
stability of the glenohumeral joint. The joint stability
required during throwing is accomplished through its
capsular ligamentous restraints and also by the dynamic contributions of the shoulder's neuromuscular
control system.

During the throwing act, the glenohumeral joint receives excessive violent stresses, which often lead to
different injuries. Angular velocities of the shoulder
joint during the acceleration phase of throwing have
been documented to exceed 7,000 degrees/s[1] (Fig. 32-
2). During this phase, the anterior translatory stress
placed on the glenohumeral joint can reach half the
thrower's body weight.[1] After ball release, deceleration
of the arm occurs, requiring vigorous posterior shoulder musculature contractions to slow the arm down
(Fig. 32-2). During this deceleration phase, the posterior shoulder muscles contract eccentrically to counteract a glenohumeral joint distraction force equal to
one times the body weight of the thrower.[1]

To facilitate the acceleration forces required during
throwing, excessive glenohumeral joint laxity is required during the cocking phase to prestretch the anterior shoulder musculature. The thrower often exhibits
in excess of 125 degrees of passive external rotation.

Because of this excessive motion seen in the thrower,
the muscular system must be capable of providing
dynamic glenohumeral joint stability. This dynamic stability is accomplished through the combined stabilizing contractions of the rotator cuff musculature and
the long head of the biceps.[3] Often when the stresses
involved in throwing exceed the capability of the muscular system to control these stresses, injury results.
This can occur due to improper mechanics, poor dynamic stability, and/or muscular fatigue. A frequent
injury-producing scenario for the throwing athlete includes the combination of abnormal high stresses that
are repeatedly applied to normal tissue, eventually resulting in tissue failure. This can be referred to as an
acquired type of repetitive microtrauma.

This chapter briefly discusses some of the common
shoulder injuries seen in the throwing athlete (Table
32-1). In the previous chapter, a thorough discussion
of the biomechanics of throwing was performed. Thus,
only specific references are made to specific biomechanics as they relate to different shoulder injuries.

## ROTATOR CUFF INJURIES

The rotator cuff is vital for normal shoulder function,
especially in the throwing athlete. It controls the movement of the humeral head and, along with the long
head of biceps, serves to steer it during different activities. The larger muscles of the shoulder are the prime
movers, which are the pectoralis major, latissimus
dorsi, and deltoid. The smaller muscles are classified
as the stabilizing muscles. These include the rotator
cuff muscles, which function to compress the humeral

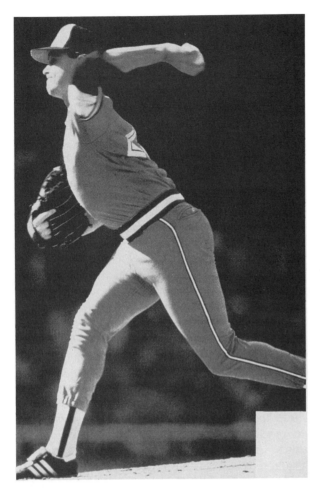

**Fig. 32-1.** During the cocking phase of throwing, the shoulder exhibits a tremendous amount of external rotation. (From Sports Illustrated, with permission.)

head into the glenoid fossa and are dynamic stabilizers.[4–6] It is this compression of the articulating surfaces that affords stability to the glenohumeral joint during the throwing motion. The subscapular and teres minor/infraspinatus muscles form a vital force couple that controls humeral head translation.[7,8] The high demands placed on the shoulder musculature during throwing may result in subsequent muscle fatigue, eccentric overload, inflammation, and eventual tendon failure. Once the rotator cuff musculature has been injured, the dynamic stabilizing ability is compromised, and additional injuries such as labral tears, capsular lesions, and osseous changes may ensue. Poor mechanics often results from this type of chronic inflammation,

producing a compensatory mechanism in the throwing act that may contribute to the injury-producing scenario. These repetitive muscular strains may result in overuse tendonitis of the rotator cuff.

*Overuse tendonitis* is commonly seen in the posterior rotator cuff muscles, the infraspinatus, and the teres minor. This occurs due to the large stress placed on the shoulder joint during the deceleration phase of throwing. As previously mentioned, the stresses applied to the posterior rotator cuff musculature effectively exceeds one times the body weight during this phase of throwing. Weakness or fatigue of the external rotators decreases the muscular efficiency required to decelerate the throwing shoulder properly leading to muscular fatigue that can result in tissue damage (Fig. 32-3). A decrease in the efficiency of the infraspinatus and teres minor muscles will affect the effectiveness of the subscapular, teres minor, and infraspinatus force couple; and humeral head translation will increase (Figs. 32-4 and 32-5). Before musculotendinous inflammation, the posterior glenohumeral capsule often becomes inflamed, which appears to act as a precursor to posterior rotator cuff tendonitis. This inflamed capsule is referred to as posterior capsulitis.

A common rotator cuff pathology seen in the thrower is a tensile lesion of the undersurface of the rotator cuff. The mechanism of injury in this instance is deceleration of the arm as the rotator cuff attempts to resist

**Table 32-1. Shoulder Injuries in Baseball**

Primary rotator cuff injuries
    Primary lesions
    Overuse tendinitis
    Tensile failure
    Compression cuff disease
    Rotator cuff tears
Secondary rotator cuff lesions
    Tensile failure secondary to laxity
    Compressive cuff disease secondary to laxity
Primary instability (nontraumatic)
    Anterior instability
    Posterior instability
    Multidirectional instability
Glenoid labral tears
Thrower's exostosis
Biceps tendon pathology
    Bicipital tendonitis
    Rupture/tears
Acromioclavicular joint degenerative changes
Suprascapular nerve entrapment
Neurovascular syndromes
Scapula disorders

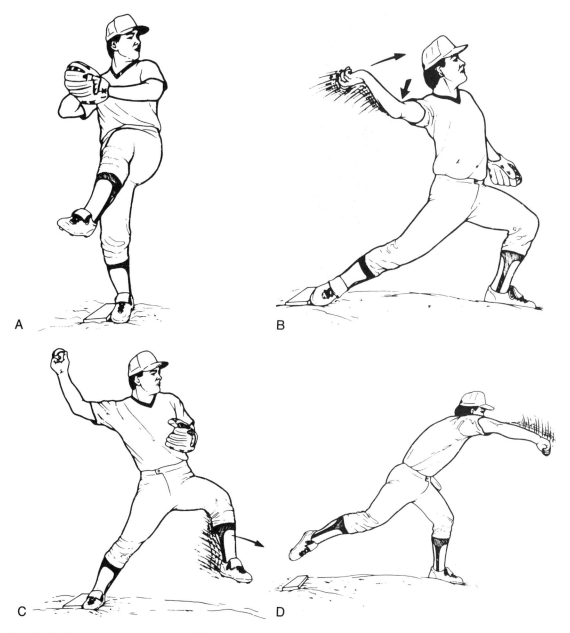

**Fig. 32-2.** Five phases of throwing: **(A)** windup, **(B)** cocking, **(C)** acceleration, **(D)** deceleration, and follow-through.

the horizontal adduction, internal rotation, and glenohumeral distraction forces placed on it. Combined, these forces result in an eccentric tensile overload failure and a partial undersurface tear of the rotator cuff caused by repetitive microtrauma.[9,10] Most commonly,

these lesions are found in the region of the supraspinatus tendon and may extend posteriorly into the infraspinatus tendon. Also, these tears may be found isolated to the infraspinatus tendon and the posterior glenohumeral capsule.

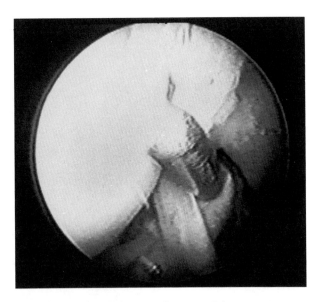

**Fig. 32-3.** Arthroscopic visualization of the posterior capsule. Note the fraying and capsular failure of the undersurface of the posterior capsule.

On physical examination, tenderness may be elicited over the supraspinatus and/or infraspinatus tendon. Obvious gross weakness of the rotator cuff usually is not present, especially in the highly skilled thrower. If weakness is present, it is most frequently found during

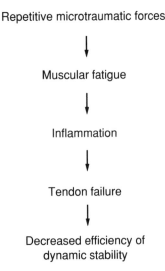

Repetitive microtraumatic forces

↓

Muscular fatigue

↓

Inflammation

↓

Tendon failure

↓

Decreased efficiency of
dynamic stability

**Fig. 32-4.** Repetitive microtraumatic forces lead to decreased efficiency of dynamic stability.

isokinetic testing of the external rotators in the 90 degree shoulder abducted position.[11] Palpation of the infraspinatus, teres minor, and posterior capsule can be helpful (Fig. 32-6). Computerized tomography (CT) or magnetic resonance imaging (MRI) may reveal a partial undersurface tear of the rotator cuff. Initially, the athlete should be placed on a rehabilitation program with emphasis on rotator cuff strengthening. If no improvement is made over a period of 3 to 6 months, an arthroscopy may be performed to debride the injured tissue and to attempt to promote a healing response.[9,12] After this procedure, an aggressive rotator cuff strengthening program must be used to minimize the risk of recurrence and maximize a return to symptom-free function. This program should emphasize eccentric strenthening of the posterior rotator cuff musculature.

Another primary rotator cuff pathology seen in the throwing athlete is that of compressive rotator cuff disease.[13] This can be a primary pathology when it is associated with a type III hooked acromion,[14] os acromiale,[15,16] degenerative acromial spurs,[17] or congenital thickening of the coracoacromial ligament.[10] Also, it can be caused by an inflamed and thickened subacromial bursa.[13] Compressive rotator cuff disease results in an "outside" type of rotator cuff tear, where the failure begins on the outer surface of the cuff and progresses inward. In contrast, the tensile overload lesion results in an "inside-out" type of rotator cuff injury.

The throwing motion requires the arm to be abducted to 90 degrees while being repetitively submitted to horizontal adduction and internal rotation motions. This repetitive motion may produce impingement symptoms.[18] Often the thrower complains of shoulder pain during activity and especially after prolonged throwing. Once the lesion becomes more severe, pain may be present during all throwing activities.

An injection of 1 percent lidocaine into the subacromial space that relieves all symptoms helps to confirm this diagnosis. Other clinical tests performed to determine the degree of involvement and differential diagnosis are specific impingement tests (Fig. 32-7). Most athletes respond successfully to a conservative program of active rest, nonsteroidal anti-inflammatory medication, and a progressive rotator cuff strengthening and stretching exercise program. In the thrower, often external rotation is excessive and internal rota-

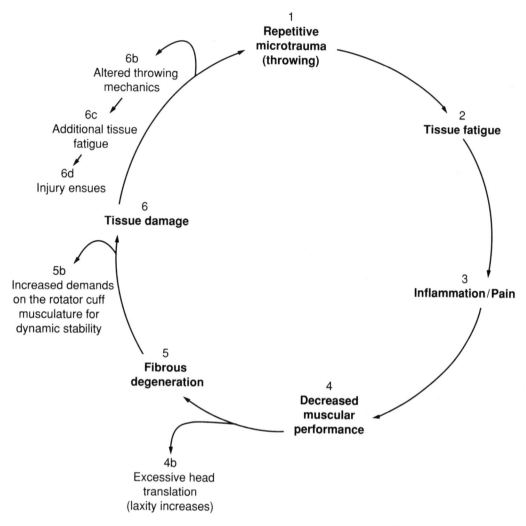

**Fig. 32-5.** Weakness or fatigue of the external rotators decreases the muscular efficiency required to decelerate the throwing shoulder, leading to muscular fatigue and tissue damage.

tion is significantly limited.[9] This limitation of internal rotation results in posterior capsular tightness, which causes the humeral head to migrate anteriorly during overhead motion.[13] The mainstays of any conservative rehabilitation program should include stretching of the posterior capsule, re-establishing normal internal rotation, and gradual aggressive strengthening of the rotator cuff musculature.[19] If the athlete's symptoms are not relieved by nonoperative measures, surgical treatment may be warranted. The surgical treatment most often performed is an arthroscopic examination to determine the structures involved and the integrity of the rotator cuff.

Full-thickness rotator cuff tears are unusual in the throwing athlete. These are usually seen late in the deterioration process of the shoulder.[20-22] This type of degenerative process begins with a small partial-thickness rotator cuff tear, which may eventually progress to a complete-thickness tear. Tears of this type can enlarge by additional trauma placed on the rotator cuff tendons during activities. Full-thickness rotator cuff tears are usually seen in older athletes; however, occa-

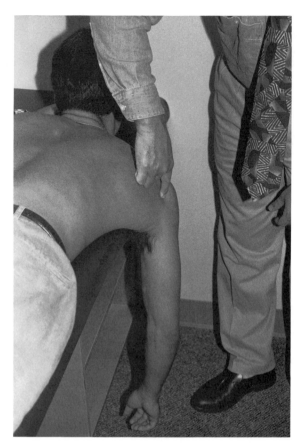

**Fig. 32-6.** Palpation of the infraspinatus, teres minor, and posterior capsule can be accomplished with the patient prone and arm hanging over the side of the examination table. This tractions the arm and allows the clinician to differentiate the various tissues accurately.

sionally, they can occur in the younger thrower (JR Andrews, personal communications). The authors have seen several throwers in the past few years who have exhibited full-thickness tears of the supraspinatus muscle (JR Andrews, personal communications).

Early recognition and treatment may prevent the progression of a partial-thickness tear to a full-thickness rotator cuff tear. Once a full-thickness tear occurs, throwing is often difficult, if possible at all. Significant weakness can be seen of the shoulder's abductors and external rotators. Often a repair of the rotator cuff is necessary to allow symptom-free return to normal daily activities.[10] The surgical procedure of choice to repair

a rotator cuff tear in a thrower uses a deltoid-splitting technique that minimizes the morbidity of the deltoid muscle. This procedure appears to allow an earlier return to functional activities and an accelerated rehabilitation program.

## SHOULDER INSTABILITY

The throwing motion requires excessive glenohumeral external rotation, which places extreme tension on the anterior stabilizing structures of the glenohumeral joint and especially the rotator cuff musculature. The identification of shoulder laxity compared with frank instability is often difficult to assess clinically. The concept of laxity is the ability of the humeral head to be passively translated on the glenoid,[23] whereas instability is a clinical condition in which unwanted translation of the humeral head on the glenoid compromises the comfort and function of the shoulder.[23] The throwing athlete must exhibit laxity to perform high-performance throwing activities. However, the rotator cuff musculature must control this laxity dynamically for symptom-free throwing. Instability ensues when the dynamic stability is altered and the rotator cuff muscles are unable to control humeral head motion within the glenoid during activities.

The previously discussed rotator cuff pathologies (compressive cuff disease and tensile failure) can occur as an indirect result of instability. Jobe et al[24,25] provided a classification to evaluate athletes presenting with this type of anterior shoulder pain.

Group I      Athletes with pure impingement
Group II     Athletes who have instability secondary to anterior ligament and labral injury with secondary impingement
Group III    Athletes who exhibit instability due to hyperelasticity and secondary impingement
Group IV     Athletes who demonstrate pure instability

In the thrower, instability is a common problem. The shoulder must be loose enough to allow the tremendous motion necessary to throw a baseball but must be tight enough to provide inherent stability. Shoulder instability is restricted by the static stabilizers, the geometry of the joint, and the ligamentous system

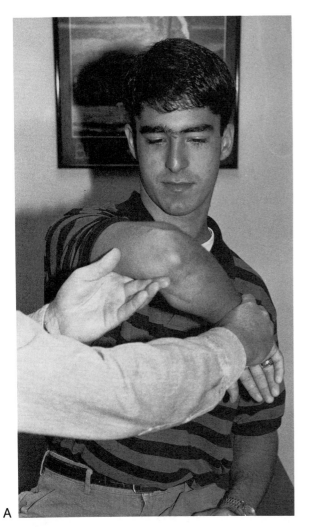

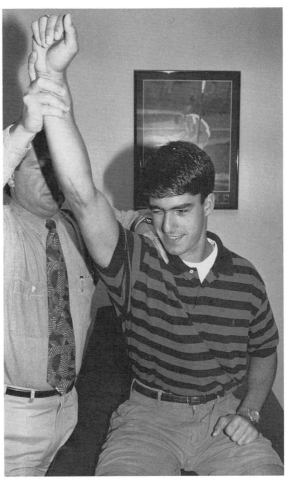

A                                                                                                 B

**Fig. 32-7.** Two clinical provocative tests for compressive cuff pathology. **(A)** Clinician passively elevates arm to 90 to 100 degrees while horizontally adducting and internally rotating arm. **(B)** Clinician passively elevates arm with internal rotation while stabilizing scapulae.

and labrum. The capsular ligaments act as a buttress to restrict humeral head translation. Repetitive overhead throwing often results in stretching of these capsular restraints and may lead to joint capsule injury. As the capsule becomes more lax, the glenohumeral joint depends on an increase in the dynamic muscular effort to provide the required functional stability required. If the dynamic stabilizers fail because of overuse, injury, or pain, underlying primary instability will result.

During the cocking and early acceleration phases of throwing, the anterior and inferior portions of the joint capsule are significantly stressed in a repeated fashion. The anteroinferior glenohumeral ligament (anterior band) provides the static stabilization for this anterior force applied with the shoulder abducted to 90 degrees[26] (Fig. 32-8). The dynamic stability required to supplement the anteroinferior glenohumeral ligament is provided through a rotator cuff muscular contraction

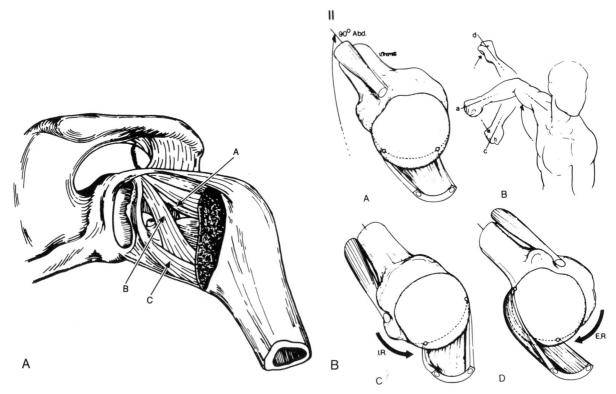

**Fig. 32-8.** **(A)** Three bands of the anterior glenohumeral ligament: (*A*) superior, (*B*) middle, and (*C*) inferior. **(B)** Note the role of the anterior band of the inferior glenohumeral ligament as the arm is abducted and externally rotated (*ER*) (*D, d*). This band acts as a buttress and restricts anterior humeral head translation *IR*, internal rotation. (Fig. B from O'Brien,[26] with permission.)

on both sides of the shoulder. Also, the inferior glenohumeral ligament complex is prone to considerable plastic deformation before ultimate failure occurs.[27] As shoulder laxity increases, labral changes commonly occur. In time, the thrower may develop a "loose shoulder joint." Because of this ensuing looseness, the thrower must rely on dynamically controlled stability and, thus, may be predisposed to overuse musculotendinous injuries, such as secondary tensile failure and/or compressive cuff disease.

Anterior instability is especially common in the thrower. The thrower may complain of anterior shoulder pain, especially during the late cocking and acceleration phases. Also, the thrower may notice clicking, popping, or early arm fatigue with competitive activities. The thrower may complain of anterior shoulder pain or posterior shoulder pain. Several clinical tests are routinely performed to determine the degree of anterior humeral head translation on the glenoid. Anterior laxity is determined with the use of a drawer test (Lachmann's test of the shoulder) (Fig. 32-9), fulcrum test (Fig. 32-10), or a relocation test (Fig. 32-11). Routinely, these tests are performed at 0, 45, and 90 degrees of shoulder abduction to test the specific bands of the anterior glenohumeral ligament. Anterior translation testing at 0 degrees of shoulder abduction tests the integrity of the superior band of the anterior glenohumeral ligament, 45 degrees of shoulder abduction tests the middle anterior glenohumeral ligament, and 90 degrees primarily the inferior anterior glenohumeral ligament.

Posterior instability also is frequently seen in the thrower. This occurs during the deceleration and follow-through phases of throwing when the arm horizontally adducts and internally rotates. During this motion, the posterior capsule is stressed and posterior labral injuries may also occur. Stretching of the posterior capsule in this fashion irritates and inflames the and neuromuscular control. Once the athlete's shoulder pain has subsided, a gradual return to throwing may begin. An example of an interval throwing program can be found in Chapter 52. If a conservative program is unsuccessful after 2 to 3 months, a surgical procedure may be warranted. An athlete with moderate-to-severe laxity and functional instability may require an arthroscopic or open stabilization procedure.

If an early Bankart lesion is present, an arthroscopic repair may be performed as described by Caspari,[28,29] Johnson,[30] Morgan and Bodenstab,[31] and Altchek et al.[32] Often an open stabilization procedure is required, using some form of a capsulolabral reconstruction or

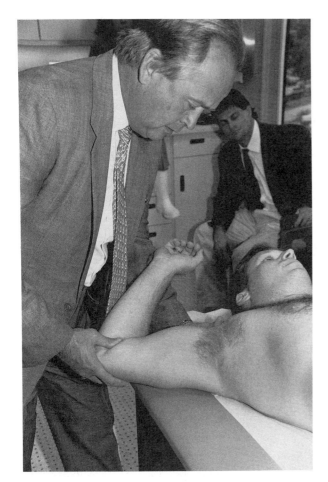

**Fig. 32-9.** Anterior drawer test to determine anterior glenohumeral joint laxity. The humeral head is passively translated on the glenoid at 0, 45, and 90 degrees of elevation.

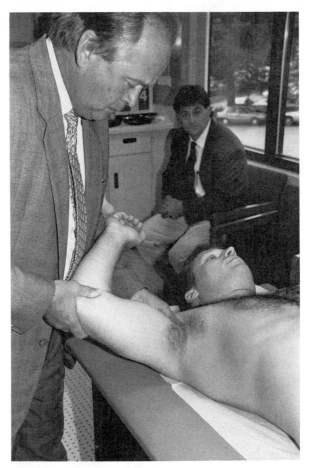

**Fig. 32-10.** Anterior fulcrum test. The arm is placed into abduction and external rotation. The distal hand horizontally abducts the humerus as the joint line head lifts up on the humerus.

capsule, which results in pain and inhibition of the posterior rotator cuff musculature. This muscular inhibition, if unaddressed, eventually results in tendon fatigue and microfailure, besides increased instability. Clinically, posterior instability can be determined through a posterior drawer test and a posterior fulcrum test. These tests are usually performed at 45 and 90 degrees of shoulder abduction.

Most athletes exhibiting glenohumeral laxity without associated labral pathology can be treated with a conservative treatment program. The program consists of temporarily decreasing the stresses from throwing, normalizing the motion of the shoulder, and improving the dynamic stability through muscular strengthening

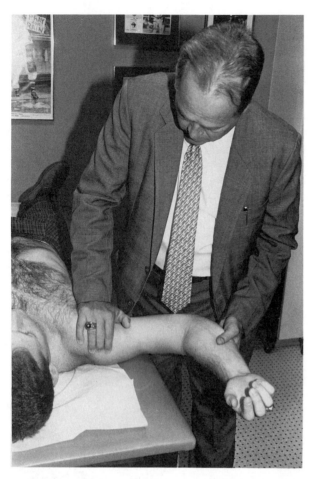

**Fig. 32-11.** The anterior relocation test for anterior instability. The arm is placed in 90 degrees abduction and maximum external rotation. If painful the opposite applies; a posterior force is applied to relocate the humeral head with the glenoid, and pain should diminish.

a capsular shift, either on the humeral or glenoid side.[25,33] In the throwing athlete, we perform a procedure referred to as a "mini-capsular shift" with or without a Bankart procedure. This mini-shift procedure is a lesser version of a capsular shift and may minimize tissue involvement. This technique uses a T incision into the glenohumeral capsule, and a longitudinal fiber-splitting incision of the subscapularis is used to gain exposure to the capsule (Fig. 32-12). After any type of surgical procedure to the throwing shoulder, an extensive and aggressive rehabilitation program must ensue for a prolonged period of time.

## GLENOID LABRAL TEARS

Glenoid labral tears are frequently seen in the throwing athlete.[34,35] During the throwing motion, the glenohumeral joint receives large compressive and shear forces, as well as distraction forces, during the movement of the humeral head anteriorly to posteriorly during the phases of throwing. These large compressive and shear forces may result in injury to the labral structure. These result in degenerative tears, frank tears, or labral detachments from the glenoid.

A common location for labral tears is in the anterosuperior portion, where the long head of the biceps attaches. During the deceleration and follow-through phase of throwing, the biceps acts at the elbow joint to decelerate the arm, slowing the extensor movement. Because of the large stabilizing muscle activity of the biceps across the glenohumeral joint, an avulsion tear of the biceps or of the biceps-labrum insertion can result.[34] Andrews and Carson[34] reported on 73 athletes with labral tears, 83 percent of whom were found to have an anterosuperior tear. After arthroscopic debridement, 88 percent exhibited a good to excellent result at an average of 13.5 months postexcision.

A frequently seen labral tear in the throwing athlete is the posterior or posterosuperior labral tear. During the follow-through phase, the humeral head translates posteriorly and may cause degenerative tearing of the labrum. Another type of labral lesion is the SLAP lesion.[36] The term *SLAP* refers to a superior labrum tear anterior and posterior in location. Snyder et al[36] classified SLAP lesions into four different types: type I, the superior labrum is frayed, no detachment; type II, the superior labrum is frayed, and the superior labrum is detached; type III, a bucket-handle tear of the labrum, labral-biceps attachments remains intact; type IV, similar to the type III, however, the labral tear extends into the biceps tendon, allowing it to sublux into the joint. It appears that SLAP lesions, posterior labral tears, and some anterior labral tears may be the result of an underlying and primary instability of the glenohumeral joint. Labral tears (other than biceps avulsion) are the result of abnormal translations of the humeral head; thus, if a labral tear is present, the clinician must carefully evaluate and treat the shoulder for instability.[37] CT-arthrography has been shown to be an accurate and noninvasive technique for evaluating the glenoid labrum.[38,39] The treatment for glenoid labral tears with-

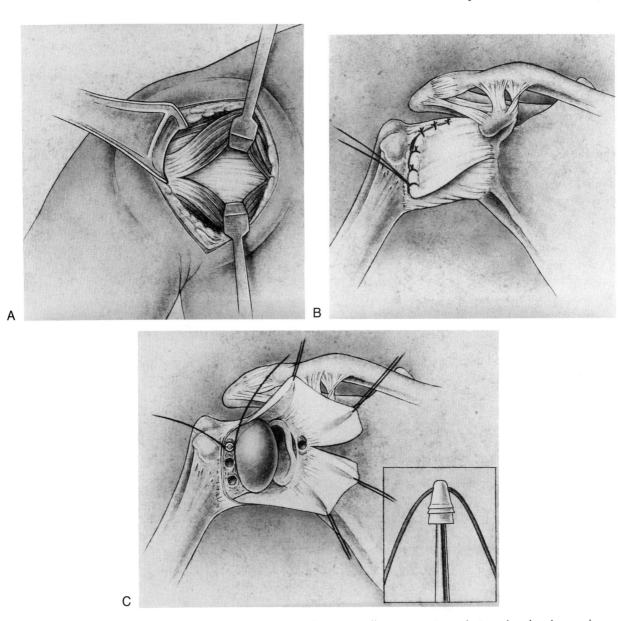

**Fig. 32-12. (A–C)** Mini-anterior capsular shift procedure. A smaller incision is made into the glenohumeral ligamentous capsule, and the shift is carried out. This procedure is commonly performed in the presence of a Bankart repair.

out glenohumeral instability is excision of the torn labrum followed by a gradual rehabilitation process and gradual return to throwing.

## THROWER'S EXOSTOSIS: "BENNETT'S LESION"

The throwing athlete who experiences persistent posterior shoulder pain may exhibit a calcification of the posteroinferior glenohumeral capsule often termed a *thrower's exostosis*. First described by Bennett in 1941,[40] this exostosis is normally located at approximately the 8 o'clock position on the right glenoid rim. This is probably a secondary reaction associated with repeated microtrauma and tearing of the posterior and inferior capsule from its glenoid insertion.[40] For years, it was believed this exostosis was a calcification of the long head of the triceps; however, on surgical inspection by the senior author (James R. Andrews), this has not been found to be true in most cases. This pathology is easily seen on plain radiographs, especially the Styker view (Fig. 32-13), and treatment is usually symptomatic relief. If pain and dysfunction persists, arthroscopic excision may be necessary.

## BICEPS BRACHII TENDON PATHOLOGY

The role of the biceps brachii during throwing is not fully understood. Jobe et al[41] reported modest biceps activity during the cocking and acceleration phase but a high level of biceps activity during the follow-through phase. During this later phase, it is believed the biceps role is in deceleration of the elbow joint. Because of the eccentric deceleration action of the biceps brachii, overuse tendinitis of the long head may occur. Also, anterosuperior shoulder stability may be enhanced and assisted by biceps activity, especially during the throwing movement. Therefore, both activities place considerable stress on the biceps musculotendinous unit and may lead to inflammation of the biceps.

If the stress is significant and applied repetitively in nature, tendon failure, biceps fraying, and/or splitting may occur. We have observed this in many throwers, an obvious split in the long head of the biceps (Fig. 32-14A). The diagnosis of biceps tendinitis is made on clinical examination through palpation, resisted muscle testing, and special tests. Palpation of the biceps tendon can be effectively performed with the patient supine, the shoulder abducted and the forearm fully

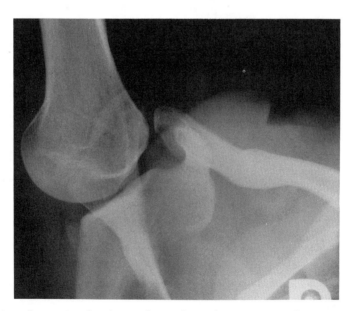

**Fig. 32-13.** Calcification of posterior glenohumeral capsule can be seen on a Styker view with plain radiograph.

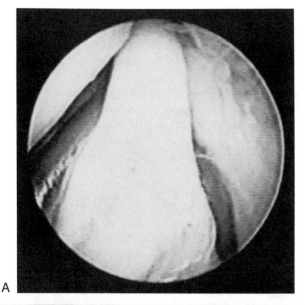

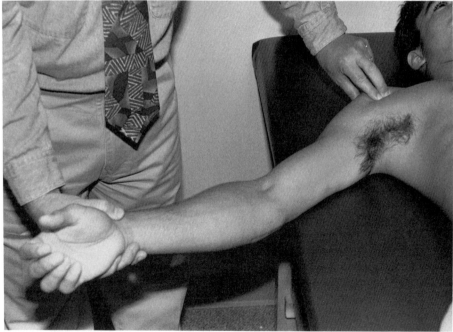

**Fig. 32-14. (A)** Arthroscopic visualization of biceps brachii tendon (long head); note fraying of the tendon and split in the tendon. **(B)** Palpation of long head of biceps brachii. Patient is supine, arm abducted approximately 45 to 60 degrees, shoulder rotated internally 30 degrees, and full forearm supination. This position clears biceps tendon from the coracoacromial arch.

supinated, and the shoulder internally rotated 30 degrees (Fig. 32-14B). This clears the biceps tendon from the coracoacromial arch, places the biceps tendon on stretch, and places the bicipital groove facing directly superiorly. The Speed's test is performed by flexing the shoulder against resistance while the elbow is extended and supinated.[42] A positive test localizes pain within the bicipital groove. The Yergasson sign is positive when biceps pain is elicited from supination against resistance with the elbow flexed.[43] MRI has proved a valuable tool in determining fluid around the tendon that may indicate inflammation of the biceps or a tear of the tendon.[44] Whatever its role in throwing, we believe the biceps should be emphasized in an appropriate exercise program using concentric and eccentric muscle contractions to control the rapid elbow extension moment during the follow-through phase.

## ACROMIOCLAVICULAR JOINT DISORDERS

Injuries to the acromioclavicular joint can occur in the throwing athlete. Sprains of the acromioclavicular joint in the thrower usually are caused by a fall or a blow to the lateral acromion. Rockwood[45] classified acromioclavicular joint sprain into six types. In the throwing athlete, most sprains are of type I or II, or minimally displaced joint. The type III acromioclavicular sprain with rupture of the coracoacromial and acromioclavicular ligaments with displacement presents a significant challenge to the physician treating the throwing athlete. On occasion, surgical intervention is considered earlier in the course of treatment for the throwing athlete compared with the general population. Fortunately, these sprains are rare in the baseball thrower.

Most acromioclavicular joint injuries in the baseball player consist of degenerative joint changes. Because of longitudinal shear and compressive forces imparted from the distal clavicle to the acromium during throwing or weight training, degenerative joint changes can occur. These changes include bony spurs, osteolysis, and osteophyte formation. The athlete usually complains of a dull ache or pain over the acromioclavicular joint. Conservative treatment is tried initially, consisting of nonsteroidal anti-inflammatory medication, physical therapy, modification of physical activity, and finally

steroid injection into the joint. If this fails, open or arthroscopic debridement of the joint may be performed by a direct superior approach. If there exists concomitant subacromial space impingement, this procedure along with a subacromial decompression is performed from below. This technique is often best performed arthroscopically. This minimizes the acromioclavicular joint dissection when compared with an open procedure. Also, the arthroscopic debridement allows a more accelerated rehabilitation process.

## NEUROVASCULAR SYNDROMES

Neurovascular syndromes are infrequently seen in the throwing athlete. The syndrome occasionally seen in the thrower is often referred to as thoracic outlet syndrome. This is a complex syndrome with diffuse, inconsistent signs and symptoms caused by compression of the nerves and vessels of the upper extremity as they pass through bony and soft tissue passageways. The three most common sites for compression of the neurovascular structures are the interscalene triangle, costoclavicular space, and in the area posterior to the pectoralis minor.[46] There are other causes for compression such as a seventh cervical rib,[46] an anomalous band,[47] and variations in the formation of muscles and vessels; but the aforementioned areas of compression are more commonly seen in the thrower.

The throwing athlete often exhibits muscular tightness of the pectoralis minor and/or the anterior and middle scalene muscles. Tightness of these muscles can cause direct compression of the neurovascular structures as they pass through the interscalene triangle or beneath the pectoralis minor. Indirectly, neurovascular compression may result via this muscular tightness because of a structural repositioning of the first rib. Thus, the throwing athlete should consistently perform a stretching program for the scalene muscles and the pectoralis minor. Also, insufficiency of the scapular suspensory muscles may contribute to this syndrome.[48] Adequate strength and flexibility of the upper trapezius, middle trapezius, rhomboids, levator scapulae, and lower trapezius are required to stabilize the scapulae adequately. Injury to the shoulder girdle muscles that produces local hemorrhage, muscle spasm, and altered shoulder girdle mechanics may also lead to neurovascular compression.

The diagnosis of this pathology is difficult because of the nonspecific inconsistent signs and symptoms localized by the thrower. Often they will complain of a dead or tired arm, numbness, weakness, a fullness or tightness in the arm, or/and a sudden change in throwing velocity. The presenting symptoms of this syndrome can be confused with shoulder instability, ulnar nerve neuropathy, rotator cuff injury, or cervical disc pathology. The diagnosis is most often made from an exhaustive workup that includes plain radiographs, electrophysiologic studies, arteriograms, and venographies. These tests are used because of the poor reliability of specific provocational tests such as the Adson maneuver.[47,49]

The clinician treating the overhead athlete is encouraged to evaluate systematically all the structures that may cause neurovascular compression. A program emphasizing stretching and strengthening of the involved structures and postural correction is often adequate in treating symptoms produced by these neurovascular syndromes. Flexibility of the scalenes, pectoralis minor, and major muscles is extremely valuable. Also, adequate posteral strength of the middle, lower trapezius, rhomboids, posterior deltoid, and levator scapulae muscles are critical in the treatment of any neurovascular syndrome of the shoulder.

## SUPRASCAPULAR NERVE ENTRAPMENT

Suprascapular nerve entrapment is a rare clinical entity and probably accounts for less than 0.4 percent of shoulder diagnoses in patients with shoulder pain.[50] The suprascapular nerve supplies both supraspinatus and infraspinatus muscles. When this nerve is compromised, there is significant atrophy of the supraspinatus and infraspinatus muscles, and the superior scapular fossa appears hollow (Fig. 32-15).

The pathomechanics of superscapular nerve entrapment can be classified into two main categories: traction injuries and compression injuries. Traction injuries can occur at the suprascapular notch as a result of excessive scapular depression or forced adduction of the upper arm. The nerve becomes "kinked" by the superior transverse scapular ligament as it passes through the scapular notch. Two other possible sites of traction injuries are the spinoglenoid notch and

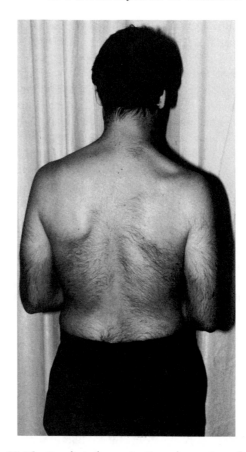

**Fig. 32-15.** On clinical examination, observation of posterior scapula indicates a hollowing of superior and inferior fossa. This indicates significant atrophy of supraspinatus and infraspinatus muscles and may be indicative of suprascapular nerve entrapment.

where the nerve inserts into the mobile infraspinatus muscle. Traction injuries at these sites appear to be caused by excessive external rotation of the arm, which places tension on the terminal portion of the suprascapular nerve. These traction-type injuries usually result in atrophy of both the supraspinatus and infraspinatus muscles.

There are several locations for suprascapular nerve compression: One of the most common sites is at the suprascapular notch by the superior transverse scapular ligament.[50,51] Other causes of compression may involve the inferior transverse scapular ligament, a congenital stenotic suprascapular notch,[52] or extrinsic masses.[53]

Often this diagnosis is overlooked because of the subtle weakness the athlete exhibits on clinical examination and because other muscles often compensate for the involved muscles. The athlete may initially complain of a poorly localized posterior shoulder girdle pain that is vague and aching in quality. The cross-arm adduction test causes tension on the suprascapular nerve and may be a provocative test in reproducing symptoms.[54] The thrower may also exhibit localized tenderness over the posterior rotator cuff musculature. The use of electromyelogram, nerve conduction velocity tests, and MRI scan is helpful in determining the site of the lesion. Once diagnosed, the treatment is focused on strengthening the infraspinatus and supraspinatus muscles and the scapular stabilizing muscles. The flexibility of the scapulothoracic articulation and glenohumeral joint are also emphasized. Occasionally, surgical dissection of the nerve is required to improve the nerve mobility about the soft tissue.

The authors have observed this pathology on several occasions in professional baseball pitchers. On isokinetic evaluation, their strength parameters were all within acceptable ranges. All the pitchers observed with this pathology pitched without difficulty or altered mechanics. They presented in clinic with symptomatic complaints of pain without obvious functional deficits. This diagnosis is often difficult to differentiate.

## SCAPULA DISORDERS

The scapula plays a vital role in the throwing athlete. The scapula functions as the proximal stable base of support, allowing distal mobility to the glenohumeral joint and hand. The scapula has some muscles attached to it. The scapula not only acts as a stable base but also must be able to move to maintain a constant length tension relationship for the rotator cuff musculature to function adequately.

During the cocking phase of throwing, the scapula must upwardly rotate. The muscles primarily responsible for this motion are the serratus anterior and middle and upper trapezius. During the acceleration phase, the scapula must forcefully protract and downwardly rotate. The muscles primarily responsible for this motion are the serratus anterior and pectoralis major and minor. The scapula must be able to rotate upwardly 60 degrees, glide 15 cm laterally, and elevate 10 to

12 cm to allow normal arm elevation.[55] Several authors have emphasized the importance of the scapular stabilizing muscles in decelerating the arm by dissipating the forces during the follow-through phase of throwing.[56,57] Several scapula pathologies are seen in the throwing athlete.

The scapula disorder termed *snapping scapula* is a pathology characterized by a loud grating and snapping sound of the scapula as it moves over the thorax. The athlete usually complains of pain in the periscapular region with overhead movements and activities. Radiographs or MRI scans are often useful to localize the lesion.[58] The treatment is most commonly conservative in nature, consisting of scapula strengthening and modalities such as heat, ultrasound, and occasional use of local steroid injections. Often as the pain subsides, the athlete will continue to notice the snapping noise; this may not warrant treatment.[58] The snapping scapula disorder is the result of an osseous or osteocartilaginous lesion of the scapula or the thorax producing this symptomatic crepitus with active scapular motion.

Scapulothoracic bursitis is a pathology closely associated with snapping scapula. In these instances, one of the scapulothoracic bursae becomes inflamed and swollen, which results in an audible and palpable crepitus with scapula motion. The crepitus is usually localized to the superomedial border of the scapula.[59] Repetitive overhead motions, such as throwing, may irritate the soft tissue of the scapulothoracic joint, producing this type of chronic overuse inflammatory reaction. Occasionally, surgery is required to excise the involved thickened bursae.[60] Most commonly, this pathology responds well to conservative management consisting of rest, analgesics, nonsteroidal anti-inflammatory medications, physical therapy, heat, and/or local steroid injections. Specific exercises designed to strengthen the scapular stabilizers and the shoulders' internal and external rotators are extremely beneficial in these instances.

## REHABILITATION

The shoulder joint complex is commonly injured in the throwing athlete. Most injuries to the throwing shoulder are from repetitive microtraumas and rarely require surgical intervention. The throwing athlete should perform specific exercises to strengthen the

**Table 32-2. Thrower's 10 Program**

1. Scaption (supraspinatus)/deltoid
2. External rotation/internal rotation (90 degrees abducted position) with exercise tubing
3. $D_2$ PNF pattern flexion and extension upper extremities
4. Shoulder horizontal abduction (prone)
5. Push-ups
6. Press-ups
7. Rowing (prone)
8. Elbow flexion/extension
9. Wrist extension/flexion
10. Forearm supination/pronation

Sit-ups
Stretch
Wall squat throws      } Daily Program
Run

different muscles of the shoulder complex. These exercises should isolate the rotator cuff, glenohumeral, and scapulothoracic muscles. Also, exercises of the muscles of the trunk and arm should be performed to strengthen all muscle groups of the kinetic chain. The exercises outlined in Table 32-2 and Figure 32-16 have been developed through the collective work of several investigators who have documented the muscle activity (electromyography) during various exercise movements.[61–67] These exercises emphasize the muscles involved in the throwing mechanics and use combined movement patterns and isolated movement patterns. In the combined movement patterns, groups of muscles are exercised to perform a movement pattern that is similar to throwing. This will assist in improving neuromuscular control, synchronized movement, and improve flexibility before throwing is begun. In the isolated movement patterns, a particular muscle or movement is isolated. Isolated movements are performed to overload a particular muscle that may be perceived as weak or plays an extremely important role in throwing. The exercises in this program have been named the "throwers' 10 program" and are prescribed to the throwing athlete as preventive exercises.[68] Also, these exercises are often prescribed as strengthening exercises after injuries and when motion and adequate strength has been achieved.

The thrower's 10 program emphasizes the muscles and muscle groups responsible for the throwing movement. The exercise program attempts to re-establish humeral head dynamic stability through rotator cuff musculature strength and neuromuscular control. Also, the prime movers of the shoulder, the accelerators or anterior shoulder muscles, are exercised using concentric and plyometric exercise drills. The posterior cuff muscles, the decelerators, are exercised using an eccentric muscular contraction. Also, the scapulothoracic joint, trunk, and legs are also conditioned in this program. A well-conditioned thrower may be less likely to sustain an injury than an unconditioned athlete.

## CONCLUSIONS

The shoulder's angular velocities during throwing often exceed 7,000 degrees/s, which results in increased muscular demands to provide the dynamic stability required by the shoulder complex. As a result of the excessive motion required to throw a baseball, laxity of the shoulder is common. The laxity perceived on clinical examination can progress to frank and symptomatic instability if the thrower is not able to exhibit adequate humeral head stabilization. Shoulder instability can lead to various pathologies including tensile rotator cuff failure, compressive rotator cuff disease, labral tears, and bicipital tendinitis. There are other injuries commonly seen in the throwing athlete other than rotator cuff injuries or instability syndromes. Glenoid labral tears, biceps tendon pathology, acromioclavicular joint disorders, scapula pain, and different neurovascular pathologies are also common in the throwing athlete. The key to injury-free throwing is proper mechanics, conditioning, and periodization in training to ensure coordinated muscular contractions of the glenohumeral and scapular muscles. The shoulder complex must exhibit excessive motion along with extraordinary strength and neuromuscular control to throw a baseball. Also, the thrower must have an adequate amount of time to ensure tissue healing between the microtraumatic injury episodes produced while throwing a baseball. Therefore, it may be necessary for the thrower to rest the arm from throwing activities for several days while rehabilitation is being performed through exercises and therapeutic modalities. This may assist in the successful return to throwing after a shoulder injury. Injuries to the throwing shoulder present the clinician with many clinical enigmas. The clinician should carefully examine the involved area with a thorough knowledge of the functional anatomy, throwing biomechanics, and the pathomechanics of the shoulder complex. An accurate diagnosis of the throwing shoulder is a significant challenge for all clinicians.

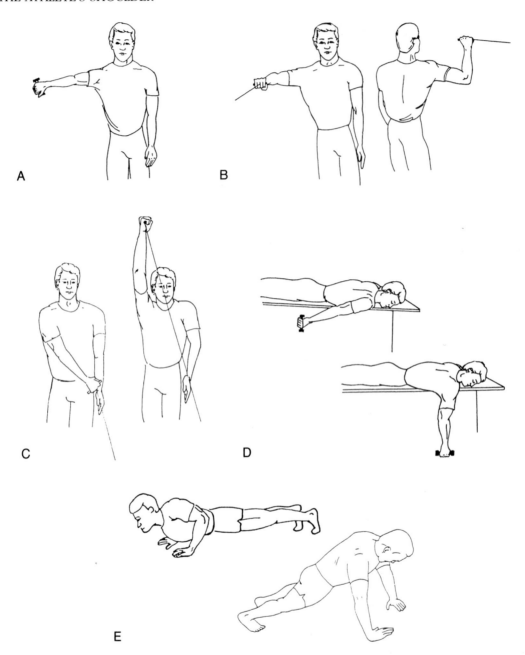

**Fig. 32-16.** **(A–J)** Throwers' 10 exercise program. **(A)** *Supraspinatus strengthening—scaption.* Stand with elbow straight and thumb down. Raise arm to shoulder level at 30-degree angle in front of the body. **(B)** *External/ internal rotation at 90-degree abduction.* Stand with shoulder abducted to 90 degrees, externally or internally rotate arm while elbow is bent to 90 degrees. **(C)** *Diagonal pattern D2 flexion.* Standing with the thumb into the opposite hip slowly elevate and rotate thumb up and outward over the shoulder. Turn palm down to reverse the movement. **(D)** *Shoulder horizontal abduction (prone).* Lying on your stomach, dumbbell in hand and palm down, slowly elevate arm to horizontal hold and slowly reverse movements. **(E)** *Push-Ups.* Place hands shoulder width apart, slowly lower body so that your nose almost touches the ground. Slowly straighten your arms to raise body. (*Figure continues.*)

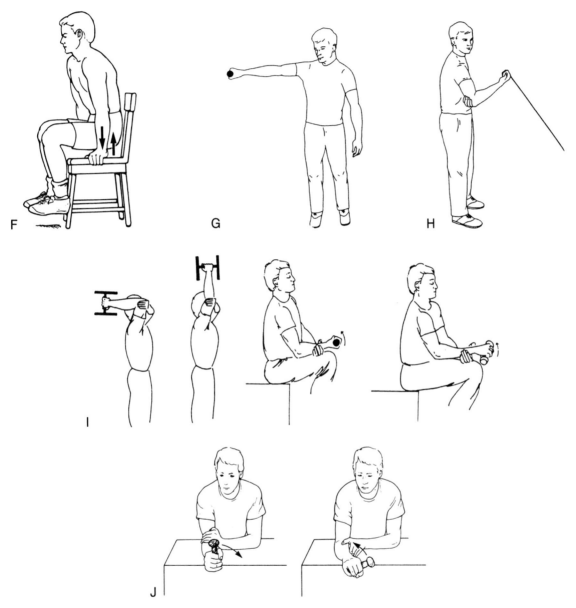

**Fig. 32-16** (*Continued*). **(F)** *Press-Ups.* Sitting in a chair with hands on each side of the chair, straighten your arm to slowly raise body off the chair; hold and slowly repeat. **(G)** *Shoulder Abduction.* Standing with arms at sides, elbow straight, and palm against side. Raise arm to the side until it reaches 90 degrees. **(H)** *Biceps Curls.* Stand with exercise tubing in hand, elbow slightly bent; slowly bend elbow to bring hand to shoulder; slowly lower. **(I)** *Triceps Extensions.* Raise arm overhead, provide support to arm by opposite hand, slowly straighten arm out. *Wrist Flexion.* Forearm supported on table with hand off edge, palm faces up; weight in hand, slowly curl hand and wrist. *Wrist Extension.* Forearm supported, palm faces downward; weight in hand, slowly extend hand upward. **(J)** *Forearm Supination/Pronation.* Forearm supported by table, dumbbell in hand and thumb up slowly rotate hand so that palm is upward and then reverse movement so that palm is downward.

# REFERENCES

1. Fleisig GS, Dillman CJ, Andrews JR: Proper mechanics for baseball pitching. Clin Sports Med 1:151, 1989

2. Wick HJ, Dillman CJ, Wisleder D et al: A kinematic comparison between baseball and fastball throwing. Sports Med Update 6:13, 1991

3. Saha AK: Dynamic stability of the glenohumeral joint. Acta Orthop Scand 42:491, 1971

4. Cain PR, Mutchler TA, Fu FH: Anterior stability of the glenohumeral joint: a dynamic model. Am J Sports Med 15:144, 1987

5. Howell SM, Galinet BJ: The glenoid-labral socket: a constrained articular surface. Clin Orthop 243:122, 1989

6. Howell SM, Imobersteg AM, Steger OH et al: Clarification of the role of the supraspinatus muscle in shoulder function. J Bone Joint Surg 68A:398, 1986

7. Basmajian JV, De Luca CJ: Muscles Alive. 5th Ed. Williams & Wilkins, Baltimore, 1985

8. Burkhart SS: Arthroscopic treatment of massive rotator cuff tears. Clin Orthop 267:45, 1991

9. Andrews JR, Angelo RL: Shoulder arthroscopy for the throwing athlete. In Paulos LE, Tibone VE (eds): Operative Techniques in Shoulder Surgery. Aspen Publishers, Rockville, MD, 1991

10. Scarpinato DF, Andrews JR, Bramhall JP: Arthroscopic management of the throwing athlete's shoulder. In Hawkins RJ (ed): Basic Science and Clinical Application in the Athlete's Shoulder. Clin Sports Med 10:913, 1991

11. Wilk KE, Andrews JR, Arrigo CA: The isokinetic muscular performance characteristics of professional baseball pitchers. Am J Sports Med 21:61, 1993

12. Andrews JR, Broussard TS, Carson WG: Arthroscopy of the shoulder in the management of partial tears of the rotator cuff. A preliminary report. Arthroscopy 1:117, 1985

13. Matsen FA, Arntz CT: Subacromial impingement. In Rockwood CA, Matsen FA (eds): The Shoulder. WB Saunders, Philadelphia, 1990

14. Bigliani LU, Morrison DSD, April EW: The morphology of the acromion and its relationship to rotator cuff tears. Orthop Trans 10:216, 1986

15. Bigliani LU, Norris TR, Fischer J, Neer CS: The relationship between the unfused acromial epiphysis and subacromial impingement lesions. Orthop Trans 7:138, 1983

16. Liberson F: Os acromial—a contested anomaly. J Bone Joint Surg 19:683, 1937

17. Peterson CJ, Gentz CF: The significance of distally pointing acromioclavicular osteophytes in ruptures of the supraspinatus tendon. Acta Scand Orthop 54:490, 1983

18. Hawkins RJ, Kennedy JC: Impingement syndromes in athletes. Am J Sports Med 8:151, 1980

19. Wilk KE, Andrews JR: Subacromial shoulder decompression; surgical treatment and rehabilitation. Orthopedics (accepted for publication)

20. Neer CS: Impingement lesions. Clin Orthop 173:70, 1973

21. Abrams JS: Special shoulder problems in the throwing athlete: pathology, diagnosis, and non-operative management. In Hawkins RJ (ed): Basic Sciences & Clinical Application in the Athlete's Shoulder. Clin Sports Med 10:839, 1991

22. Cofield RH: Rotator cuff disease of the shoulder. J Bone Joint Surg 67A:974, 1985

23. Matsen FA, Harryman DT, Sidles JA: Mechanics of glenohumeral instability. In Hawkins RJ (ed): Basic Science & Clinical Application in the Athlete's Shoulder. Clin Sports Med 10:783, 1991

24. Jobe FW, Tibone JE, Jobe CM et al: The shoulder in sports. p. 961. In Rockwood CA, Matsen FA (eds): The Shoulder. WB Saunders, Philadelphia, 1990

25. Jobe FW, Glousmann RE: Anterior capsulolabral reconstruction. Techniques in Orthopaedics—the Shoulder. 3:29, 1985

26. O'Brien SJ, Neves MC, Arnoczky SP et al: The anatomy and histology of the inferior glenohumeral ligament complex of the shoulder. Am J Sports Med 18:449, 1990

27. Pollack RG, Bigliani LU, Flatow EL et al: The mechanical properties of the inferior glenohumeral ligament. Presented at the Annual Meeting of the American Shoulder and Elbow Surgeons, New Orleans, LA, 1990

28. Caspari RB: Arthroscopic reconstruction for anterior shoulder instability. In Paulos LE, Tibone JE (eds): Operative Techniques in Shoulder Surgery. Aspen Publishers, Rockville, MD, 1991

29. Caspari RB, Savoie FH: Arthroscopic shoulder reconstruction; Bankart repair. p. 514. In McGinty JB (ed): Operative Arthroscopy. Raven Press, New York, 1990

30. Johnson LL: Shoulder arthroscopy. In Johnson LL (ed): Arthroscopic Surgery, Principles and Practices. CV Mosby, St Louis, 1986

31. Morgan CD, Bodenstab AB: Arthroscopic Bankart suture repair. Technique and early results. Arthroscopy 3:111, 1987

32. Altchek DW, Warren RF, Skyhar MJ: Shoulder arthroscopy. p. 276. In Rockwood CA, Matsen FA (eds): The Shoulder. WB Saunders, Philadelphia, 1990

33. Neer CS, Foster CR: Inferior capsular shift for involuntary inferior and multidirectional instability of the shoulder. J Bone Joint Surg 62A:897, 1980

34. Andrews JR, Carson WG: The arthroscopic treatment of glenoid labrum tears in the throwing athlete. Orthop Trans 8:44, 1984

35. Andrews JR, Carson WG, McLeod WD: Glenoid labrum

tears related to the long head of the biceps. Am J Sports Med 13:337, 1985

36. Snyder SJ, Karzel RP, Del Pizzo W et al: SLAP lesions of the shoulder. Arthroscopy 6:274, 1990

37. Pappas AM, Gross TD, Kleinman PK: Symptomatic shoulder instability due to lesions of the glenoid labrum. Am J Sports Med 11:279, 1983

38. Wilson AJ, Totty WG, Murphy WA et al: Shoulder joint. Arthrographic CT and long term follow-up with surgical correlation. Radiology 173:329, 1989

39. Bigliani LU, Singson R, Feldman F et al: Double contrast CT arthrography in the evaluation and treatment of shoulder instability. Surg Rounds Orthop 1:37, 1987

40. Bennett GE: Elbow and shoulder lesions of the professional baseball pitcher. JAMA 8:510, 1941

41. Jobe FW, Moynes DR, Tibone JE: An EMG analysis of the shoulder in pitching. A second report. Am J Sports Med 12:218, 1984

42. Crenshaw AH, Kilgore WE: Surgical treatment of bicipital tenosynovitis. J Bone Joint Surg 48A:1496, 1966

43. Michele AA: Bicipital tenosynovitis. Clin Orthop 18:261, 1960

44. Vellet AD, Munk PL, Marks P: Imaging techniques of the shoulder: present perspectives. Clin Sports Med 10:721, 1991

45. Rockwood CA, Young DC: Disorders of the acromioclavicular joint. p. 413. In Rockwwod CA, Matsen FA (eds): The Shoulder, WB Saunders, Philadelphia, 1990

46. Leffert RD: Thoracic outlet syndrome and the shoulder. Symposium on injuries to the shoulder in the athlete. Clin Sports Med 2:439, 1983

47. Roos DB: The thoracic outlet syndrome is underrated. Arch Neurol 47:327, 1990

48. Britt LP: Nonoperative treatment of the thoracic outlet syndrome symptoms. Clin Orthop 51:45, 1967

49. Wright IS: The neurovascular syndrome produced by hyperabduction of the arms. Am Heart J 157:1, 1945

50. Post M, Mayer J: Suprascapular nerve entrapment. Clin Orthop 223:126, 1987

51. Callahan JD, Scully TB, Shapiro SA et al: Suprascapular nerve entrapment. J Neurosurg 74:893, 1991

52. Rengachary SS, Burr D, Lucas S et al: Suprascapular entrapment neuropathy; clinical, anatomical and comparative study. Neurosurgery 5:447, 1979

53. Fritz RC, Helms CA, Steinbach LS et al: Suprascapular nerve entrapment—evaluation with magnetic resonance imaging. Radiology 182:437, 1992

54. Thompson WA, Kopell HP: Peripheral entrapment neuropathies of the upper extremity. N Engl J Med 260:1261, 1959

55. Kapandji IA: The Physiology of the Joints. 5th Ed. Vol. 1. Churchill Livingstone, New York, 1982

56. Kibler WB: Rule of the scapula in the overhead throwing motion. Contemp Orthop 22:525, 1991

57. Glousman RE, Jobe FW, Tibone JE et al: Dynamic electromyographic analysis of the throwing shoulder with glenohumeral instability. J Bone Joint Surg 70:220, 1988

58. Milch H: Snapping scapula. Clin Orthop 20:139, 1961

59. Bigliani LU: Shoulder injuries in athletics. Presentation at Advances of the Shoulder and Knee, Hilton Head, SC, May 30, 1992

60. Sisto DJ, Jobe FW: The operative treatment of scapulothoracic bursitis in professional pitchers. Am J Sports Med 14:192, 1986

61. Moseley JB, Jobe FW, Pink M et al: EMG analysis of the scapular muscles during a shoulder rehabilitation program. Am J Sports Med 20:128, 1992

62. Townsend H, Jobe FW, Pink M, Perry J: Electromyographic analysis of the glenohumeral muscles during a baseball rehabilitation program. Am J Sports Med 19:264, 1991

63. Blackburn TA, McLeod WD, White B: EMG analysis of posterior rotator cuff exercises. Athl Training 25:40, 1990

64. Blackburn TA: Off-season program for the throwing arm. p. 277. In Zarins B, Andrews JR, Carson WG (eds): Injuries to the Throwing Arm. WB Saunders, Philadelphia, 1985

65. Jobe FW, Bradely JP: Rotator cuff injuries in baseball: prevention and rehabilitation. Sports Med 6:378, 1980

66. Jobe FW, Moynes DR: Delineation of diagnostic criteria and a rehabilitation program for rotator cuff injuries. Am J Sports Med 10:336, 1982

67. Pappas AM, Zawacki RM: Rehabilitation of the pitching shoulder. Am J Sports Med 13:223, 1985

68. Wilk KE, Arrigo C, Courson R et al: Preventive and Rehabilitative Exercises for the Shoulder and Elbow. 3rd Ed. American Sports Medicine Institute, Birmingham, AL, 1991

# 33
# Shoulder Injuries in Football

*JUDY L. SETO*
*CLIVE E. BREWSTER*
*CLARENCE L. SHIELDS, Jr.*

Football is a high-contact sport and collisions are an inherent aspect of the game. The probability of a player sustaining an injury sometime during his career has been reported to be between 50 and 80 percent.[1-6] Canale et al[4] documented the injuries of 265 intercollegiate football players over a 5-year period. They reported a 46.6 percent chance for an athlete to sustain an injury during any 1 year period. The likelihood of injury escalated as the years of experience increased. In contrast, Powell[6] followed 6,544 high school football players and found that although 37 percent of the football players were injured at least one time, there was little relationship between the percentage of injury and years of experience. Athletes who played 1 full year comprised 28 percent of the injuries, whereas 31 percent of the reported injuries were to players with 3 years of experience.

Although the possibility of sustaining an injury is high, studies show that most injuries are mild[4,6,7] and consist of sprains, strains, and contusions.[6-10] The National Athletic Injury/Illness Reporting System[8] defines a mild injury as one in which the athlete is able to return to participation within 1 week from the day of injury onset. A moderate injury is one in which the player returns to participation within 8 to 21 days. An athlete with a major injury returns to participation after 21 days. Permanently disabling injuries are classified as severe.

The shoulder complex, including both the glenohumeral and acromioclavicular joints, is second only to the knee as the area most injured.[4,7,9-14] Injuries are defined as direct, a force directly applied to the injured area, and indirect, a force transmitted from its point of application and concentrated at another point. Direct injuries include contusions, acute subacromial bursitis, acromioclavicular and sternoclavicular joint sprains or dislocations, and fractures of the clavicle and humerus. Indirect injuries consist of major muscle strains (i.e., deltoid, pectoralis major), shoulder dislocations, and proximal humeral fractures.[15] The mechanism of injury occurring in most shoulder injuries involves direct forces. Powell[6] reported that 43.9 percent of high school football injuries resulted from direct impact, three times greater than injuries resulting from any other cause.

## ACROMIOCLAVICULAR JOINT
### Anatomy

The acromioclavicular joint is a diarthroidial joint containing a fibrocartilaginous intra-articular disc. The joint capsule is surrounded by the superior and inferior acromioclavicular ligaments, which act as the primary structures resisting posterior displacement of the clavicle.[16] The deltoid and trapezius muscles, along with fibers from the superior acromioclavicular ligament, attach to the superior aspect of the clavicle and acromion process.[17] These muscles assist the acromioclavicular ligaments in providing joint stability.

Another structure essential in acromioclavicular joint stability is the coracoclavicular ligament, which is composed of two components. The conoid ligament originates on the posteromedial aspect of the coracoid process, inserting onto the conoid tubercle of the clavicle.[17] This cone-shaped ligament restricts anterior and superior displacement of the lateral aspect of the clavicle.[16] The trapezoid ligament attaches on the coracoid process, just anterior and lateral to the conoid ligament, and rises superiorly to insert on the inferior surface of the clavicle.[17] This ligament acts against medial scapular displacement.[16]

The acromioclavicular joint has two degrees of motion and augments the motion at the glenohumeral joint. The motions occurring at this joint are elevation, depression, retraction, protraction, and rotation. Inman et al[18] reported that clavicular motion is essential in allowing shoulder motion. In a cadaver study, a pin was inserted into the clavicle, and when clavicular rotation was restricted, overhead elevation was limited. However, studies have shown that in cases of acromioclavicular joint arthrodesis, full shoulder range of motion may still be attained.[19,20]

## Mechanism of Injury

The most common mechanism of acromioclavicular joint injury is by a direct force resulting in subluxation or dislocation. The athlete falls on the point of the shoulder with his arm by his side in an adducted and internally rotated position, thereby depressing the acromion process and clavicle. If the clavicle does not fracture, the first soft tissue structure to absorb the force is the acromioclavicular ligament followed by the coracoacromial ligament. With additional force, the deltoid and trapezoid muscles may also be disrupted.[17,21–23]

Acromioclavicular joint injuries may also occur because of an indirect force. The athlete falls onto an outstretched hand with the glenohumeral joint positioned in flexion and abduction. The force is transmitted through the humerus and concentrated on the acromion process.[17,24] The joint capsule may become stretched or torn, the acromioclavicular ligament sprained, and the acromioclavicular joint partially separated. This type of injury is less common than injuries related to a direct force.

## Classification of Injury

Acromioclavicular joint injuries may be classified as mild, moderate, or severe (Table 33-1). In the type I injury, there is a mild sprain of the acromioclavicular ligament. The coracoclavicular ligament remains intact, and the acromioclavicular joint is stable. Tearing of the acromioclavicular ligament and joint capsule indicate a type II injury, or moderate sprain. The coracoclavicular ligament still remains intact. A type III, or severe, injury refers to a complete disruption of the acromioclavicular and coracoclavicular ligaments. Visible deformity is evident as the acromioclavicular joint is dislocated with possible tearing of the deltoid and trapezius muscles away from the distal end of the clavicle. Rockwood and Young[17] also described additional classifications of injuries, each one involving complete disruption of the acromioclavicular and coracoacromial ligaments. A type IV injury occurs when the acromioclavicular joint is dislocated and the clavicle travels posteriorly and superiorly, piercing into or through the trapezius muscle. A type V injury involves an exaggerated separation of the clavicle from the scapula. When the clavicle dislocates inferiorly under the coracoid process, it is classified as a type VI injury.

## Treatment

There is a consensus as to the recommended treatment after acute type I and II injuries. The upper extremity should be supported with a sling during the initial 2 to 3 weeks, accompanied by rest and ice. After the early stage, gentle range of motion may be performed within the limits of pain.[21,23,25] Strengthening exercises with

**Table 33-1.** Classification of Injury

| Structure | Type I | Type II | Type III | Type IV | Type V | Type VI |
|---|---|---|---|---|---|---|
| Acromioclavicular ligament | Sprain | Disrupted | Disrupted | Disrupted | Disrupted | Disrupted |
| Acromioclavicular joint | Intact | Separated | Dislocated | Dislocated, clavicle displaced posteriorly into/through trapezius | Dislocated | Dislocated, clavicle displaced inferiorly to acromion or coracoid process |
| Coracoclavicular ligament | Intact | Sprain | Disrupted | Disrupted | Disrupted | Disrupted |
| Coracoclavicular joint space | Intact | Slight increase | Increased | Displaced | Gross disparity between clavicle & scapula | Clavicle inferior to acromion or coracoid process |
| Deltoid/trapezius | Intact | Intact | Detached | Detached | Detached | Detached |

emphasis on the deltoid muscles are gradually added as tolerated.

If symptoms of pain consistent with degenerative joint disease occur at a later stage, excision of the distal clavicle (Mumford procedure) is recommended.[21] Controversy exists when determining the treatment of choice after an acute type III injury. Studies have shown that the results subsequent to a conservative course are as successful as operative treatment in terms of patient satisfaction, return to function, time of recovery, and shoulder strength and endurance.[23,26-30] The conservative route also avoids complications related to the implanted hardware and infection. The fabrication of an acromioclavicular pad (see Chapter 53) may help to facilitate the painfree return to football participation.

## Clavicular Fracture

Allman[31] classifies clavicular fractures into three groups based on the fracture location. Group I consists of fractures in the middle third of the clavicle. This is the most common type of clavicular fracture, with the mechanism of injury as falling onto an outstretched hand in a position of shoulder flexion and abduction. This indirect force is transmitted up the humerus, through the glenohumeral joint, and to the clavicle, resulting in clavicular fracture. In group II, fractures occur in the outer third of the clavicle, distal to the coracoacromial ligaments. This type of fracture is sustained from falling by the point of the shoulder, forcing the humerus and scapula inferiorly and levering the distal clavicle. Fractures in group III occur in the proximal clavicle and are caused by a direct force applied to the lateral aspect of the shoulder. Football players sustain a greater percentage of type I injuries than type II. Type III injuries are typically seen among athletes susceptible to direct blows to the shoulder, such as in hockey or lacrosse.[32]

# GLENOHUMERAL JOINT

## Anatomy

The glenohumeral joint is a ball-and-socket synovial joint capable of multidirectional motion. As a result of its high degree of mobility, there is an inherent amount of biomechanical instability. This joint relies on the static and dynamic stability afforded to it by the ligamentous attachments and surrounding musculature rather than bony congruency. The large spherically shaped humeral head articulates approximately one-third of its surface with a shallow glenoid fossa. The glenoid labrum, a fibrocartilaginous ring, lines the rim of the glenoid fossa, thereby contributing to glenohumeral joint stability.

## Anterior Instability

Anterior shoulder instability, a common injury in football, may be caused by indirect or direct forces. In the case of an indirectly applied force, the athlete falls onto an outstretched arm in a position of abduction and external rotation. As the humerus is forced into horizontal abduction, the humeral head is levered anteriorly. Less frequently, anterior shoulder instability is caused by a direct force when a direct blow is placed to the posterior aspect of the shoulder, forcing the humeral head forward.[33,34] The soft tissue structures resisting anterior motion of the humeral head are the subscapularis muscle and the inferior and middle glenohumeral ligaments.[35] These structures vary in levels of importance in resisting anterior instability depending on the degree of abduction.

Conservative treatment after an anterior instability injury consists primarily of restoring normal range of motion while protecting the anterior joint capsule from further stress. If needed, a sling is used for 1 to 2 weeks to allow for pain reduction and permit the traumatized structures to heal. Emphasis is placed on strengthening not only the anterior cuff musculature but also the posterior cuff to restore normal joint mechanics. Occasionally it may be necessary to place the player in a shoulder brace to restrict abduction and external rotation (see Chapter 53). This is only possible in players who do not require full shoulder motion, such as interior linemen.

## Posterior Instability

Posterior shoulder instability among football players typically occurs because of indirect forces applied when the shoulder is positioned in flexion, adduction, and internal rotation.[24,36-38] As the humeral head is pushed posteriorly, the posterior joint capsule is stretched or disrupted. Schwartz et al[38] reports that the diagnosis of posterior dislocation may be missed 60 to 80 percent of the time on the initial examination because of a reliance on anteroposterior radiograph without obtaining lateral or axillary views. Clinically, the athlete maintains a position of shoulder adduction and internal rotation. Pain is elicited with attempted abduction or external rotation from a neutral or internally rotated position.[37,38]

During the initial phase after posterior shoulder subluxation or dislocation, the patient uses a sling for 1 to 2 weeks to reduce the stress on the posterior cuff structures. Modalities are used to decrease inflammation and pain. Range of motion and strengthening exercises are progressively added while protecting the posterior joint capsule. Modifications to the strengthening exercises include limiting the range of motion during internal shoulder rotation, horizontal abduction, and horizontal adduction.

## SHOULDER POSTERIOR RECONSTRUCTION

If surgery is required to repair the damage that transpired during posterior dislocation, reconstruction of the posterior shoulder is performed. The patient is placed on the operating table in the lateral decubitus position with the involved shoulder superior. The patient is held in position with an inflatable Olympic Vac-Pac Surgical Positioning System "bean bag" and kidney rest. The operating table itself is placed on a slightly reversed Trendelenburg position.

A saber incision is made at the superior aspect of the shoulder. This incision starts at the acromioclavicular joint and extends posteriorly approximately 8 cm into the posterior axillary fold. The subcutaneous tissues are undermined to expose the deltoid muscle attachment to the acromion and the spine of the scapula. Next, the fascial raphe between the middle and posterior third of the deltoid muscle is identified and slit distally and posteriorly up to 4 cm. In doing so, care should be taken to avoid the axillary nerve that enters the deltoid muscle at the interior border of the teres minor muscle. Using sharp dissection, the deltoid is reflected from the scapular spine and posterior aspect of the acromion. The deltoid attachment adheres to the infraspinatus attachment to the spine of the scapula. Thus, it is easier to find the place between these two muscles by starting out laterally in the area of the acromion with the sharp dissection.

After the deltoid muscle is reflected, the teres minor and infraspinatus muscles are encountered below the fascia of the deltoid. The infraspinatus is a bipennate muscle with a raphe between its two heads. This raphe can be confused with the interval between the infraspinatus and teres minor muscles. The true interval between the infraspinatus and teres minor muscles is below this raphe, which is below the inferior head of the infraspinatus.

With blunt dissection in line with its fiber, the interval between the teres minor and infraspinatus muscles is developed by exposing the posterior shoulder capsule. An arthrotomy in the posterior capsule is made in the same direction as the fibers of the infraspinatus and teres minor muscles. This allows inspection of the glenohumeral joint.

At this point, any bone spurs on the posterior glenoid are debrided. A posterior anchored lesion is usually found with the labrum detached from the posterior glenoid. The posterior capsule is striped further off the posterior glenoid and the labrum. If the labrum is torn, it should be moved.

The bone on the posterior glenoid labrum is roughened with curettes and rongeurs, and the two leaves of the posterior capsule are held with Kocher's clamps while a barbed Richards' 1-in. staple is positioned. It is usually necessary to make drill holes through the cortex of the posterior glenoid with a 7/64-in. drill bit to allow the staple to be positioned. The holes should be marked with a staple before drilling.

The staple is placed approximately 1 cm from the glenoid rim and directed slightly medially to avoid entering the joint. The reason for this approach is the glenoid, which is usually anteverted in relationship to the sagittal place of the body. Next, the posterior capsule is fixed to the posterior glenoid with the staple, and the capsule is closed with horizontal mattress sutures by using no. 1 Vicryl suture.

If there is inferior instability as well as posterior instability, the inferior capsule is developed and advanced as far superiorly as possible to eliminate the inferior capsule and advanced as far superiorly as possible to eliminate the inferior capsular pouch. No sutures are needed between the teres minor and infraspinatus muscles, and these muscles are not imbricated. The deltoid muscle is repaired into the bone of the spine and the acromion with no. 1 Ethibond sutures on a small cutting needle. Finally, the skin and subcutaneous tissues are closed in routine fashion, and a compressive dressing is applied.

## SHOULDER IMPINGEMENT AND ROTATOR CUFF TENDONITIS

The impingement syndrome is a common shoulder disorder often associated with periods of repetitive overhead activities. Among athletes, it is typically seen among baseball pitchers but may also be present in football quarterbacks. The mechanics of throwing a football are not unlike the mechanics involved in baseball pitching. This impingement syndrome may occur when the rotator cuff and subacromial bursa become trapped between the greater tuberosity and coracoacromial arch.[39,40] The coracoacromial arch is formed by the acromion, acromioclavicular joint, and coracoacromial ligament. The subacromial bursa buffers the rotator cuff and biceps tendons as the greater tuberosity glides underneath the coracoacromial arch during overhead motions.[39] A decrease in this joint space may impinge on the underlying soft tissues. Abnormal bony prominences, fibrotic thickening of the subacromial bursa, and alteration in the biomechanics of the shoulder secondary to muscle weakness and joint laxity may all contribute to restrictions of the underlying soft tissues and present symptoms similar to an impingement syndrome. Supraspinatus point tenderness, biceps tendon inflammation, and painful overhead motions are the commonly presented symptoms.

Conservative management may include anti-inflammatory medication and corticosteroid injection into the subacromial space and acromioclavicular joint.[39,41] Because the primary problem causing impingement is excessive anterior translation of the humeral head, emphasis is placed on restoring the dynamic joint stability. If the posterior joint capsule is tight, the humeral head is unable to move posteriorly and will ride up anteriorly and superiorly.[35] Joint mobilization techniques and posterior cuff stretches are used to restore normal joint biomechanics. Also, rhomboid and levator scapulae tightness will contribute to increased downward scapular rotation and prevent normal scapulohumeral rhythm. Strengthening exercises are performed accentuating the rotator cuff muscles and modified to minimize stress on the anterior joint capsule. However, if this condition continues to persist, chronic shoulder pain may develop, resulting in rotator cuff tears.[40,41]

## ROTATOR CUFF REPAIR

The surgical technique in repairing the rotator cuff involves a saber-type incision over the acromioclavicular joint. The posterior limb extends to the posterior angle of the acromion process and tapers anteriorly toward the deltopectoral groove. The skin is undermined a distance of 1 to 2 cm medial to the acromioclavicular joint and laterally to the posterolateral corner of the acromion. The periosteum of the deltoid muscle is incised with a scalpel blade on an electrocautery knife over the acromion and the distal end of the clavicle. In this area, the periosteum is too adherent for the use of the periosteal elevator. Once the periosteum is elevated to the lateral border of the acromion process, the deltoid tendon fibers that insert underneath the anterior acromion at the tendon bone junction are released. This will preserve the maximum amount of tendon tissues for later reapproximation of the deltoid to the acromion.

Once the deltoid is released in a semicircle from the acromion process, scissors are used to make an incision through the deltoid along one of the anterior raphe. The deltoid muscle may then be retracted medially and laterally to improve exposure of the rotator cuff and the undersurface of the acromion.

The subacromial bursa is carefully resected because it is usually adherent to the defect in the rotator cuff. If it is not immediately seen, the humerus should be rotated internally or externally to bring the extent of the tear into view.

It is important to spend time dissecting medially along the infraspinatus and supraspinatus. This maneuver will assist in maximal lateral movement of the retracted tendons. The tendon ends are not excised in these large tears. The goal is to attempt to close the defect from side to side with no. 1 Ethibond suture. The tendon is inserted laterally into a trough made in the natural sulcus between the greater tuberosity and the articular surface of the humeral head. It is attached through drill holes with the nonabsorbable Ethibond suture.

Frequently, the rotator cuff tear cannot be reapproximated without placing the arm into abduction. If this is the case, the arm is splinted in abduction via a pillow or splint postoperatively. If the tear is extremely large, the rotator cuff tissues are contracted so that they cannot be reapproximated. The deltoid muscle is split a little further anteriorly to mobilize the upper portion of the subscapularis muscle and tendon to bring it posteriorly to close the gap. The V-shaped defect in the subscapularis can be partially or completely closed with interrupted absorbable sutures.

If the rotator cuff defects are quite large and the contracted tissues cannot be mobilized or are too in-elastic to allow reapproximation, the margins of the tear should be debrided. Care must be taken with the supraspinatus slide procedure as there is a high incidence of injury to the suprascapular nerve. Sacrificing the biceps tendon for a graft has been advocated; however, this should be done with caution because the biceps functions as an abductor in rotator cuff tears. A 1-mm Gore-Tex soft-tissue patch may be fashioned and sutured into the defect. A traumatic needle with a non-absorbable suture is passed through the graft and through the defect in the rotator cuff using multiple interrupted sutures. This graft should allow fibrous ingrowth into its substance and provide adequate coverage of the previously exposed humeral head. However, because the rotator cuff muscle length is short-ened, the repair may not result in an increase in strength. Once the rotator cuff defect is closed, the very important reattachment of the deltoid muscle is accomplished by using Ethibond sutures on a cutting needle and passing them through drill holes in the acromion process. Each stitch should exit along the flattened surface and then pass inferiorly through the substance of the deltoid tendon. The periosteal flap thereby pulls the deltoid more to the superior surface of the acromion process and not to the undersurface. This alleviates the possibility of soft tissue impingement against the underlying rotator cuff.

## SUMMARY

The shoulder is second only to the knee as the area most commonly injured in football. Most injuries result from a direct force as opposed to indirect impact. Mild injuries (athlete returns to participation within 1 week of injury) predominate. Common acromioclavicular joint injuries consist of ligament sprains and clavicular fractures, whereas injuries to the glenohumeral joint primarily consist of anterior and posterior joint insta-bilities. Occasionally the use of an acromioclavicular

pad or shoulder brace may assist the player to a pain-free return. All players who have sustained a shoulder injury should be placed on a shoulder motion and strengthening program.

## REFERENCES

1. Blyth CS, Mueller FO: Football injury survey: when and where players get hurt. Phys Sportsmed 2:45, 1974
2. Blyth CS, Mueller FO: Football injury survey: identifying the causes. Phys Sportsmed 2:71, 1974
3. Blyth CS, Mueller FO: Football injury survey: injury rates vary with coaching. Phys Sportsmed 2:45, 1974
4. Canale ST, Cantler ED, Sisk TD, Freeman BL: A chronicle of injuries of an American intercollegiate football team. Am J Sports Med 9:384, 1981
5. Garrick JG, Requa RK: Injuries in high school sports. Pediatrics 61:465, 1978
6. Powell J: 636,000 injuries annually in high school football. Ath Train 22:19, 1987
7. Shields CL, Zomar VD: Analysis of professional football injuries. Contemp Orthop 4:90, 1982
8. Alles WF, Powell JW, Buckley W, Hunt EE: The national athletic injury/illness reporting system 3-year findings of high school and college football injuries. J Orthop Sports Phys Ther 1:103, 1979
9. Halpern B, Thompson N, Curl WW et al: High school football injuries: identifying the risk factors. Am J Sports Med 15:316, 1987
10. Zemper ED: Injury rates in a national sample of college football teams: a 2-year prospective study. Phys Sportsmed 17:100, 1989
11. Dagiau RF, Dillman CJ, Milner EK: Relationship between exposure time and injury in football. Am J Sports Med 8:257, 1980
12. Goldberg B, Rosenthal PP, Robertson LS, Nicholas JA: Injuries in youth football. Pediatrics 81:255, 1988
13. Hill JA: Epidemiologic perspective on shoulder injuries. Clin Sports Med 2:241, 1983
14. Olson OC: The Spokane Study: high school football injur-ies. Phys Sportsmed 7:75, 1979
15. Cofield RH, Simonet WT: The shoulder in sports. Mayo Clin Proc 59:157, 1984
16. Fukuda K, Craig EV, An K et al: Biomechanical study of the ligamentous system of the acromioclavicular joint. J Bone Joint Surg 68A:434, 1986
17. Rockwood CA Jr, Young DC: Disorders of the acro-mioclavicular joint. p. 413. In Rockwood CA Jr, Matsen FA III (eds): The Shoulder. Vol. 1. WB Saunders, Philadel-phia, 1990

18. Inman VT, Saunders JB, Abbott LC: Observations on the function of the shoulder joint. J Bone Joint Surg 26:1, 1944
19. Caldwell GD: Treatment of complete permanent acromioclavicular dislocation by surgical arthrodesis. J Bone Joint Surg 25:368, 1943
20. Kennedy JC, Cameron H: Complete dislocation of the acromioclavicular joint. J Bone Joint Surg 36B:202, 1954
21. Cook DA, Heiner JP: Acromioclavicular joint injuries. Orthop Rev 19:510, 1990
22. Cox JS: The fate of the acromioclavicular joint in athletic injuries. Am J Sports Med 9:50, 1981
23. Dias JJ, Gregg PJ: Acromioclavicular joint injuries in sport. Sports Med 11:125, 1991
24. Hoyt WA Jr: Etiology of shoulder injuries in athletes. J Bone Joint Surg 49A:755, 1967
25. Neviaser RJ: Injuries to the clavicle and acromioclavicular joint. Orthop Clin North Am 18:433, 1987
26. Galpin RD, Hawkins RJ, Grainger RW: A comparative analysis of operative versus nonoperative treatment on grade III acromioclavicular separations. Clin Orthop 193:150, 1985
27. Imatani RJ, Hanlon JJ, Cady GW: Acute complete acromioclavicular separation. J Bone Joint Surg 57A:328, 1975
28. Larson E, Bjerg-Nielsen A, Christensen P: Conservative or surgical treatment of acromioclavicular dislocation. J Bone Joint Surg 68A:552, 1986
29. Skjeldal S, Lundbald R, Dullerud R: Coracoid process transfer for acromioclavicular dislocation. Acta Orthop Scand 59:180, 1988
30. Walsh WM, Peterson DA, Shelton G, Neumann RD: Shoulder strength following acromioclavicular injury. Am J Sports Med 13:153, 1985
31. Allman FL: Fractures and ligamentous injuries of the clavicle and its articulations. J Bone Joint Surg 49A:774, 1967
32. Silloway KA, McLaughlin RE, Edlich RC, Edlich RF: Clavicular fractures and acromioclavicular joint dislocations in lacrosse: preventable injuries. J Emerg Med 3:117, 1985
33. Aronen JG: Anterior shoulder dislocations in sports. Sports Med 3:224, 1986
34. O'Brien SJ, Warren RF, Schwartz E: Anterior shoulder instability. Orthop Clin North Am 18:395, 1987
35. Turkel SJ, Panio MW, Marshall DVM, Girgis FG: Stabilizing mechanisms preventing anterior dislocation of the glenohumeral joint. J Bone Joint Surg 63A:1208, 1981
36. May VR: Posterior dislocation of the shoulder: habitual, traumatic, and obstetrical. Orthop Clin North Am 11:271, 1980
37. Norwood LA, Terry GC: Shoulder posterior subluxation. Am J Sports Med 12:25, 1984
38. Schwartz E, Warren RF, O'Brien SJ, Fronek J: Posterior shoulder instability. Orthop Clin North Am 18:409, 1987
39. Kerr R: Shoulder impingement syndrome. Orthopedics 10:637, 1987
40. Neer CS: Impingement lesions. Clin Orthop 173:70, 1983
41. DePalma AF: Surgery of the Shoulder. 3rd Ed. JB Lippincott, Philadelphia, 1983

# 34

# Shoulder Injuries in Tennis

## TODD S. ELLENBECKER

The inherent characteristics of the game of tennis produce specific physiologic and mechanical stresses to the musculoskeletal system. This is particularly evident in the upper extremity. The repetition required for initial skill acquisition and subsequent practice and competition at all levels of play can subject the shoulder to overuse injury.

## ETIOLOGY

In a survey of 84 world-class tennis players, Priest and Nagel[1] reported that 74 percent of men and 60 percent of women had a history of shoulder or elbow pain on the dominant arm that affected tennis play. Injuries to both the shoulder and elbow of the dominant arm were reported by 21 and 23 percent of the world-class male and female players, respectively. Another survey by Priest et al[2] of 2,633 recreational tennis players found the incidence of tennis elbow to be 31 percent. One specific finding was the 63 percent greater incidence of shoulder injury among those players reporting tennis elbow injury. These epidemiologic studies clearly show the demands placed on the entire upper extremity kinetic chain.

Most injuries to the shoulder in tennis players are classified as overuse[3] and involve the rotator cuff and/or biceps tendon.[4] Because of the overhead nature of the tennis serve, the rotator cuff and biceps tendon can be placed in a compromised position between the humeral head and coracoacromial arch, resulting in subacromial impingement.[5,6] The progression of shoulder impingement from tendinitis to partial- and full-thickness tearing of the rotator cuff has been reported in the literature.[5,7]

Recent reports, however, have focused on the intrinsic tendon overload[8,9] from the high-intensity decelerative function of the posterior rotator cuff as well as anterior shoulder instability[7] as the primary mechanisms for shoulder overuse injury in the overhead athlete. Anterior instability of the glenohumeral joint can be caused by insufficiency of the static (inferior glenohumeral ligament and anterior inferior glenoid labrum) and dynamic (rotator cuff complex) stabilizers. Progressive attenuation of the static stabilizers is reported with overhead activities such as the tennis serve and overhand throw.[10] The increased role of the dynamic stabilizers of the glenohumeral joint can lead to microtraumatic tendon injury and further compromise joint stability and overhead function. It is the challenge of the rehabilitation professional to enhance the dynamic stabilizers of the shoulder without compromising the static stabilizing mechanisms. The enhancement of the dynamic stabilizers is particularly challenging during prevention and treatment of overuse shoulder injury in the tennis player because of the physiologic and anatomic demands caused by repetition and high-velocity decelerative function required for biomechanically acceptable tennis play. A review of the epidemiology of shoulder injuries in both recreational and highly skilled tennis players is presented in Table 34-1.

Evaluation and treatment of the tennis player with a shoulder injury requires a total upper extremity approach. An understanding of the sport-specific biomechanical demands placed on the upper extremity with tennis play is of paramount importance. The goal of this chapter is to outline the inherent muscular activity patterns and joint kinematics incurred with tennis play. The specific anatomic upper extremity adaptations

**Table 34-1.** Epidemiology of Shoulder Injuries in Tennis Players

| Population | Age (years) | Sample Size | Incidence (%) | Source |
|---|---|---|---|---|
| Elite juniors | 11–14 | 97 | 14 | Kibler et al, 1988[11] |
| Elite juniors | 16–20 | — | 8 | Reece et al, 1986[4] |
| Danish elite professional players | 14–48 | 104 | 17 | Winge et al, 1989[3] |
| Competitive | | 2,481 | 9 | Nigg et al, 1986[12] |
| Competitive | 14–63 | 534 | 36 | Hang & Peng, 1984[13] |
| Competitive/ recreational | 10–60+ | 260 | 8 | Kamien, 1989[14] |
| Recreational adults | 25–55+ | 2,633 | 7 | Priest et al, 1980[2] |
| Elite juniors | 12–19 | — | 24 | Lehman, 1988[15] |

found in musculoskeletal evaluation and research in tennis players are presented, followed by application of this information to treatment of the tennis player with overuse shoulder injury.

## ANALYSIS OF THE SHOULDER JOINT IN TENNIS-SPECIFIC MOVEMENTS
### Muscular Activity Patterns

The high-velocity dynamic muscular contractions present in the tennis serve and groundstrokes have been studied in minimally skilled and elite-level tennis players. Yoshizawa et al[16] recorded the peak and median muscular activity patterns of the shoulder and forearm muscles during the serve and groundstrokes. They found significantly higher muscular activity levels during the serve, indicating that it is the most strenuous stroke in tennis from an upper extremity muscular standpoint.

The serve can be broken down into four stages. The windup phase is characterized by the initiation of the serving stance to the toss of the ball by the contralateral extremity. There is very low electromyogram (EMG) activity during this phase in the muscles surrounding the shoulder.[17] The second phase of the serving motion is the cocking phase, which begins after the ball toss and terminates at the point of maximal external rotation of the glenohumeral joint of the racquet arm. Muscular activity during this phase is moderately high in the supraspinatus, infraspinatus, subscapularis, biceps brachii, and serratus anterior. Muscular activity levels expressed as a percentage of the maximum voluntary isometric contraction (MVC) were 53, 41, 25,

39, and 70 percent, respectively.[17] The stabilizing and approximating role of the rotator cuff identified by Inman et al[18] is clearly shown in the cocking phase of the tennis serve. The moderately high activity during this phase shows the importance of both anterior and posterior rotator cuff strength as well as scapular stabilization for proper execution of the required mechanics.

The third phase of the tennis serve is acceleration. This phase begins at maximal external rotation and terminates at ball impact. Consistent with EMG recordings during the acceleration phase of throwing,[19] high muscular activity was found in the pectoralis major, subscapularis and lattisimus dorsi, and serratus anterior during the forceful concentric internal rotation of the humerus.[17] EMG research published by VanGheluwe and Hebbelinck[20] using intermediate tennis players and by Miyashita et al[21] using skilled and unskilled tennis players also found high activity levels of the pectoralis major, as well as the deltoid, trapezius, and triceps, during the acceleration phase. Both reports showed a relative silence of electrical activity in the accelerating musculature during impact with peak levels of muscular activity occurring just before impact. One exception is the stabilizing contribution of the infraspinatus, which remained active during impact.[20]

The fourth and final phase occurs after impact and is termed the follow-through. This phase is characterized by moderately high activity of the posterior rotator cuff, serratus anterior, biceps brachii, deltoid, and latissimus dorsi. After the electrical silence of the shoulder musculature during impact or collision,[20,21] forceful eccentric muscular contraction is necessary to decelerate the humerus and maintain glenohumeral joint congruity.

A relatively consistent pattern of muscular activity is reported for skilled tennis players. The presence of increased, as well as overlapping, muscular activity patterns across the outlined stages in the tennis serve has been reported by untrained[16] and less skilled[21] tennis players. This increase in the muscular contribution during the serving motion in less-skilled players is a perfect example of how nonoptimal timing and a lack of whole-body contributions to force generation and deceleration subject an individual's shoulder to overuse injury. The contribution of the larger muscle groups in the lower extremities and trunk via proper biomechanical energy transfer during the tennis serve protect the player from injury and optimize performance.[22–24]

The forehand and backhand groundstrokes can be broken down into three phases: preparation, acceleration, and follow-through. EMG activity during the preparation phases of both the forehand and backhand is relatively low. Acceleration during the forehand involves very high activity in the subscapularis, biceps brachii, pectoralis major, and serratus anterior with a percentage of MVC of 102, 86, 85, and 76, respectively.[17] Acceleration during the backhand stroke consists of high muscular activity levels in the middle deltoid, supraspinatus, and infraspinatus with percentage of MVC of 118, 73, and 78, respectively. Again the serratus anterior and biceps musculature was active during acceleration for both the forehand and backhand strokes.

The follow-through phase of the forehand groundstroke produced moderately high activity of the serratus anterior, subscapularis, infraspinatus, and biceps musculature.[17] The continued activity of the infraspinatus was evident during impact and continued into the follow-through phase of the forehand groundstroke.[20] Follow-through activity during the backhand was moderately high in the biceps, middle deltoid, supraspinatus, and infraspinatus, but this level of activity was significantly lower than during the acceleration phase.

A sound understanding of the shoulder and scapular muscle function during tennis play is imperative for implementation of preventative and rehabilitative exercise programs for the shoulder girdle. It is beyond the scope of this chapter to review the complex interaction of the musculature of the lower extremities, trunk, and distal upper extremities required during functional performance.

## Joint Kinematics

To further understand the demands placed on the upper extremity, analysis of shoulder joint angular velocities and ranges of motion incurred during tennis play are indicated. Angular velocities incurred during the serving motion necessitate high-velocity muscular stabilization outlined above. Biomechanical study of the tennis serve has produced data measuring the speed of internal rotation of the humerus during acceleration. Shapiro and Stine[25] filmed 14 highly skilled male tennis players and reported a maximum internal rotation velocity of 1,074 to 1,514 degrees/s. Slightly faster velocities were reported by Dillman[26] in a pilot study of professional tennis players with maximal internal rotation velocities up to 2,300 degrees/s. Comparable velocities of internal rotation during the acceleration phase of throwing have been reported to exceed 7,000 degrees/s.[8]

Demands placed on the dominant shoulder during the tennis serve are also high with respect to range of motion. Dillman[26] reported maximal external rotation values of 154 degrees. Abduction angles at the shoulder in elite Australian players were reported to average 83 degrees during the cocking phase at the time of 90 degrees of elbow flexion.[27]

These range of motion characteristics have definite implications for overuse shoulder injury. Repeated maximal external rotation during the cocking phase of the tennis serve produces adaptations of the glenohumeral joint range of motion on the dominant arm.[28,29] Greater external rotation of the glenohumeral joint may come at the expense of anterior capsular attenuation and is similar to the range of motion and anterior laxity patterns found in highly skilled baseball players.[10]

The degree of glenohumeral joint abduction during cocking and acceleration is of prime importance in proper mechanical serve execution. Increases in glenohumeral joint abduction can lead to placement of the shoulder in a position of subacromial impingement. Initial observation of a highly skilled player's service motion shows an apparent vertical orientation of the arm to contact the ball overhead. Closer observation reveals that highly skilled players have significant contributions from contralateral trunk lateral flexion and scapular abduction. These components allow for a midrange of glenohumeral joint abduction throughout the four phases of the tennis serve.

Analysis of joint angular velocities during forehand groundstrokes shows maximal internal rotation at the shoulder to be between 364 and 746 degrees/s.[25] This finding will again have implications in determining appropriate exercises for prevention and rehabilitation of shoulder injuries. Groppel[22,30] outlined the rationale and methodology for generation of topspin to the forehand ground stroke. Topspin is a desired characteristic used to improve both velocity and control of a shot and has been taught by coaches emphasizing a low backswing during preparation and a high follow-through. This creates a low to high stroke path. This requires proper timing and body segment positioning and preparation.[24] Many unskilled and intermediate players use a method of "rolling over" the ball to achieve topspin. This effect increases the pronatory influence of the distal upper extremity and also increases internal rotation acceleration during the stroke.[23] The close association between pronation of the forearm and internal rotation of the shoulder has been reported during the serve.[31] Distal upper extremity pronatory acceleration and internal rotation compensation to incorrectly produce topspin increase the demand on the posterior rotator cuff musculature during the follow-through as the external rotators contract to counteract the internally rotating humerus after impact.

Angular velocities of external rotation during the backhand stroke in highly skilled tennis players range between 328 and 1640 degrees/s.[25] Rotation of the shoulders into a position perpendicular to the net is of vital importance to optimize the contribution of torso rotation and lower extremity input to force generation.[30] Use of a two-handed backhand has been recommended for players with upper extremity injury, particularly tennis elbow, because of bilateral upper extremity force generation and load sharing.[32]

## ANATOMIC ADAPTATIONS OF THE DOMINANT SHOULDER

It is beyond the scope of this chapter to comprehensively cover a full shoulder evaluation, but specific clinically relevant anatomic adaptations found in the tennis player are summarized.

## Postural

A characteristic postural adaptation that Priest and Nagel[1] found in clinical evaluation of 84 world-class tennis players is drooping or depression of the dominant shoulder. Priest and Nagel believe that the eccentric stretching of the posterior shoulder and scapular musculature and the increased weight of the playing arm because of muscular hypertrophy causes this adaptation. Presence of the "tennis shoulder" was reported in all 56 senior tennis players evaluated by Kulund et al.[33] The competitive players in their study had an average of greater than 50 years of playing experience and ranged in age from 60 to 85 years. The downward rotation of the scapula and resultant change in glenoid and acromial positioning may have implications for injury with repeated elevation of the glenohumeral joint. No definitive relationship has been formed regarding this postural adaptation and shoulder injury.

## Anthropoemetric

Circumferential measures are commonly used in sport science research to determine externally the presence of hypertrophic muscular development through bilateral comparisons. In a study of 84 world-class players, Chinn et al[34] found significantly greater dominant arm proximal humerus girth when compared bilaterally for male and female players. Similar results are reported by Vodak et al[35] in 50 middle-aged above-average players. A study of Australian elite junior male and female tennis players found greater upper arm circumference on the dominant arm in female tennis players, with no significant difference between extremities in the male tennis players.[36] Muscular adaptation of the dominant arm at both distal and proximal margins supports the EMG findings of dynamic repetitive muscular work required for successful tennis play.

## Range of Motion

The kinematic analysis presented earlier in this chapter showed the extremes of external rotation required for highly skilled tennis players' stroke execution. Several clinical studies have presented active range of motion measures of elite tennis players. Chandler et al[28] measured active range of motion of the shoulder internal and external rotators in 90 degrees of abduction in 86

**Table 34-2.** Internal and External Rotation Active Range of Motion Measures[a] Taken at 90 Degrees of Glenohumeral Joint Abduction in 26 Elite Male and Female Junior Tennis Players Aged 11 to 14 Years

| Group | No. | Dominant Arm | | | Nondominant Arm | | | Significance |
|---|---|---|---|---|---|---|---|---|
| | | mean | SD | range | mean | SD | range | |
| External rotation | | | | | | | | |
| Male | 12 | 110 | 10.6 | (95–135) | 101.25 | 11.7 | (80–125) | .008 |
| Female | 14 | 111 | 10.0 | (95–130) | 109.64 | 10.4 | (95–130) | .504 |
| Internal rotation | | | | | | | | |
| Male | 12 | 58.3 | 11.3 | (40–80) | 67.92 | 13.3 | (50–90) | .012 |
| Female | 14 | 65.3 | 7.9 | (50–75) | 71.43 | 10.2 | (60–100) | .023 |

[a] All measures in degrees.

junior elite tennis players between the ages of 12 and 21 years. They found significantly less mean internal rotation range in the dominant arm compared with the nondominant arm (65 versus 76 degrees). The dominant shoulder also had significantly greater external rotation active range of motion (100 versus 103 degrees). Similar findings were reported by Ellenbecker[29] in a study of 26 elite junior players aged 11 to 14 years. Data from this study are presented in Table 34-2. Significantly greater external rotation was found on the dominant arm of male tennis players only, with both male and female players showing less internal rotation active range of motion on the dominant arm.

Active range of motion measurement of 83 world-class tennis players by Chinn et al[34] also found significantly less internal rotation on the dominant arm in male players (58 versus 52). Less dominant arm internal rotation was present in the female players (62 versus 50) as well. Greater external rotation range of motion was measured on the dominant arm in male players but not in the female players in 90 degrees of glenohumeral joint abduction.

A consistent pattern of range of motion is present in the literature[28,29,34] showing decreased internal rotation and increased external rotation on the dominant shoulder when compared bilaterally. As with other anatomic and mechanical characteristics of the tennis shoulder, this finding has implications for both the prevention and rehabilitation of overuse injury. The increased external rotation may indicate anterior and inferior capsular laxity and identify the potential for anterior subluxation without adequate dynamic stabilization from the rotator cuff.[10] The decrease in internal rotation with probable causation from posterior capsular tightness has also been shown to increase anterior translation of

the humeral head in the glenoid with elevation[37] as well as with a cross-body/internal rotation maneuver similar to a forehand ground stroke follow-through.[38]

## Strength

Objective measurement of shoulder strength has been performed in elite and recreational tennis players.[29,39,40,41] Concomitant with range of motion, specific relationships in shoulder strength have been identified in the tennis player that again have implications for the development of preventative and rehabilitative exercise programs.

Ellenbecker[40] used a Cybex II isokinetic dynamometer to measure both shoulder internal and external rotation and flexion/extension in 22 highly skilled male adult tennis players. Ellenbecker found significantly greater dominant arm internal rotation, extension, and flexion compared with the nondominant extremity. No difference between extremities was found in shoulder external rotation. Significantly lower external/internal rotation unilateral strength ratios were reported for the dominant arm, showing a relative external rotation strength deficit on the tennis playing shoulder.

Similar results were found in elite junior tennis players tested isokinetically for internal and external rotation strength with 90 degrees of abduction.[29] Significantly greater dominant arm internal rotation strength was measured with no difference between extremities in external rotation strength. The decrease in unilateral strength ratios on the dominant arm was also present at all three testing speeds.

A study by Koziris et al[41] tested collegiate female tennis players on a Cybex II at 180 degrees/s. The consistent pattern of dominant shoulder strength and relative external rotation strength imbalance were also reported in this population.

The previously reported isokinetic research assessed concentric muscular performance in 90 degrees of abduction of the rotator cuff in highly skilled tennis players. A 6-week training study of concentric or eccentric isokinetic exercise was performed on a KinCom using 22 collegiate tennis players.[39] Results of the pre- and post-testing showed statistically significant increases in concentric and eccentric internal and external rotation strength in the concentric training group. Subjects in this group also showed a significant increase in maximal serve velocity. The eccentric isokinetic training group also showed significant increases in concentric internal and external rotation strength but did not show eccentric strength gains or an increase in functional performance. Results from this study[39] provide rationale for inclusion of isokinetic training of the rotator cuff in rehabilitation and preventative conditioning.

Isokinetic research presented in this chapter clearly shows specific patterns found in the dominant arm of highly skilled tennis players. Care must be taken, however, in the use of normative isokinetic strength data presented in these studies. Research has indicated that isokinetic parameters are both apparatus-specific[42,43] and specific to the position of the shoulder joint during the testing procedure.[44,45]

## APPLICATION OF TENNIS RESEARCH TO THE TREATMENT OF SHOULDER INJURIES

The review of epidemiology presented earlier in this chapter showed the overuse nature and common occurrence of rotator cuff and bicipital tendinitis in the tennis player's shoulder.

### Evaluation

Before treatment of the injured tennis player, a thorough tennis-specific subjective evaluation is indicated. This is consistent with orthopaedic and sports physical therapy shoulder evaluation[46]; however, the exact relationship between the injured shoulder and tennis play must be determined. Specific questions regarding the player's tennis history, skill level, stroke mechanics,

play frequency and duration, and tournament schedule as well as current racquet type and string tension are of paramount importance. Consistent with most musculoskeletal overuse injuries in athletes, a change, however small, has usually been made in one or more of the aforementioned factors before the injury. Often a particular tennis stroke or phase of the stroke can be identified with the onset of injury or with exeracerbation of symptoms.

### Reduction of Overload/Total Arm Rehabilitation

The initial goal of overuse shoulder rehabilitation includes the reduction of pain and inflammation in the involved tissues. Although many methods are appropriate, including physical therapy modalities and anti-inflammatory medications,[47,48] the injured extremity must be protected from further stress or overload but not from full function. Specific or complete cessation of tennis play is indicated. Compensation by the upper extremity kinetic chain in individuals with shoulder pathology can lead to overuse injury in the elbow, forearm, and wrist.[32] Avoidance of overhead movements in activities of daily living and cross-training activities is also recommended.

During the initial phase of shoulder overuse rehabilitation, stresses imparted to the injured tissues are minimized. Early stress of the distal upper extremity in the form of isotonic eccentric and concentric elbow, forearm, and wrist exercise is indicated to preserve the important distal musculature. Adaptation of the distal upper extremity in the form of hypertrophy is a consistent finding in the dominant arm of highly skilled tennis players.[34,35]

### Protection and Restoration of Joint Arthrokinematics

Presented earlier in this chapter were specific shoulder range of motion patterns in elite junior[28,29] and adult[34] tennis players. Thorough evaluation of shoulder stability via assessment of the static and dynamic stabilizers must be performed to appropriately base the progression of exercise and range of motion during rehabilitation. Use of the load and shift test,[49] subluxation relocation test,[10] and other testing to assess the passive anterior, posterior, and inferior translation of the glenohumeral joint are integral parts in determining the causation of the overuse injury. These findings also provide the framework for the use or lack of use of range of motion/mobilization techniques in rehabilitation.

The increased external shoulder rotation and reduced internal rotation can indicate anterior capsular laxity and the potential for anterior subluxation.[50] Therefore, use of stretching or mobilization techniques to further increase external rotation range of motion by attenuating the anterior capsule are not indicated. Posterior capsular mobilization and stretching techniques for the posterior musculature address the lack of glenohumeral joint internal rotation and have been recommended in treatment of unilaterally dominant upper extremity athletes.[51]

## Promotion of Upper Extremity Strength Balance and Local Muscular Endurance

As the inflammation and pain levels decrease in the injured tissues, early submaximal resistive exercise is initiated. As in the rehabilitation of other musculotendinous injuries, the presence or lack of pain in the joint or over the affected tendon determines the progression or regression of resistive exercise. Research on muscle activity patterns in the tennis strokes highlight concentric as well as eccentric muscle work in the rotator cuff and scapular stabilizers. Treatment of rotator cuff pathology either from primary impingement or secondary to intrinsic tensile overload or joint instability necessitates specific emphasis on strengthening the dynamic stabilizers of the glenohumeral joint. The force couple outlined by Inman et al[18] and precise function of the deltoid, infraspinatus, supraspinatus, and teres minor delineated by Weiner and MacNab[52] reinforce this author's emphasis on isolated rotator cuff strengthening for the above-mentioned overuse shoulder injuries. Figure 34-1 illustrates the approximating role of the supraspinatus and inferior or caudal role inherent in muscular contraction of the infraspinatus and teres minor.

Progression of the isolated rotator cuff exercises is predicated on patient signs and symptoms and begins briefly with the isometric and manual resistance mode

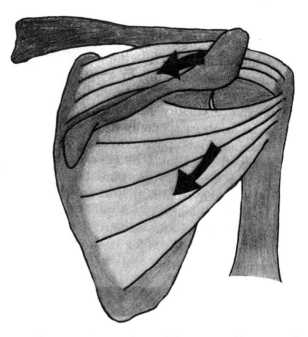

**Fig. 34-1.** Approximate lines of force exerted by supraspinatus (*top arrow*) and infraspinatus and teres minor (*bottom arrow*) as the approximating and inferior components of the force couple system.

and progresses rapidly to isotonic concentric and eccentric exercise. Four isotonic exercises are recommended for overuse shoulder rehabilitation caused by the increased rotator cuff activity reported in EMG studies.[53,54] These exercises are the "empty can" (shoulder elevation in the scapular plane with internal rotation), sidelying external rotation, prone extension, and prone horizontal abduction with external rotation. These exercises are performed via a pain-free range of motion and were chosen because of noncompromising glenohumeral joint positions and high EMG activity of the rotator cuff mechanism. A low-resistance high-repetition format is advocated. This emphasizes local muscle endurance[55] and will begin to prepare the athlete for the repetitive nature of the muscular work during tennis play and stroke execution. Concentric and especially eccentric biceps brachii exercise is also emphasized throughout rehabilitation. This is indicated throughout rehabilitation because of the stabilizing nature of the biceps musculature shown in the muscle activity research on tennis strokes. Increased bicep activity has also been reported in overhand throwing of patients with glenohumeral joint instability.[56] Early emphasis is also given to the scapulothoracic musculature, particularly the serratus anterior, rhomboids, and trapezius. Again exercises using noncompromising ranges of glenohumeral joint motion and a low-resistance high-repetition format are followed.

Application of isokinetic research on highly skilled tennis players to rehabilitation of overuse shoulder injury assists in determining focal muscle groups necessary to obtain strength balance. The relative absence of a strength enhancement of the external rotators on the dominant shoulder of highly skilled tennis players highlights the need for specific external rotation strength training to balance the external/internal rotation strength relationship. Isokinetic research also shows dominant arm strength 15 to 30 percent greater than the nondominant arm,[40] indicating a need for postinjury isokinetic strength levels to exceed the healthy, contralateral limb.

Continued use of isotonic exercise with weights and surgical tubing is recommended in shoulder rehabilitation with a progression to the isokinetic form of resistance once a pain-free range of motion and isotonic exercise tolerance are shown. Initial submaximal isokinetic exercise in the modified neutral position[51,57] for internal and external rotation at intermediate contractile velocities is used. Specific emphasis continues on the external rotators because of their important role in functional activities[17,20] and in the maintenance of dynamic anterior glenohumeral joint stability.[58]

Rapid progression from intermediate to fast contractile velocities is recommended because of the fast joint kinematic characteristics of the tennis strokes.[25] Progression from the modified neutral isokinetic internal and external rotation position to the 90 degree abducted position is recommended, with tissue tolerance being the limiting factor. The functional nature of this isokinetic training position is outlined in the joint kinematic section of this chapter.[27,59]

Isokinetic and manual strength assessments are only two methods used in determining the patient's readiness to return to tennis play. Isokinetic strength of the internal and external rotators equal to the contralateral limb have been one minimum criterion used by this author for functional return. Again a goal of achieving a strength level 15 or even 20 percent greater on the dominant extremity is set based on the literature.[29,40]

Presence of a full pain-free range of forward flexion and abduction without subacromial impingement, as well as full pain-free internal and external rotation at 90 degrees of abduction, are other important determinants in the progression to functional activity.

## Return to Functional Activity

Analysis of the patient's objective strength and range of motion status predicate the return to tennis play. A submaximal and graded return to tennis is used and is similar to the interval return programs for throwing.[8,60] The initial trial of tennis play includes both stroke simulation without ball contact as well as forehand and backhand ground stroke execution with a lightweight foam ball. Proper stroke mechanics are emphasized throughout the interval tennis program. Once a tolerance has been shown with stroke simulation and foam ball contact, the patient is progressed to a standard tennis ball.

The basic concept applied in the interval tennis program is the progression from situations with low or decreased preimpact ball velocity to situations with functional preimpact ball velocity. Application of this concept is evidenced by the initiation of ground stroke execution from the baseline via ball feeds hit by a partner from the net. This initial activity is built on by progressing to controlled baseline to baseline rallying with forehand and backhand ground strokes. Partner feeding from the net ensures a controlled and slower preimpact ball velocity, which minimizes impact stress to the injured extremity. A backboard is not initially used because of the fast and continual rebound characteristics that encourage continued, noninterrupted muscle work in the upper extremity.

Once several trials of pain-free ground strokes are achieved, the forehand and backhand volley are initiated. Repetitions of ground strokes and volleys used in the early stages of the interval program are as low as 15 to 30, with gradual progression as signs and symptoms allow. Pain-free volley and ground stroke execution are prerequisites for progression to the serve and overhead smash.

A submaximal trial is initiated with the serving motion using stroke simulation and foam ball impact. Initial velocity on progression to a standard tennis ball is as low as 30 to 40 percent preinjury levels. The player's velocity and serving repetitions are gradually increased as muscular strength and endurance as well as subjective tolerance allows.

Evaluation of the player's equipment is also indicated during the return to tennis. Research indicates that lower string tensions allow for greater postimpact ball velocity[61] and hence greater power with lower stroke effort from the player. Lowering the racquets string tension by several pounds has been recommended in the treatment of tennis elbow.[32,46] Although a definitive relationship between racquet head size or stiffness and upper extremity injury has not been delineated, sports medicine professionals have recommended a midsize racquet head and medium flexibility rating for patients with lateral and medial epicondylitis.[47] Optimal racquet grip size has been discussed relative to upper extremity injury and muscle activity.[62] Proper grip size had been described by Nirschl,[48] using a measurement from the distal tip of the ring finger along the radial border to the proximal palmar crease.

## SUMMARY

Thorough knowledge of the mechanical and physiologic demands and subsequent sport-specific adaptations in the upper extremity of the tennis player are required for optimal rehabilitation, as well as performance enhancement. Implementation of the total arm strength program presented in this chapter, integrated with proper stroke mechanics and equipment, is a critical component of rehabilitating and preventing overuse shoulder injuries in the tennis player.

## REFERENCES

1. Priest JD, Nagel DA: Tennis shoulder. Am J Sports Med 4:28, 1976
2. Priest JD, Braden V, Gerberich SG: An analysis of players with and without pain. Physician Sports Med 8:81, 1980
3. Winge S, Jorgensen U, Nielsen AL: Epidemiology of injuries in Danish championship tennis. Int J Sports Med 10:368, 1989
4. Reece LA, Fricker PA, Maguire KF: Injuries to elite young tennis players at the Australian Institute of Sport. Australian J Sci Med Sport 18:11, 1986
5. Bigliani LU, Kimmel J, McCann PD, Wolfe I: Repair of rotator cuff tears in tennis players. Am J Sports Med 20:112, 1992
6. Neer CS: Impingement lesions. Clin Orthop 173:70, 1983
7. Jobe FW, Kvitne RS: Shoulder pain in the overhand or throwing athlete: the relationship of anterior instability and rotator cuff impingement. Orthop Rev 18:963, 1989
8. Andrews JR, Kupferman SP, Dillman CJ: Labral tears in throwing and racquet sports. Clin Sports Med 10:901, 1991
9. Nirschl RP: Shoulder tendinitis. Upper extremity injuries in athletes, American Academy of Orthopaedic Surgeons Symposium, Washington, D.C. CV Mosby, St. Louis, 1986
10. Jobe FW, Bradley JP: The diagnosis and nonoperative treatment of shoulder injuries in athletes. Clin Sports Med 8:419, 1989
11. Kibler WB, McQueen C, Uhl T: Fitness evaluation and fitness findings in competitive junior tennis players. Clin Sports Med 7:403, 1988
12. Nigg BM, Frederick EC, Hawes MR, Luethi SM: Factors influencing short term pain and injuries in tennis. Int J Sport Biomech 2:156, 1986
13. Hang YS, Peng SM: An epidemiological study of upper extremity injury in tennis players with a particular reference to tennis elbow. J Formosan Med Assoc 83:307, 1984
14. Kamien M: The incidence of tennis elbow and other injuries in tennis players at the Royal Kings Park Tennis Club of Western Australia from October 1983 to September 1984. Aust J Sci Med Sport 21:18, 1989
15. Lehman RC: Shoulder pain in the competitive tennis player. Clin Sports Med 7:309, 1988
16. Yoshizawa M, Itani T, Jonsson B: Muscular load in shoulder and forearm muscles in tennis players with different levels of skill. In Jonsson B (ed): Biomechanics X-B. Human Kinetics, Champaign, IL, 1987
17. Rhu KN, McCormick J, Jobe FW et al: An electromyographic analysis of shoulder function in tennis players. Am J Sports Med 16:481, 1988
18. Inman VT, Saunders JB de CM, Abbot LC: Observations on the function of the shoulder joint. J Bone Joint Surg 26A:1, 1944
19. Bradley JP, Tibone JE: Electromyographic analysis of muscle action about the shoulder. Clin Sports Med 10:789, 1991
20. VanGheluwe B, Hebbelinck M: Muscle actions and ground reaction forces in tennis. Int J Sport Biomech 2:88, 1986
21. Miyashita M, Tsunoda T, Sakurai S et al: Muscular activities in the tennis serve and overhand throwing. Scand J Sports Sci 2:52, 1980
22. Groppel JL: Tennis for Advanced Players: And Those Who Would Like to Be. Human Kinetics, Champaign, IL, 1984
23. Groppel JL: The utilization of proper racket sport mechanics to avoid upper extremity injury. In Pettrone FA (ed): Proceedings of the Symposium on Upper Extremity

Injuries: Sponsored by the Academy of Orthopaedic Surgeons. Mosby Publications, St. Louis, 1986

24. Groppel JL: High Tech Tennis. Human Kinetics, Champaign, IL, 1992

25. Shapiro R, Stine RL: Shoulder rotation velocities. Technical report submitted to the Lexington Clinic, Lexington, KY, 1992

26. Dillman CJ: Presentation on the upper extremity in tennis and throwing athletes. United States Tennis Association National Meeting, Tucson, Arizona, March 1991

27. Elliot B, Marsh T, Blanksby B: A three dimensional cinematographic analysis of the tennis serve. Int J Sport Biomech 2:260, 1986

28. Chandler TJ, Kibler WB, Uhl TL et al: Flexibility comparisons of junior elite tennis players to other athletes. Am J Sports Med 18:134, 1990

29. Ellenbecker TS: Shoulder internal and external rotation strength and range of motion of highly skilled junior tennis players. Isokinetics Exerc Sci 2:1, 1992

30. Groppel JL: The biomechanics of tennis: an overview. Int J Sport Biomech 2:141, 1986

31. VanGheluwe B, DeRuysscher I, Craenhals J: Pronation and endorotation of the racket arm in a tennis serve. In Jonsson B (ed): Biomechanics X-B. Human Kinetics, Champaign, IL, 1987

32. Nirschl RP: Tennis elbow. Prim Care 4:367, 1977

33. Kulund DN, Rockwell DA, Brubaker CE: The long-term effects of playing tennis. Physician Sports Med 7:87, 1979

34. Chinn CJ, Priest JD, Kent BE: Upper extremity range of motion, grip strength, and girth in highly skilled tennis players. Phys Ther 54:474, 1974

35. Vodak PA, Savin WM, Haskell WL, Wood PW: Physiological profile of middle-aged male and female tennis players. Med Sci Sports Exerc 12:159, 1980

36. Carlson JS, Cera MA: Cardiorespiratory, muscular strength and anthropoemetric characteristics of elite Australian junior male and female tennis players. Aust J Sci Med Sport 16:7, 1984

37. Matsen FA III, Arntz CT: Subacromial impingement. In Rockwood CA Jr, Matsen FA III (eds): The Shoulder. 1st Ed. WB Saunders, Philadelphia, 1990

38. Harryman DT, Sidles JA, Clark JM et al: Translation of the humeral head on the glenoid with passive glenohumeral motion. J Bone Joint Surg 72A:1334, 1990

39. Ellenbecker TS, Davies GJ, Rowinski MJ: Concentric versus eccentric isokinetic strengthening of the rotator cuff: objective data versus functional test. Am J Sports Med 16:64, 1988

40. Ellenbecker TS: A total arm strength isokinetic profile of highly skilled tennis players. Isokinetics Exerc Sci 1:9, 1991

41. Koziris LP, Kraemer WJ, Triplett NT et al: Strength imbalances in women in tennis players (abstr). Med Sci Sports Exerc 23:253, 1991

42. Francis K, Hoobler T: Comparison of peak torque values of the knee flexor and extensor muscle groups using the Cybex II and Lido 2.0 isokinetic dynamometers. J Orthop Sports Phys Ther 8:480, 1987

43. Gross MT, Huffman GM, Phillips CN, Wray A: Intramachine and intermachine reliability of the Biodex and Cybex II for knee flexion and extension peak torque and angular work. J Orthop Sports Phys Ther 13:329, 1991

44. Hageman PA, Mason DK, Rydlund KW, Humpal SA: Effects of position and speed on eccentric and concentric isokinetic testing of the shoulder rotators. J Orthop Sports Phys Ther 11:64, 1989

45. Soderberg GJ, Blaschak MJ: Shoulder internal and external rotation peak torque production through a velocity spectrum in differing positions. J Orthop Sports Phys Ther 8:518, 1987

46. Davies GJ, Gould JA, Larson RL: Functional examination of the shoulder girdle. Physician Sports Med 9:82, 1981

47. Nirschl RP, Sobel J: Conservative treatment of tennis elbow. Physician Sports Med 9:43, 1981

48. Nirschl RP: Tennis injuries. In Nicholas JA, Hershman EB (eds): The Upper Extremity in Sports Medicine. CV Mosby, St. Louis, 1990

49. Abrams JS: Special shoulder problems in the throwing athlete: pathology, diagnosis, and nonoperative management. Clin Sports Med 10:839, 1991

50. Warner JJP, Micheli LJ, Arslanian LE et al: Patterns of flexibility, laxity, and strength in normal shoulders and shoulders with instability and impingement. Am J Sports Med 18:366, 1990

51. Ellenbecker TS, Derscheid GL: Rehabilitation of overuse injuries of the shoulder. Clin Sports Med 8:583, 1989

52. Weiner DS, MacNab I: Superior migration of the humeral head. J Bone Joint Surg 52B:524, 1970

53. Blackburn TA, McLeod WD, White B, Wofford L: EMG analysis of posterior rotator cuff exercises. Athletic Training 25:40, 1990

54. Townsend H, Jobe FW, Pink M, Perry J: Electromyographic analysis of the glenohumeral muscles during a baseball rehabilitation program. Am J Sports Med 19:264, 1991

55. Fleck S, Kraemer W: Designing Resistance Training Programs. Human Kinetics, Champaign, IL, 1987

56. Glousman R, Jobe FW, Tibone JE et al: Dynamic electromyographic analysis of the throwing shoulder with glenohumeral joint instability. J Bone Joint Surg 70A:220, 1988

57. Davies GJ: A compendium of isokinetics in clinical usage. S & S Publishing, LaCrosse, WI, 1984

58. Cain PR, Mutschler TA, Fu F, Lee SK: Anterior stability of the glenohumeral joint. A dynamic model. Am J Sports Med 15:144, 1987

59. Elliot BC: Biomechanics of the serve in tennis: a biomedical perspective. Sports Med 6:285, 1988

60. Seto JL, Brewster CE, Randall CC, Jobe FW: Rehabilitation following ulnar collateral ligament reconstruction of athletes. J Orthop Sports Phys Ther 14:100, 1991

61. Brody H: Physics of the tennis racquet. Am J Phys 6:482, 1979

62. Adelsberg S: An EMG analysis of selected muscles with rackets of increasing grip size. Am J Sports Med 14:139, 1986

# 35

# Shoulder Injuries in Swimming

## TIMOTHY C. MURPHY

At the recreational level, swimming is an extremely popular activity, with more than 120 million Americans reporting that they swim regularly, although most of these undoubtedly could be classed as bathers rather than individuals who are actively involved in swim training at the fitness or competitive levels. More than 165,000 regularly competing swimmers are registered with United States Swimming, Inc., and organized competitive swimming is also available through summer leagues, YMCA/YWCA programs, high school and college swimming programs, Masters Swimming, and Special Olympics.[1-5]

Interest in competitive swimming has grown considerably in the past several decades, as media coverage of national and international competition has improved and swimming personalities have become better known to the public. The popularity of triathalons has also had an impact on the growth of swimming as a fitness activity. Interestingly, as a result of the surge in triathalon training, many previously unskilled swimmers have begun to train for distance events, with predictable overuse consequences.

Swimmers compete in four strokes.[6-8] The freestyle (front crawl) stroke is the most widely used and preferred stroke. It is characterized by alternating overhead stroking of the arms with alternating (flutter) kicking of the legs. The backstroke (back crawl) is similar to freestyle but is performed with the swimmer on his or her back. Breaststroke is performed by symmetric movements of the arms and legs without breaking the plane of the water. The most demanding of the four is butterfly, which involves the simultaneous movement of the arms over the water, accompanied by concurrent kicking of the legs (dolphin kick).

Today's successful competitive swimmer can look forward to training 10 to 11 mo/yr in a competitive career, which may last as long as 10 to 15 years (Tables 35-1 and 35-2). Some swimmers practice twice a day and may average, at the elite high school and collegiate levels, as high as 8,000 to 20,000 yd (11.4 miles)/day. Based on an average of six to 10 stroke cycles per 25-yd pool length, a swimmer completing a 10,000-yd freestyle workout performs 2,400 to 4,000 overhead strokes per arm per session. This figure does not account for the fact that the swimmer, as he or she fatigues and stroke efficiency declines, must take additional strokes to complete each pool length.

Age group swimming usually begins with competitive events for 6 to 8 year olds, although competition at an exhibition level may begin as early as 4 to 5 years of age. The life span of the competitive swimmer may extend into the sixth and seventh decades with the advent of active Masters swimming programs and competition.

It is estimated that up to 40 to 60 percent of competitive swimmers experience shoulder pain (Fig. 35-1) to the extent that their training is interrupted.[1,9-14] Interestingly, this applies to all swimmers regardless of stroke preference or specialty. The reason for this appears to be the relatively high amount of freestyle as a training stroke. Nonfreestylers may swim as much as

**Table 35-1. Recommended Daily Training Yardage for Age-Group Swimmers Based on Competitive Level**

| Age Group (yr) | Novice (yd) | Experienced (yd) |
|---|---|---|
| 8 & younger | 400–800 | 1,000–1,500 |
| 10 & younger | 600–1,200 | 1,500–3,000 |
| 11–12 | 1,000–2,000 | 4,000–5,000 |
| 13–14 | 2,000–4,000 | 6,000–12,000 |

(From Maglischo,[7] with permission.)

411

**Table 35-2. Recommended Daily Training Yardage for Senior Swimmers Based on Competitive Level, Season, and Event Category**

| Season/Category | Novice (yd) | Experienced (yd) |
|---|---|---|
| Early season | | |
| Sprinters | 3,000–5,000 | 8,000–12,000 |
| Middle distance | 4,000–6,000 | 10,000–15,000 |
| Distance | 6,000–8,000 | 12,000–18,000 |
| Competitive season | | |
| Sprinters | 5,000–6,000 | 7,000–11,000 |
| Middle distance | 7,000–9,000 | 8,000–12,000 |
| Distance | 8,000–10,000 | 12,000–18,000 |

(From Maglischo,[7] with permission.)

60 to 90 percent of their workouts in freestyle, depending on the nature of training or the relative fatigue of their primary stroke (e.g., butterfly). For this reason, most overuse problems relate in some way to the freestyle stroke.

## TRAINING THE COMPETITIVE SWIMMER

The single most important factor in training the competitive swimmer is technique.[6,7] Swimmers with poor basic technique may expend enormous amounts of

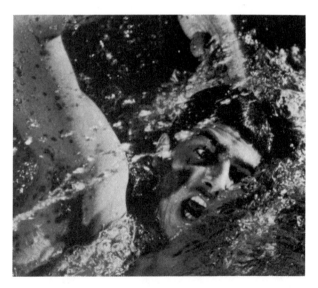

**Fig. 35-1.** Shoulder is primary site of pain and dysfunction in swimmers. (From Counsilman,[30] with permission.)

energy to propel themselves through the water. In some cases, performance may actually be diminished as effort increases. Even in swimmers with good basic technique, muscular fatigue may be a factor in the deterioration of stroke mechanics over the course of a long workout. In other words, a swimmer with excellent technique but with poor local muscular endurance may become a swimmer with poor technique (and attendant biomechanical overuse stresses) as specific areas of weakness develop during a fatiguing workout.

Poor technique is a particularly important factor in the evolution of overuse problems that are commonly seen in the swimming athlete. High school and collegiate swimming coaches frequently "inherit" athletes with firmly ingrained stroke errors or deficiencies that quickly lead to injuries when rigorous training programs are implemented. Proper technique development is very important in youth swimming, because of the remarkable motor learning skills available to youngsters. For this reason, the development of good stroke mechanics should be one of the primary coaching goals in youth swimming programs.

Recommended daily training distance for age group and senior swimmers varies from 400 to 18,000 yards,[7] depending on many factors (see Tables 35-1 and 35-2), although considerable controversy has developed over the use of "quality" versus "quantity" training. Many coaches favor keeping the total training yardage to a minimum to avoid overuse injuries among their swimmers. Decisions regarding the daily training distance may be made by the coach based on age, the competitive level of the swimmer (novice versus advanced), and the desired distance and intensity of the event for which the athlete is training.

Increasing emphasis is being placed on the physiology of swimming in the development of training programs, although significant misperceptions remain in the swimming community with respect to training distances and workout intensity. Councilman[6] suggested that swimming and running be equated on a 4 : 1 ratio based on the performance times in the 440-yd dash and the 100-yd freestyle. This ratio would suggest that swimming 1 mile is roughly the equivalent of running 4 miles, and so on. When the maximum training distances of elite swimmers are taken into consideration, the swimmer performing 16,000 yd (10 miles)/day equates to similar performance by the runner of 40 miles/day! Although the significant weight-bearing stresses of the runner are not present in swimming, the repetitive overhead mechanical stresses of the swimmer cannot be ignored.

A great deal of effort in training is expended on strengthening of those muscles that exert force in the actual pull-through phase of the swimming stroke. For this reason, exceptional emphasis is placed on shoulder internal rotation, extension, and adduction, along with elbow extension. Little, if any, emphasis is generally placed on shoulder external rotation, flexion, and abduction or on elbow flexion.

Imparting resistance to the pull-through muscles in a relatively sport-specific manner may involve any or all the following techniques:

1. Isolated pull-through exercises are performed against free weights, machine weights, or isokinetic devices such as the Mini-Gym or Biokinetic Swim Bench. They are also almost universally performed against surgical tubing pull cords.
2. Pull buoys and kick boards are used to selectively eliminate legs or arms respectively to place all propulsive stress on the other.
3. Drag is a frequently used training tool. It is routine for the swimmer to wear two to five bathing suits, along with old panty hose or other clothing, to increase the resistance to movement through the water and thus the training intensity. A drag suit may

also be used to create resistance to movement in the water through the use of parachute-like pockets. Drag may also be provided through swimming against (away from) an elastic tether. This forces the hands actually to move through the water with high resistance, rather than pulling the body past a given point in the water.

4. Hand paddles may be used to increase the resistance to the pull-through muscles (Fig. 35-2). Several sources have attempted to link the use of hand paddles to the incidence of shoulder problems in swimmers.[15] Although the use of hand paddles may not directly cause shoulder pain, it may contribute to shoulder girdle fatigue and the attendant changes in stroke mechanics that lead to different overuse pathologies.

## BIOMECHANICS OF SWIMMING

Upper extremity propulsive force in the primary competitive strokes (freestyle, backstroke, butterfly, and breaststroke) comes about specifically by some combination of shoulder extension, adduction, and internal rotation (Fig. 35-3) during the pull phase in the water.[6–8,14] The swimmer attempts to pull him- or herself past a given point in the water rather than simply moving the arms through the water. As the hand enters the water at the beginning of the pull phase (the catch), the swimmer sets the hand to "grasp" the water. The hand is then pulled past the body using a sculling motion that combines movements of the shoulder, elbow, wrist, and hand. This pull-through phase makes up about 65 percent of the swimming stroke (both arms are actually in the water at the same time for about one-third of the cycle) and is the main emphasis of muscular strength and muscular endurance training for most swimmers (Fig. 35-4).

The remaining 35 percent of the stroke cycle consists of the recovery phase, which returns the arm to the starting position for the next pull-through. Although recovery is not a productive part of the stroke in terms of propulsion, it is the topic of increasing interest on the part of coaches and sports medicine professionals as a potential contributing factor in many of the overuse problems associated with swimming.[1–4,12,14,16] For the swimmer's arm to provide consistent power over many repetitions, the recovery must continue to place the

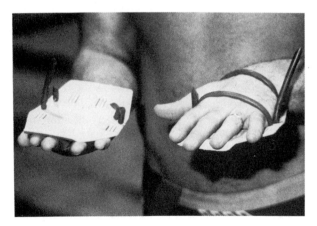

**Fig. 35-2.** Hand paddles are frequently used to increase resistance during pull phase of swimming. Use of hand paddles may accelerate fatigue-related changes in stroke mechanics. (From Falkel and Murphy,[14] with permission.)

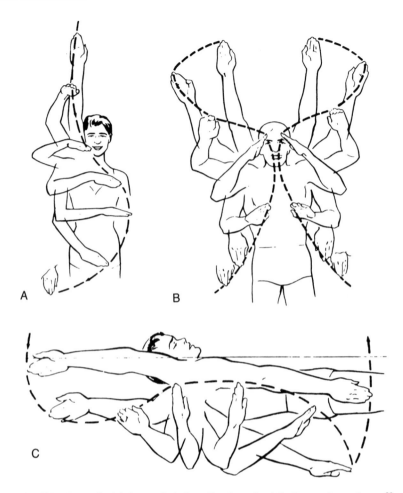

**Fig. 35-3.** Phases of pull for freestyle (*A*), butterfly (*B*) and backstroke (*C*). (From Counsilman,[30] with permission.)

arm in an optimal position for initiating the pull-through phase time after time. The muscles that perform the recovery generally do not hold the highest priority in most training programs, because of the heavy emphasis on the pull-phase muscles. It is fairly predictable then that a breakdown in the mechanics of stroke recovery is one of the first observable fatigue-related changes in the stroke during a long workout.

The pull-through phase (Table 35-3) begins with hand entry, continues through mid pull-through, and is terminated with the shoulder fully internally rotated, adducted, and extended as the elbow reaches terminal extension.[1,8,14] The recovery phase begins with the elbow lift as the hand leaves the water. External rotation begins immediately and passes the rotational "midposi-

tion" by the middle point in recovery (Fig. 35-5). The degree of external rotation achieved before the midpoint in recovery and decrements in the amount of external rotation achieved as the swimmer fatigues may be factors in the incidence of subacromial impingement stress over time.

## Humeral Rotation/Depression

The rotational position of the humerus is critical with respect to impingement of the subacromial structures by the greater tuberosity. If the glenohumeral joint is internally rotated, the greater tuberosity is in closer approximation to the coracoacromial arch, and mechanical impingement of the subacromial structures is

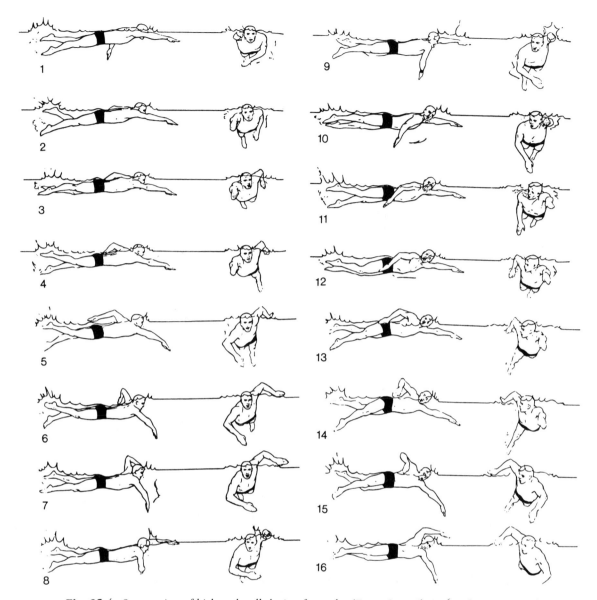

**Fig. 35-4.** Sequencing of kick and pull during freestyle. (From Counsilman,[6] with permission.)

**Table 35-3. Biomechanical Description of the Stroke Phases in Freestyle**

| Stroke Phases | Description |
| --- | --- |
| Pull-through | |
|    Hand entry | Shoulder externally rotated and abducted; body roll begins |
|    Mid pull-through | Shoulder at 90° abduction and neutral rotation; body roll is at maximum of 40°–60° from horizontal |
|    End of pull-through | Shoulder internally rotated and fully abducted; body returned to horizontal position |
| Recovery phase | |
|    Elbow lift | Shoulder begins abduction and external rotation; body roll begins in opposite direction from pull-through |
|    Midrecovery | Shoulder abducted to 90° and externally rotated beyond neutral; body roll reaches maximum of 40°–60°; breathing occurs by turning head to side |
|    Hand entry | Shoulder externally rotated and maximally abducted; body roll has returned to neutral |

(From Richardson et al,[20] with permission.)

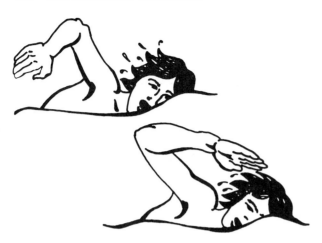

**Fig. 35-5.** Degree of external rotation during recovery will affect amount of subacromial impingement. (From Falkel and Murphy,[14] with permission.)

more likely. This is particularly true during the abduction component of recovery.[1,8,14]

The action of humeral head depression by the rotator cuff and biceps tendon mechanisms (and by the latissimus dorsi when the shoulder is flexed/abducted) has been well documented.[8] This depression serves to minimize the degree of subacromial impingement as overhead movement occurs and allows the humeral head to seek out the broader articular surface of the lower glenoid.

## Hand Placement and Position

Proper hand placement allows for the correct setting of the hand at the catch and assists in establishing optimal shoulder and elbow position to begin pull-through. Poor stroke mechanics during the recovery phase may lead to unfavorable hand placement at the moment of the catch and therefore reduce pull efficiency.[6,7,14]

Cross-over placement of the hand at entry or moving across the midline during the early stages of pull-through places the shoulder in a position of horizontal adduction, flexion, and internal rotation that creates a mechanical impingement of the biceps long head as well as a vascular impingement of the biceps and supraspinatus tendons (Fig. 35-6). This position of midline crossing in early pull-through has been cited as the position of greatest discomfort by many swimmers[14]

and would appear to be the position of greatest mechanical impingement on the biceps long head.

## The Kick

The kick is unquestionably an important component in the overall propulsive force of the swimming stroke, although it is secondary by far to the arm force in all competitive strokes. The kick also serves to "smooth" out the intermittent surges of the arms during both alternating and symmetric upper extremity stroke patterns.

Besides its propulsive role, the kick also serves to keep the body horizontal in the water to optimize streamlining and thereby improves the efficiency of the arm stroke. The kick serves as an anchoring mechanism for body roll, further maintaining the body in an optimal position for efficient use of the arms.[6,7]

## Body Roll and Rotation

Body roll of 40 to 60 degrees during the recovery phase minimizes the amount of horizontal abduction necessary for initiating the recovery and allows the overhead movement of the arm to occur with the necessary external rotation to avoid mechanical and vascular impingement stress.[1,8,14,17] This positioning also allows for abduction more within the plane of the scapula with an associated reduction in soft tissue tension related to the overhead movement.

Excessive roll will lead to a cross-over entry and/or cross-over during the propulsive phase. Lack of body roll in the recovery phase restricts the achievement of full external rotation, increases the degree of mechanical stress, and provides for an abnormal hand placement during entry.

## Head Position and Breathing Patterns

An exaggerated head-down position will lead to a deeper arm pull as well as promote malalignment during the pull-through and recovery phases. Conversely, an exaggerated head-up position will result in concomitant lowering of the hips in the plane of the water and result in excessive drag.[6,7]

The side of pain has been inconsistently correlated to the side of breathing in a number of studies, and thus no consensus of opinion is prevalent in the literature at

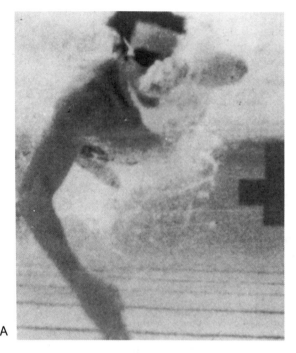
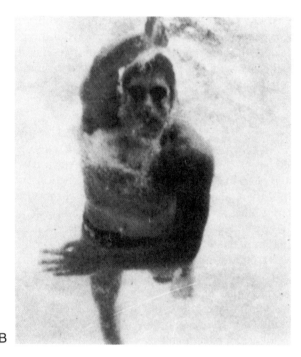

A                                          B

**Fig. 35-6.** Examples of mid pull-through to midline (**A**) and crossing the midline (**B**). Midline crossing may be associated with mechanical and vascular impingement. (From Counsilman,[30] with permission.)

this time.[14] Incomplete body roll to the nonbreathing side can certainly increase the horizontal abduction component of the nonbreathing arm and thereby increase impingement stresses. Clinical experience has revealed fewer impingement problems in that population that incorporates a bilateral breathing pattern, presumably as a function of greater symmetry in body roll related to breathing to both sides.

## PATHOMECHANICS OF SHOULDER INJURY IN SWIMMERS

### Mechanical Impingement

Improper or deteriorated stroke mechanics are presumably the greatest single precursor to impingement stresses at the shoulder during the excessive overhead repetitive motion encountered by swimmers.[18–20]

The problem of mechanical subacromial impingement is compounded by the fatigue and functional decrement of the rotator cuff muscles in their role as humeral head depressors as well as external rotators.

Fatigue of the shoulder muscles during swimming leads to deterioration of normal mechanics, particularly during recovery. In this case, external rotation during recovery is either incomplete or occurs late in abduction, with attendant subacromial impingement by the greater tuberosity.

Besides mechanical changes in the stroke with fatigue, the swimmer must also take more strokes to go a given distance as a function of central and local fatigue. This increases the number of overhead repetitions at a time when those movements are increasingly incorrect.

Primary mechanical impingement of the supraspinatus occurs between the greater tuberosity of the humerus and the middle and posterior portions of the coracoacromial arch. This transpires primarily during the recovery phase, and the swimmer experiences discomfort during the recovery as well as the early portion of the catch and pull-through.

Impingement of the biceps long head occurs against the anterior portion of the coracoacromial arch during late recovery and early pull-through. Clinically, individuals with biceps impingement seem to complain of symptoms from the early to midportions of the pull-through. Fatigue in the power stroke muscles may lead to a crossing of the midline with the arm during mid pull-through and subsequent anterior impingement of the biceps long head.

## Vascular Insult

Studies of the microvasculature of the rotator cuff[17] suggested that during glenohumeral abduction, there is nearly complete filling of the vessels in the distal supraspinatus tendon. There is a point, however, with the arm adducted at the side, at which the supraspinatus tendon becomes poorly supplied with blood distally because of the mechanical "wringing out" of the tendon as it passes over the head of the humerus. This occurs approximately 1 cm proximal to the insertion into the greater tuberosity and has become known as the "critical zone" because of the extremely high incidence of rotator cuff tears at that site.[1,4,18,21–23]

There is a similar response with shoulder flexion and horizontal adduction, a position of critical importance during mid pull-through. This vascular impingement is exaggerated by midline crossing (Fig. 35-6) and dropped elbow associated with arm fatigue (Fig. 35-7). The biceps long head demonstrates a similar pattern of avascularity (to that of the supraspinatus) as it passes over the head of the humerus.[17]

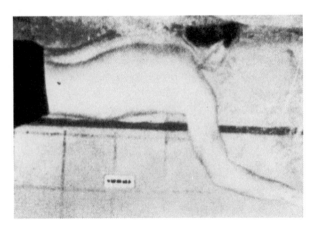

**Fig. 35-7.** Dropped elbow during pull-through, whether caused by fatigue or poor stroke mechanics, may be associated with impingement as well as decreased pull efficiency. (From Counsilman,[30] with permission.)

Besides the positionally defined vascular impingement described here, there is a mechanical vascular impingement associated with the compression of the subacromial structures while the arm is overhead.

## Fatigue-Related Overuse

Because of the small muscle mass of the external rotators and the prevailing lack of strength/endurance training for these muscles, it is not uncommon to see overuse syndromes associated with the external rotators as they attempt to provide not only their primary role but that of accessory stabilization of the scapula. This is particularly true of the infraspinatus and teres minor as they pass over the posterior glenohumeral joint capsule.

Frequently, there is involvement of the suprascapular and medial periscapular musculature in overuse syndromes associated with poor dynamic control of the scapula. Clinically, these problems are usually unilateral or asymmetric and are seen more frequently in unilateral breathers. There may also be a history of previous "scapulocervical" dysfunction, particularly associated with resolved traumatic strains that have been poorly rehabilitated.

These annoying conditions lead to pain throughout the recovery phase as well as pain with passive elongation and resisted contraction. They may occur independently or in conjunction with impingement syndromes and may, in fact, come about as a result of stroke compensatory changes that the swimmer creates in an effort to avoid impingement pain.

## Glenohumeral Instabilities

Anterior glenohumeral laxity is not an infrequent finding in swimmers of all strokes, but it seems to be much more prevalent in backstrokers.[1,9,12,14] These swimmers may experience a spectrum of symptoms with their strokes that ranges from anterior shoulder pain to palpable subluxation and even frank dislocation.

Trouble points in the backstroke include the catch (immediately after hand entry) when the shoulder is externally rotated, flexed, and horizontally abducted maximally, as well as the turn. Here there is a rapid force into horizontal abduction and external rotation through a closed kinetic chain when the hand hits the wall at the initiation of the turn.

These forces may result clinically in anterior capsular laxity to the extent that the anterior inferior glenohumeral ligament may become "incompetent." There may also be a tendency toward degenerative changes or tearing of the anterior portion of the glenoid labrum with attendant anterior instability.[1,9,12,14]

## Body Roll/Breathing Pattern

Asymmetries in body roll may lead to excessive horizontal abduction during recovery and associated increases in impingement stress. Body roll may be seen to decrease in response to fatigue and may be added to the growing list of noxious stresses acting on the tired swimmer.

Unilateral breathing is generally associated with asymmetric body roll and its attendant problems as noted previously. Bilateral breathers seem clinically to have fewer impingement problems, presumably as a function of the more symmetric body roll brought about by turning the head to either side regularly.

## Postural Faults and Muscular Asymmetries

Although specific "abnormal" postural sets have not been consistently applied to swimmers, those swimmers with underlying postural faults may be at risk for progressive associated overuse problems.

Frequent postural problems that have yielded clinical shoulder problems in swimmers include scoliosis, forward shoulder posturing with associated pectoralis minor tightness and thoracic outlet symptoms, and gross scapular instability.

The exact role of scapular stabilization is a difficult one to determine. It is certainly biomechanically important to provide proximal stability for distal function, and a large proportion of swimmers may appear to have scapular winging and instability. Yet is also important to encourage scapular mobility to allow for a reduction in glenohumeral and subacromial impingement forces during repetitive overhead motions.

The shoulder complex, in summary, may be seen to experience a series of mechanical and vascular insults by the very nature of the involved motions, made more abusive by progressive failure of the component functions as the swimmer fatigues. This process is very logical, yet it is rarely apparent to a swimmer in a proactive fashion and is usually discovered retrospectively.

## IN-SEASON MANAGEMENT CONSIDERATIONS

Historically, swimmer's injuries have been difficult to manage in the face of continued training and competition. It has not been uncommon for the swimmer to receive "damage control" treatment until the end of the swimming season, when it was hoped that the swimmer would cooperate and reduce training. For many swimmers with competitive training lasting 10 to 11 mo/yr, this is clearly an unrealistic expectation. Management has generally consisted of therapeutic modalities, medication, and rest, with occasional attempts at management through steroid injection or surgical decompression. Unfortunately, the swimmer usually has experienced some recurrence of the same problems shortly after returning to training, because of the renewal of the abnormal or excessive behaviors and physical stresses that initiated the problems in the first place.[1,9,14,24]

The "key" to in-season management of swimmers' problems, which are mostly of an overuse nature, is to identify not only the pathology but to recognize the source of the overuse and remediate it as well. In this manner, the swimmer should be able to return to full participation in a reasonable period and may even be able to continue training during treatment.[14]

### Evaluation

Besides evaluating the clinical signs and symptoms about the shoulder, it is important to ascertain what, if any, factors in the swimming stroke or training relate to the problem. Of special interest here (which may need to be discussed with coach) are daily training distance and intensity, along with recent pertinent changes in distance, stroke technique, underlying stroke mechanical faults, fatigue-related stroke changes, and goals for upcoming participation.[10]

### Clinical Treatment

Successful clinical treatment is dependent on elimination of most of the predisposing factors. Therapeutic heat and cold, with positioning respect for the vascularity of the involved structures, along with ultrasound (phonophoresis) and electrical stimulation, may assist in the inflammatory symptomatic management of the problem. Iontophoresis of anti-inflammatory agents may also be beneficial in the management of several of the superficial inflammatory problems in the swimmer's shoulder, as is local steroid injection, if coupled with some consideration for the cause of the problem and subsequent remediation.

The key to clinical management in early progressive initiation of rotational exercises is based on evaluation findings of weakness or fatigue problems (Fig. 35-8). Because most of the overuse problems with swimmers are related to very specific fatigue factors, elimination of these factors is paramount to eliminating exacerbating forces on return to training. The real goals of clinical management are to reduce the symptoms and to give the swimmer the "capacity" to endure the stresses of the stroke.

One unique management tool consists of the use of an upper arm strap[1,14,25] in tendinitis or impingement of the biceps long head, as well as subacromial impingement. Similar to a tennis elbow strap, this device is worn above the proximal muscle belly of the biceps (Fig. 35-9). It is thought to stabilize the biceps tendon in the intertubercular groove, thus reducing irritating friction in the groove. It is also thought to assist, through compression in the groove, the biceps tendon role in humeral head depression, thus the indication for use with subacromial impingement. Clinically, greater than 80 percent (author's unpublished data) of individuals with biceps tendon pathology report at least some reduction in shoulder discomfort within several days after beginning to use the strap.

## Training Modification

The training recommendation to the swimmer should be to continue swimming to whatever extent is asymptomatic and progress slowly (within symptom limitations) back to regular levels. For example, a swimmer who usually performs 7,000 yd/day and notes progres-

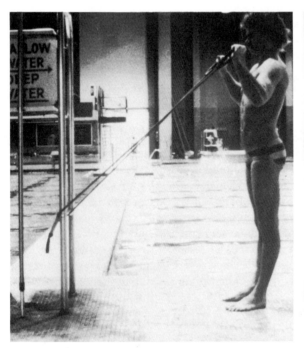
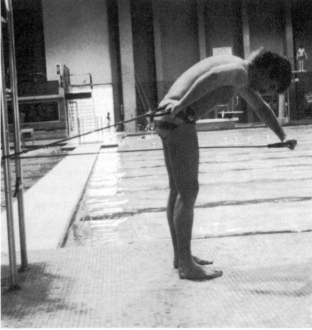

**Fig. 35-8.** Elastic pull cord exercises are very effective in improving muscular endurance of external rotators as well as scapular stabilizers. (From Falkel and Murphy,[14] with permission.)

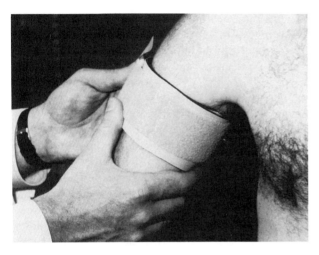

**Fig. 35-9.** Upper arm strap. (From Falkel and Murphy,[14] with permission.)

sive pain that begins after the midpoint of the workout may be placed on a remedial program of 3,000 yd/day with several short rest breaks to avoid fatigue changes. They may also be counseled to complete the same daily distance as usual but in several sessions instead of one. The swimmer may also be advised to perform cross-training or specific dry land workouts in an effort to "break up" the swimming routine. Incorporation of arm ergometry allows for relatively safe reproduction of resistance and pacing components and should definitely be considered as an adjunctive training tool.

There is a natural tendency for the health care provider to attempt to change the swimmer's stroke pattern in an effort to avoid the stresses discussed here. In fact, as has been presented throughout this chapter, it is the series of changes brought about by fatigue or repetition that accounts for most of these problems. The goal of rehabilitation should be to provide the swimmer with the "ammunition" to combat overuse in the form of the ability to maintain good mechanics rather than the manipulation of the basic techniques of the sport.

It is not uncommon to observe swimmers posting personal best performances shortly after returning to participation after in-season management. This may account for continued compliance with rehabilitation. It may also encourage other swimmers to adopt training techniques that are beneficial in avoiding injury.

## PREVENTION OF SWIMMER'S SHOULDER INJURIES

### Muscular Strength and Endurance

Because the external rotators of the shoulder have been implicated in most of the impingement considerations presented here, it follows that improvement in strength, and particularly endurance, of these muscles is critical in both rehabilitation and prevention (Fig. 35-8).

The objective for strength and endurance training is to achieve a closer balance between internal and external rotators by incorporating exercises for both. Specific exercises for the supraspinatus and biceps long head are particularly important as well. Biceps training has been eliminated from many training programs, presumably so the swimmer would not become "muscle-bound" and to give greater emphasis to the triceps. The biceps long head is an important mover in early pull-through, and ignoring it during training may leave the swimmer susceptible to overuse.

The principle of training specificity suggests that is most appropriate to train an athlete in a way that most closely duplicates the stresses of his or her sport activity. In competitive swimming, although there are many stroke specialists, almost all competitive swimmers perform most of their workout in freestyle. For this reason, the particular stresses of freestyle should always be kept in mind.

### Flexibility

Swimmers are frequently too flexible, as opposed to being inflexible (Fig. 35-10). For that reason, a clinical judgment should be made by the coach or therapist/trainer before placing the swimmer on a remedial flexibility program. Generally, anterior shoulder flexibility is not a problem, although stretches that address the rotator cuff and biceps may be extremely helpful.[26] Some earlier references to the management of shoulder problems in swimmers have suggested that anterior capsular tightness and inflexibility of the anterior musculature were responsible for most shoulder problems in swimmers.[26] Subsequent clinical experience with detailed flexibility programs has fallen short of consistent application of these suggestions in most swimmers with shoulder problems.[27]

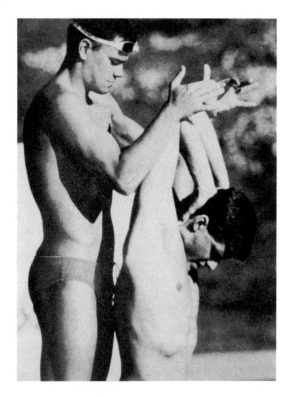

**Fig. 35-10.** Excessive shoulder flexibility in swimmers. (From Counsilman,[30] with permission.)

The exception to this is the swimmer with anterior shoulder girdle tightness related to forward shoulder posture. This anterior tightness may be associated with subacromial impingement by restricting scapular retraction and/or external rotation during recovery. It may also be associated, particularly in the case of compensatory tightness of the pectoralis minor, with significant thoracic outlet symptoms. Remediation of this problem may preclude early return to swimming until the recovery phase of the stroke can be achieved with appropriate scapulohumeral freedom.

## Stroke Mechanics

Videotape analysis has revealed that it is not only the degree of external rotation but the timing as well that impacts the impingement process. Recent experiences have revealed that external rotation is generally complete by the halfway point in the freestyle recovery in swimmers with no shoulder pain. Others may display similar mechanics that subsequently break down later

in the workout.[28] Slow motion analysis of fluoroscopic videos reveals that impingement contact between the greater tuberosity and the coracoacromial arch occurs at about 90 degrees of abduction when the humerus is internally rotated, essentially reproducing the "impingement sign,"[11,14] while external rotation during the first 90 degrees allows the tuberosity to roll posteriorly and clear the arch.[8,14] This reinforces the necessity of maintenance of local muscular endurance of the external rotators.

Coaching awareness of the mechanical sources of overuse is, without a doubt, an effective tool in contending with a pathologic failure in stroke mechanics. Generally, a breakdown in external rotation manifests itself as the elbow leading the hand during recovery. Experienced coaches are able to recognize this fault without difficulty,[29] whereas those with less experience may need to rely on videotape.

Maintenance of proper stroke mechanics throughout the workout is potentially a responsibility for delegation, as clinical experience has shown that most swimmers are acutely aware of the specific changes that occur in their stroke mechanics through the workout. With proper coaching, the swimmer may be able to modify the workout at the point of stroke breakdown to spare impingement stress.

## Training Intensity

Quality workouts are being recommended by some coaches now as an alternative to the ultralong distance workouts that were in favor in the past. Coaches are beginning to address the energy systems required for improving performance, with respect to the physiologic demands of particular swimming events, by incorporating higher-intensity interval training methods with a reduction in total training yardage. The net effect this has on the swimmer is to diminish the number of overhead motions and associated impingement stress over the course of a workout.

The swimmer should be counseled to "mix up" his or her workouts to minimize shoulder fatigue. This may include such things as kickboard, pull buoy, and stroke variation. Bilateral breathing is also useful in maintaining optimal body roll patterns.

As with many sports, many swimming injuries are related, at least in part, to training errors. Progressing too far, too fast, and/or too soon may be associated with significant overuse. Midseason training reductions, coupled with other therapeutic measures, have recently been shown to be of benefit in the in-season management of shoulder pain in swimmers.[1,4,14]

Given the usually more than adequate shoulder flexibility demonstrated by most swimmers, aggressive flexibility exercises during the warm-up period are probably not necessary, and a light stretching routine followed by a low-level swim of at least several hundred yards should be sufficient as workout preparation.

Dry land training should be as sport-specific as possible, incorporating resisted training of the power stroke (extension/adduction/internal rotation), as well as the external rotation/flexion and abduction of the recovery phase. This may be accomplished through the use of stretch cords, isokinetic exercise, and manual resistance.

## SUMMARY

The most effective course of managing the unique shoulder problems of the swimmer is to be aware of the stresses brought about by participation in this sport as well as the mechanisms most likely to be responsible for such specific patterns of overuse. Management of the mechanism of the injury along with the symptoms is most likely to provide a satisfactory solution to the swimmer's problems, and incorporation of this type of program on a prophylactic basis is likely to improve performance as well as avoid injury.

## REFERENCES

1. Johnson JE, Sim FH, Scott SG: Musculoskeletal injuries in competitive swimmers. Mayo Clin Proc 62:289, 1987
2. Pettrone FA: Shoulder problems in swimmers. In Zarins B, Andrews JR, Carson WG (ed): Injuries to the Throwing Arm. WB Saunders, Philadelphia, 1985
3. Aronen J: Swimmers shoulder. Swimming World 25:43, 1985
4. Cuillo JV: Swimmer's shoulder. Clin Sports Med 5:115, 1986
5. Cuillo JV, Stevens GC: The prevention and treatment of injuries to the shoulder in swimming. Sports Med 7:182, 1989
6. Councilman JE: The Science of Swimming. Prentice Hall, Englewood Cliffs, NJ, 1968
7. Maglischo EW: Swimming Faster: A Comprehensive Guide to the Science of Swimming. Mayfield Publishing Co., Mountain View, CA, 1982
8. Richardson AB: The biomechanics of swimming: the shoulder and knee. In Cuillo JV (ed): Swimming. Clin Sports Med 5:103, 1986
9. Kennedy JC, Craig AB, Schneider RD: Swimming. In Schneider RC, Kennedy JC, Plant ML (ed): Sports Injuries: Mechanisms, Prevention and Treatment. Williams & Wilkins, Baltimore, 1985
10. McMaster WC: Painful shoulder in swimmers: a diagnostic challenge. Phys Sportsmed 14:108, 1986
11. McMaster WC: Diagnosing swimmer's shoulder. Swimming Technique (Feb–Apr):17, 1987
12. Falkel JE: Swimming injuries. p. 477. In Sanders B (ed): Sports Physical Therapy. Appleton & Lange, Norwalk, CT, 1990
13. Nuber GW, Jobe FW, Perry J et al: Fine wire electromyography analysis of muscles in the shoulder in swimming. Am J Sports Med 14:7, 1986
14. Falkel JE, Murphy TC: Swimming injuries. In Malone T (ed): Sports Injury Management Series. Williams & Wilkins, Baltimore, 1988
15. Hall G: Hand paddles may cause shoulder pain. Swimming World 21:9, 1980
16. Murphy TC, Riester JN: Managing the young swimmer: a practical approach to prevention and treatment. Student Athlete 1:4, 1988
17. Rathbun RB, McNab I: The microvascular pattern of the rotator cuff. J Bone Joint Surg 52B:544, 1970
18. Blatz D: Swimmer's shoulder. Swimming World 25:41, 1985
19. Fowler P: Swimmer problems. Am J Sports Med 7:141, 1979
20. Richardson AB, Jobe FW, Collins HR: The shoulder in competitive swimming. Am J Sports Med 8:159, 1980
21. Andrews JR, Carson WG: Operative arthroscopy of the shoulder. In Zarins B, Andrews JR, Carson WG (eds): Injuries to the Throwing Arm. WB Saunders, Philadelphia, 1985
22. Arnheim DD: Modern Principles of Athletic Training. Times Mirror/Mosby College Publishing, St. Louis, 1985
23. Hawkins RJ, Kennedy JC: Impingement syndrome in athletes. Am J Sports Med 8:151, 1980
24. Penny JN, Smith C: The prevention and treatment of swimmer's shoulder. Can J Appl Sport Sci 5:195, 1980
25. Blatz D: Upper arm strap. Swimming World Feb 25:43, 1985
26. Greipp JF: Swimmer's shoulder: the influence of flexibility and weight training. Phys Sportsmed 13:92, 1985
27. Beach ML, Whitney SL, Dickoff-Hoffman SA: Relationship of shoulder flexibility, strength and endurance to shoulder pain in competitive swimmers. J Orthop Sports Phys Ther 16:262, 1992

28. Falkel JE, Murphy TC, Murray TF: Prone positioning for testing shoulder internal and external rotation on the Cybex II isokinetic dynamometer. J Orthop Sports Phys Ther 8:368, 1987

29. Magee D: Care and prevention of injuries. In: Coaching the Championship Swimmer: Level III National Coaching Certification Program. Canadian Amateur Swimming Association, Vanier City, Ottowa, Ontario, 1982

30. Counsilman JE: Competitive Swimming Manual. Counsilman, Inc., Bloomington, MN, 1977

# 36

# Shoulder Injuries in Gymnastics

*KATHRYN P. HEMSLEY*

Shoulder injuries in gymnasts occur more frequently from overuse than from any specific traumatic episode. This reflects the training intensity inherent in this particular sport. The incidence of shoulder pathology is higher with male gymnasts because of the stress imposed by the weight-bearing demands on the upper extremities in executing the rings and high-bar skills unique to the men's events. Improper technique used in performing their demanding skills or inadequate strength to support the normal shoulder flexibility necessary to execute the skills are some predisposing factors to the injuries addressed in this chapter.

## INCIDENCE OF INJURY

A review of literature reveals several epidemiologic studies that implicate the particular population as well as particular events involved in higher rates of shoulder injury. Mandelbaum et al[1] cited an National College Athletic Association study that ranks the relative frequency of gymnastic injuries as those found in wrestling, football, and lacrosse. Several authors[1-3] found that the incidence and severity of injury actually increase with the gymnasts' skill and experience. The difficult demands of the advanced skill execution in terms of strength, flexibility, and complexity in coordination also place the gymnast at frequent risk for more severe injuries. Training intensity obviously expands the exposure time of the gymnast to injury. Pettrone and Ricciardelli[2] reported a positive correlation between duration and frequency of practice with higher injury rate. Gymnasts who train more than 20 h/wk are also a greater risk to both acute and chronic injury. Competitive gymnasts invest at least 20 h/wk to their

sport and their pursuit knows no "off season." Much like swimmers, training can consume 50 weeks of the year, a standard in this sport.

Although Lowry and LeVeau[3] cited a higher incidence of traumatic (64.5 percent) than chronic-type injuries (35.5 percent), Snook's[4] study reported a disproportionately greater number of upper extremity lesions resulting from overuse stress pathomechanism. Of the traumatic injuries he documented, none involved the shoulder joint. However, of the chronic injuries catagorized, approximately 50 percent involved the shoulder.

Radiographically documented evidence of osteoarticular changes indicating chronic stress characterized 52 gymnasts of the study of Szot et al.[5] Such changes in the shoulder joint were found in 59.8 percent of this population. Fulton et al[6] also found cortical reaction at the insertion of the pectoralis major at the proximal humerus in 50 percent of the gymnasts studied. Permanent radiographic changes were not accompanied by pain, a point that tends to underscore the long-term, chronic etiologic nature of these lesions.

## CAUSATIVE FACTORS

Perhaps in no other athletic endeavor are biomechanical demands on the upper extremity so unyielding than in gymnastics. Successful execution of apparatus skill events of the high bar and the rings require a delicate and masterful management of forces through the upper extremities (Fig. 36-1). The shoulder links the appendicular to the axial skeleton and is literally a pivotal area for translation of compressive, rotational, shear, and distractive forces.

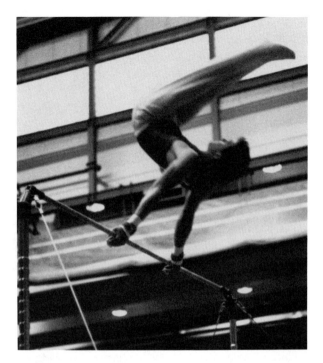

**Fig. 36-1.** Apparatus skill events such as the high bar require masterful control of forces through the upper extremities and reflect the extreme biomechanical demands inherent in gymnastics.

Several extrinsic and intrinsic factors are integral in management of these forces. A healthy gymnastic career with any longevity requires a sensitive, finely tuned neuromuscular system that has reached and maintained a critical balance between extrinsic and intrinsic factors. A specific injury to the shoulder and its etiologic pathomechanics is inevitably rooted in a disturbance of the critical balance between these factors.

Extrinsic factors include the apparatus skill demands on the gymnast and the equipment used to meet those demands. Apparatus skill execution on the rings and high bar particularly require proper technique for force management. In an attempt to analyze force generation and control in terms of gymnastic skill techniques, as well as to quantify the magnitude of forces, Cheetham et al[7] studied developmental level gymnasts' technique on the rings. Thirteen gymnasts were videotaped while executing a series of three "dislocates." Considered a basic skill to be executed by 10- to 12-year-old gymnasts as a precursor to the shoot to handstand through a giant swing, proper technique requires that each dislocate enhance in magnitude. The greater the velocities produced, the greater the performance level is considered to be. The authors gathered video-

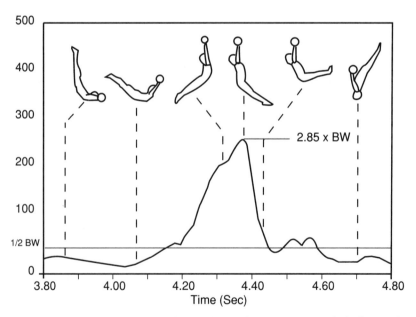

**Fig. 36-2.** A closer analysis of the last of three dislocates shows that gymnast A, with the best technique, dissipates the least energy in excess moves and shows only one peak (Modified from Cheetham et al.,[7] with permission.)

tape observations simultaneously with the data from a force transducer placed on one of the two rings.

Analysis of the data revealed that the ideal performance was produced by gymnast A (Fig. 36-2). He demonstrated a smooth rise to 5.7 times his body weight but with a minimal drop-off between peaks. This was thought to represent the least dissipation of energy and concomitantly minimal impact on the gymnasts' shoulders. Comparatively, gymnast B (Fig. 36-3) produced a two-peak curve by a more dramatic drop on the downswing of 3.8 times body weight force to rise to 5.4 times body weight and to finish with force generation up to 7.9 times body weight. The peak and

drop was thought to represent a significant loss of energy, necessitating a greater demand of overall force produced and two impacts of force to complete the skill. This technique was considered improper in the inefficient translation of energy and especially stressful to the shoulders. The authors hypothesized that this and similar disparities in quality of fundamental skill execution of developmental components early in the gymnastic career is a predisposing factor in the incidence of chronic shoulder injuries.

The authors commented that such high force generation seen in the gymnast using improper techniques would not have been possible without use of dowel

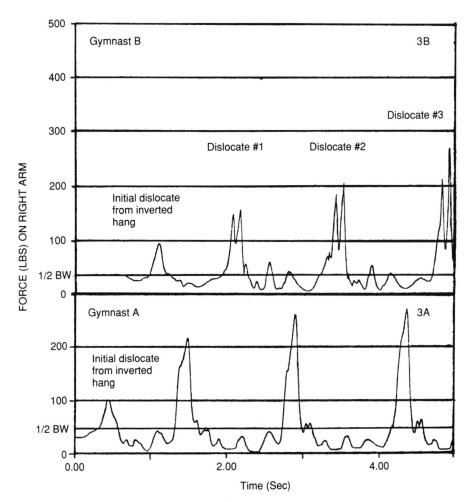

**Fig. 36-3.** Force profiles for an entire sequence of dislocates from two gymnasts show that dislocates for gymnasts B and A were gaining in magnitude from one to the next. (Modified from Cheetham et al.,[7] with permission.)

grips (Fig. 36-4). These grips are an important equipment factor to be considered in an analysis of shoulder injury pathomechanics specific to apparatus skills, demands. Such demands may not be met by the gymnast without using these grips. For the most part, such grips are used solely on the rings and high bar; but many female gymnasts are using them on the uneven parallel bars if the bars are circular and not oval. Use of the grips allows the gymnast greater capability in performing difficult skills by increasing the depth and surface area of the grip. Therefore, duration of contact time on the apparatus is increased and greater velocities and forces result from the product of the mass of the gymnast and his or her body length. This enhanced capability may also result in less true grip strength required to perform a skill and conversely may enable a gymnast to attempt skills more difficult than that which he or she has the adequate strength to execute safely. When considering the magnitude of forces generated on apparatus that is elevated several feet above the floor, the risk for injury is understated.

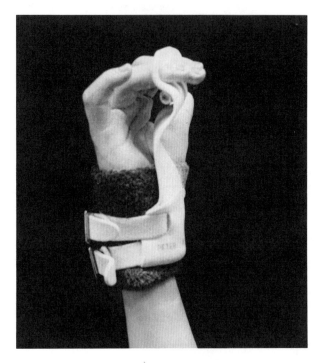

**Fig. 36-4.** Greater depth, stability, and duration of grip is afforded the gymnast using the "dowel grip." Production of greater velocities and forces required to execute the difficult skills are made possible with their use.

Adequate strength has been an important factor in the production and translation of forces for skill execution, but it is an equally important intrinsic factor in providing stability at the shoulder for optimal mobility. Gymnasts have truly optimal mobility. Few other sports require such "normal" hypermobility for force development, skill execution, and aesthetic value. Perhaps no other joint has such inherent ligamentous laxity as the shoulder. In the light of this inadequate static stability, another critical balance to be mastered by these athletes is controlling their mobility with sufficient dynamic stability. Such dynamic stabilizers are constantly used in skill-specific training to produce, control, and prevent motion; to sustain rapid compressive and distractive forces; and to produce isometric force when movement is counterproductive. Young's[8] study of the grip and shoulder positions needed to sustain the familiar iron cross position revealed that internal shoulder rotation produced the greatest torque (203.27 Nm). This underscores the need for proximal stability, particularly involving the serratus anterior, which has the longest moment arm of the involved musculature. Of equal importance is the balance of the rotator cuff with the rhomboids, levator scapulae, and lower trapezius. The rotator cuff must be finely tuned to offset the high shear forces produced by the deltoid during abduction. Loss of adequate humeral head depression by the rotator cuff and its resultant impingement is perhaps the most common form of chronic overuse shoulder injuries presented by this population. As one appreciates the nature of this sport both in the closed kinetic chain position of the upper extremities and in the ranges of motion in which maneuvers must be executed through and above the transverse plane, the challenge of injury prevention and rehabilitation is obvious.

Last to be considered in causative factors is physiologic in nature. Elite-level female gymnasts are almost invariably prepubescent in their physiology if not chronology. Prepubescence affords a body type of narrow hips and a relatively higher center of gravity, which is more readily managed by the upper extremity strength at this stage than through puberty or postpubescence. The inevitable change in their physiology is often career ending, perhaps accounting for their shortened longevity when compared with a male gymnast who typically sustains a career into his third decade.

Although both male and female gymnasts start their

training at an early age of 5 years, the female gymnast must reach the apex of skill development before the onset of puberty. This perception may explain the intensity of their gymnastic sessions. Elite female gymnasts train for two 4-hour sessions daily, 6 days a week, 50 weeks a year. Although they perform in four events compared with six for the male gymnasts, the female gymnasts typically execute each routine in its entirety including stressful dismounts each event, both compulsory and optional routines, several times each session. Their male counterparts of the elite level train one 4-hour session each day and perform portions of their routine focusing on specific aspects of their movement repertoire. For both groups the cumulative stress of landings from difficult dismounts is often buffered with multiple mats or use of a pit filled with foam cushions. Male gymnasts seem to reach their peak late in their collegiate or postgraduate years. Perhaps their relatively older metabolism, coupled with the longer career and stress of six events, two of which place a great deal of stress on the upper extremity, is thought to help explain the higher incidence of overuse injuries to the shoulder in the male population.

# INJURIES

Improper or inadequate warm-up, use of improper technique, and/or a break in concentration can open the door to injury, ensuing inflammation, and pain. Aronen[9] documented the "vicious cycle" with the impingement mechanism, the most common form of chronic shoulder injury. The pain produced reflexively inhibits muscle action and weakness results. The efficiency of the rotator cuff as a counterbalance to the deltoid is lost, allowing continued impingement if the inflammation is not controlled and the weakness eliminated. This cycle, coupled with Aronen's astute observation of the perception pervasive in the gymnastic community (i.e., pain and inflammation are consequences of the gymnast's pursuit and not an injury until the athlete is unable to compete) may help explain the frequency of this type of injury. This tendinitis can clinically present with insidious onset of discomfort and tightness. Episodes of deep-seated pain at the supraspinatus insertion can radiate to the deltoid tubercle and may be relieved by external rotation of the shoul-

der. Pain can be elicited with a Hawkins sign, placing the greater tuberosity against the anteroinferior acromion. Pain is associated with overhead skills. Specific to gymnastics is a phenomenon that allows the gymnast to function with less pain after warming up on the high bar. By performing giant swings, the gymnast milks the swelling out of the suprahumeral space using the coracoacromial arch. After cessation of activity, swelling and pain return.

The second most common inflammatory structure is the proximal biceps tendon. This too can become impinged, but more often the inflammation results from rotational movements that impose stress on the tendon as it is seated in the bicipital groove. A common traumatic episode tearing the transverse ligament can allow the tendon to subluxate out of its groove. Such an episode is not in itself debilitating, but repeated episodes are inevitable granted the forces involved in gymnastics, and such frequency of trauma can lead to eventual tendon fraying and rupture caused by persistent irritation and compromise of blood supply. Clinically, pain is reproduced with contractile testing of forearm supination; a positive Yergason's test may elicit a catching sensation with flexion and external rotation. Pain with a passively insufficient position of the biceps may also be elicited.

Acromioclavicular joint inflammation may also be considered a chronic problem in this population. This joint can incur inflammation from chronic irritation associated with impingement mechanisms. With the repetitive and ballistic movements inherent in gymnastics, the humeral head, when either in a neutral or externally rotated position, can impinge against the anteroinferior acromion process as the shoulder elevates forward in its functional arc as described by Neer.[10] Whereas with an internally rotated humeral head, the suprahumeral structures are impinged against the coracoacromial ligament, particularly through the 70 to 120 degree arc of elevation.

Pathogenesis for this joint inflammatory process warrants evaluation for altered joint mechanics at the sternoclavicular joint. Combined movements at both the acromioclavicular and sternoclavicular joints account for the 60 degrees of upward scapular rotation inherent in glenohumeral abduction. This rotation not only provides the appropriate length–tension relationship of the muscles that control the glenohumeral joint but also controls the position of the glenoid fossa in relationship to the humeral head. The implication for glenohumeral joint stability is apparent.

The musculature that controls this rotation must also be evaluated. The serratus anterior and trapezius provide the force couple that produces this scapular rotation. These two muscles, with the rhomboids and levator scapulae, provide dynamic scapular stability especially during abduction. Both static and dynamic components to scapular movement and control must be analyzed and subsequently addressed for therapeutic intervention when acromioclavicular joint inflammation is clinically presented.

The gymnast will be symptomatic with the myriad of skills that places him or her in horizontal adduction, forward flexion with abduction above 90 degrees, and horizontal adduction with internal rotation. Parallel bar routines that require the gymnast to sustain repetitive compression forces with the shoulder in a horizontally adducted position with forward flexion may initiate if not exacerbate symptoms consistent with acromioclavicular joint inflammation.

Rarely do gymnasts find this inflammatory process debilitating, and they continue to train and compete. Although symptomatic relief can allow the gymnast to continue, chronic inflammation can encourage altered joint mechanics: joint hypermobility that can affect glenohumeral abduction and/or sternoclavicular joint motion.

Glenohumeral joint laxity is not uncommon in this population; hypermobility is, in fact, the rule. Because of the finely tuned quality and high degree of dynamic stabilization inherent in these athletes, dysfunctional hypermobility is rarely a problem. However, this joint laxity, as exhibited in the gymnasts' ability to perform beyond the extremes of normal glenohumeral joint motion, can predispose athletes for labral fraying. The labrum may come into jeopardy if insufficient dynamic stability or ineffective recruitment patterns fail to manage rapid deceleration forces. This failure can cause the joint to distract enough to place the humeral head off center of the glenoid onto the labrum. This allows the shoulder to sublux as well as affording the opportunity for portions of the labrum to become fixed between articulating surfaces of the shoulder. Labral tears and further degeneration may ensue.

Clinically, the gymnast will convey discomfort that may range from a vague ache to stabbing transient pain. They are able to relate positions or moves that "catch" or loosen or describe a painful click, locking, and/or a concomitant loss of strength. Gymnasts may state that relief is obtained by "shaking the shoulder" to relieve the sensation.

## TREATMENT PRINCIPLES AND APPLICATIONS

Particularly in this population, which knows no off season and for whom an injury is merely a given consequence of sport and is not subject to therapeutic intervention until it renders them incapable of continued training, it is imperative to initiate treatment as soon as the most minor dysfunction is detected. Educating the athlete and coach as to the value of relative rest is imperative to successful inflammation management while maintaining the fitness level of the gymnast.

Clinically soft tissue inflammation involving suprahumeral tissues or the acromioclavicular joint implicated in an impingement syndrome is managed with liberal use of ice. In acute stages, ice is used 20 minutes of every 2 hours, four to five times a day. In chronic cases, ice after the workout is the standard.

Use of high-voltage electric stimulation with short-pulse duration for comfort and high peak current for greater penetration is effective.[11] However, edema control using rhythmic muscle contraction through pulsed, modulated alternating current at a phase duration greater than 100 seconds is well documented.[12]

Nonsteroidal anti-inflammatory medication such as salicylate or analgesic preparations such as lidocaine are applied topically through iontophoresis or phonophoresis and are particularly effective as applicable to subcutaneous tendon or bursa sites.[12]

Chronic tendinitis may be effectively treated with transverse friction massage after pre-icing/anesthetizing the area of concern and following with postmassage icing.

Restoring range of motion and capsular mobility is rarely a problem in this population, which is normally hypermobile. However, it is important to maintain the great degree of flexibility required of this sport, particularly in the anterior chest wall, as forward shoulder posture is frequently evident in gymnasts.

As the acute inflammatory process is controlled and normal joint mechanics are restored to the sternoclavicular, acromioclavicular, scapulothoracic joints as well as the cervical and thoracic spine, strengthening and muscle re-education must be addressed. The treatment plan should take into consideration the present status of strength as well as the demands that the shoulder must meet to return to full but protected function. Controlled movements at slow speeds with isometrics held submaximally throughout a nonimpingement range is considered the initial step to elevating the athlete's tolerance to imposed contractile demands. This initial progression must be pervasive in that it focuses on restoration of the force couples providing the needed balance to this joint complex. The scapulothoracic stabilizers must be trained to afford controlled distal mobility through the glenohumeral joint. This involves shrugs for the trapezius and levator scapulae, and protraction and retraction for the serratus anterior, midtrapezius, and rhomboids. The rotator cuff must be restored in balance with the deltoid. Training these muscles in the modified neutral position of the functional plane of the scapula allows for optimal vascularity.

Proprioceptive neuromuscular facilitation techniques involving hold/relax and contract/relax as well as slow reversal hold methods are especially effective in coordinating contractile input and rotational position of the limb. These techniques, applicable to both glenohumeral and scapulothoracic musculature, afford the rehabilitation specialist immediate feedback for ongoing evaluation and program modification. In early stages, it is the optimal tool to impose/elicit graded isometric, concentric, and eccentric contractions throughout the entire upper kinetic chain in specific ranges of motion. However, caution should be exercised when using D1 patterns above the transverse plane when treating impingement syndromes. Pain-free contractile tolerance must be established through use of proprioceptive neuromuscular facilitation techniques, upper body ergometry, resisted isotonic work using light free weights, surgical tubing, or TheraBand in specific positions to train rotator cuff, deltoid, and scapular stabilizers.

Higher-speed activities such as isokinetics can then be instituted. Short arc work, avoiding symptomatic ranges, is performed in intermediate speeds initially. Progression expanding the symptomless range through which isokinetics are performed both in rotation in a modified neutral position up to 90 degrees abduction, as well as the diagonal patterns through overhead work, is gradually implemented. No time table is offered here because the criteria for progression is the gymnast's tolerance for contractile demands as evidenced in absence of inflammatory signs and symptoms.

# FUNCTIONAL PROGRESSION

Upper extremity weight-bearing and, therefore, more functional exercises that mimic the positions and gradual stress of gymnastic routines need to be rapidly instituted as part of the isometric-isotonic stress through nonimpingement ranges. Restoration of proprioception is best provided through upper extremity weight-bearing. Proprioceptive neuromuscular facilitation techniques using rhythmic stabilization at varying angles and with variable forces throughout pain-free ranges stimulate kinesthesia. Initially, proximal hand placement can shorten the resistance arm, allowing less force to be overcome by the gymnast. Gradually elongating this resistance arm increases the challenge and more closely mimics the performance position for apparatus involving high bar and rings.

Closed kinetic chain activities start with hand weight-bearing shifts on a table both in standing and in quadruped to triped to bipedal positions. Resisting the uninvolved limbs through protraction to retraction is also used to tax the weight-bearing stability of the involved limb. A progression that involved holding a table while performing bridges with both feet hooklying to one leg raised to overcoming resistance at the pelvis are steps that can be used early on.

Progression and diversion using upper extremity balance skills while supported over the Bobath ball or using hand weight-bearing on a Fitter or Baps Board are commonly used.

Specific gymnastic weight-bearing skills use cut-down pommel horse handles for dips, push-ups, and handstands and isometric holds with increasing weight-bearing percentage used as the athlete tolerates. The rocker bar (Fig. 36-5) affords the added dimension of balance training to increased upper extremity weight-bearing stabilization capability. Devices such as the ring trainer and inversion machines as well as the harness play an important intermediary role in return to full gymnastic activity.

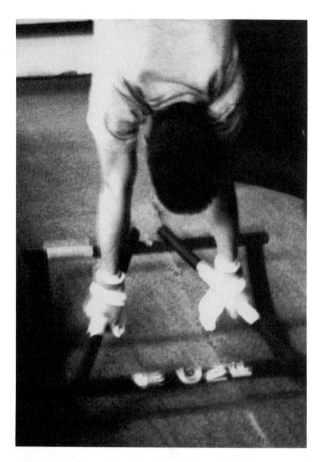

**Fig. 36-5.** The rocker bar affords the added dimension of balance training to increased upper extremity weight-bearing stabilization.

## INJURY PREVENTION

However, the most important role played in this critical time between modified and full activity is that of the gymnastic coach. Truly, there is no substitution for gymnastic activity, and the rehabilitation specialist must establish an understanding with the gymnastic coach in terms of establishing and maintaining protected function during this time. No other professional has the knowledge base of the imposed demands specific to every gymnastic maneuver than this individual. Their grasp of functional lead-up strength exercises, best witnessed in their training of young developmental gymnasts, provides a tremendous insight regarding the same rehabilitation progression necessary to return the older gymnast to full activity. In lieu of athletic trainers working with most of these athletes, the coach must not only insist on proper technique and strength to perform the skills safely but must exhibit the wisdom to minimize training errors in frequency, intensity, and duration of apparatus and strength workouts. This often proves to be the unrecognized key to full recovery for the athlete.

Finally, by gradually restoring the self-confidence of the gymnast in his or her ability to perform with restored strength, adequate flexibility, and normal timing in skill execution, the gymnast totally concentrates on the tasks at hand. Thereby, optimal performance using the ability to protect themselves from injury is possible.

## REFERENCES

1. Mandelbaum BR, Bartolozzi AR, Daus CA et al: Wrist pain syndrome in the gymnast. Am J Sports Med 17:305, 1989
2. Pettrone FA, Ricciardelli E: Gymnastic injuries: the Virginia experience. Am J Sports Med 15:59, 1987
3. Lowry CB, LeVeau BF: A retrospective study in gymnastic injury to competitors and noncompetitors in private clubs. Am J Sports Med 110:237, 1982
4. Snook GA: A review of women's collegiate gymnastics. Clin Sports Med 20:31, 1985
5. Szot Z, Boron Z, Galaj Z: Overloading changes in the motor system occurring in elite gymnastics. Int J Sports Med 6:36, 1985
6. Fulton MN, Albright JP, El-Khoury GY: Cortical desmoid-like lesion of the proximal humerus and its occurrence in gymnasts (ringman's shoulder lesion). Am J Sports Med 7:57, 1979
7. Cheetham PJ, Sreden HI, Mizoguchi H: The gymnast on rings—a study of forces. SOMA April:30, 1987
8. Young WR: A study of the effects of varying the amount of humeral rotation on torque development in the iron cross position. Masters Thesis, Pennsylvania State University, 1984
9. Aronen JG: Shoulder rehabilitation. Clin Sports Med 4:477, 1985
10. Neer CS: Impingement syndrome. Clin Orthop 173:70, 1983
11. Sobel J: Shoulder rehabilitation: rotator cuff tendinitis, strength training and return to play. p. 338. In Pettrone FA: Upper Extremity Injuries in Athletes (AAOS). CV Mosby, Princeton, 1986
12. Snyder-Mackler LS, Robinson A: Electrophysiology. Williams & Wilkins, Baltimore, 1989

# SUGGESTED READINGS

Allman F: Impingement, biceps and rotator cuff lesions. p. 158. In: Injuries to the Throwing Arm. WB Saunders, Philadelphia, 1985

Bowerman JW: Gymnastics. p. 200. In: Radiology and Injury in Sport. Appleton-Century-Crofts, East Norwalk, CT, 1977

Cahill BR: Understanding shoulder pain. In: Instructional Course Lectures (AAOS). Vol. 34. CV Mosby, St Louis, 1985

Hageman PA, Mason DK, Rydlund KW, Humpal SA: Effects of position and speed on eccentric and concentric isokinetic testing of the shoulder rotators. J Orthop Sports Phys Ther 11:64, 1989

Hart DL, Carmichael SW: Biomechanics of the shoulder. J Orthop Sports Phys Ther 6:229, 1985

Hawkins RJ, Hobeika PE: Impingement syndrome in the athletic shoulder. Clin Sports Med 2:391, 1983

Hesson J: Three ways to stronger shoulders. Int Gym 28:44, 1986

Jobe FW: Serious rotator cuff injuries. Clin Sports Med 2:407, 1983

Kirby RL, Simms FC, Dymington BA, Garner JB: Flexibility and musculoskeletal symptomatology in female gymnasts and age-matched controls. Am J Sports Med 9:160, 1981

McLeod WD, Andrews JR: Mechanism of shoulder injuries. Phys Ther 66:1901, 1986

Nitz AJ: Physical therapy management of the shoulder. Phys Ther 66:1912, 1986

Penny JN, Welsh RP: Shoulder impingement syndromes in athletes and their surgical management. Am J Sports Med 9:11, 1981

Perry J: Anatomy and biomechanics of the shoulder in swimming, gymnastics and tennis. Clin Sports Med 2:247, 1983

Pfoerringer W: Sportartspezifische Schulterlaesionen. Dtsch Z Sportsmed 36:137, 1985

Redmond CJ: Gymnastic injuries: recognition and management. Runner 17:28, 1979

Richardson AB: Overuse syndromes in baseball, tennis, gymnastics, and swimming. Clin Sports Med 2:379, 1983

Steele VA, White JA: Injury prediction in female gymnasts. Br J Sports Med 31, 1986

Tullos HS, Bennett JB: The shoulder in sports. p. 110. In: Principles of Sports Medicine. Williams & Wilkins, 1984

# 37

# Neuromuscular Control Exercises for Shoulder Instability

## STEVEN A. DICKOFF-HOFFMAN

The concept of shoulder instability has received a significant amount of attention in the literature in recent years.[1-5] With regard to the athletic shoulder, two basic types of instability have been identified: static and dynamic (frequently referred to as functional instability).[4,6,7]

Static instability is defined as insufficiency of the static restraining structures, such as the glenohumeral capsule, glenoid labrum, and supporting ligaments. A shoulder that is statically unstable can be subluxed during clinical examination and does not function well athletically because the fine coordinated action of the rotator cuff is unable to be maintained because of the loss of static support.

Dynamic instability differs from static laxity in that the inert noncontractile structures are basically intact. Dynamic or functional instability is a result of an imbalance between antagonistic muscle groups (i.e., the internal/external rotators), which can result in a loss of proprioceptive control, kinesthesia, and ultimately subluxation.[1,2,6] Clinical manifestations of this subluxation phenomenon resulting from muscle imbalance range from relatively "minor" inflammatory changes in the subdeltoid bursa and rotator cuff to more serious rotator cuff tears and glenoid labrum pathology. In the throwing shoulder, fine coordinated action of the glenohumeral and scapulothoracic stabilizers are important for facilitating synchronous function of the glenohumeral joint. Without proper neuromuscular control, muscles fire asynchronously, which can result in suprahumeral elevation, eventual impingement, rotator cuff pathology, and dysfunction.[4,5,7-9]

The purpose of this chapter is to review some of the basic concepts of neuromotor control and how they relate to functional instability. Paramount in understanding the role of kinesthesia and proprioception in the throwing shoulder is understanding the act of throwing. A brief review of the throwing sequence will lead to a description of exercises that can be used to enhance neuromuscular control. These exercises are useful in facilitating dynamic stability of the glenohumeral and scapulothoracic joints, which can help to prevent the functional subluxation phenomenon.

## NEUROMOTOR CONTROL

Payton et al[10] defined neuromotor control as a purposeful act initiated at the cortical level. They stated that "motor control is an involuntary associated movement organized subcortically and results in a well learned skill operating without conscious guidance." With reference to the shoulder, subcortical control of the muscles responsible for throwing results in a fine coordinated action, which can propel a ball rapidly and in a controlled direction. The basic component of neuromotor control is the ability to discriminate joint position and movement, which is defined as proprioception or kinesthesia. Freeman and Wyke[11] identified muscle and joint afferents, which are present in ligaments and synovial tissue. Newton[12] described kinesthesia as "the ability to discriminate joint position, relative weight of body parts, and joint movement including direction, amplitude, and speed." Joint pro-

435

**Table 37-1. Characteristics of Joint Receptors**

| Type | Location | Physiologic Function |
|------|----------|----------------------|
| I | Stratum fibrosum of ligaments | Active at rest and during movement |
| II | Junction of synovial and fibrosum of capsule | Active at onset and termination of movement |
| III | Collateral ligaments | Active at end of joint range |
| IV | Ligaments, capsule | Active only to extreme mechanical irritation |

(Adapted from Freeman and Wyke,[11] with permission.)

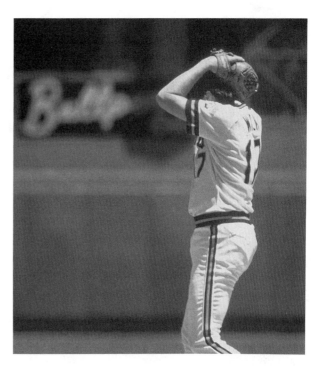

**Fig. 37-1.** Windup phase. (From the Pittsburgh Pirates Baseball Club, ©Dave Arrigo, used with permission.)

prioceptors are responsible for signaling a stretch reflex when the shoulder capsule becomes taut and prevent translation at extremes of motion. The mechanism of throwing a ball requires that joint proprioceptors be active, because motor control does occur at the subcortical level and the neuromuscular component must be activated to control ball propulsion and enhance joint stability. A summary of the typical joint receptors found in ligaments and synovial capsule is presented in Table 37-1.

## REVIEW OF THE THROWING ACT

The throwing act requires a concerted effort between the rotator cuff and scapulothoracic muscles. It is divided into five distinct phases: windup, cocking (early and late), acceleration, ball release, and deceleration or follow-through.

### Windup

The windup is a preliminary act that results in little or no electromyographic activity of major consequence.[13] It is the point at which the pitcher gathers the ball into his or her glove, initiates trunk rotation, and prepares for the more active phases of throwing (Fig. 37-1).

### Cocking

The cocking phase follows the windup by continuing with trunk rotation. As the throwing hand leaves the glove, the shoulder elevates to 90 degrees and externally rotates. This phase can be divided into two distinct subphases, early and late. Early cocking begins with a period of shoulder abduction and external rotation and ends when the forward foot strikes the ground (Fig. 37-2). Late cocking begins with forward foot contact and ends with maximum external rotation of the shoulder. During the late cocking phase of throwing,

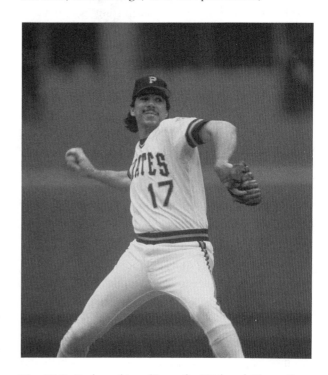

**Fig. 37-2.** Early cocking. (From the Pittsburgh Pirates Baseball Club, ©Dave Arrigo, used with permission.)

NEUROMUSCULAR CONTROL EXERCISES FOR SHOULDER INSTABILITY   437

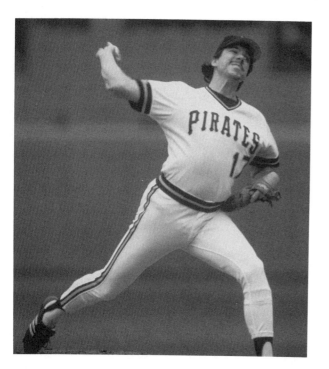

**Fig. 37-3.** Late cocking. (From the Pittsburgh Pirates Baseball Club, ©Dave Arrigo, used with permission.)

the shoulder internal rotators are eccentrically active, attempting to maintain glenohumeral stability and prevent anterior humeral translation (Fig. 37-3). The scapular stabilizers (serratus anterior, trapezius, levator scapula) are maximally active to maintain a stable base of support for the scapulothoracic joint. The late cocking phase ends at the point of maximum glenohumeral external rotation. Passive external rotation must exceed 140 degrees for trunk recoiling and concentric internal rotation activity to result in a smooth internal rotation movement without protraction of the shoulder.[7,14,15] A lack of passive external rotation can result in "short-arming the ball," a mechanical flaw in which the shoulder protracts and the arm lags behind the trunk. This flaw in technique can create an anterior subluxating force on the glenohumeral joint, which can microtraumatize the suprahumeral structures.

## Acceleration

The acceleration phase is initiated as soon as the arm propels forward and internally rotates. It requires a burst of activity in the internal rotators and scapular

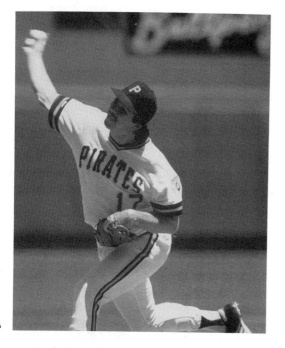

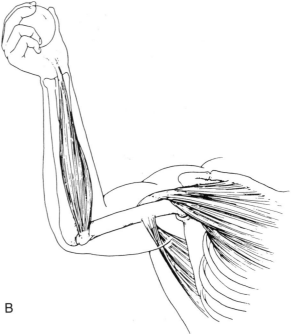

A    B

**Fig. 37-4. (A)** Acceleration. (Fig. A from the Pittsburgh Pirates Baseball Club, ©Dave Arrigo, used with permission.) **(B)** Proximal support of the scapulothoracic joint results in strong rotator cuff action during acceleration. (Fig. B from Tullos and Bennett,[22] with permission.)

stabilizers to provide proximal stability and allow the arm to act as a lever to complete its external rotation movement. During this phase, the pectoralis major, latissimus dorsi, and serratus anterior are maximally active.[9,13] At this point, the scapula is acting as a fulcrum and the arm as a lever (Fig. 37-4). The concept of "proximal stability for distal mobility" is evident, as the scapulothoracic and glenohumeral joints act in synchrony to provide neuromuscular control for ball propulsion.

### Ball Release

Ball release occurs directly after acceleration as the hand relinquishes the ball slightly anterior to the ear level (Fig. 37-5).

### Deceleration or Follow-Through

The deceleration phase is the most violent phase of throwing. After ball release, the arm decelerates through space at a velocity between 6,000 and 9,000

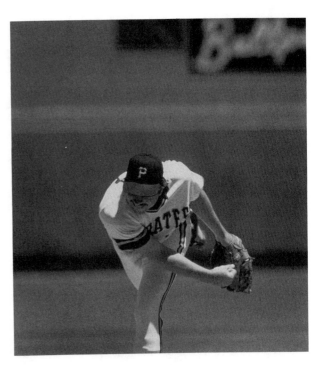

**Fig. 37-6.** Deceleration or follow-through. (From the Pittsburgh Pirates Baseball Club, ©Dave Arrigo, used with permission.)

degrees/s.[13,15] The posterior rotator cuff must contract eccentrically to decelerate the arm and reduce anterior translational forces (Fig. 37-6). Maximum electromyographic activity during this phase is noted in the infraspinatus, teres minor, serratus anterior, and posterior head of the triceps.[7,9,13,14] Weakness of the scapular stabilizers can create an anterior subluxating force on the shoulder during the deceleration phase of throwing, because a stable base must be controlled neuromuscularly for the posterior rotator cuff to contract eccentrically to slow the arm.

## KINESIOLOGY OF NEUROMUSCULAR CONTROL OF THE SHOULDER

The shoulder is composed of four independent articulations that move synchronously via a force-couple arrangement between muscles attaching to these joints. These joints are (1) glenohumeral, (2) acromioclavicular, (3) sternoclavicular, and (4) scapulothoracic. An

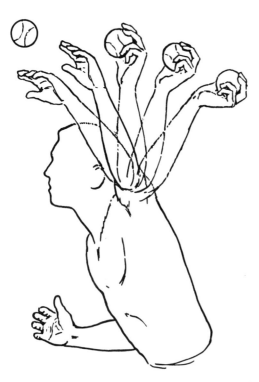

**Fig. 37-5.** Ball release. (From Tullos and Bennett,[22] with permission.)

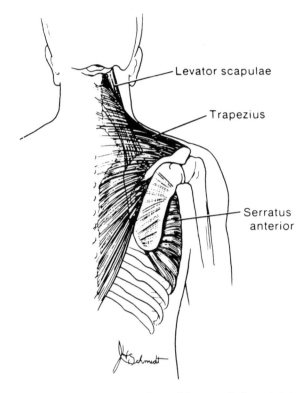

**Fig. 37-7.** Anatomy/kinesiology of the scapulothoracic joint. (From Tullos and Bennett,[22] with permission.)

of the arm does change the length–tension relationship of the capsule. Research has shown that the 90 degree position of elevation is the one that promotes maximum stability of the glenohumeral joint.[14,17] Because muscle weakness can result in abnormal compression and shear forces, they must be balanced to create stability of the humeral head in the glenoid fossa. A favorable balance between compression and shear forces makes the shoulder position of 90 degrees elevation the optimal position for joint stability.[5,7,10,14,16,17] Therefore, when evaluating the throwing mechanism, one can observe that all throwers, regardless of style and technique, maintain a 90-degree position of glenohumeral elevation relative to the horizontal surface.

Dynamic control of the glenohumeral joint is dependent on the strength of the rotator cuff and biceps tendon.[1,7,14] The biceps tendon acts to depress and anteriorly stabilize the glenohumeral joint, whereas the rotator cuff compresses and rotates the humerus throughout the dynamic phases of throwing. Without adequate control of the rotator cuff and biceps tendon, the glenohumeral joint can become unstable, resulting in an abnormal throwing pattern. The purpose, therefore, of neuromuscular conditioning and control of the glenohumeral joint, is to facilitate dynamic coordination of the rotator cuff and scapulothoracic stabilizers.

abnormal movement pattern of these joints caused by static or dynamic imbalances can result in excessive stress being placed on soft tissue, manifesting in an inflammatory process. This joint "interdependence" creates a very unique method for maintaining neuromuscular control of the shoulder.

The scapulothoracic joint is controlled by the levator scapulae, trapezius, rhomboids, and serratus anterior muscles (Fig. 37-7). Without adequate control of the scapulothoracic joint, the glenohumeral jont can become dynamically unstable.[6–8,16]

## TORQUE, FORCE, AND LEVERAGE

Torque is defined as a force that is applied around an axis of rotation. Leverage of the glenohumeral joint is greatest at 90 degrees elevation, with muscle force and torque being dependent on lever arm[17] (Fig. 37-8). Because articulation and compression of the glenohumeral joint are also dependent on lever arm, position

## EXERCISES TO ENHANCE NEUROMUSCULAR CONTROL

When establishing a program for the dynamically or functionally unstable shoulder, the following goals should be in mind:

1. Proximal stability for distal mobility
2. Glenohumeral control at the desired angle
3. Eccentric rotator cuff strength
4. Flexibility of the internal rotators
5. Compressive stability and force-couple enhancement
6. Rapid acceleration/deceleration
7. Progressive overload
8. Arm position relative to function

The purpose of an exercise program for neuromuscular conditioning is to maintain dynamic muscle balance and flexibility. This program incorporates the SAID principle (specific adaptation for imposed de-

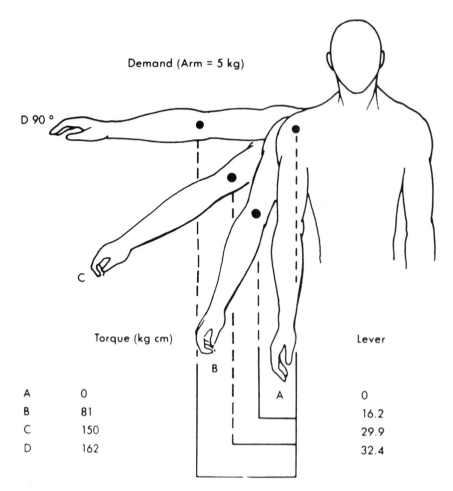

**Fig. 37-8.** Leverage and torque of the glenohumeral joint at varying degrees of abduction. (From Rowe,[24] with permission.)

mand). Specificity refers to the concept that to be proficient at a skill or task, that specific task must be practiced. Demand means that the system must be stressed beyond its normal limits for an improvement in skill to occur. This directly relates to the concept of "overload."

The following exercises combine eccentric loading, plyometrics, closed/open chain facilitation to enhance dynamic stability and compression/shear force balance, and repetition.

## Stability Exercises

Stability exercises can be performed in both an open and closed chain position. Closed-chain training enhances static stability by facilitating compression of the glenohumeral capsule and stimulating neuromuscular proprioceptors to provide static control. Examples of a closed-chain stability exercise progression, including wall, table, and floor push-ups, unilateral balance, oscillations on a fitter, and sitting push-ups, are outlined in Figures 37-9 to 37-15.

Open-chain exercises facilitate dynamic control and kinesthetic awareness. Examples of open-chain exercises for neuromuscular control are shown in Figures 37-16 to 37-21.

## Flexibility Exercises

Flexibility of the capsule and rotator cuff is important because of the necessity to obtain at least 140 degrees of external rotation during the late cocking phase of

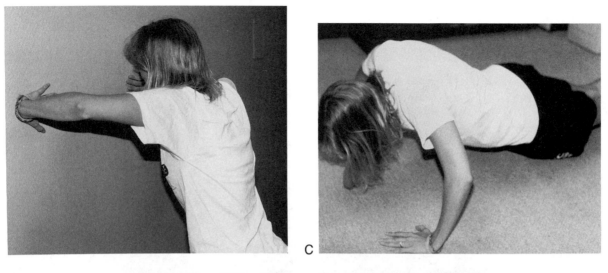

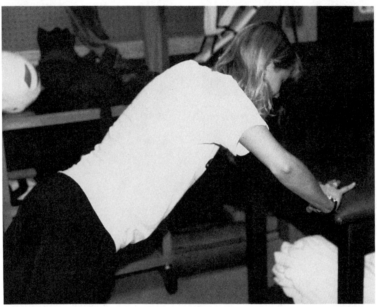

**Fig. 37-9.** (**A–C**) Progressive push-up from the wall, a table, the floor. These exercises enhance strength of scapular stabilizers.

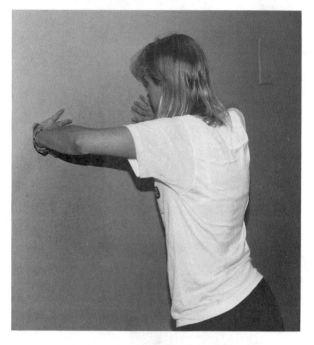

**Fig. 37-10.** Wall push-up in a 90-degree abducted position.

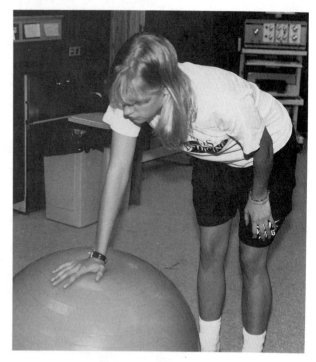

**Fig. 37-12.** Unilateral balance on a ball.

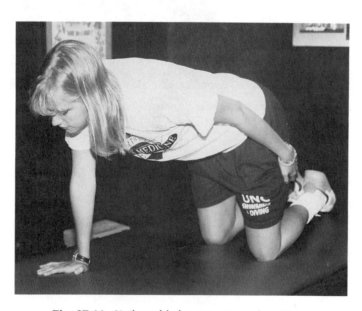

**Fig. 37-11.** Unilateral balance in a tripod position.

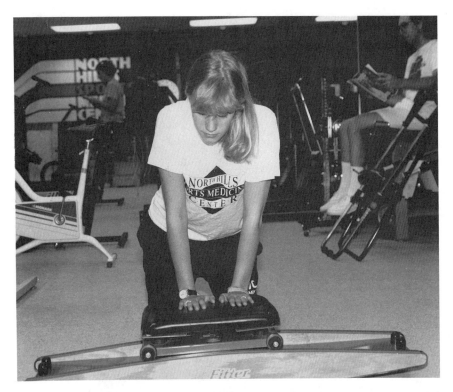

**Fig. 37-13.** Balancing on the Profitter (Fitter International, Calgary, Alberta, Canada.)

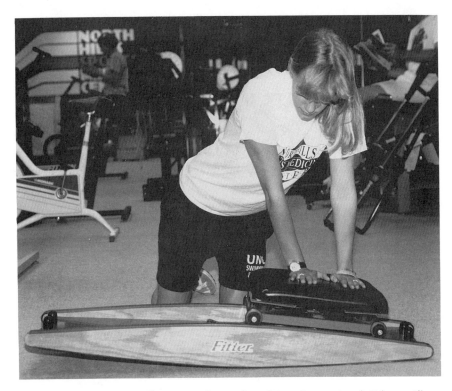

**Fig. 37-14.** Compressions and oscillations on the Profitter (Fitter International, Calgary, Alberta, Canada.)

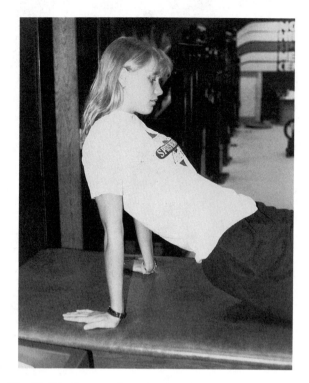

**Fig. 37-15.** Sitting push-up for scapular depression strength.

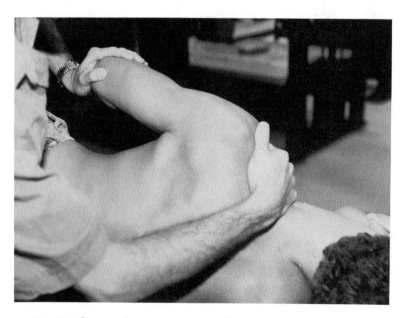

**Fig. 37-16.** Manual resistance to scapular depression and elevation.

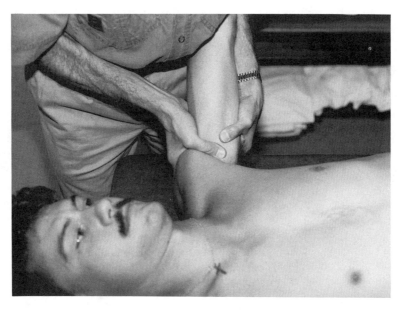

**Fig. 37-17.** Manual glenohumeral compression to facilitate co-contraction isometric stability.

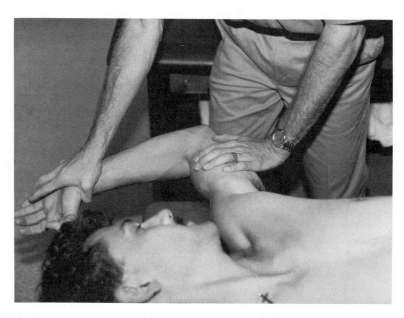

**Fig. 37-18.** Eccentric resistance to the anterior rotator cuff (for strength during late cocking).

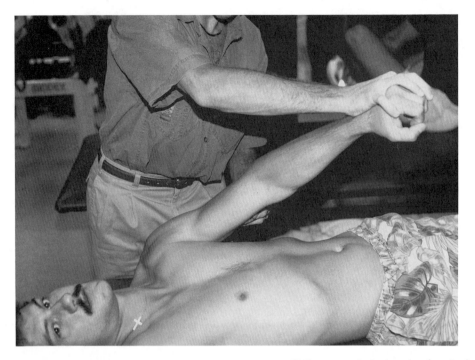

**Fig. 37-19.** Eccentric resistance to the posterior rotator cuff (for strength during deceleration).

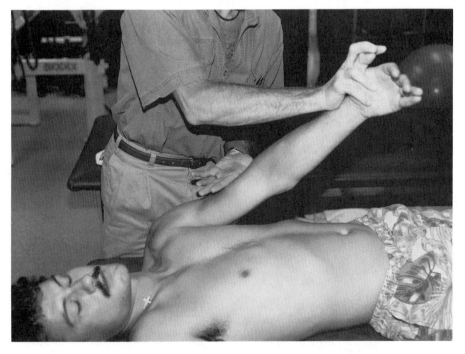

**Fig. 37-20.** Manually resisted proprioceptive neuromuscular facilitation diagonal 2 (mimics direction of arm during deceleration and can be resisted eccentrically).

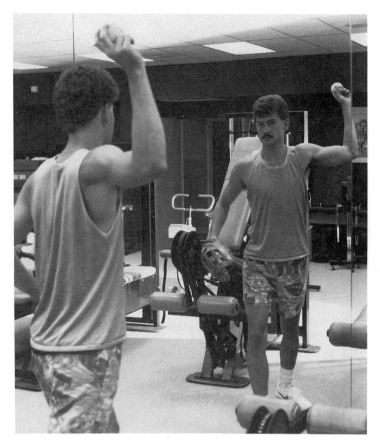

**Fig. 37-21.** Mirroring the pattern of motion helps to enhance joint position and proprioceptive sense.

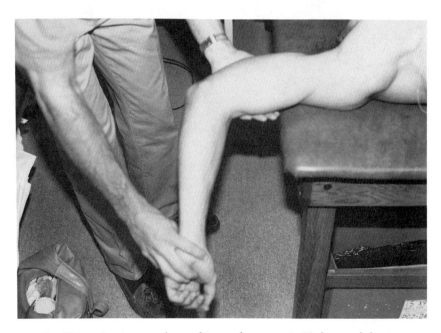

**Fig. 37-22.** Passive stretching of internal rotators in 90-degree abduction.

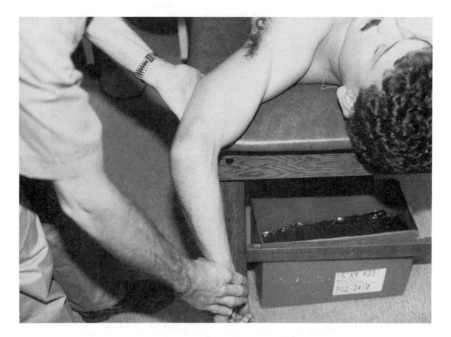

**Fig. 37-23.** Passive stretching of internal rotators in 135-degree abduction.

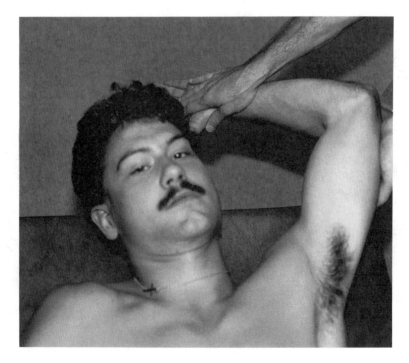

**Fig. 37-24.** Passive stretching of the internal rotators in 180-degree abduction.

throwing. It is also important for facilitating a normal stretch reflex, thus equating to an improvement in neuromotor control (Figs. 37-22 to 37-24).

## CONCLUSION

Dynamic instability of the shoulder during the throwing act is the result of a lack of proprioception/kinesthesia, inflexibility, and muscle weakness. These parameters can be trained by applying the SAID principle, which specifically encourages repetition and training that mimics the functional activity that is going to be performed. Because throwing involves quick acceleration/deceleration, rapidity of movement is a necessity. The physiologic factors of speed and reaction time need to be considered to enhance neuromuscular control. Exercising in the position of function is necessary to "educate" the receptors, which would result in a well-learned skill operating without conscious guidance. The summation of all these activities would result in a fine-coordinated glenohumeral and scapulothoracic joint acting in concert and thus creating a fine-tuned mechanism for throwing without any sensation of dynamic instability.

## REFERENCES

1. Cain PR, Mutschler TA, Fu FH: Anterior stability of the glenohumeral joint: a dynamic model. Am J Sports Med 15:144, 1987
2. Norwood LA, DelPizzo W, Jobe FW, Kerlan RK: Anterior shoulder pain in baseball players. Am J Sports Med 6:103, 1978
3. Pappas AM, Gross TP, Kleinman PK: Symptomatic shoulder instability due to lesions of the glenoid labrum. Am J Sports Med 1:279, 1983
4. Rowe CR, Zarins B: Recurrent transient subluxation of the shoulder. J Bone Joint Surg 63A:863, 1981
5. Smith RL, Brunolli J: Shoulder kinesthesia after anterior glenohumeral joint dislocation. Phys Ther 69:106, 1989
6. Albright JA, Jokl P, Shaw R et al: Clinical study of baseball pitchers: correlation of injury to the throwing arm with method of delivery. Am J Sports Med 6:15, 1978
7. Atwater AE: Biomechanics of overarm throwing movements and of throwing injuries. Exerc Sport Sci Rev 7:43, 1979
8. Andrews JR, Carson WG, McLeod WD: Glenoid labrum tears related to the biceps. Am J Sports Med 13:337, 1985
9. Jobe FW, Moynes DR, Tibone JE et al: An EMG analysis of the shoulder in pitching. A second report. Am J Sports Med 12:218, 1984
10. Payton OD, Hirt S, Newton RA (eds): Scientific Bases for Neurophysiologic Approaches to Therapeutic Exercise. FA Davis, Philadelphia, 1977
11. Freeman MAR, Wyke B: The innervation of the knee joint: an anatomical and histological study in the cat. J Anat 101:505, 1967
12. Newton R: Joint receptor contributions to reflexive and kinesthetic responses. Phys Ther 62:22, 1982
13. Jobe FW, Tibone JE, Perry J et al: An EMG analysis of the shoulder in throwing and pitching. A preliminary report. Am J Sports Med 11:3, 1983
14. Dillman CJ, Fleisig GS, Werner SL, Andrews JR: Biomechanics of the shoulder in sports: throwing activities. Post Graduate Studies in Physical Therapy. Forum Medicum, Pennington, NJ, 1990
15. Pappas AM, Zawacki RM, Sullivan TJ: Biomechanics of baseball pitching. A preliminary report. Am J Sports Med 13:216, 1985
16. Nicholas JA, Hershman EB (eds): The Upper Extremity in Sports Medicine. CV Mosby, St Louis, 1990
17. Siewert MW, Ariki PK, Davies GJ et al: Isokinetic torque changes based on lever arm placement. Phys Ther 65:715, 1985
18. Sanders B (ed): Sports Physical Therapy. Appleton & Lange, East Norwalk, CT, 1990
19. Scott NW, Nisonson B, Nicholas JA: Sports Medicine. Williams & Wilkins, Baltimore, 1984
20. Wyke B: Articular neurology: a review. Physiotherapy 58:94, 1972
21. Zarins B, Andrews JR, Carson WG: Injuries to the Throwing Arm. WB Saunders, Philadelphia, 1985
22. Tullos HS, Bennett JB: The shoulder in sports. p. 116. In Norman SW, Niconson B, Nicholas JA (eds): Sports Medicine. Williams & Wilkins, Baltimore, 1985
23. Perry J, Glousman R: Biomechanics of throwing. p. 735. In Nicholas JA, Hershman EB (eds): The Upper Extremity in Sports Medicine. CV Mosby, St Louis, 1990
24. Rowe CR: The Shoulder. p. 735. Churchill Livingstone, New York, 1988

# 38

# Proprioceptive Neuromuscular Facilitation for the Shoulder

*ROBERT P. ENGLE*

Proprioceptive neuromuscular facilitation (PNF) is an integrated pattern of rehabilitation techniques and procedures that have become widely used for neurologic and orthopaedic patients. These techniques, developed in the 1940s, are based on the classic neurophysiologic principles of Sherrington,[1] Kabat,[2] and others. Designed to improve neurologic response to exercise, this therapeutic system focuses on diagonal and spinal patterns of movement that use rotational pivots about a joint. Employing these movements in rehabilitation provides a useful array of functional treatment exercises for the shoulder complex. Modifications to the original patterns of movement of Knott and Voss[3] can be performed for selected shoulder pathologies while considering the same neurophysiologic concepts.[1]

This chapter discusses the principles and describes the techniques and patterns of PNF. The descriptions are those we commonly use in shoulder rehabilitation along with pattern modifications based on my experience.

## PRINCIPLES

PNF is based on a definition of various principles—directions for the basic treatment techniques. They require the therapist to have a basic scientific knowledge of anatomy, biomechanics, neurophysiology, motor development, and neuromuscular function. Treatment programs using PNF require the clinician to understand dysfunctional patterns of movement. The principles defined below are applied to all patients to improve their orthopaedic pathology.

## Manual Contacts

Hand pressure stimulates skin and other receptors, enhancing neuromuscular response. It provides the patient with direct sensory input to gain a specific motor output in a desired direction of motion. The use of manual contacts provides a hands-on technique that differs from traditional resistive exercise devices. Manual pressure in the opposing direction also serves as a cue for the patient to move in the specific resisted position.

## Appropriate Resistance

Appropriate resistance is the amount of resistance applied by the physical therapist to gain the specific motor response. Resistance can be submaximal or maximal depending on the situation. Johnson and Saliba[4] discussed three uses of appropriate resistance: (1) to teach and increase awareness of a movement, (2) to stimulate appropriate irradiation from strong to weak components, and (3) to reinforce weak patterns by irradiation from strong patterns.

## Traction and Approximation

The use of joint traction (separation) of approximation compressive forces further stimulates facilitation of the desired response through the joint receptor system. Stimulation of these mechanoreceptors helps to signal the muscle for a response. This is critical in the shoulder for both enhancing stability (approximation) and mobility (traction).

## Quick stretch

This uses the stretch reflex for excitation of a specific movement response. The shoulder joint is taken into a position to apply a controlled manual stretch to all components of the movement.

## Verbal Stimuli

The use of verbal communication further enhances the facilitation process by increasing patient excitation. Direction to patients is also more clearly defined. Verbal tone may also be important to monitor, as it may again serve an excitation role.

## Visual Stimuli

Visual cues and stimuli help the patient learn movement patterns more easily, coordinating the head, trunk, and extremities.

## Patterns of Facilitation

Spiral and diagonal patterns of movement for both lower and upper extremities and trunk are included. There are four shoulder patterns: (1) flexion/abduction/external rotation, (2) extension/adduction/internal rotation, (3) flexion adduction/external rotation, and (4) extension/abduction/internal rotation.

## Timing

The sequencing of motions associated with normal timing is distal to proximal of a freely moving segment and proximal to distal with a fixed segment. Changes in normal timing can be used, however, to emphasize a specific component of the movement pattern. It is important to correct proximal dysfunctions, then process to distal dysfunctions, unless one is already normal.

## TECHNIQUES

Understanding the basic principles allows the therapist to apply them to specific techniques. These techniques require the therapist to control the patient's muscular effort, movement patterns, and joint position. The patterns of movement are designed to stimulate rhythmically the agonist of the movement while causing relaxation to the antagonist.

## Rhythmic Initiation

The pupose of rhythmic initiation is to apply unidirectional concentric contraction to initiate and control a muscular contraction through a specific motion. It aids the patient's ability to learn a direction of motion that is supposedly normal.

## Repeated Quick Stretch

In repeated quick stretch, the therapist applies a stretch force to invoke a reflex to further stimulate muscular contraction. The stretch mechanism stimulates a response by the gamma system in the musculotendinous unit. This technique is helpful in cases of fatigue and specific areas of inhibition.

## Combination of Isotonics

The use of concentric, eccentric, and maintained isotonic techniques facilitates control of movement.

## Reversal of Antagonists

Reversal of antagonists is crucial in normal function to allow a movement to occur without excessive resistance of the antagonistic muscle. It consists of reciprocal isometric (stabilizing reversal) or isotonic (isotonic reversal) contractions through the desired range of motion. The goal is to work on facilitation of the agonist and antagonist.

## Relaxation Techniques

Relaxation of synergistic muscle groups stimulates the agonist and inhibits the antagonist to increase range of motion. Hold, relax, and contract–relax techniques can be used.

# COMMON PROCEDURES FOR SHOULDER PATHOLOGIES

Performance of PNF revolves around specific spiral and diagonal patterns that include three integrated mechanical motions: flexion/extension, abduction/adduction, and internal/external rotation. The patterns for the shoulder will involve combining the above motions, resulting in the whole extremity being exercised. By exercising the extremity in mass, the therapist must apply resistance, allow muscle shortening and lengthening, permit proper sequencing of muscle contraction, invoke a stretch response, and reproduce normal biomechanical joint function.

Patterns for the upper extremities can isolate joint movements and muscle groups or employ movement and facilitation that include the cervical spine, shoulder complex, trunk, and lower extremities. Movements about the shoulder for PNF combine flexion/extension with abduction/adduction, external rotation with flexion, and internal rotation with extension. The possible combinations of all of these patterns are beyond the scope of this chapter. Readers are referred to other sources.[2,3,5]

Instead, those patterns most commonly used by the author for the throwing athlete will be presented. This includes movement patterns that are not part of the PNF "system," but which are based on the same principles and techniques.

## Scapular Patterns

The scapula is a crucial proximal stabilizer of the shoulder complex and upper quarter. Concentric, eccentric, and maintained isotonic techniques should be emphasized when deficiencies are recognized, as well as appropriate approximation and traction. Range of motion of the scapula is also important to evaluate because shortening of the upper trapezius and levator scapula can lead to muscle imbalances, which affect the scapulohumeral relationship.

Initially, four isolated diagonal patterns can be incorporated, including anterior elevation, posterior elevation, anterior depression, and posterior depression (Figs. 38-1 to 38-4). These procedures are performed sidelying where they can also be combined with pelvic patterns (Fig. 38-5). The sitting position can use the uninvolved side for cross facilitation with both symmetric and asymmetric patterns (Figs. 38-6 to 38-7).

Linear patterns are sometimes necessary postoperatively when scapula/clavicle rotation produces pain at the rotator cuff, acromioclavicular joint, or capsular restraints. They can also help when diagonal patterns are limited by soft tissue and myofascial restrictions secondary to chronic postural dysfunction (Fig. 38-8). Prone scapular adduction can assist with upper quarter alignment. Resistance of the shoulder extensors at end range of the extension/abduction pattern can enhance scapular adduction facilitation (Figs. 38-9 to 38-10).

The serratus anterior can be facilitated by resisting scapular abduction with a combination of isotonic techniques at multiple angle positions. Supine with a bilateral technique for cross facilitation in shoulder elevation in the plane of the scapula is effective. A bar of various weights can offer resistance in addition to that provided by the physical therapist (Fig. 38-11).

Input to the rotator cuff can be increased by having the patient hold the shoulder isometrically at one point in the range of motion while performing synergistic scapular movements. For example, scapular elevation patterns with the shoulder maintained in 40-degree abduction in the plane of the scapula includes the deltoid and supraspinatus in the exercise pattern with the serratus anterior and upper trapezius/levator scapula (Fig. 38-12).

Adjunctively to the manual techniques, scapular exercises can be performed with dumbbell weights or elastic cords (Fig. 38-13). Individual components of the scapula in throwing movements can be facilitated (Fig. 38-14). After reestablishing normal scapular mobility, strength, and stability in this manner, the scapula treatment can be integrated with the glenohumeral joint.

## Shoulder Patterns

Knott and Voss[3] describe four basic diagonal patterns for the shoulder and upper extremity: (1) flexion/abduction/external rotation, (2) extension/adduction/internal rotation, (3) flexion/adduction/external rotation, and (4) extension/abduction/internal rotation. For many clinicians this is the extent of their knowledge regarding PNF for the shoulder. These patterns can be altered by choosing among unilateral/bilateral, symmetric/asymmetric, elbow straight/flexion-extension,

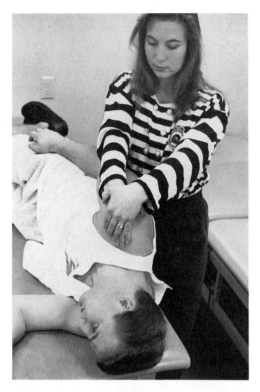

**Fig. 38-1.** Scapular anterior elevation sidelying.

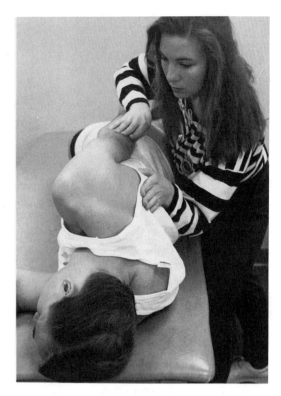

**Fig. 38-2.** Scapular posterior depression sidelying.

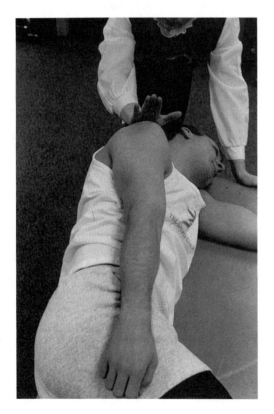

**Fig. 38-3.** Scapular posterior elevation sidelying.

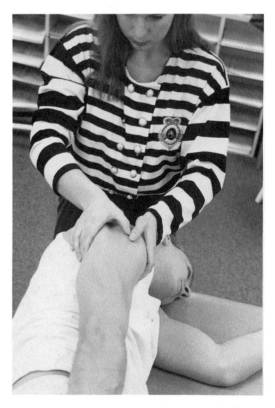

**Fig. 38-4.** Scapular anterior depression sidelying.

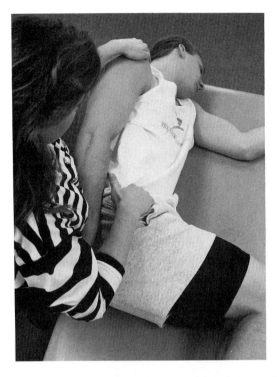

**Fig. 38-5.** Scapular anterior elevation with pelvic anterior elevation.

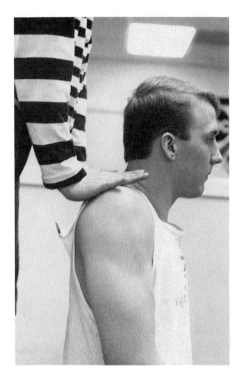

**Fig. 38-6.** Scapular posterior elevation sitting.

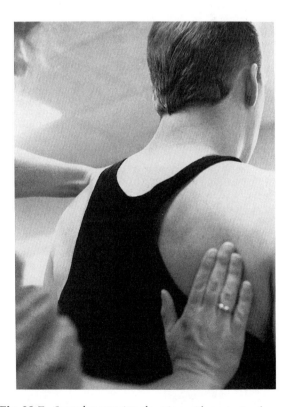

**Fig. 38-7.** Scapular anterior elevation with posterior depression on the contralateral side sitting.

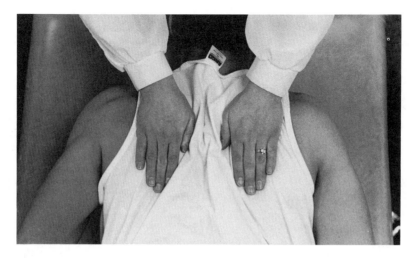

**Fig. 38-8.** Scapular adduction prone.

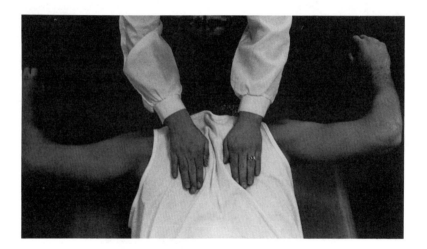

**Fig. 38-9.** Scapular adduction prone with extension/abduction and external rotation.

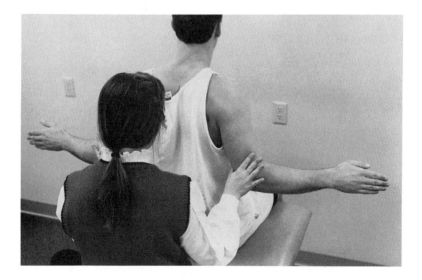

**Fig. 38-10.** Scapular adduction sitting with end range extension/abduction.

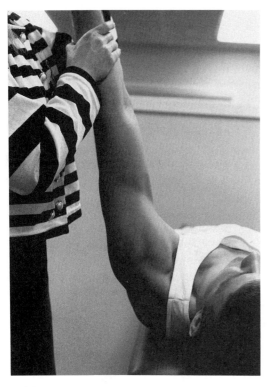

**Fig. 38-11.** Serratus anterior facilitation.

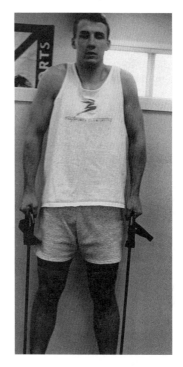

**Fig. 38-13.** Scapular elevation with elastic cord.

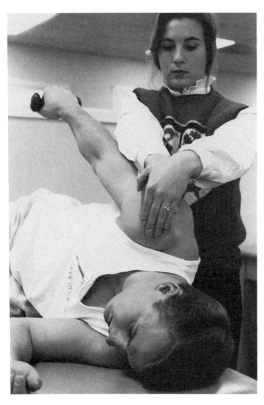

**Fig. 38-12.** Scapular elevation with shoulder isometrically held at 40 degrees abduction.

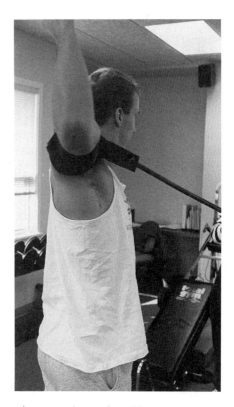

**Fig. 38-14.** Resisted scapular adduction in throwing using elastic cord.

timing for emphasis, submaximal/maximal efforts, or full range/partial range of motion. If the choices above are integrated into the treatment, they become extensive and extremely varied. They influence the shoulder components by facilitating the synergistic scapular musculature.

Each exercise technique and pattern must have a specific goal, and the therapist must consider its effect on various structures (primarily the rotator cuff, capsulo-ligamentous stabilizers, acromioclavicular joint, and upper quarter). This demands a thorough understanding of shoulder anatomy and biomechanics, meticulous clinical examination, and detailed knowledge of pathologies and surgical procedures before initiating therapeutic exercises. Specific application yields very specific results.

The flexion/abduction/external rotation and extension/adduction/internal rotation diagonals are the most commonly used PNF diagonals for athletes.

Resistance to external rotation motion in the *flexion/abduction/external rotation pattern* can be modified to be isometric as well as isotonic. This is especially important in cases of infraspinatus tendonitis or partial tears in which overload must be avoided. Full glenohumeral elevation can create subacromial impingement of the rotator cuff against the coracoacromial arch. Predictably, this leads to far greater problems than it solves, especially in patients with partial or full rotator cuff tears, history of classic impingement syndrome, and encroachment of the supraspinatus outlet secondary to acromial morphology or bony changes. When applied appropriately, this pattern can be extremely useful in facilitation of the shoulder elevators (Figs. 38-15 to 38-17). Supine, prone, or upright positioning of the patient can be used as well as bilateral and asymmetric techniques. Slight modification of this pattern can put the patient in an elevation/plane of the scapula movement which is also very effective and usually less stressful to the rotator cuff than beginning from an adducted position (Fig. 38-18). Bilateral techniques for cross facilitation and positioning the glenohumeral joint in mid-ranges from a supine position are good starting points for scapular/rotator cuff stabilization in elevation.

*Extension/adduction/internal rotation* is the diagonal pattern opposite to flexion/abduction/external rotation. It has mechanical characteristics similar to the

acceleration, follow-through, and deceleration phases of throwing. Again, as in the flexion/abduction/external rotation diagonal, rotation can be isometrically or isotonically resisted (Fig. 38-19). This pattern is excellent for subscapularis facilitation in conjunction with other glenohumeral components. Patients with posterior shoulder instabilities must be monitored carefully to avoid subluxation and overloading of the capsulo-ligamentous restraints. Supine, standing, and sitting positions can also be used for this exercise.

In the throwing athlete the *flexion/adduction/external rotation–extension/abduction/internal rotation* is more important for the glove or non-throwing side since that extremity functions oppositely of the throwing side. End range flexion/adduction can create overcompression or repetitive microtrauma at the acromioclavicular joint.

The end range of extension/abduction resisted in an upright position with trunk rotation can assist in facilitation of the posterior glenohumeral, scapular adductor/depressor, and trunk rotator muscle groups (Fig. 38-20) used during the course of the throwing motion. From this same position reciprocal shoulder flexion/extension motions can be facilitated with concentric and eccentric techniques through an appropriate range of motion synergistically with trunk rotation (Fig. 38-21).

Facilitation of the shoulder rotators in isolated patterns is extremely important because the rotator cuff muscles are directly affected. Initially, the shoulder is positioned slightly abducted in the plane of the scapula (approximately 30 degrees forward flexion at 70 degrees abduction). This position has recently been shown by Greenfield et al[6] to be optimal for rotational strengthening over the more traditionally neutral arm at the side position (Figs. 38-22 and 38-23). Also, isometric resistance to adduction for isotonic internal rotation and isometric abduction for isotonic external rotation can be given to "lock" the shoulder and provide overflow facilitation from a stronger source. These are not PNF patterns as described by Knott and Voss[3] but modifications made to avoid positions of impingement and instability while taking advantage of manually applied techniques and principles.

Similarly, the shoulder can be manually resisted for both internal and external rotation at 90 degrees abduction (Figs. 38-24 and 38-25). This position is associated

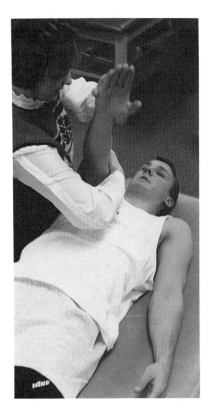

**Fig. 38-15.** Flexion/abduction/external rotation diagonal supine.

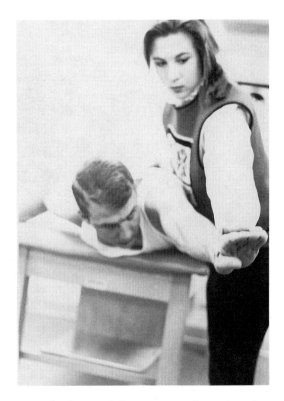

**Fig. 38-16.** Flexion/abduction/external rotation diagonal prone.

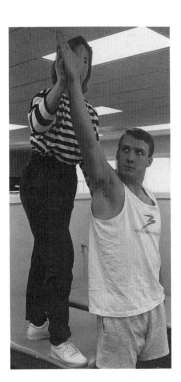

**Fig. 38-17.** Flexion/abduction/external rotation diagonal standing.

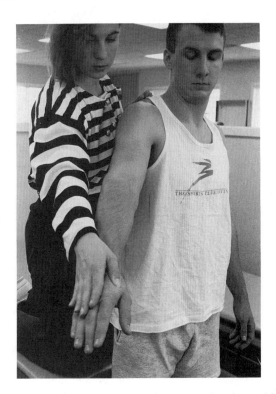

**Fig. 38-18.** Starting position of elevation in the plane of the scapula.

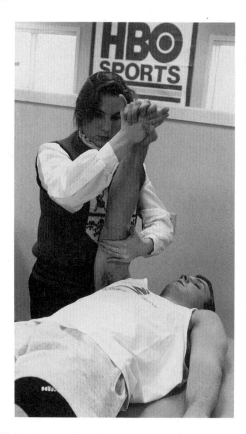

**Fig. 38-19.** Extension/adduction/internal rotation diagonal supine.

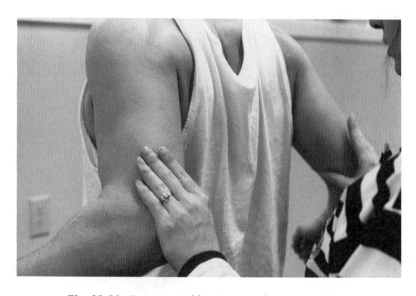

**Fig. 38-20.** Extension/adduction at end range in sitting.

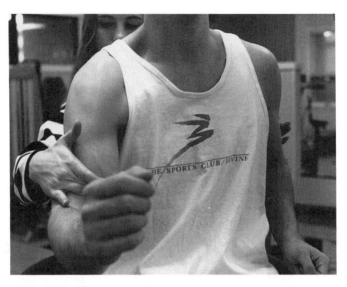

**Fig. 38-21.** Shoulder flexion/extension sitting.

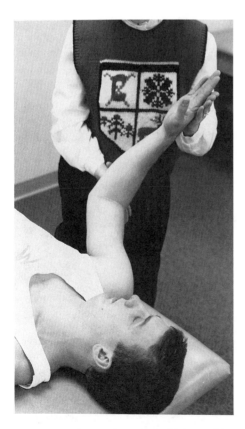

**Fig. 38-22.** External rotation in neutral/plane of the scapula position.

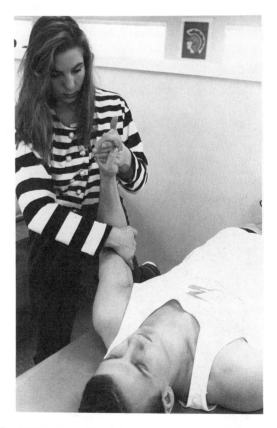

**Fig. 38-23.** Internal rotation in neutral/plane of the scapula position.

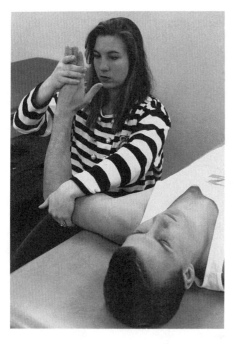

**Fig. 38-24.** External rotation at 90 degrees abduction.

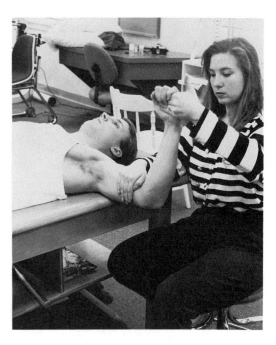

**Fig. 38-25.** Internal rotation at 90 degrees abduction.

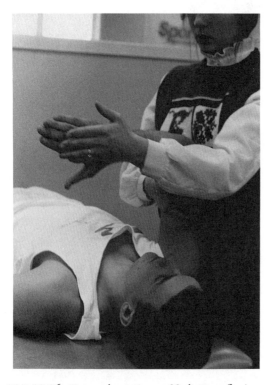

**Fig. 38-26.** External rotation at 90 degrees flexion.

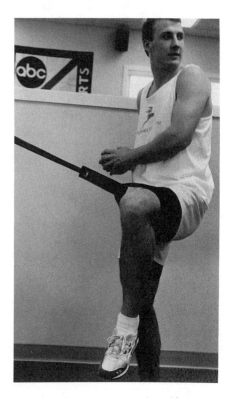

**Fig. 38-27.** Pelvic resistance to trunk and lower extremities using Sportcord (SPORT, Vail, CO).

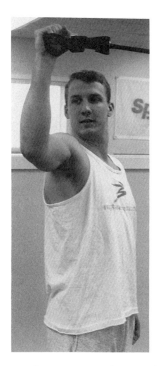

**Fig. 38-28.** External rotation at 90 degrees abduction standing, using elastic cord.

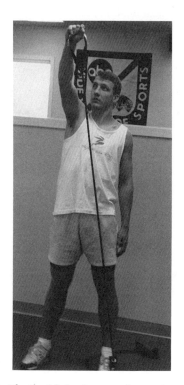

**Fig. 38-29.** Flexion/abduction standing, using elastic cord.

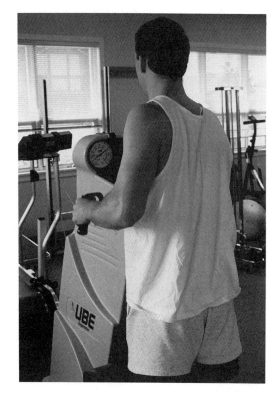

**Fig. 38-30.** Upper body ergometry emphasizing reciprocal scapular/shoulder movements (Cybex, Ronkonkoma, NY).

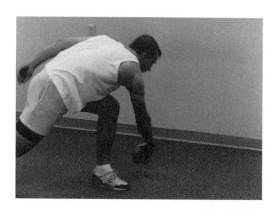

**Fig. 38-31.** Plyometrics using a medicine ball at end range extension/adduction.

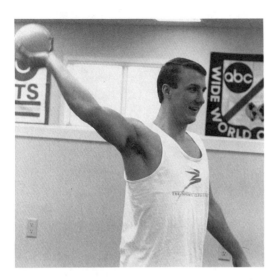

**Fig. 38-32.** Plyometrics using a medicine ball at end range external rotation.

with anterior instability and is used for strengthening the subscapularis as described in many rehabilitation programs with multiple exercise devices (i.e., weights, tubing, mechanical weights). External rotation in this position is associated with cocking phases of throwing and can be important for facilitation of the posterior rotator cuff. Maximal external rotation at 90 degrees abduction, however, stresses the inferior glenohumeral ligament complex, which is the main restraint to anterior instability and is often associated with patient apprehension.

External rotation at 90 degrees flexion is a component of the flexion/abduction diagonal. Flexion/abduction is isometrically resisted at 90 degrees flexion while working isotonically in external rotation (Fig. 38-26). Maximal internal rotation range of motion will impinge the rotator cuff against the coracoacromial arch and is a contraindication. Over-resistance to a weak external rotator group should also be avoided. Infraspinatus/teres minor strengthening in this pattern is an effective technique for the posterior subluxation patient when applied correctly.

## Trunk and Neck Patterns

Patterns that include the upper extremities with the trunk and neck provide a higher functional level of neuromuscular training and movement reeducation. These procedures, however, demand a higher degree of skill on the part of clinician and patient. Normal functional activity includes whole body involvement, making this type of treatment pattern very valuable in patient rehabilitation programs.

## Adjunctive Procedures

The principles and specific techniques presented may be enhanced by using more effective exercise devices as well as manual techniques. On the market today are a variety of elastic cords, weights, resistive exercise machines, and other equipment that can be modified for rehabilitation of the shoulder patient (Figs. 38-27 to 38-30). Plyometric exercise activities can also be applied in diagonal patterns and other components of shoulder complex motion. The goal of the addition of resistance is to build strength, endurance, stabilization, and coordination at higher velocities, which are considered more functional (Figs. 38-31 and 38-32).

## SUMMARY

Shoulder rehabilitation has developed into a very complex process. As part of an integrated approach, PNF treatment techniques offer advantages for the clinician treating shoulder pain and dysfunction. Its concepts are built on basic neurophysiology and provide a sound scientific basis for their application. The hands-on manual procedures allow for specific input to the central nervous system and provide greater control over patient movement reeducation. Resistance through applying concentric, eccentric, and isometric contractions can be emphasized.

Patterns include the rotational components of joint movement and can isolate individual muscle groups or work patients across many segments, integrating upper and lower extremities, trunk, and neck. Also, the traditional patterns can be modified using the same neurophysiologic principles to account for common pathologies.

This chapter has attempted to provide a useful foundation for the clinician to apply PNF techniques for shoulder rehabilitation as part of holistic approach.

# REFERENCES

1. Sherrington C: The Integrative Action of the Nervous System. (Reprinted Ed.) Yale University Press, New Haven, 1961
2. Kabat H: Proprioceptive facilitation in therapeutic exercise. p. 327. In: Therapeutic Exercises. Waverly Press, Baltimore, 1965
3. Knott M, Voss DE: Proprioceptive Neuormuscular Facilitation. Harper & Row, New York, 1968
4. Johnson G, Saliba V: PNF I and II Course Notes. Institute of Physical Art, San Anselmo, CA, 1987
5. Sullivan PE, Markos PD, Minor MAD: An Integrated Approach to Therapeutic Exercise: Theory and Clinical Application. Reston Publishing Co., Reston, VA, 1982
6. Greenfield BH, Donatelli, R, Wooden MJ, Wilkes J: Isokinetic evaluation of shoulder rotational strength between the plane of scapula and the frontal plane. Am J Sports Med 18:124, 1990

# 39

# Mobilization of the Shoulder*

## ROBERT A. DONATELLI

In the past decade, mobilization has been shown clinically to be an important part of rehabilitation and assessment of restricted joint movement. Clinical application is based on an understanding of joint mechanics, connective tissue histology, and muscle function. Mobilization has developed into a clinical science, requiring the therapist to understand anatomic and histologic characteristics of synovial joints. Significant advancement have been made in describing the benefits of passive movement. Thanks to the hard work and dedication of such researchers as Akeson, Woo, Matthews, Amiel, and Peacock,[1-3] we have a better understanding of joint stiffness and wound healing. As clinicians, we can take this knowledge and apply our mobilization techniques during critical stages of wound healing to influence the extensibility of scar tissue and reduce the development of restrictive adhesions. We can also use this knowledge to prevent and treat joint stiffness by applying the appropriate stress to the muscles and connective tissue, promoting homeostasis.[4] It is through an understanding of normal tissue function, tissue changes during immobilization, and the structure of scar tissue that we can establish the criteria for mobilization.

This chapter discusses mobilization from a basic science approach. The mobilization techniques for the shoulder are described, with emphasis on the mechanical and neurophysiologic effects.

---

* From Donatelli RA: Mobilization of the shoulder. In Donatelli RA (ed): Physical Therapy of the Shoulder. 2nd Ed. Churchill Livingstone, New York, 1991, with permission.

## DEFINITION

Several terms must be defined when mobilization is discussed. Articulation, oscillation, distractions, manipulation, and mobilization all describe a specialized type of passive movement.

Articulatory techniques are derived from the osteopathic literature. They are defined as passive movement applied in a smooth rhythmic fashion to stretch contracted muscles, ligaments, and capsules gradually.[5] They include gentle techniques designed to stretch the joint in each of the planes of movement normal to it.[5] The force used during articulatory techniques is usually a prolonged stretch into the restriction or tissue limitation.

Oscillatory techniques are best defined by Maitland,[6] who describes oscillations as passive movements to the joint, which can be of a small or large amplitude and applied anywhere in a range of movement and which can be performed while the joint surfaces are held distracted or compressed. There are four grades of oscillations: grade I is a small amplitude movement performed at the beginning of range; grade II is a large amplitude movement performed within the range but not reaching the limit of the range; grade III is a large amplitude movement up to the limit of range; and grade IV is a small amplitude movement performed at the limit of range.[6] Grades I and II are used for the neurophysiologic effects, and grades III and IV are designed to initiate mechanical changes in the tissue.

Distraction is defined as "separation of surfaces of a joint by extension without injury or dislocation of the parts."[7] Distractive techniques are designed to separate the joint surface attempting to stress the capsule.

*Manipulation* is defined by *Dorland's Illustrated Medical Dictionary* as "skillful or dextrous treatment by the hand. In physical therapy, the forceful passive movement of a joint beyond its active limit of motion."[8] Maitland[6] described two manipulative procedures. Manipulation is a sudden movement or thrust, of small amplitude, performed at a speed that renders the patient powerless to prevent it. Manipulation under anesthesia is a medical procedure used to restore normal joint movement by breaking adhesions.

*Mobilization* is defined as "the making of a fixed or ankylosed part movable. Restoration of motion to a joint."[7,8] To the clinician, mobilization is passive movement that is designed to improve soft tissue and joint mobility. It can include oscillations, articulations, distractions, or manipulations.

*Mobilization,* in this chapter, is defined as a specialized passive movement, attempting to restore the arthrokinematics and osteokinematics of joint movement. It includes articulations, oscillations, distractions, and thrust techniques. The techniques are built on active and passive joint mechanics. They are directed at the periarticular structures that have become restricted secondary to trauma and immobilization. These same techniques can be effective tools in the evaluation of joint movement.

## ROLE OF MOBILIZATION

The main goal of the physical therapist is to restore normal function. The normal mechanics of synovial joints include a combination of arthrokinematics (the intimate mechanics of joint surfaces), osteokinematics (the movement of bones), and muscle function.[9]

*Gray's Anatomy* describes the intimate joint mechanics as roll, spin, and slide. These movements occur during active movement between articular surfaces.[9] Besides the active movements, there are accessory movements, two types of which are described in *Gray's Anatomy*. The first type occurs only when resistance is encountered during active movement (e.g., metacarpophalangeal joint rotation can only occur when a solid object is grasped by the hand).[9] The second type of accessory movement is purely a passive motion produced by an outside force[9] (e.g., if muscles surrounding the shoulder joint are relaxed, a distractive force can separate the head of the humerus from the glenoid cavity).

The combination of the active movements of roll, spin, and slide plus the accessory movements constitute joint mobility. For example, from 0 to 30 degrees—and often from 30 to 60 degrees—of glenohumeral joint abduction the humeral head moves upward on the glenoid face by approximately 3 mm. Thereafter, the excursion of the humeral head during elevation is 3 mm in a superior and inferior direction.[9a] Previously, joint arthrokinematics was believed to be a result of joint surface geometry. Research has demonstrated that the direction and amount of the humeral head translation may be primarily a function of tissue tension.[9b]

## EFFECTS OF PASSIVE MOVEMENT

Normal joint motion includes a dynamic combination of arthrokinematics, sufficient periarticular tissue extensibility, osteokinematics, and normal muscle function. Joint stiffness results from a loss or change in one or all the components of joint mobility. Passive movement has its most therapeutic effect in the treatment of joint stiffness secondary to immobilization and trauma. Continuous passive movement has been shown to be effective in reducing wound edema and joint effusion, eliminating joint restrictions after trauma.[4] Franks and associates[4] found that continuous passive movement resulted in increased patient comfort and shorter hospital stays. Passive movement has been shown to provide proprioceptive feedback to the central nervous system by maintaining tension in the muscle.[4] It has also been hypothesized that stimulation of the proprioceptors interferes with transmission of pain through the central nervous system.[4] The nociceptive afferents (pain fibers) have a much higher threshold of excitation than do the mechanoreceptor afferents,[10,11] and there is evidence that the stimulation of peripheral mechanoreceptors blocks the transmission of pain to the brain.[10] Wyke[10] explained this phenomenon as a direct release of inhibitory transmitters within the basal spinal nucleus, inhibiting the onward flow of incoming nociceptive afferent activity. Mobilization is one method of enhancing the frequency of discharge from the mechanoreceptors, thereby diminishing the intensity of many types of pain. If the mechanoreceptor stimulation is of high enough frequency and is maintained long enough, the pain may be abolished.[10]

An important aspect of passive movement is in the prevention and treatment of the complications resulting from immobilization. The lack of stress to connective tissue results in changes in normal joint mobility. The periarticular tissue and muscles surrounding the joint show significant changes after periods of immobilization. Akeson et al have subtantiated a decrease in water and glycosaminoglycans (the fibrous tissue lubricant), an increase in fatty fibrous infiltrates (which may form adhesions as they mature into scar), an increase in abnormally placed collagen cross-links (which may contribute to the inhibition of collagen fiber gliding), and the loss of fiber orientation within ligaments (which significantly reduces their strength).[1,4] Passive movement or stress to the tissues can help to prevent these changes by maintaining tissue homeostasis.[4] The exact mechanisms of prevention are uncertain.

## EFFECTS OF PASSIVE MOVEMENT ON SCAR TISSUE: INDICATIONS AND CONTRAINDICATIONS FOR MOBILIZATION

Research indicates that mobilization is most effective in reversing the changes that occur in connective tissue after immobilization.[4] Conversely, mobilization after trauma must be carefully analyzed. When is it safe to apply stress to scar tissue? How much stress should be applied to the scar to promote remodeling? In what direction should the stress be applied? These important questions must be answered before we can determine the indications for mobilization of scar tissue.

Research has shown that stress applied early to healing wounds is important in establishing the characteristics of scar tissue. The production of scar tissue begins on the fourth day of wound healing and increases rapidly during the first 3 weeks.[2,12] Peacock[2] substantiated this peak production of scar by the increased quantities of hydroxyproline. Hydroxyproline is a by-product of collagen synthesis.[2,13] New collagen is deposited in the scar, at a rate higher than normal connective tissue, for up to 4 months. Research indicates that early stress to scar tissue influences the remodeling process. The collagen fibers are initially deposited within the scar in a random fashion. This random order changes as the tissue begins to remodel. The new collagen fibers align with the pre-existing fibers, and the assimilation of the new fibers is part of the remodeling process. Scar tissue begins to resemble the previous normal tissues by the process of maturation.[2,12] Another

important aspect of remodeling is the ability of the collagen fibers to glide. If this does not occur, the scar tissue can cause limitations in the mobility of the normal tissue.

The collagen fibril in its early stages is very weak. Intermolecular and intramolecular cross-linking of collagen molecules develop, designed to resist tensile forces.[2,13] The tensile strength of the collagen fibers continues to develop linearly for at least 3 months.[2,12] Arem and Madden[14] demonstrated that after 14 weeks of scar maturation, elongation of the scar was no longer possible. In contrast, the 3-week-old scar was significantly lengthened when subjected to tension.[14] It is evident that as scar tissue matures, it develops the capability to resist tensile forces. Peacock[2] hypothesized that the mechanism by which the length of the scar is increased becomes critical for the restoration of the gliding mechanism. Stretching, or an increase in length of the scar, is a result of straightening or reorientation of the collagen fibers, without a change in their dimensions.[2] For this to occur, the collagen fibers must glide on each other. This gliding mechanism is hampered in unstressed scar tissue by the development of abnormally placed cross-links and a random orientation of the newly synthesized collagen fibrils.[1] Clinically, this can mean limited joint movement.

Joint stiffness results from immobilization and/or trauma. The limitations in movement result from the changes that occur in the periarticular tissues as described above. Mobilization is indicated when the lack of extensibility of the periarticular structures limits the arthrokinematic movement of joint surfaces. This limitation will produce compensations in normal motion and changes in muscle function. The patient experiences pain and limited movement of the involved joint. The therapeutic effects of mobilization on scar and immobilized tissue is important in re-establishing normal active range of motion. Mobilization of the immobilized tissue stimulates the production of glycosaminoglycans, which is important for lubrication and maintaining a critical distance between collagen fibers to allow for the gliding mechanism to occur.[1,3] It also assures an orderly deposition of new collagen fibrils, thereby preventing abnormal cross-link formation.[1,3] Enneking and Horowitz[15] and Evans et al[16] documented that forceful manipulation breaks intracapsular fibrofatty adhesions that may have formed within the joint during immobilization.

As previously mentioned, early stress to scar tissue determines the tissue flexibility. Arem and Madden[14] advocated stressing the tissue as early as the third week of scar tissue production. Tissue flexibility is enhanced by passive movement of the young scar, and this is accomplished by promoting alignment of new collagen fibers with pre-existing fibers, preventing the development of obstructive adhesions, and enhancing fiber glide. The direction, velocity, duration, and magnitude of the stress to scar tissue needs further investigation. The exact effects mobilization has on the remodeling process have not been determined. The forces applied during application of the mobilization techniques are controlled by the pain tolerance of the patient and tissue resistance. The direction of stress applied to connective tissues should be determined in the evaluation by the location of tissue resistance and assessment of joint mobility.

It is easier to understand the contraindications of mobilization by becoming aware of the common abuses of passive movement. The abuses of passive movement can be broken down into two categories: creation of excessive trauma to the tissues and the causing of "undesired" or abnormal mobility.[4]

Improper techniques, such as extreme force, poor direction of stress, and excessive velocity, may result in serious secondary injury or damage to the tissues surrounding the joint that is mobilized. Also, mobilization to joints that are moving normally or that are hypermobile can create and/or increase joint instabilities.

Ultimately, selection of a specific technique will determine contraindications. For example, the very gentle grade I oscillations, as described by Maitland, rarely have contraindications. These techniques are mainly used to block pain. They are of small amplitude and controlled velocity. In contrast, manipulative techniques have many contraindications. Haldeman[17] described the following conditions as major contraindications for thrust techniques: arthritides, dislocation, hypermobility, trauma or recent occurrence, bone weakness and destructive disease, circulatory disturbances, neurologic dysfunction, and infectious disease.

In summary, connective tissue heals by formation of scar tissue. Peak production of scar occurs within the first 3 weeks of wound healing.[18] Between 3 weeks and 6 weeks, there is a decrease in fibroblast numbers. Controlled stress at this early stage is important in realignment of collagen fibers. At 14 weeks, scar length appears to be maximal. Influencing the mobility of the scar at this stage may be difficult, requiring a greater magnitude of force. The mechanical properties of untreated scar tissue were inferior to normal ligament tissue after 40 weeks of healing.[18] The ligament "scar" was found to be structurally abnormal chemically and mechanically at long-term follow-up.[18] Tipton et al[19] clearly showed that increased or decreased levels of systematic exercise will markedly influence the strength of ligaments. Exercise was found to increase the number of collagen fibrils and to alter their arrangement and thickness. Also, ligaments from trained animals had a significantly higher hydroxyproline content than ligaments from immobilized animals.[19] Therefore, normal maturation of scar tissue is dependent on stress at early stages.

## PRINCIPLES OF MOBILIZATION TECHNIQUES

The mobilization techniques are designed to restore intimate joint mechanics. Several general principles should be remembered during application of the techniques.

### Hand Position

The mobilization hand should be placed as close as possible to the joint surfaces, and the forces applied should be directed at the periarticular tissues. The stabilization hand counteracts the movement of the mobilizing hand by applying an equal but opposite force or by preventing movement at surrounding joints.

### Direction of Movement

The direction of forces to the joint should be away from pain and into resistance. The resistance represents the direction of capsular or joint limitation. Movement into the restriction is an attempt to make mechanical changes within the capsule and its surrounding tissue. The mechanical changes may include breaking up of adhesions, realignment of collagen, or increasing fiber glide. Certain movements stress specific parts of the capsule. It has been substantiated through arthrogram studies that external rotation of the glenohumeral joint stresses the anterior recess of the capsule.[20]

The direction of movement should not exceed the normal limits of the joint. When applying the mobilization techniques, the therapist must be aware of the joint's movement within the body planes (degrees of freedom) and the contour of the joint surfaces. The glenohumeral joint has three degrees of freedom, or it is capable of moving in all three body planes (frontal, sagittal, and transverse).[9] Also, movement occurs at the joint surface. For example, Poppen and Walker[21] established that during the first 30 to 60 degrees of shoulder elevation, the head of the humerus moves upward approximately 3 mm. Thereafter, it moves 1 or 2 mm upward and downward between each successive position.[21] The earlier works of Saha[22] demonstrated the movements of roll, spin, and slide of the humeral head during elevation of the shoulder. For the therapist to determine the direction of force, there must be an understanding of joint movement and the location and nature of the joint restriction.

## Body Mechanics

It is important for the therapist to maintain good body mechanics during the application of mobilization techniques. The therapist should stand as close as possible to the patient. The therapist's hands and arms should be positioned to act as fulcrums and levers, and the therapist's position should allow for the most efficient application of techniques.

## Duration and Amplitude

Several studies have been performed to determine the most effective technique for obtaining permanent elongation of collagenous tissue, using different loads and loading time. The studies used rat tendons to demonstrate the elongation of tissue under varied loads. The treatments included low load and a long duration using 5 g and stretch for 15 minutes. High-load, short-duration treatment used 105 to 165 g for 5 minutes.[23,24] The results indicated that low-load long-duration stretch was more effective in obtaining a permanent elongation of the tissue. Several studies also indicated further improvement with the use of heat before or during the stretch and ice immediately afterward.[25,26]

In a recent study, healthy subjects received 3 40-minute treatments, using low-load prolonged stretch (LLPS) to increase shoulder external rotation across a 5-day period. The conclusions of the study indicated that applying heat in conjunction with a LLPS to a non-pathologic shoulder is a clinically superior method of improving flexibility, compared with using LLPS alone. Furthermore, LLPS associated with the use of heat, ice, or a combination of both facilitated greater long-term improvements in shoulder flexibility, compared to controls.[29]

# GLENOHUMERAL JOINT TECHNIQUES

## Inferior Glide of the Humerus (Fig. 39-1)

*Patient position:* supine, with the involved extremity close to the edge of the table. A strap stabilizes the scapula. The extremity is abducted to the desired range.

*Therapist position:* facing the lateral side of the upper arm. Left hand is into the axilla as close as possible to the joint line. The web space of the right hand is over the superior humeral head as close as possible to the acromion. The left hand maintains the abducted position while applying a distractive force. The right hand pushes the head of the humerus inferiorly, attempting to stress the axillary pouch or inferior portion of the glenohumeral capsule. Oscillatory techniques using grades III and IV are effective. For more aggressive stretching to the inferior capsule, a prolonged stretch and manipulations are effective with the patient's arm held in 60 degrees of abduction or less.

## Longitudinal Distraction—Inferior Glide of the Humerus (Fig. 39-2)

*Patient position:* supine, with the involved extremity as close as possible to the edge of the table.

*Therapist position:* facing the joint, with the right hand into the axilla attempting to hold the glenoid. The left hand grips the epicondyles of the humerus, applying a downward traction on the humerus and stressing the inferior capsule. A prolonged stretch is effective with this technique.

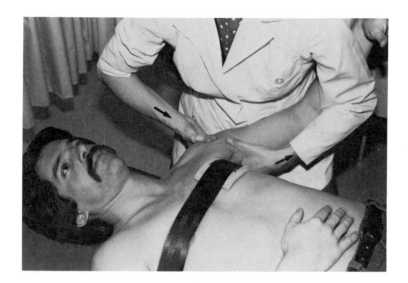

**Fig. 39-1.**

## Caudal Glide of the Humerus
### (Fig. 39-3)

*Patient position:* supine, with the involved extremity flexed to 90 degrees at the shoulder.

*Therapist position:* as close as possible to the involved extremity, with both hands grasping the humerus as close as possible to the head of the humerus. The hands pull the humerus inferiorly, stressing the inferior aspect of the glenohumeral capsule. A prolonged stretch is most effective.

## Posterior Glide of the Humerus
### (Fig. 39-4)

*Patient position:* supine, with the involved extremity as close as possible to the edge of the table. A wedge is placed under the dorsal scapula. The extremity is flexed and horizontally adducted to the desired range. The elbow is flexed.

*Therapist position:* facing cranially, with the right hand maintaining the flexed and adducted position and the left hand over the elbow with the forearm

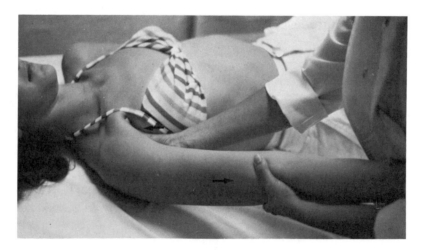

**Fig. 39-2.**

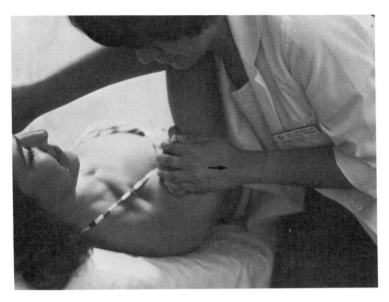

**Fig. 39-3.**

parallel to the patient's forearm. The force is applied through the elbow, pushing the humerus posteriorly and stressing the posterior aspect of the glenohumeral capsule and the tendinous portion of the subscapularis. A prolonged stress or oscillatory techniques is useful.

## Lateral Distraction of the Humerus (Fig. 39-5)

*Patient position:* as close as possible to the edge of the table, with the involved extremity flexed at the elbow

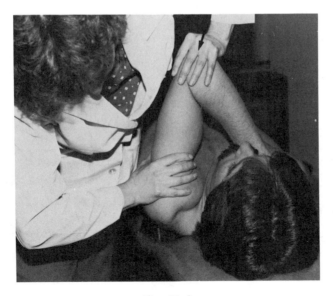

**Fig. 39-4.**

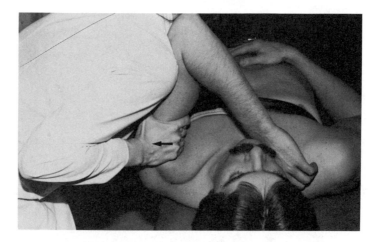

**Fig. 39-5.**

and glenohumeral joint. The extremity rests on the therapist's shoulder. A strap stabilizes the scapula.

*Therapist position:* facing laterally, both hands grasp the humerus as close as possible to the joint. The force is a lateral pull to the humerus, stressing the anterior, posterior, superior, and inferior aspect of the capsule. A prolonged stretch is most effective.

## Anterior Glide of the Humerus (Fig. 39-6)

*Patient position:* prone, with the involved extremity as close as possible to the edge of the table. The head of the humerus must be off the table. A wedge is placed just medial to the joint line under the coracoid process. The extremity is abducted in the plane of the scapula.

*Therapist position:* distal to the abducted part, facing cranially. The left hand applies an inferior pull to the humerus. The right hand moves the head of the humerus anteriorly, stressing the anterior recess and capsule. The tendinous portion of the subscapularis is also stressed with this technique. A prolonged stretch with oscillations at the end of the available range is very effective.

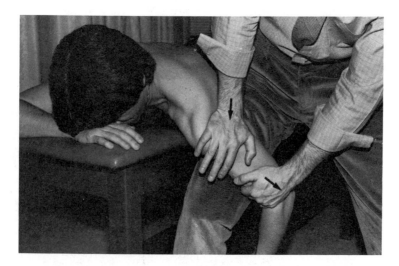

**Fig. 39-6.**

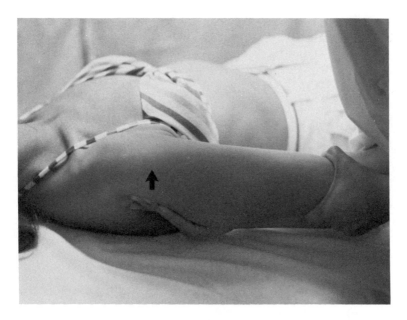

**Fig. 39-7.**

## Anterior Glide of the Head of the Humerus (Fig. 39-7)

*Patient position:* supine, with the involved extremity as close as possible to the edge of the table. A strap may be used to stabilize the scapula (see Fig. 39-5).

*Therapist position:* facing cranially, with the right hand holding the head of the humerus as close as possible to the joint line. The left hand stabilizes the distal humerus, applying a slight distractive force. The force of the right hand moves the head of the humerus in an anterior direction, stretching the anterior capsular structures and the tendinous portion of the subscapularis. A prolonged stretch is most effective.

## Anterior/Posterior Glide of the Head of the Humerus (Fig. 39-8)

*Patient position:* prone, with the involved extremity over the edge of the table abducted to the desired range. A strap may be used to stabilize the scapula.

*Therapist position:* facing laterally in a sitting position, with the forearm of the involved extremity held between the therapist's knees. Both hands grasp the head of the humerus and apply an up-and-down movement, oscillating the head of the humerus. Grades I

and II are mainly used with this technique to stimulate mechanoreceptor activity.

## Anterior/Posterior Glide of the Head of the Humerus (Fig. 39-9)

*Patient position:* supine, with the involved extremity supported by the table. A towel roll or wedge is placed under the elbow to hold the arm in the plane of the scapula (abduction anterior to the frontal plane).

*Therapist position:* facing laterally in a sitting position. The fingertips hold the head of the humerus while a gentle up-and-down movement is applied. This technique is used with grades I and II oscillations.

## External Rotation of the Humerus (Fig. 39-10)

*Patient position:* supine, with the involved extremity supported by the table. The arm is held in the plane of the scapula.

*Therapist position:* facing laterally, with the right hand grasping the distal humerus; the heel of the left hand is placed over the lateral aspect of the head of the humerus. The force is applied through both hands. The right externally rotates the humerus. The left

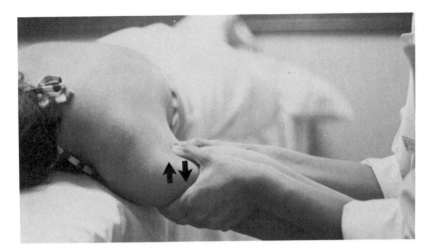

**Fig. 39-8.**

pushes on the most lateral aspect of the humeral head in a posterior direction, promoting external rotation of the humerus. A long-axis distractive force is applied during this technique. Graded oscillations or a thrust technique can be used.

### External Rotation/Abduction/Inferior Glide of the Humerus (Fig. 39-11)

*Patient position:* supine, with the involved extremity supported by the table. The arm is abducted in the plane of the scapula.

*Therapist position:* facing laterally, with the right hand holding the distal humerus and the heel of the left hand over the head of the humerus. The forces are applied simultaneously. The right hand abducts the arm and externally rotates the humerus while maintaining the plane of the scapula position. The left hand simultaneously pushes the head of the humerus into external rotation and an inferior glide. The force applied can be a thrust or a prolonged stretch, both occurring at the end of the available range.

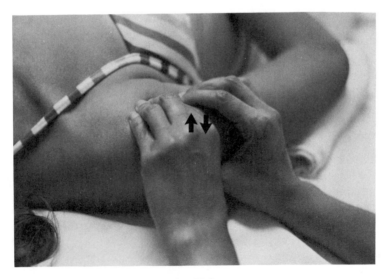

**Fig. 39-9.**

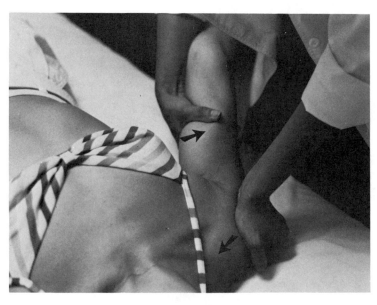

**Fig. 39-10.**

## SCAPULOTHORACIC TECHNIQUES

A prolonged stretch is used with all the scapulothoracic techniques.

### Scapula External Rotation
### (Fig. 39-12)

*Patient position:* sidelying, with the involved extremity accessible to the therapist.

*Therapist position:* facing the patient, with the left arm under the involved extremity through the axillary

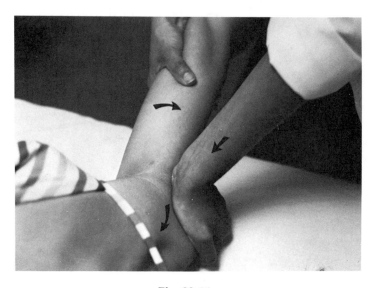

**Fig. 39-11.**

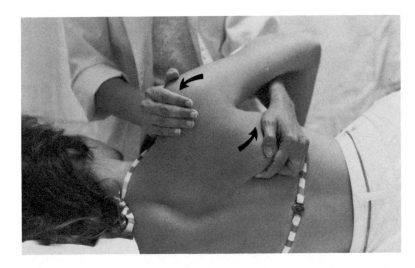

Fig. 39-12.

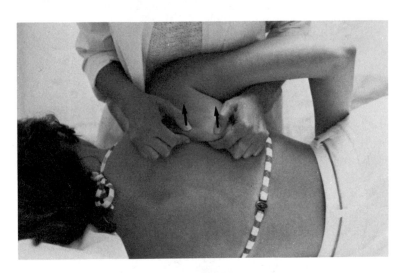

Fig. 39-13.

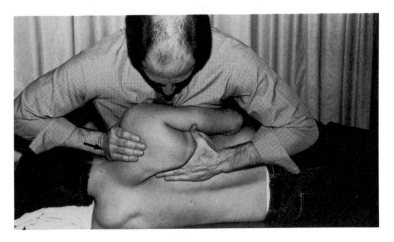

Fig. 39-14.

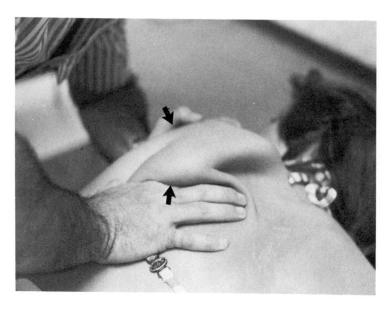

**Fig. 39-15.**

area. This allows the left hand to grasp the inferior angle of the scapula. The right hand holds the superior aspect of the scapula. The force is applied simultaneously, producing an external rotation of the scapula.

## Scapula Distraction (Fig. 39-13)

*Patient position:* same as in Figure 39-12.

*Therapist position:* facing the patient, with the left hand grasping the inferior angle of the scapula and the right hand grasping the vertebral border of the scapula. Both hands tilt the scapula up and away from the thoracic wall. Stabilization of the humerus anteriorly by the therapist's upper body is important. This technique is beneficial because it stretches the subscapularis.

## Inferior Glide of the Scapula (Fig. 39-14)

*Patient position:* same as Figure 39-12.

*Therapist position:* facing the patient, with the left web space surrounding the inferior angle of the scapula. The right hand holds the superior aspect of the scapula with a lumbrical grip. The right hand pushes in a caudal direction while the left hand moves under the inferior angle of the scapula.

## Scapula Distraction, Prone (Fig. 39-15)

*Patient position:* prone, with the involved extremity supported by the table.

*Therapist position:* facing cranially, with the left hand under the head of the humerus and the right web space under the inferior angle of the scapula. The forces are applied simultaneously. The left hand lifts the humerus while the right web space moves the inferior angle of the scapula.

# STERNOCLAVICULAR AND ACROMIOCLAVICULAR TECHNIQUES

## Superior Glide of the Sternoclavicular Joint (Fig. 39-16)

*Patient position:* supine, with the involved extremity close to the edge of the table.

*Therapist position:* facing cranially. The volar surface of the left thumb pad is placed over the inferior surface of the most medial aspect of the clavicle. The right thumb reinforces the dorsal aspect of the left thumb. Both thumbs push the clavicle superiorly. The graded oscillations are most successful with this technique.

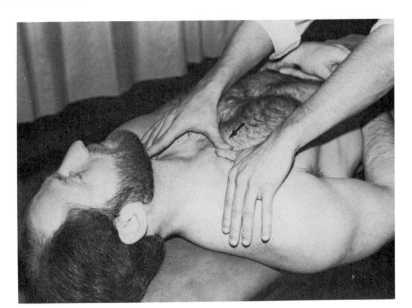

**Fig. 39-16.**

## Anterior Glide of the Acromioclavicular Joint (Fig. 39-17)

*Patient position:* supine and at a diagonal to allow the involved acromioclavicular joint to be over the edge of the table.

*Therapist position:* with the dorsal surface of the thumbs together, the therapist places the distal tips of the thumbs posteriorly to the most lateral edge of the clavicle. Both thumbs push the clavicle anteriorly. The graded oscillations are mainly used with this technique.

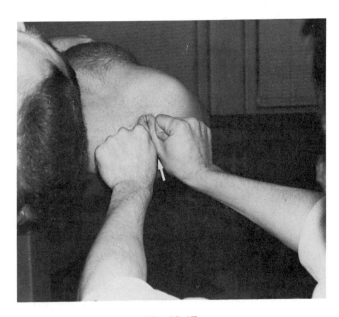

**Fig. 39-17.**

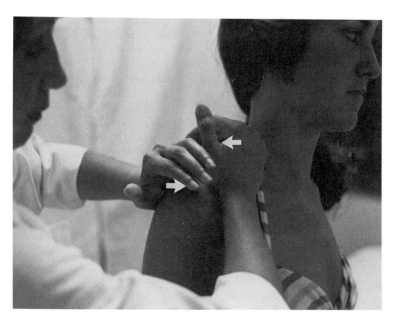

**Fig. 39-18.**

## Gapping of the Acromioclavicular Joint (Fig. 39-18)

*Patient position:* sitting close to the edge of the table.

*Therapist position:* facing laterally, with the heel of the left hand over the spine of the scapula and the thenar eminence of the right hand over the distal clavicle. The force is applied simultaneously. Both hands push the bones in opposite directions, obtaining a general stretch to the capsular structures of the acromioclavicular joint. Oscillations or a prolonged stretch are used with this technique.

The duration and amplitude of force suggested with each technique is based on my clinical experience.

## SUMMARY

This chapter has reviewed several important mechanical, histologic, and neurophysiologic effects of mobilization. The shoulder joint is a complex organ. Mobilization is one aspect of treatment. The application of the mobilization techniques for the shoulder are dependent on the evaluation and assessment of the therapist. The indications and contraindications must be based on an understanding of the histology of immobilized and traumatized connective tissue. Remodeling of scar tissue is far more difficult than reversing the effects of short periods of immobilization. The most recent research indicates that early passive movement is important in the rehabilitation of joint restrictions. However, the velocity, amplitude, duration, and direction of force needed to produce a therapeutic effect requires further investigation. The role of mobilization in the future will be determined by the clinical research performed over the next decade.

## ACKNOWLEDGMENTS

I thank William Boissonnault, M.S., R.P.T., Zita Gonzalez, R.P.T., and Amy Sowinski for their assistance with the technique pictures and extend special thanks to Christy Moran and Helen Owens-Burkhart for their assistance with this chapter.

## REFERENCES

1. Akeson WH, Amiel D, Woo SL-Y: Immobility effects on synovial joints. The pathomechanics of joint contracture. Biorheology 17:95, 1980

2. Peacock EE, Jr: Wound Repair. 3rd Ed. WB Saunders, Philadelphia, 1984

3. Woo S, Matthews, JV, Akeson WH et al: Connective tissue response to immobility: correlative study of biomechanical and biochemical measurements of normal and immobilized rabbit knees. Arthritis Rheum 18:257, 1975

4. Franks C, Akeson WH, Woo S et al: Physiology and therapeutic value of passive joint motion. Clin Orthop 185:113, 1984

5. Stoddard A: Manual of Osteopathic Technique. Hutchinson, London, 1959

6. Maitland GD: Peripheral Manipulation. Butterworth, London, 1970

7. Clayton L (ed): Taber's Cyclopedic Medical Dictionary. FA Davis, Philadelphia, 1977

8. Friel J (ed): Dorland's Illustrated Medical Dictionary. 25th Ed. WB Saunders, Philadelphia, 1974

9. Warwick R, Williams P (eds): Gray's Anatomy. 35th British Ed. WB Saunders, Philadelphia, 1973

9a. Poppen NK, Walker PS: Normal and abnormal motion of the shoulder. J Bone Joint Surg 58:195, 1976

9b. McClure PW, Flowers KR: Treatment of limited shoulder motion: case study based on biomechanical considerations. Phys Ther 72:97, 1992

10. Wyke BD: The neurology of joints. Ann R Coll Surg Engl 41:25, 1966

11. Wyke BD: Neurological aspects of pain therapy: a review of some current concepts. p. 1. In Swerdlow M (ed): The Therapy of Pain. MTP Press, Lancaster, England, 1981

12. Kelly M, Madden JW: Hand surgery and wound healing. p. 49. In Wolfort FG (ed): Acute Hand Injuries: A Multispeciality Approach. Little, Brown, Boston, 1980

13. Cohen KI, McCoy BJ, Diegelmann RF: An update on wound healing. Ann Plast Surg 3:264, 1979

14. Arem AJ, Madden JW: Effects of stress on healing wounds: intermittent noncyclical tension. J Surg Res 20:93, 1976

15. Enneking W, Horowitz M: The inter-articular effects of immobilization on the human knee. J Bone Joint Surg 54A:973, 1972

16. Evans E, Eggers G, Butler J, Blumel J: Immobilization and remobilization of rats' knee joints. J Bone Joint Surg 42A:737, 1960

17. Haldeman S: Modern Developments in the Principles and Practice of Chiropractic. Appleton-Century-Crofts, East Norwalk, CT, 1980

18. Frank C, Woo SL-Y, Amiel D et al: Medial collateral ligament healing: a multidisciplinary assessment in rabbits. Am J Sports Med 11:379, 1983

19. Tipton CM, James SL, Mergner W, Tcheng, T: Influence of exercise on strength of medial collateral knee ligament of dogs. Am J Physiol 218:814, 1970

20. Kummel BM: Spectrum of lesion of the anterior capsule mechanism of the shoulder. Am J Sports Med 7:111, 1979

21. Poppen NK, Walker PS: Normal and abnormal motion of the shoulder. J Bone Joint Surg 58A:195, 1976

22. Saha AK: Theory of Shoulder Mechanism: Descriptive and Applied. Charles C Thomas, Springfield, IL, 1961

23. Light LE, Nuzik S, Personius W, Barstrom A: Low-load prolonged stretch vs. high-load brief stretch in treating knee contractures. Phys Ther 64:330, 1984

24. Warren CG, Lehman JF, Koblanski NJ: Elongation of rat tail tendon: effects of load and temperature. Arch Phys Med Rehabil 52:465, 1971

25. Warren CG, Lehman JF, Koblanski JN: Heat and stretch tech-procedure: an evaluation using rat tail tendon. Arch Phys Med Rehabil 57:122, 1976

26. Lehman JF, Masock AJ, Warren CG, Koblanski JN: Effects of therapeutic temperatures on tendon extensibility. Arch Phys Med Rehabil 51:481, 1970

27. Lentell G, Hetherington T, Eagan J, Morgan M: The use of thermal agents to influence the effectiveness of a low-load prolonged stretch. Orthop Sports Phys Ther 5:200, 1992

# 40

# Alternative Techniques for the Motion-Restricted Shoulder

ROBERT E. MANGINE
TIMOTHY HECKMANN
MARSHA EIFERT-MANGINE

## TREATMENT OF ARTHROFIBROSIS

Loss of motion of the glenohumeral joint caused by the development of arthrofibrosis occurs frequently after injury or surgery of the shoulder. Establishing range of motion after a joint trauma is the earliest goal of rehabilitation. When treating the motion-restricted shoulder, it does not take long to realize that many possible pathologies are associated with this complication. The most common pathologies correlating to "frozen shoulder" include the following[1-8]:

1. Adhesive capsulitis
2. Periarthritis
3. Painful shoulder syndrome
4. Periarticular adhesions
5. Short rotator tendinitis
6. Bicipital tenosynovitis
7. Subacromial bursitis
8. Fibromyositis
9. Supraspinatus tendinitis
10. Reflex sympathetic dystrophy

These pathologies would be considered primary diagnoses, which may lead to a motion complication; therefore, adequate differential diagnosis is critical in determining the primary lesion. To attempt and progress the patient into the strength or functional activities portion of the program may lead to exacerbation of the motion restriction. All too often clinicians intervene with strengthening exercises as a means to establishing motion, with the reverse effect as the end result. To understand motion complications, the therapist must consider the causal factors:

1. Arthrokinematic disruption in the direction of the restriction
2. Biomechanics of surgical intervention
3. Adaptation of musculotendonous fibers in a shortened position
4. Scar tissue development involving capsular or ligamentous tissue
5. Pathomechanics involved within the joint

Following a logical progress of evaluation, the above indications will help the therapist initiate a treatment program to prevent the secondary diagnosis from occurring. The secondary diagnoses include those associated with loss of joint range of motion (i.e., frozen shoulder or adhesive capsulitis) or those associated with abnormal response to pain (i.e., reflex sympathetic dystrophy).

Review of the motion-restricted shoulder requires detailing the following concepts:

1. Historic perspective of motion loss theories
2. General factors associated with range of motion loss

3. Postoperative complications leading to motion loss
4. Manual therapy principles of restriction
5. The patient's clinical response
6. The connective tissue's response to factors associated with restricted motion

## HISTORICAL PERSPECTIVE

To provide an adequate treatment approach to the motion-restricted shoulder, it is necessary to identify structures involved in the injury process. A review of the literature provides a capsulized version of the advanced research performed. Codman[1] in 1934 identified the concept of the "frozen shoulder." He attributed the decrease in range of motion to the painful, stiff shoulder associated with a short rotator tendinitis. McLaughlin[2] in 1938 used surgical exploration of frozen shoulders to reveal no histologic evidence of inflammation. The loss of range of motion was correlated to a loss of elasticity in the redundant fold of the inferior capsule. Shortening of the rotator cuff kept the humeral head position tight in the glenoid, and with prolonged disuse of the shoulder, it appeared to precede the stiff shoulder. Changes in the periarticular connective tissue collagen were believed to be related to the effects of immobility.

Lippman[3] in 1943 performed surgical examination to diagnose frozen shoulders. He observed tenosynovitis of the long head of the biceps and thickening of the sheath as well as edema of the tendon, which was roughened and adherent to the sheath. As the condition advanced, it was associated with increased adhesions. An upward spread of the tenosynovitis into the shoulder created intracapsular adhesions of the tendon.

Work by Neviaser[4] in 1945 revealed decreased synovial fluid glenohumeral space and associated thickening of the auxiliary fold of the capsule. The capsule became adherent to the humeral head, thus defining the term *adhesive capsulitis.*

Simmonds[5] in 1949 suggested that a loss in range of motion was associated with rotator cuff inflammation. Impingement of the supraspinatus tendon created degenerative changes within the tendon caused by impaired circulation. Further impingement of this decreased vascular area was cause for partial tears of the rotator cuff.

In 1966 Reeves[6] substantiated the concept of the capsular pattern with the use of the arthrogram. Contrast dye was used to show an increased depositing of the dye in the posterior aspect of the shoulder. The joint capsule size was reduced, and the inferior capsular fold, subscapularis bursa, and biceps sheath were obliterated. By assessing the arthrokinematics, joint motion restrictions became clear. Involvement of the anterior capsule results in loss of external rotation. Further, the decrease in abduction is consistent with inferior capsular involvement.

Turek[7] in 1977 indicated that repetitive trauma of the rotator cuff and biceps tendon against the acromion results in degeneration and inflammation. With persistent trauma, granular scar tissue occurs during healing, which leads to fibrous adhesions of the rotator cuff, biceps, subacromial bursa, and capsule. The resulting scar lesions lead to a decrease in range of motion.

Last, DePalma[8] in 1983 suggested that a frozen shoulder involves a fibrous capsule. The capsular tissues shrink and become nonelastic. As the inflammatory process progresses, it involves the synovial fluid, fascia, rotator cuff, biceps tendon, biceps sheath, and subacromial bursa. The inferior redundant fold of the capsule becomes constrained initially. The synovial lining thickens and becomes hypervascular. The coracohumeral ligament also thickens. The subscapularis, infraspinatus, and supraspinatus become tight and also lead to decreased rotation.

## ETIOLOGIC CONSIDERATIONS ASSOCIATED WITH MOTION LOSS

Factors associated with motion loss can be addressed on both a nonsurgical and surgical basis. Nonsurgical factors include

1. Severity of the injury
2. Joint effusion
3. Pain
4. Upper extremity swelling
5. Joint inflammation
6. Patient compliance
7. Delayed mobilization
8. Muscle weakness

Postsurgical factors include

1. Type of surgery performed (i.e., arthroscopy versus arthrotomy)
2. Postoperative hemarthrosis
3. Pain
4. Reflex sympathetic dystrophy
5. Muscle shutdown
6. Infection
7. Postoperative neuropraxia
8. Patient compliance

## CLINICAL PRESENTATION

The clinical presentation of patients with arthrofibrosis or motion restrictions displays a capsular pattern (restricted external rotation greater than abduction greater than internal rotation).[9] However, other pathologies may mimic these capsular patterns. Therefore, a differential diagnosis must be made to rule out a myeloma, reflex sympathetic dystrophy, arthritis, intra-articular lesions, and capsular inflammatory lesions.

Stage I restrictions are those in which the complaints of pain are limited to the shoulder region. The patient exhibits no pain at rest and limited pain with movement. The patient is able to sleep or lie on the involved shoulder. With passive range of motion, the capsular end feel is a soft springy restriction that is encountered before eliciting the pain response. Muscle spasm is limited and does not interfere with range of motion.

Stage II restrictions are evident by several combinations of one or more of the symptoms in Stage I (i.e., positive rest pain, an inability to sleep or lie on the involved side, and/or pain to the elbow). Also passive movement, pain is elicited at the same time the capsular restriction is achieved. Muscular spasm may also limit range immediately on entering the restricted range.

Stage III restrictions are exhibited by the patient's complaint of radiating pain into the entire distal segment. The patient also has pain at rest and occasional waking pain. Finally, with passive movement, pain increases before the capsular restriction is reached. Once the end range is reached, a hard leathery end feel stops movement. If pain becomes disproportionate to the pathology, it is crucial to evaluate for other neurologic problems.

## CONNECTIVE TISSUE RESPONSE

The connective tissue elasticity will be decreased in response to immobilization. With immobilization, structural and cellular alterations are seen that result in decreased range of motion. In 1972 Enneking[11] described an increase in proliferation of fibrofatty tissue within the joint space. Second, during immobilization, the ground substance of connective tissue undergoes water depletion, reduced glycosoaminoglycans, and a decreased lubricating action.[10] This results in alteration of the gel–fiber ratio, correlating to joint stiffness. Range of motion is important to maintain the normal glycosoaminoglycans buffer between the collagen fibers.

Another tissue response to restricted motion is to have random collagen alignment secondary to loss of stress application during normal motion. This leads to adhesions within the connective tissue. Again, fibrofatty deposits within the joint interfere with normal joint range of motion.[11]

Last, muscle shortening is also associated with prolonged immobilization. This is evidenced by a decrease in the number of sarcomeres present.[12] This process also appears to be correlated with age. Muscle response can be reversed by initiating an active range of motion program. This may be one of the advantages with continuous passive motion postsurgery. Unfortunately, if immobilization is left unchecked, the result is continued movement dysfunction, which typically leads to a vicious cycle of pain/decreased range of motion/muscle spasm.[13] The clinician must define the physiologic component for a motion complication. Total joint range of motion is controlled by noncontractile versus contractible elements. The range of motion is defined by arthrokinematic versus osteokinematic movement. The noncontractile soft tissue component that limits range of motion includes all the periarticular structures that came under stress during movement of the joint. The second component controlling joint motion is the contractile component of the muscle-tendon unit.[14] Joint motion results in the muscle-tendon unit adapting to a lengthened state to allow the joint or series of joints to move freely.

After trauma or surgery, changes in either component of the surrounding soft tissue may result in a motion complication. Early motion intervention is crucial to avoid tissue length changes and development of bridge adhesions in the inferior glenohumeral capsule. The small acromioclavicular and sternoclavicular joints require motion for normal glenohumeral motion. Because the total amount of joint laxity at these joints is small, they can become easily involved. Structural changes, which commonly occur to joints with immobilization, need to be reversed as soon as possible. The physiologic alterations associated with motion limitation include

1. Collagen length decreases in the shortened tissue position[15]
2. Fibrofatty infiltration into the capsular recesses[11]
3. Ligament atrophy resulting in decreased stress absorption[16]
4. Collagen bands bridging across recesses[11]
5. Collagen production that is random in orientation[17]
6. Altered sarcomere number in muscle tissue (increase in sarcomes in the lengthened tissue, decreased sarcomes in the shortened)[15]

## MOTIONS OF RESTRICTIONS

In the shoulder with loss of motion, specific patterns of range loss in external rotation, abduction, and flexion are associated with the complication. This is a physiologic response secondary to the position of immobilization and comfort on the part of the patient. Restrictions in these patterns of motion can begin as soon as 24 hours after the onset of immobilization, with or without an injury or surgical procedure. Therefore, early intervention of a motion program to place tension on the periarticular structures should be used. A successful approach after surgery is the use of continuous passive motion. This allows gentle motion to be placed across the healing tissue and avoids high stresses.

Manual therapy as a treatment technique for motion complications is also well established in the literature. These techniques are divided into tractions (prolonged holds) or oscillations. Treatment intervention by manual therapy is meant to apply passive movement to restricted joints. Techniques are often based on clinical trials and kinematic knowledge. The mobilization technique chosen by the therapist is based on clinical evaluation, primary cause of motion restriction, and the primary diagnosis that led to the motion restriction.

A crucial factor for the clinician during manual therapy is force application. Unfortunately, the literature is subjective in reference to the amount of force applied during mobilization technique. The clinician applies a force correlated to the degree of motion in the joint. This occurs through evaluating the amount of accessory motion glide obtained in the normal shoulder or based on preoperative evaluation. An example of motion versus restriction correlation is displayed in Fig. 40-1.

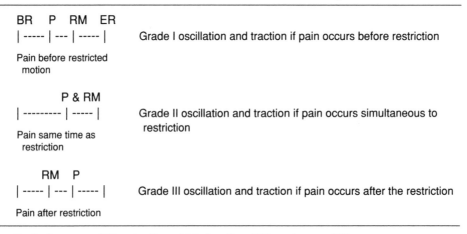

Beginning range, BR; pain, P; restricted motion, RM; end range, ER.

**Fig. 40-1.** Range of motion versus restriction stages.

**Table 40-1. Mobilization Grades**

| Grade I Minimal | Grade II Moderate | Grade III Severe | Grade IV Maximum Overpressure |
|---|---|---|---|
| Range limited by 25% | Range limited by 25–75% | Range <75% | Range 90–<100% |
| Pain after restriction | Pain restricted simultaneous | Pain before restrictions | Pain after restriction |
| Muscle spasm minimal | Muscle spasm moderate | Muscle spasm severe | Muscle spasm may limit range |
| Soft end point | Hard end point after restriction encountered | Hard end point as restriction encountered | Hard end point |

When moving a joint through accessory motion glides, the total amount of displacement may be broken into four ranges, as described in the literature. An initial amount of force is needed to move the joint the first 10 percent of its available displacement (Grade I motion). The second grade of motion is to move the joint up to 50 percent of the total displacement. Grade III motion is to move it up to 75 percent of displacement and grade IV is to the maximum. Force application beyond this is grade V, or manipulation.

The second factor the clinician accounts for is end feel of periarticular tissue at the end range. Patterns to end feels in patients with contractures include[9,14]

1. Soft leathery: tissue that is resisting movement but may respond well to manual techniques
2. Spasm: secondary muscular protection, or internal impingement
3. Hard leathery: tissue that is resisting motion but may require a high force or longer periods of mobilization

In the first part of the range when applying small traction or oscillation forces, the clinician is primarily affecting the neurologic system or mechanoreceptors.[18] These small amplitude forces may cause relaxation of the surrounding musculature through the type I and type II receptors. In the beginning range, it is considered the elastic end of the range where capsular tissue easily elongates and returns. This is an excellent clinical treatment that can be used regardless of what stage of restriction the patient feels (Tables 40-1 and 40-2).

Grade I treatment movements can be implemented within the first 3 weeks after immobilization, and only 25 percent of the range is restricted. Grade I and II mobilization forces may occur for up to 50 percent of the treatment time. Stage I restrictions can occur very quickly and are not always associated with injury or

surgery. This will frequently occur even with simple overuse syndrome injuries.

Grade II movements take the joint into the 50 percent point of the range and apply a force on the collagen into a stretched position. If the joint shows restrictions to 50 percent of the range, a moderate amount of force will be needed to accomplish this. Postcapsular shift patients often show restrictions into this range.

Grade III restrictions are generalized by greater than 50 percent motion loss with muscle guarding and a

**Table 40-2. Treatment Stages**

Stage I Treatment
    Moist heat
    Grade I and II oscillation
    Pulley program
    Pendulum motions
    Cane program
    Isometrics, shortened range
    Muscular strengthening
    Light-resistance exercises
    Muscular stretching
    Ice in the stretch position

Stage II Treatment
    Moist heat in stretch position
    Grade I oscillation or traction
    Passive motion devices with overpressure (i.e., Biodex)
    Grade II and III mobilization
    Pulley program
    Cane program
    Isometrics shortened range with electrical muscle stimulus
    Muscular strengthening
    Grade I oscillation
    Ice in the stretch position

Stage III Treatment
    Moist heat in the stretch position
    Grade I oscillation and traction
    Passive motion devices with overpressure (i.e., Biodex)
    Electrical muscle stimulus in shortened position
    Grade II and III mobilization once pain is controlled
    Pulley program
    Iosmetrics in shortened position
    Muscle strength
    Grade I oscillation
    Ice in the stretch position

painful examination. The restriction is highlighted by a hard leathery end feel, which results in pain as the restriction is entered. Aggressive mobilization may only cause a secondary muscular response of spasm to protect the joint. Low force, to moderate pain, with long hold periods is generally used to avoid the muscular response. Care must be taken to avoid triggering an inflammatory response of the synovial tissue with treatment.

## Mobilization Positions and Direction

### Single-Plane Movements

The simplest of all mobilization techniques are single plane. These movements are designed to follow the arthrokinematics of the joint. The movements revolve around the following positions.

*Distraction*

Distraction is a movement in which the therapist applies a traction in the long-axis direction of the lever arm (Fig. 40-2).

*Anterior/Posterior Glide*

Anterior/posterior glide is a movement in the sagittal plane. The common position for the therapist to stabi-

lize the arm is 30 degrees of flexion and 70 degrees of abduction. A slight amount of distraction is applied to the joint before the gliding movement (Fig. 40-3).

*Inferior Glide*

Inferior glide is a movement in the coronal plane. Again, the arm is stabilized in 30 degrees of flexion, and 70 degrees of abduction while distraction is applied before moving into the inferior direction (Fig. 40-4).

*Internal/External Rotation*

Internal/external rotation is a movement in the transverse plane. The therapist may elect to perform these movements in the 90 degree/90 degree position. Slight distraction is applied before beginning to mobilize. Further, the therapist can choose between long-axis or short-axis force application. It is important to recognize that long-axis forces may result in a higher joint force because of the lever arm (Fig. 40-5).

### Multiplane Movement

During the past 10 years, the scientific knowledge of collagen tissue adaptation and stress capabilities has become well established. Work by Butler et al[19] defined the structural matrix of collagen and the effects of single-plane versus multiple-plane force application (Fig. 40-6). Based on this and soft tissue healing (extra-

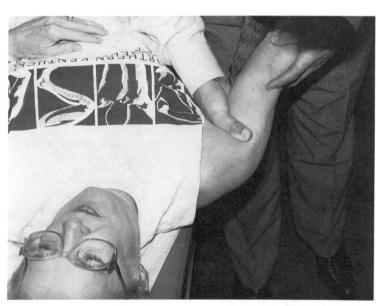

**Fig. 40-2.** Distraction technique with shoulder held in 30 degrees of forward flexion and 70 degrees of abduction.

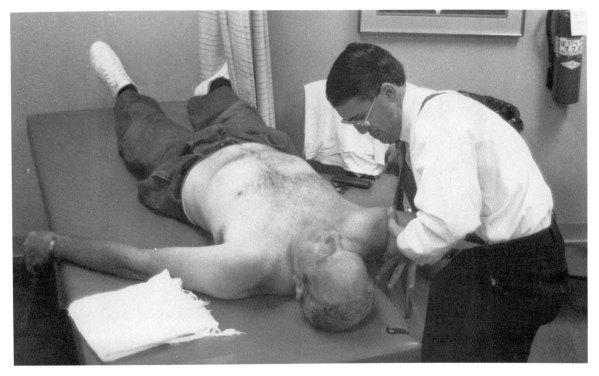

**Fig. 40-3.** Anterior and posterior glide with arm abducted to 70 degrees and neutral flexion.

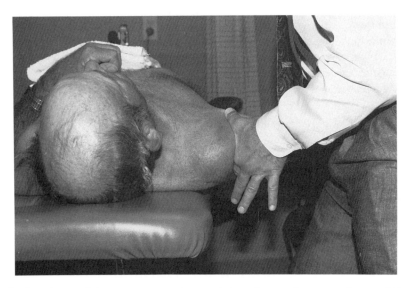

**Fig. 40-4.** Inferior glide movement with arm abducted to 70 degrees and neutral flexion.

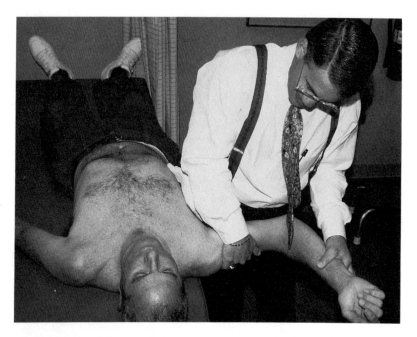

**Fig. 40-5.** External rotation in 90-degree abduction. Distraction and inferior glide are simultaneously being applied.

articular) and scar remodeling, the amount of force and positions may need to be varied in the late stages of motion complications. Therefore, the senior author developed a series of mobilization positions defined as multiplane.

The purpose of these movements is to replicate normal arthrokinematic motions that occur at the joint articular surface. Also, by applying multiplane movements, the amount of force needed can be lower based on adaptation of collagen tissue as shown in laboratory study.[19]

Many patients who are at this stage of treatment are into stage II or III restriction and are a long time into their motion restriction. Single-plane techniques often work well in the initial phase of manual therapy, and excellent results to regain motion are seen. However, these techniques often result in a plateau effect after 2 or 3 weeks. The therapist must now be able to apply a greater force to maintain motion gains using single-plane techniques. Because collagen will respond to lower forces if multi-plane movements are used, the patient can be treated more comfortably to reach the same goal.

By this stage of treatment, the key factors are force and time of application. Studies have shown the need for long periods of manual techniques in order to be effective. In congruence with manual techniques in the clinic, the patient must also be placed on a home program to maintain motion between manual treatment bouts. The patient is asked to perform this home program four to six times per day between clinic visits.

1. Position 1: Distraction, anterior glide, external rotation. The patient's arm is placed at an end range (where restriction is first encountered). Distraction is the initial force, followed by anterior glide and finally an external rotation force. Both oscillations and holds are applied, and low force is applied first, followed by high force (Fig. 40-7).
2. Position 2: Distraction, posterior glide, internal rotation (Fig. 40-8). Again the arm is placed at the end of the available range, and distraction is applied. A

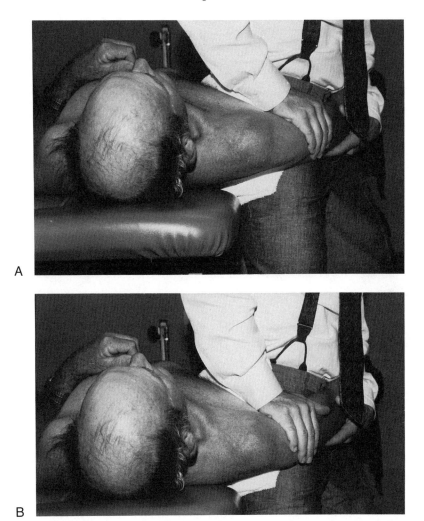

**Fig. 40-6.** Amount of distraction and posterior glide that can be accomplished by using low-force multiplane techniques. **(A)** Unloaded; **(B)** three directions of load, distraction, posterior glide, and external rotation.

posterior glide force is followed by internal rotation. This is a position that is infrequently used because internal rotation is often not limited.

3. Position 3: Distraction, inferior glide, and external rotation. In some patients, scarring in the subdeltoid space can lead to motion complications secondary to impingement. This maneuver is useful to facilitate inferior capsule mobilization. The patient's arm is in a flexed position. Distraction is applied in the long axis, inferior glide is next applied, and finally, external rotation is applied. Care is taken with this position because pain can easily be elicited and a low force is used to avoid secondary muscular spasm (Fig. 40-9).

Again it is important for the clinician to recognize that these techniques are end-stage treatment methods. They are used in a motion complication in which scar-

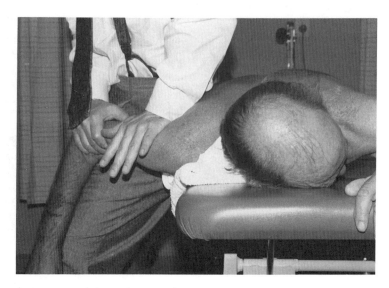

**Fig. 40-7.** Distraction, anterior glide, and external rotation being applied at 70 degrees abduction. External rotation is applied by upward force on arm by the thigh.

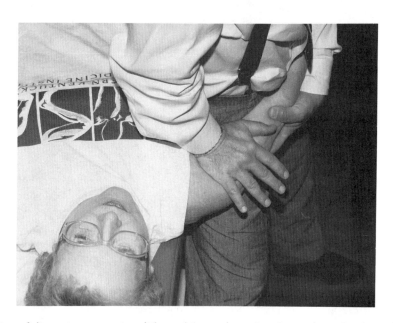

**Fig. 40-8.** Position of distraction, posterior glide, and internal rotation. Internal rotation is applied by therapist with distal hand placement and slight trunk rotation.

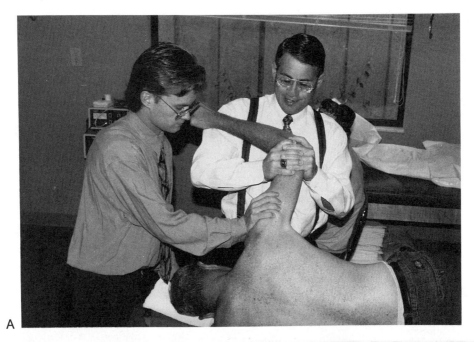

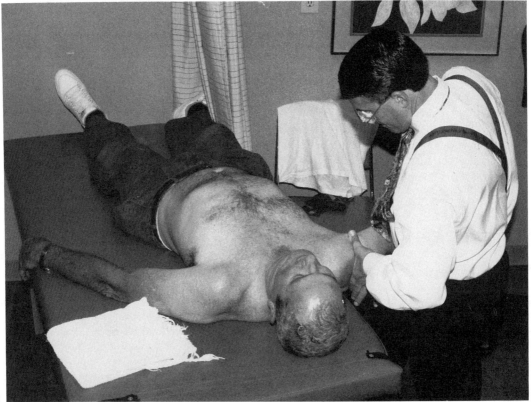

**Fig. 40-9. (A)** Distraction, external rotation, and inferior glide with assistance for application of inferior glide.
**(B)** Same technique in 70-degree abducted position and with only the therapist applying force.

ring is the primary cause of motion loss. The scar that is encountered by this time period is maturing but may have a random orientation of the collegen fibers requiring higher stresses in multiple planes.

## CONCLUSION AND SUMMARY

The most effective treatment of arthrofibrosis of any joint is prevention. In today's protocols, faster, more efficient, and highly scientific levels of knowledge are used. The clinician must be in a position to evaluate the patient as soon as possible after injury or surgery and recognize the early motion complication. In this scenario, effective patient management can be implemented to avoid the progressive stages of motion complications.

The therapist must also be able to communicate the patient's needs to the physician for early intervention once problems are recognized. Treatment of these conditions require input from the entire health care team to provide the most effective care for the patient.

The outcome of the program is a functional joint, able to achieve full range of motion without substitution of the normal arthrokinimatics, normal tissue length of capsule and other extra-articular tissues, functional length of the musculotendonous structures without reflex spasm, and correct management of the primary diagnosis if other than adhesive capsulitis. The focus of this program is to evaluate, recognize, communicate, treat, and educate.

## REFERENCES

1. Codman EA: The Shoulder. Robert E. Kreiger, Malabar, FL, 1934
2. McLaughlin HL: The "frozen shoulder." Clin Orthop 20:126, 1961
3. Lippmann RK: Frozen shoulder; periarthritis; bicipital tenosynovitis. Arch Surg 47:283, 1943
4. Neviaser JS: Adhesive capsulitis of the shoulder: study of pathological findings in periarthritis of the shoulder. J Bone Joint Surg 27:211, 1945
5. Simmonds FA: Shoulder pain with particular reference to the "frozen" shoulder. J Bone Joint Surg 31B:426, 1949
6. Reeves B: Arthrographic changes in frozen shoulder and post-traumatic stiff shoulders. Proc Soc Med 59:827, 1966
7. Turek S: Orthopaedics. Principles and Their Application. JB Lippincott, Philadelphia, 1977
8. DePalma AF: Surgery of the Shoulder. JB Lippincott, Philadelphia, 1983
9. Cyriax J: Textbook of Orthopaedic Medicine. 7th Ed. Vol. 1. Bailliere Tindall, London, 1978
10. Lundberg BJ: Glycosaminoglycans of the normal and frozen shoulder-joint capsule. Clin Orthop 69:279, 1970
11. Enneking WF, Horowitz M: The intra-articular effects of immobilization on the human knee. J Bone Joint Surg 54A:973, 1972
12. Akeson WH, Woo SLY, Amiel D et al: Biomechanical and biochemical changes in the periarticular connective tissue during contracture development in the immobilized rabbit knee. Connect Tissue Res 2:315, 1974
13. Donatelli R: Physical Therapy of the Shoulder. 2nd Ed. Churchill Livingstone, New York, 1991
14. Zachazewski JE: Improving flexibility. p. 698. In Scully RM, Barnes MR, (eds): Physical Therapy. JB Lippincott, Philadelphia, 1989
15. Lavigne AB, Watkins RP: Preliminary results of immobilization-induced stiffness in monkey knee joints and posterior capsule. p. 177. In: Perspectives in Biomedical Engineering: Proceedings of a Symposium, Biological Engineering Society, University of Strathyclyde, Glasgow, Scotland. University Park Press, Baltimore, 1972
16. Noyes FR, Butler DL, Paulos LE et al: Intra-articular cruciate reconstruction: Part I. Perspectives on graft strength, vascularization and immediate motion after replacement. Clin Orthop 712:71, 1983
17. Wojtys EM, Noyes FR, Gikas P: Patella Baja syndrome. Presented at the Annual Meeting of the AAOS, New Orleans, February 1986
18. Newton RA: Joint receptor contributions to reflexive and kinesthetic responses. Phys Ther 62:22, 1982
19. Butler DL, Grood ES, Noyes FR et al: Biomechanics of ligaments and tendons. Exerc Sports Sci Rev 6:144, 1979

# 41

# The Role of the Scapula in the Shoulder

*RUSSELL M. PAINE*

The role of the scapula has received renewed interest recently as knowledge of the shoulder and surrounding structures has increased. The scapulothoracic joint is dependent on the surrounding musculature to provide dynamic stability. The scapular muscles provide a stable base that dynamically positions the glenoid so that efficient glenohumeral rotation occurs. Proper positioning of the glenoid allows the instant center of rotation to follow humeral rotation. A breakdown of normal mechanics caused by scapular weakness may be associated with pathologies such as instability, impingement, and scapular winging.

This chapter describes the anatomy, biomechanics, evaluation, and treatment of the scapula and surrounding musculature.

## FUNCTIONAL ANATOMY AND BIOMECHANICS

### Serratus Anterior

Motions of the scapula are defined by the direction the glenoid moves. When describing scapular movement, the glenoid is the point of reference. The serratus anterior is an important scapular stabilizing muscle. The serratus anterior is supplied by the long thoracic nerve, which arises from the ventral rami of the 5th and 7th cranial nerves. The function of the serratus is to pull the scapula forward around the thoracic cage and to stabilize the scapula during elevation. Advancement of the scapula to an anterior position on the thoracic cage is termed *protraction* or *scapular abduction*. The term *protraction* is more frequently used to avoid confusion with shoulder abduction. Protraction is involved with pushing and punching motions.

An important force couple exists to allow forward rotation of the scapula. A force couple is the action of two forces acting in opposite directions to impose rotation about the axis.[1] The lower fibers of the serratus draw the lower angle of the scapula forward to couple with the trapezius and levator scapulae in forward rotation.[1] Inman et al[2] also described the relation of the levator scapulae and upper trapezius in assisting with upward rotation of the scapula. They described the levator scapulae as the upward force unit rather than the lower fiber of the serratus. The lower force unit is described as consistent activity of the fourth and fifth digitations of the serratus anterior. The seventh and eigth digitations display less activity in the last degrees of abduction, which allows the angle to remain in the coronal plane. This coupling effect was confirmed by Moseley et al[3] by performing electromyographic (EMG) analysis during several scapular exercises (Table 41-1). This force couple provides an extremely important function to the upward rotation of the acromion, making the serratus, upper trapezius, and levator scapulae vital components in movements overhead.

As the serratus, trapezius, and levator scapulae provide upward rotation of the scapula, the deltoid is able to assert its action on the humerus and not the scapula.[4] Carrying weights in front of the body causes the serratus to contract strongly to prevent the backward rotation of the scapula. This position can be helpful in demonstrating scapular winging during clinical evaluation of the shoulder.

495

**Table 41-1. Most Efficient Exercises for Specific Muscles**[a]

| Muscle | Exercise | % MMT | Function |
|---|---|---|---|
| Upper trapezius | Rowing | 75 | Retraction |
| Middle trapezius | Horizontal abduction (neutral) | 78 | Retraction |
| Lower trapezius | Rowing abduction | 50 | Retraction |
| | | 50 | Upward rotation |
| Levator scapulae | Rowing | 30 | Retraction |
| Rhomboids | Rowing | 30 | Retraction |
| | Horizontal abduction | 33 | Retraction |
| Middle serratus anterior | Flexion | 69 | Upward rotation & protraction |
| Lower serratus anterior | Push-ups with a plus | 67 | Upward rotation & protraction |
| Pectoralis minor | Press-ups | 75 | Depression |

[a] Values reported were expressed as a percentage of a maximum isometric muscle test (MMT) performed for each muscle. (From Moseley et al,[3] with permission.)

Scapular winging can be exhibited by having the patient push against the wall with hands lowered just below waist (Fig. 41-1). The scapula will backwardly rotate or wing if the serratus and other stabilizers are weak. I have found another method to demonstrate scapular winging by having the patient forward flex with rubber tubing to 90 degrees (Fig. 41-2). This demonstrates the dynamic ability of the serratus to stabilize the scapula during elevation. Winging of the scapula will be observed if there is a weakness of the stabilizing musculature. Bilateral examination is of utmost importance, as slight winging may be normal in individuals that present with normal hypermobility. If the serratus is not stabilizing, the most dramatic effect will be observed in the first 45 degrees of elevation as the scapula is seeking the most stable position to allow for proper glenohumeral rotation. This is the stage in which the scapula and surrounding scapular muscles act together to stabilize and allow normal mechanics to proceed with glenohumeral and scapulothoracic articulation occurring in proper synchrony. This active scapular test proves helpful in examining throwing athletes. The eccentric phase or return to starting position of this activity also maximally demonstrates scapular winging. This test may also be used as a screening test for any patient with rotator cuff tendinitis, impingement, or instability to observe possible unilateral scapular muscle weakness during an active movement.

The function of the serratus as the most important stabilizer of the scapula is dramatically presented in patients with damage to the long thoracic nerve. This injury may be caused by a direct blow and resultant

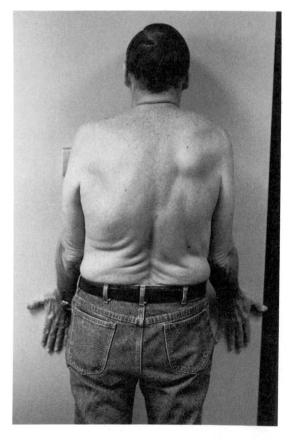

**Fig. 41-1.** Position shows winging of the scapula by having the patient push into the wall with the hands below the waist. The serratus anterior contracts to prevent backward rotation of the scapula. If weakness is present unilaterally, winging will be observed.

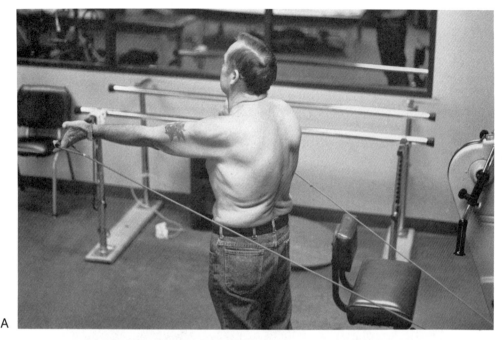

A

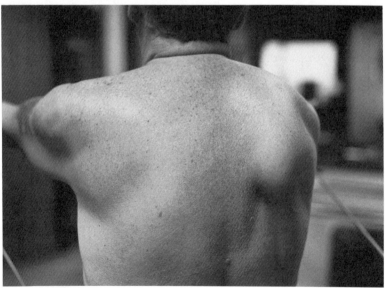

B

**Fig. 41-2. (A & B)** This technique allows the clinician to view scapular winging during dynamic elevation of the arm. Resistance from the rubber tubing forces maximum contraction of the serratus anterior to stabilize the scapula. Weakness will be observed unilaterally as scapular winging.

injury to the brachial plexus or by prolonged repetitive trauma that may lead to resultant scapular weakness.[5]

Neuralgic amyotrophy is thought to be the commonest cause of scapular winging.[5,6] The clinical presentation is onset of shoulder pain with associated night pain. After the pain is resolved, the patient is left with a flaccid paralysis and resultant winging of the scapula. The etiology is unknown but is thought to be a viral infection. This condition will be painless but may take 18 to 24 months to recover.

## Rhomboids

The rhomboids (major and minor) function to stabilize the medial border of the scapula. The rhomboids contribute to medial stabilization of the scapula during abduction or elevation of the humerus. The rhomboids are especially active in scapular adduction or retraction. This is defined as the backward rotation of the scapula toward the vertebral column. Strengthening of the rhomboids is vital in the throwing athlete. If there is weakness of the rhomboids, the scapula is unable to achieve full retraction. Inability to achieve the fully retracted position during pitching could lead to increased stress to anterior structures of the shoulder.[7] Full retraction is also required to perform swimming strokes such as the crawl effectively. Activities that require pulling may also be affected by a lack of rhomboid strength. EMG analysis showed a high level of rhomboid activity during the acceleration phase of pitching.[8] This suggests the rhomboids are contracting eccentrically to provide stability to the medial border of the scapula during acceleration.[8] There is also a high degree of EMG activity of the rhomboids during follow-through to absorb or "brake" the energy released during acceleration.[8] Moseley et al[3] found a high level of EMG activity of the rhomboids during rowing, one of the most effective exercises to strengthen the scapular musculature (Table 41-1).

## Upper Trapezius/Levator Scapulae

The upper trapezius muscle is a suspensory muscle of the scapula. Besides suspensory function, the upper trapezius and levator scapulae upwardly rotate the scapula in synchrony with the serratus anterior, as previously described. The upper trapezius is a key muscle of elevation. If the suspensory/upward rotation of the scapula is not effective, subacromial impingement may occur because of failure to produce sufficient lateral or upward rotation during elevation. Upper trapezius EMG activity has been found to be very high during the acceleration phase of throwing.[8] The upper trapezius is partially responsible for suspension of the scapula along with the muscle mass of the levator scapulae.[9] Minimum upper trapezius EMG activity has been reported during quiet standing.[10] Adding a weight to the hand or elevation of the scapula initiates contraction of both the upper trapezius and levator scapula.[11] The upper trapezius has also been shown to be constantly active during ambulation to perform its suspensory role.[12]

The middle trapezius acts in conjunction with the rhomboids. The lower trapezius is active during depression of the scapula.

In summary, there must be a coordination of all scapular stabilizers to allow normal motion of the shoulder. Weakness of these anchor muscles may lead to altered biomechanics of the glenohumeral joint and resultant excessive stress to the rotator cuff musculature.[7] The scapula must be stabilized in proper position for efficient glenohumeral rotation and sliding. Patients who have chronic pathologies or undergo surgical procedures of the shoulder may have atrophy and weakness of the scapula rotators as well as weakness of the rotator cuff. To treat shoulder dysfunction effectively, attention must be given to strengthening these deficits as well as strengthening the rotator cuff.

## EXERCISE TECHNIQUES

The following discussion reviews specific exercise techniques of strengthening the scapular muscles. Moseley et al[3] described EMG patterns that were recorded for 16 rehabilitation exercises (Table 41-1).

### Serratus Anterior

Figure 41-3 describes push-ups with a plus. This exercise has been shown by Moseley et al[3] to be an effective strengthening exercise for the serratus anterior. The exercise is performed by doing a push-up and fully protracting the scapula at the top of the push-up with an extra push toward the ceiling. If the patient is unable to tolerate this position, he or she may begin the push-up with a plus in the standing position with hands

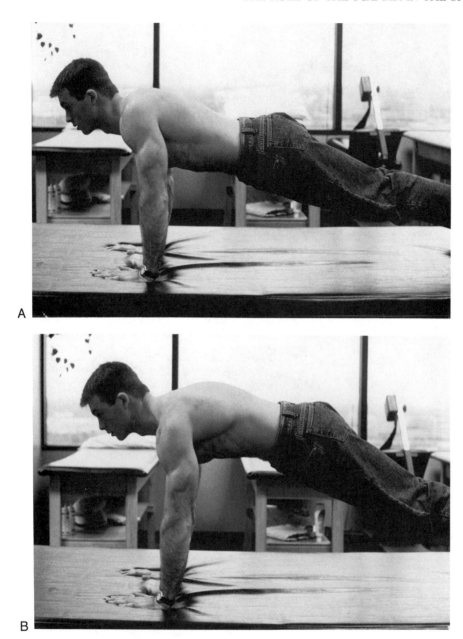

**Fig. 41-3.** (**A & B**) Push-ups with a plus. This exercise was shown by Moseley to have the highest EMG activity for the serratus anterior. The exercise is performed by executing a normal push-up followed by an extra "push" to the ceiling to allow full protraction. The digitations of the serratus can be observed in the "plus" position.

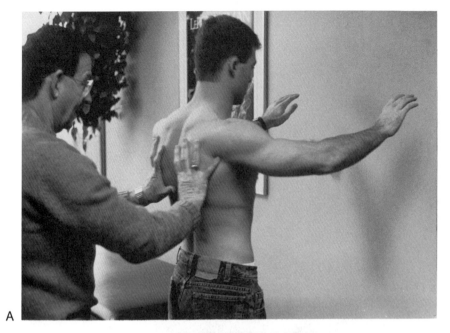

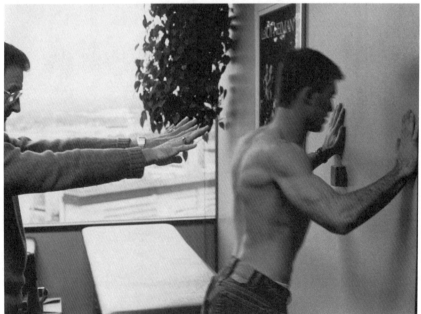

**Fig. 41-4.** (**A & B**) Push-offs allow the patient to perform a closed kinetic chain exercise. This exercise will strengthen all muscles of the shoulder girdle with emphasis on the pectoralis major. Progression to assisted wall push by the therapist forces the patient to perform both concentric and eccentric contractions.

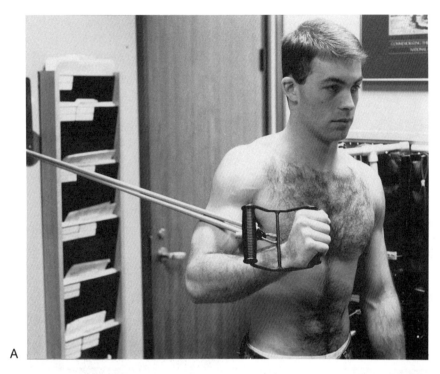

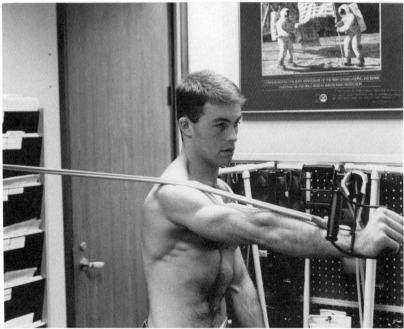

**Fig. 41-5. (A & B)** A punching motion in standing position will strengthen the serratus anterior muscle. Patient is instructed to protract the scapula fully by reaching forward.

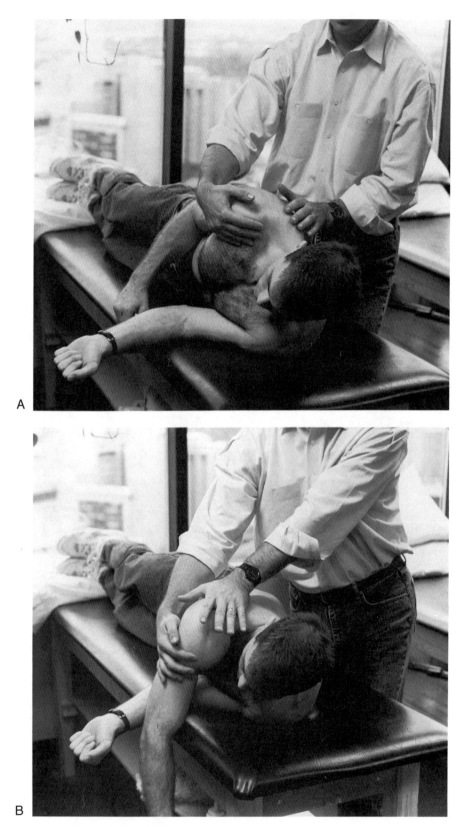

**Fig. 41-6.** (**A & B**) Manual resisted protraction and retraction allows isolation of the proximal muscles. Hand placements are the anterior aspect of the shoulder and the distal spine of the scapula.

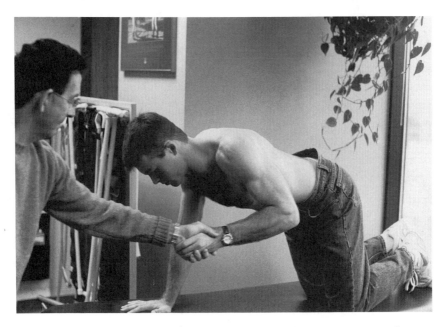

**Fig. 41-7.** Quadruped stabilization. This exercise is another closed chain activity. Patient focuses on controlling the scapula of the weight-bearing limb while the therapist manually resists elbow flexion and extension.

against the wall. Wall push-offs are another way to exercise the serratus (Fig. 41-4). Progression allows the therapist to push the patient gently into the wall, and the patient "catches" him- or herself to provide an effective eccentric exercise. The punching (supine or standing) exercise is also an effective exercise for serratus strengthening. This is performed with the use of rubber tubing or dumbbells. The patient elevates the arm to 90 degrees, with the elbow extended, and performs a punching motion to allow maximum protraction (Fig. 41-5). Manual techniques using manual contacts on the anterior portion of the shoulder and the spine of the scapula allow the most aggressive and isolated form of serratus/rhomboid strengthening. This exercise allows isolation of the scapular muscles and maximally fatigues the scapular muscles by diminishing action of the rotator cuff musculature (Fig. 41-6). Quadruped stabilization is another "closed kinetic chain" exercise that stimulates proper stabilization of the scapula (Fig. 41-7). The goal of this exercise is for the patient to try to control any winging that is present while the therapist provides manual resistance to the opposite arm (Fig. 41-7).

## Rhomboid/Middle Trapezius

Initial strengthening of rhomboids may begin with simply setting the rhomboid by pinching the shoulder blades together and pushing out the chest while holding rubber tubing resistance (Fig. 41-8). The seated row exercise showed highest EMG activity[3] (Fig. 41-9). The seated row is performed by using a scapular strengthening device (BREG Corp., Vista, CA) that simulates rowing through use of rubber tubing. Proper technique is important so that full protraction and retraction are allowed (Fig. 41-9). Isolation of rhomboid strengthening is maximized by the manual resisted technique as previously described (see Fig. 41-6). A high-level strengthening exercise for rhomboid strengthening is the bent-over lateral raise (Fig. 41-10).

## Upper Trapezius/Levator Scapulae

The trapezius muscle may be exercised by performing shrugs or manually resisting elevation (Figs. 41-11 and 41-12).

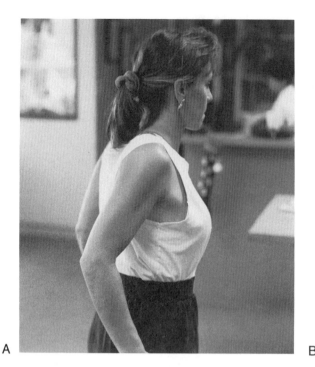
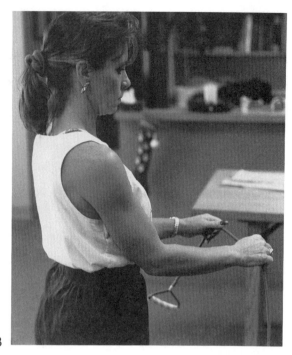

A B

**Fig. 41-8.** (**A & B**) Rhomboid sets are performed early in rehabilitation of any pathology. This activity is executed by having the patient pinch shoulder blades while protruding the chest. Use of rubber tubing allows resistance for this activity. Care must be taken so that elbows remain tucked to the sides.

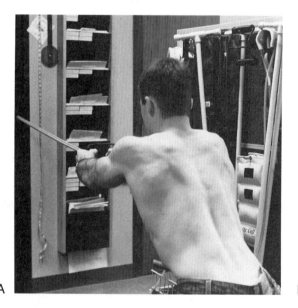
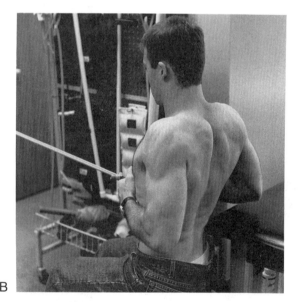

A B

**Fig. 41-9.** The seated row exercise is excellent for aggressive strengthening of the rhomboids. This device is a home product (scapular strengthening kit—BREG Corp., Vista, CA) that assists in developing scapular strength. Proper technique is important. (**A**) Subject reaches forward to allow full protraction followed by full retraction of the shoulder blades. (**B**) Elbows must remain tucked and the handle is pulled into the chest as the shoulder blades are pinched.

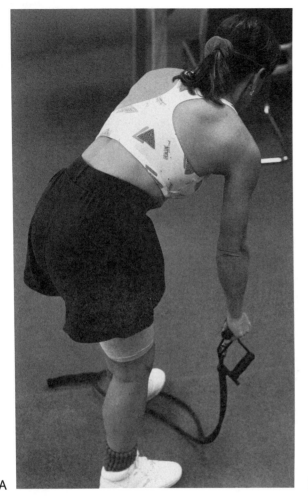
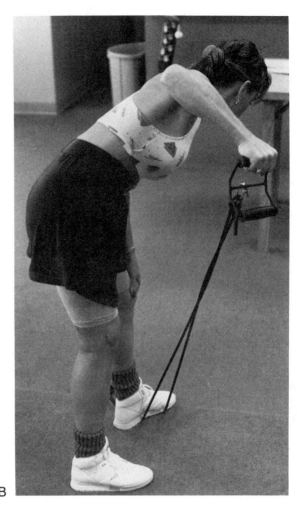

**Fig. 41-10. (A & B)** Lateral raise exercise also provides strengthening of the rhomboids. This exercise is similar to a sawing-type motion.

### Lower Trapezius/Pectoralis Minor

Moseley et al[3] found a high level of EMG activity in the lower trapezius when the press-up exercise is performed (Fig. 41-13).

## LOSS OF NORMAL S-T/G-H ARTICULATION

Factors other than muscular weakness can be related to a lack of normal scapulohumeral rhythm. One of these factors is a loss of normal scapulohumeral motion

resulting from adhesive capsulitis. This loss of motion is primarily related to a loss of glenohumeral motion. The scapulohumeral rhythm relationship is complex. This ratio has been studied by several authors and results vary according to arm position/rotation.[1,2,13–16] The overall consensus is that for every 1 degree of scapular rotation there are 2 degrees of glenohumeral rotation. The S-H ratio also varies according to arm position/rotation.

Inman et al[2] showed that there was irregular motion of the scapula between 30 and 60 degrees of arm elevation, depending on the scapular position at rest. There-

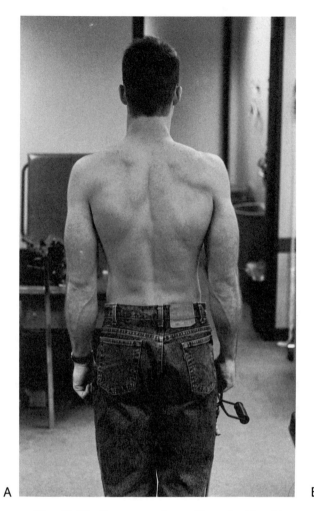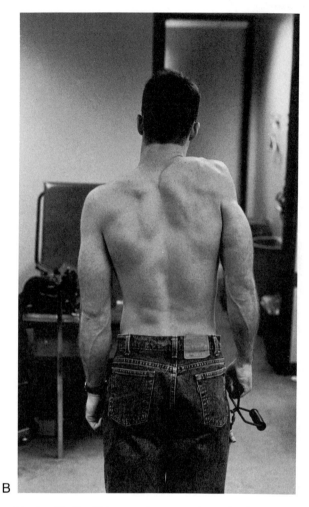

A   B

**Fig. 41-11.** Shrugs may be performed with tubing or with dumbbells. This exercise strengthens the levator scapulae and the upper trapezius.

after, the 2 : 1 ratio of G-H to S-T motion was found to be uniform.[2]

Doody et al[14] showed that by adding a small weight in the hand, the scapulothoracic motion increased during the early stages of arm elevation. This was probably due to the increased stabilization of the scapula that is required when lifting a weight.

If this normal synchrony of movement is disrupted because of capsular adhesions, restoring the normal synchrony should be a goal of treatment. I believe that the lack of G-H rotation during elevation in patients with adhesive capsulitis is primarily due to a loss of the inferior capsular recess as described by Nichol-

son.[17] The loss of the inferior capsular recess has been shown in several studies. The inferior capsular recess actually "glues" to itself, creating a lack of mobility during elevation (Fig. 41-14). This can be observed from behind as the patient actively elevates in the scapular plane. When these patients are viewed from behind, it can be seen that the primary contribution to arm elevation is the scapulothoracic forward rotation. When the scapulothoracic joint has reached its maximum forward/upward rotation, elevation stops because of restriction of the G-H joint rotation. Muscle spasms on the vertebral border and upper trapezius may be detected because of the overcompensating of

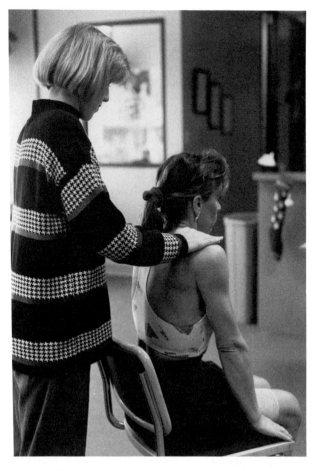

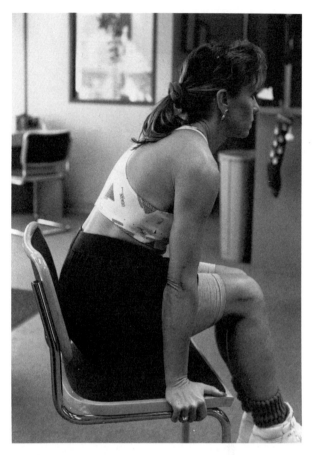

**Fig. 41-13.** Press-ups while sitting in a chair will exercise the lower trapezius.

**Fig. 41-12.** Manual resisted elevation may be performed to strengthen upper trapezius and levator scapulae.

the scapular muscles and are a frequent complaint of patients with loss of G-H motion.

Nicholson[17] noted that inferior glide of the head of the humerus is the most restricted motion in patients with adhesive capsulitis. Increasing inferior glide of the head of the humerus is another mobilization technique to loosen the inferior capsular restriction. This is performed with the arm in loose pack position (Fig. 41-15). A distraction force is given as inferior displacement of the humerus occurs with manual pressure from the mobilizing hand of the therapist.

Techniques for increasing this lack of motion are shown in Figure 41-16. The manual technique is exhibited with the patient sidelying on the normal side. The involved scapula is held down with one hand while

the therapist mobilizes the inferior capsular recess by passively moving the arm away from the body while maintaining pressure on the lateral border of the scapula (Fig. 41-16). The goal of this technique is to restore the glenohumeral rotation that is lost with a loss of the normal capsular spaces.

## SNAPPING SCAPULA

Grinding, popping, and snapping sounds are symptoms that have been described and related to the so-called snapping scapula. Milch[18–20] described three scapular sounds. Froissement is a general friction sound caused by normal muscular function and is con-

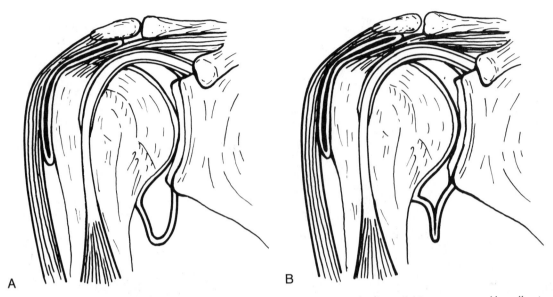

**Fig. 41-14.** (**A & B**) Normal inferior capsular recess is present, along with a loss of this space caused by adhesions. Mobilizations to increase inferior glide help to loosen this structure and increase glenohumeral rotation. (From Murnaghan,[26] with permission.)

sidered to be physiologic and asymptomatic in most cases. Froittemant, described as a snapping or grating sound, in somewhat louder and may be pathologic. Craquemont is a loud, snapping sound frequently associated with pain and decreased function. Butters[21] did not believe there was a parallel between the intensity of the sound and the severity of the symptoms nor that it indicated a diagnosable anatomic entity. Milch[18] found normal scapular sounds in 70 percent of the normal population and noted that abnormally loud sounds were rare.

Causes for the snapping scapula could be changes in the bony structure of either the undersurface of the scapula or the opposing ribs. For the snapping to be present, the serratus anterior must be functioning properly to adhere the scapula to the rib cage. Milch[18] believed a large mass at the site of a healing rib fracture could also cause snapping.

Soft tissue changes may also cause snapping scapula but are difficult to document. Bateman[22] described a soft tissue lesion as periosteal microtears with medial muscle attachment. Rockwood[23] described a procedure in which a rhomboid muscle avulsion flap was excised with elimination of snapping and pain. Scapular sounds have been observed in the young female

patient who has lost an excessive amount of weight and thus loses the cushioning effect between the scapula and ribs. As Butters[21] described, the snapping is usually voluntarily produced, may be painful, and often is bilateral.

Treatment for this condition varies from modalities such as heat, ultrasound, Marcaine, and steroid injection applied to the subscapular region. Exercise may include shoulder shrugs and scapular retraction exercises. As Butters[21] described, the treatment of choice is rehabilitation, unless an exostosis is clearly seen or a rib deformity is present.

## THE SCAPULA AND THROWING

The scapula has been described by several authors as being a vital component in the overhead throwing motion.[3,7,8] Kibler[7] studied the position of the scapula and believed that alteration of the normal position of the scapula can lead to altered biomechanics of the shoulder. Kibler believed that there must be a coordinated firing pattern during the throwing motion that contributes to the stability of the joint. Efficient concentric and eccentric activity of the shoulder muscles is

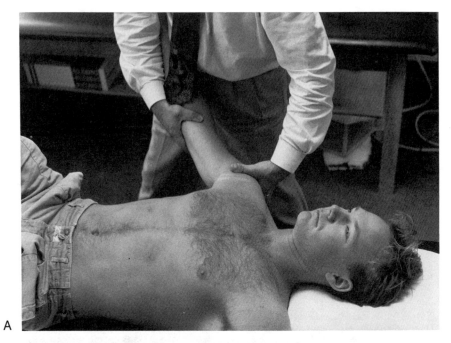

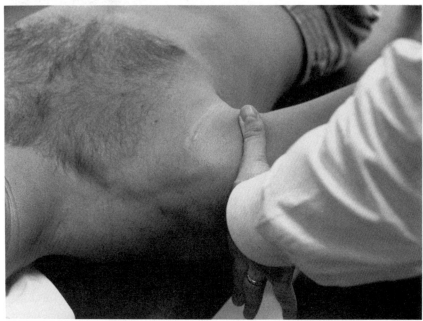

**Fig. 41-15.** (**A & B**) To increase inferior glide of the head of the humerus, the patient is positioned supine, with the arm abducted 45 degrees from the body. The therapist applies a distraction force along with an inferior glide force with the mobilizing hand.

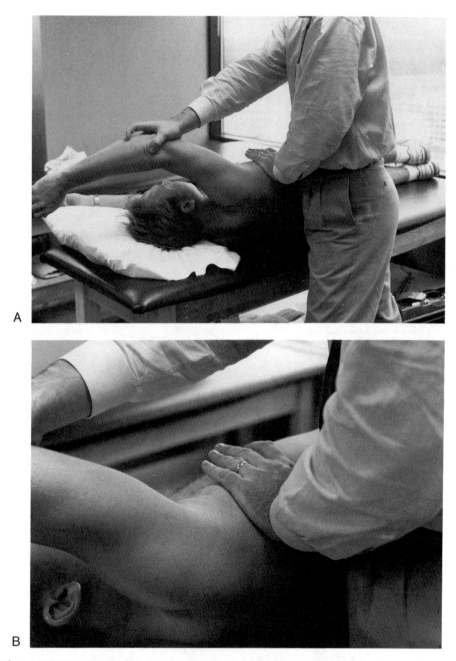

**Fig. 41-16. (A & B)** To mobilize the glenohumeral joint and restore the normal synchrony of movement, patient is positioned sidelying. The scapula is held stationary while the arm is moved away from the body. The aim of this mobilization is to loosen adhesions in the inferior capsular recess.

dependent on having strong anchor muscles to stabilize the scapula. During the windup and cocking phases, maximum retraction of the scapula is mandatory. Kibler described the pretensing of the anterior muscles that allows maximum stored energy to be released through acceleration and follow-through. As described by Jobe et al[24,25] the scapular muscles are shown to be active on EMG analysis during the entire throwing motion. During early windup and cocking, the rhomboids contract strongly to retract the scapula fully.[8] In acceleration and follow-through, the scapular stabilizers contract eccentrically to allow smooth force dissipation.[8] In follow-through, the stabilizers continue to contract eccentrically to absorb the generated forces of acceleration.[8]

Kibler[7] believed that excessive lateral slide of the scapula may cause the orientation of the glenoid to become "more antetilted," which may cause the anterior structures of the shoulder to see excessive strain. Saha[15] also described the antetilted position to be a possible component of the subluxation/dislocation complex in patients that have undergone repetitive microtrauma such as may occur during throwing activities.

## OBJECTIVE MEASUREMENT OF SCAPULAR INSTABILITY

Current treatment techniques to increase scapular stability have been developed and positive clinical results have been observed. The most dramatic effect has been seen in the patient with obvious scapular winging during examination. The limiting factor in objectifying these results is inability to document accurately this instability or weakness of the scapula. Kibler[7] described the lateral slide measurement test, which measures the ability of the scapular stabilizers to control the medial border of the scapula during three positions of the arm. An increase of 1 cm or more side to side was reported to correlate with symptoms of pain and decreased shoulder function. Isokinetic testing of protraction and retraction is currently under investigation at our facility and reproducibility of day-to-day testing has been promising. Proper stabilization of the trunk is important so that isolation of protraction and retraction will be maximized (Fig. 41-17).

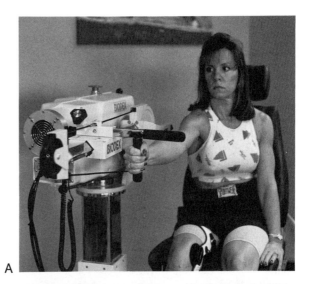

A

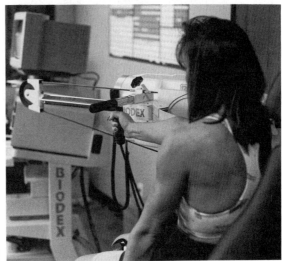

B

**Fig. 41-17.** (**A & B**) Isokinetic protraction and retraction performed with the closed chain attachment (Biodex, Shirley, NY). This may help to document weakness of the serratus and rhomboid musculature.

## CONCLUSION

The shoulder is no longer to be considered as one joint. As has been outlined, the function of the scapula and surrounding musculature are vital components to normal function of the shoulder. Advancements in knowledge of biomechanics and EMG patterns of the shoulder have allowed us to develop strengthening exercises that maximally strengthen these "anchor" muscles. Maintenance of the normal scapulohumeral rhythm is also a factor that must be addressed in restoring normal shoulder function. Although the scapula is a vital component, treatment of the shoulder must include the rotator cuff musculature and a thorough evaluation of the entire shoulder complex. Through proximal strengthening, many shoulder problems can be improved.

# REFERENCES

1. Kent B: Functional anatomy of the shoulder complex. A review. Phys Ther 51:867, 1971
2. Inman JT, Saunders M, Abbott L: Observations on the function of the shoulder joint. J Bone Joint Surg 26:1, 1944
3. Moseley BJ, Jobe FW, Pink M et al: EMG analysis of the scapular muscles during a rehabilitation program. Am J Sports Med 20:128, 1992
4. Copeland SA, Howard RC: Thoracoscapula fusion for fascio-scapulo-humeral dystrophy. J Bone Joint Surg 60B:547, 1978
5. Devathasan G, Tong HI: Neuralgic amyotrophy: criteria for diagnosis and a clinical with electromyographic study of 21 cases. Aust N Z J Med 10:180, 1980
6. Parsonage MJ, Aldren Turner JW: Neuralgic amyotrophy. The shoulder girdle syndrome. Lancet 1:973, 1948
7. Kibler BW: Role of the scapula in the overhead throwing motion. Contemp Orthop 22:525, 1991
8. DiGiovine NM, Jobe FW, Pink M, Perry J: An electromyographic analysis of the upper extremity in pitching. J Shoulder Elbow Surg 1:15, 1992
9. Weber EF: Ueber die langenderhaltnisse der fleischfasen der muskeln im allgemeinen. Berlin Verh K Sach Ges Wissensch Math-Phys 63, 1851
10. Shoo MJ, Perry J: The shoulder girdle muscles in transfer, an electromyographic study. Resident Seminars, Rancho Los Amigos Hospital, Downey, CA, 1978
11. De Freitas V, Vitti M, Furlani J: Electromyographic study of levator scapulae and rhomboideus major muscles in movements of the shoulder and arm. Electromyogr Clin Neurophysiol 20:205, 1980
12. Ballesteros MLF, Buchthal F, Rosenfalck P: The pattern of muscular activity during the arm swing of natural walking. Acta Physiol Scand 63:296, 1965
13. Freedman L, Munro RR: Abduction of the arm in the scapular plane: scapular and glenohumeral movements. Aroentgenographic study. J Bone Joint Surg 48A:1503, 1966
14. Doody SG, Freedman L, Waterland JC: Shoulder movements during abduction in the scapular plane. Arch Phys Med Rehabil 51:595, 1970
15. Saha AK: Mechanics of elevation of glenohumeral joint. Its application in rehabilitation of flail shoulder in upper brachial plexus injuries and poliomyelitis and in replacement of the upper humerus by prosthesis. Acta Orthop Scand 44:668, 1973
16. Poppen NK, Walker PS: Normal and abnormal motion of the shoulder. J Bone Joint Surg 58A:195, 1976
17. Nicholson CG: The effects of passive joint mobilization on pain and hypomobility associated with adhesive capsulitis of the shoulder. J Orthop Sports Phys Ther 6:238, 1985
18. Milch H: Snapping scapula. Clin Orthop 20:139, 1961
19. Milch H: Partial scapulectomy for snapping in the scapula. J Bone Joint Surg 32A:561, 1950
20. Milch H, Burgman MS: Snapping scapula and humerus varus. Arch Surg 26:570, 1933
21. Butters KC: The Scapula. p. 335. In Rockwood CA, Matsen FA III (eds): The Shoulder. Vol. 1. WB Saunders, Philadelphia, 1990
22. Bateman JE: The Shoulder and Neck. 2nd Ed. WB Saunders, Philadelphia, 1978
23. Rockwood CA: Management of fractures of the scapula. J Bone Joint Surg 10:219, 1986
24. Jobe FW, Moynes DR, Tibone JE et al: An EMG analysis of the shoulder in pitching. Am J Sports Med 11:3, 1983
25. Jobe FW, Moynes DR, Tibone JE: An EMG analysis of the shoulder in pitching; a second report. Am J Sports Med 12:218, 1984
26. Murnaghan PJ: Frozen shoulder. p. 837. In Rockwood CA, Jr., Matsen FA III (eds): The Shoulder. Vol. 2. WB Saunders, Philadelphia, 1990

# 42

# Special Considerations in Shoulder Exercises: Plane of the Scapula

*BRUCE GREENFIELD*

Implementing exercises during shoulder rehabilitation is influenced by the interaction of exercise mode (open versus closed kinetic chain positions), contraction type, speed of motion, and joint angle. A functional exercise progression is therefore a result in a constant interplay of exercise variables applied with proper timing to coincide with soft tissue healing and improvement in the patient's motoric capabilities. The clinician assumes the responsibility for effective and creative rehabilitation by using a wide range of treatment options and strategies. This chapter presents a treatment strategy for shoulder rehabilitation with the upper limb positioned in the plane of the scapula (POS).

## THEORY

Different shoulder pathologies present different treatment challenges and strategies, but an essential element to rehabilitate the shoulder is to re-establish the force couple at the glenohumeral joint.[1-5] A force couple is defined as two forces of equal magnitude but of opposite direction that produce rotation on a body.[6] The force couple at the glenohumeral joint results in a balance between the rotator cuff muscles (supraspinatus, infraspinatus, teres minor, and subscapularis muscles) and the deltoid muscle.

Contraction of the rotator cuff muscles results in an inward force and downward glide of humeral head within the glenoid fossa, whereas contraction of the deltoid muscle elevates the upper limb. Inman et al[7] calculated the magnitude and direction of forces within the glenohumeral joint during abduction of the upper limb in the frontal plane. The total forces produced within the glenohumeral joint during elevation of the upper limb in the frontal plane were the summation of three forces: (1) contraction of the rotator cuff muscles; (2) contraction of the deltoid muscle; and (3) the mass of the upper limb, acting along the center of gravity of the limb. The forces necessary to establish the upper and lower components of the rotatory force couple were equal but opposite in direction to maintain equilibrium of forces within the glenohumeral joint. Inman et al calculated that the maximum force within the glenohumeral joint occurred between 60 and 90 degrees of elevation and measured approximately 10 times the weight of the upper limb. Electromyographic activity of the deltoid muscle in this range of motion was maximum to produce upward shear of the humeral head along its line of pull above the axis of rotation of the glenohumeral joint. The electromyographic activity of the rotator cuff muscles increased linearly above 60 degrees of humeral elevation, which provided an inward and downward pull on the humeral head that balanced the upward shear produced by the deltoid muscle. Without the balance between these muscle groups, an impingement may potentially occur between the humeral head and the corocohumeral ligament and anterior acromion.[8] The painful arc described by Cyriax[9] occurs within the range of 60 to

513

**Table 42-1. Comparisons of Upper Extremity Muscle Torque**

| Study | Subjects | Speeds (°/s) | Flexion/Extension (%) | Abductors/Adductors (%) | External Rotation/Internal Rotation (%) |
|---|---|---|---|---|---|
| Cook et al[12] | Male pitchers and nonpitchers | 180 | 70–81 76–99 | NA | 80–81 81[a] |
| Soderberg & Blaschak[13] | Males, nonathletes | 60, 180, 300 | NA | NA | 57–69 |
| Davies[14] (Ch. 12) | 20 Males and females | 60 and 300 | 60 Males, 48 females | 66 Males, 52 females | 64[a] |
| Ivey et al[15] | 31 Normals, mixed activity | 60 and 180 | 66 Males, 73 females | 61 Males, 57 females | 67[a] |
| Alderink & Kuck[16] | 24 Males, high school and college pitchers | 90, 120, 180, and 300 | 48–55 | 50–57 | 66–76[a] |
| Hinton[17] | 26 Pitchers, high school | 90 and 240 | NA | NA | 56–62[a] |
| Connelley-Maddux et al[18] | 21 Males, 20 females | 60 | NA | NA | 63 Males, 71 females |

NA, not available.
[a] Data from 90° shoulder abducted position.
(Modified from Albert and Wooden,[26] with permission.)

120 degrees of humeral elevation and probably represents an imbalance in the glenohumeral force couple. Saha[10] described the important function of the rotator cuff muscles as "steerers" of the humeral head.

The study of Inman et al was seminal because it indicated that a balance must exist within the shoulder muscles for normal function. As a result, several studies examined relative strength ratios of the muscles at the shoulder.[11–18] Reid et al[11] performed a series of isokinetic strength tests using a Cybex II isokinetic dynamometer (Cybex, Ronkonkoma, NY). Abduction and adduction were tested with the subject in a supported sitting position, and external and internal rotation were tested with the subject standing and lying and the limb at the side (neutral) and abducted to 90 degrees, respectively. All data were reported at 60 degrees/s, using the best

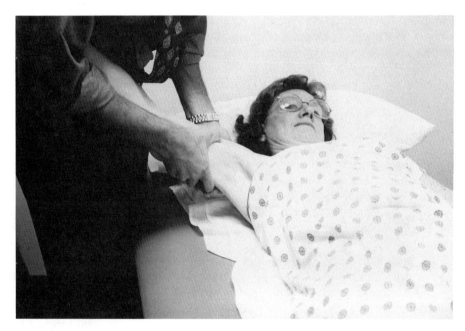

**Fig. 42-1.** Manual mobilization to anterior glenohumeral joint capsule performed in POS. Clinician cradles patient's upper limb in clinician's axilla to maintain POS position.

of three trials. Forty healthy subjects were tested for a total of 80 shoulders. The strongest muscle group was the adductors, being about twice as strong as the abductors. If the adductors, being the strongest, were considered as 100 percent, the abductors were approximately 50 percent. The internal rotators were approximately 45 percent of the adductors, and the external rotators were approximately 30 percent of the adductors when the upper limb was at 90 degrees of abduction and 45 percent when the limb was in the neutral position. The external to internal rotation ration was approximately 80 percent. A study completed by Fowler (unpublished data) found the external to internal strength ratio to be 80 percent with the upper limb in 90 degrees abduction but reported a ratio of 65 percent with the limb in the neutral position. Table 42-1 illustrates torque comparisons of muscles around the shoulder performed with the upper limb in different positions and moving at different angular velocities.

A review of these studies indicates that muscle torque comparisons were performed with the upper limb in either the frontal or sagittal planes. However, Poppen and Walker[19] and Johnston[20] suggested that the true plane of movement in the glenohumeral joint occurs in the POS, which is angled 30 to 45 degrees anterior to the frontal plane. Kondo et al[21] devised a method for taking radiographs to define the POS during elevation of the limb. The medial tilting angle was used to define the POS from the resting position to 150 degrees of elevation. The medial tilting angle refers to tilting of the scapula toward the sagittal plane. The glenoid fossa faced in an anterior and lateral direction as the medial tilting angle increased. The increase in the medial tilting angle represented the movement of the scapula around the thoracic cage. Kondo et al showed that the medial tilting angle was constant at 40 degrees anterior to the frontal plane throughout elevation of the limb. Therefore, with the limb oriented in the POS, the mechanical axis of the glenohumeral joint is in line with the mechanical axis of the scapula. The result of this alignment is that the glenohumeral capsule is lax, and the deltoid and rotator cuff muscles are optimally positioned to elevate the limb.

Because rotator cuff muscle attachment is from the scapula to the humerus, reorienting the humerus into the POS increases the length of these muscles and improves their length–tension relationship, a result that will presumably facilitate optimal muscle force.[22]

The scapular attachment of the infraspinatus and teres minor muscles is more posterior than normal to the glenohumeral joint axis in the POS to result in greater external rotatory force and less compressive force.

A study by Greenfield et al[23] examined rotational muscle force in the POS. Isokinetic shoulder rotational strength was evaluated in 20 healthy subjects. Using the MERAC (Universal Gym Equipment Inc., Cedar Rapids, IA), test data were gathered in the right shoulder in 45 degrees abduction, at a speed of 60 degrees/s, in the POS and the frontal plane. Intraexaminer test–retest reliability was established across tests using a Pearson

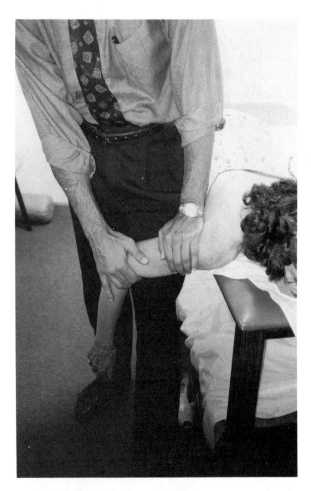

**Fig. 42-2.** Alternative method to stretch anterior glenohumeral joint capsule. Patient is placed prone, and upper limb is "dropped" inferiorly into POS. Patient's upper limb is then stabilized across clinician's knee, and clinician applies a downward force to stretch anterior capsule.

coefficient of correlation at .87. The MERAC computer analyzed peak torque to body weight (PT:BW) data. A paired *t*-test was used to examine the difference in means of internal and external rotation between the two positions. The results indicated no significant difference between the two positions for shoulder internal rotation strength values. However, shoulder external rotation PT:BW values in the POS were statistically significantly higher than in the frontal plane ($P \le .001$). A study performed by Wooden et al[24] examined pitching velocity and PT:BW values in high school baseball players after high-speed and individualized dynamic isotonic training on the MERAC. The subjects were trained with the upper limb abducted to 90 degrees and in the POS. The results germane to this discussion showed statistically significant increases in external PT:BW rotation strength values but no change in PT:BW internal rotation strength values in all subjects across all test conditions. Both studies performed in the POS showed an increase in external rotation strength and supported the hypothesis presented by Poppen and Walker and by Johnston that the POS enhances rotator cuff muscle force. Interestingly, neither study found that the POS influences the strength output

of the internal rotators, which may indicate that the larger internal rotators including the pectoralis major or latissimus dorsi are less affected by subtle changes in limb position than the smaller external rotators.

## CLINICAL APPLICATION

The following section reviews the clinical application and specific techniques for shoulder rehabilitation in the POS. Techniques may be modified based on individual clinical preference, differences in pathology and dysfunction, the type of available exercise equipment, and considerations for specificity of exercise.

Irrespective of the pathology, the initial goals for most shoulder rehabilitation programs are to restore passive range of motion in the glenohumeral joint and to increase strength in rotator cuff muscles. Figures 42-1 to 42-3 illustrate mobilization and stretching techniques performed in the POS to restore glenohumeral joint range of motion. Multiple angle isometrics are a useful and safe method in early postsurgical patients to increase external rotators' strength and are performed manually in the POS, as illustrated in Figure 42-4.

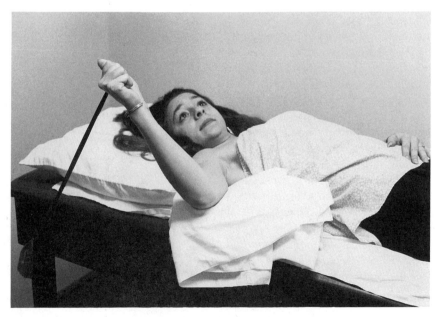

**Fig. 42-3.** Example of prolonged low-load stretch to gain external rotation using a surgical tubing-type material. Patient's upper limb is positioned on sheets into POS. Amount of abduction is varied, depending on portion of capsule that is tight.

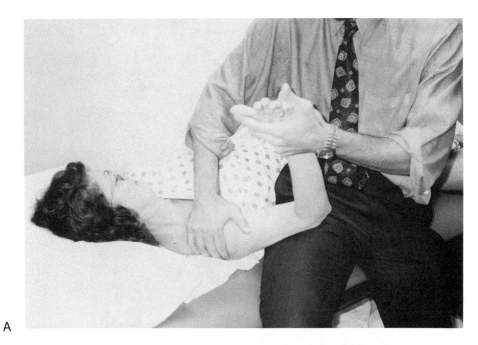

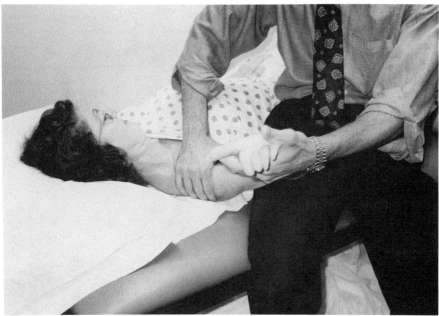

**Fig. 42-4.** Manual multiple angle isometrics used during early rehabilitation to increase external rotation strength. (**A**) Starting position with shoulder in 45 degrees abduction and positioned on clinician's knee in POS. (**B**) End position. Notice that clincian's free hand stabilizes patient's scapula to avoid compensatory scapula elevation.

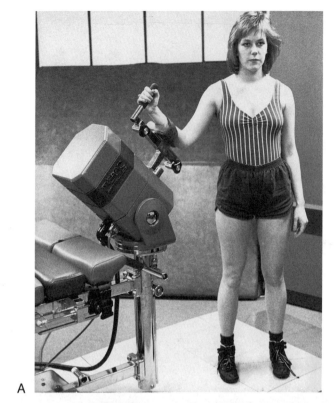

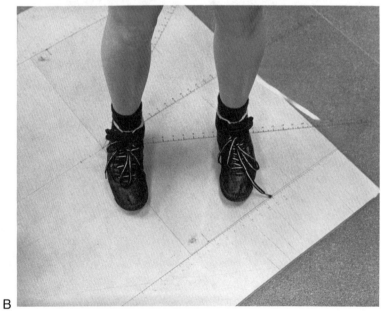

**Fig. 42-5.** Isokinetic rotational strengthening in POS. (**A**) MERAC dynamometer is tilted to 45 degrees. (**B**) A square of Plexiglass, measuring 30 × 30 in., with three lines marked at ½-in. intervals, was constructed. The center line is oriented along frontal plane at 90 degrees to dynamometer. The two remaining lines were oriented at 30-degree angles from the apex of frontal line and represent POS. A plumb line is dropped from axis of glenohumeral joint, and the apex of the Plexiglass is oriented so that the apex of all three lines were positioned where the plumb line touches the ground. Patient then stood on POS line for rotational training. (From Greenfield et al,[23] with permission.)

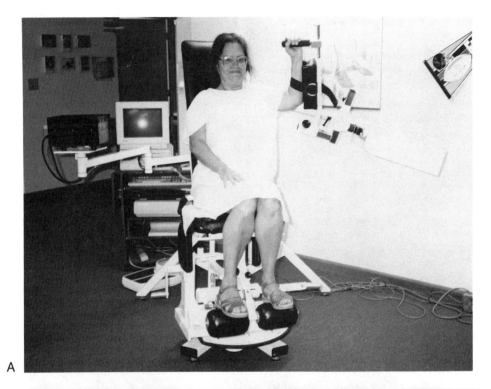

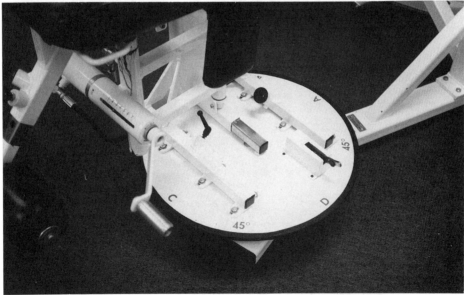

**Fig. 42-6.** Hydraulic training on Omnitron (Hydra-Gym Athletics, Inc., Belton, TX). (**A**) Patient is performing rotational training with shoulder abducted to 90 degrees and 30 degrees in POS. (**B**) Omnitron seat is on a swivel base that allows seat to rotate into POS.

During the intermediate phase of shoulder rehabilitation, the goals of treatment are to restore rotator cuff muscle strength and to increase the strength of the elevatory muscles of the upper limb. Initially, proprioceptive neuromuscular facilitation, including D2 (flexion-abduction-external rotation) of the upper limb, is performed manually with the patient supine. For most postsurgical cases, isokinetic glenohumeral rotation strengthening is implemented at 4 to 6 weeks. Figure 42-5 illustrates isokinetic rotator cuff strengthening in the POS, which was modified from a technique developed by Freedman and Munro.[25] Figure 42-6 illustrates an alternative technique for glenohumeral rotational strengthening using hydraulic resistance on the Omnitron system (Hydra-Gym Athletics, Inc., Belton, TX). Active isokinetic elevatory strengthening (Fig. 42-

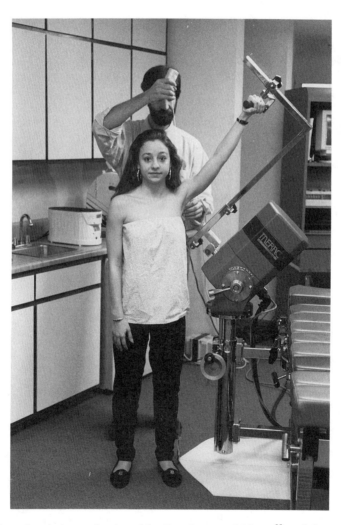

**Fig. 42-7.** Modification of techniques developed by Freedman and Munro[25] and Greenfield et al.[23] A plastic overlay was cut at 30-degree angles. Patient is standing and a plumb line is dropped from glenohumeral joint to center line; the apex of the plastic overlay is located on this point. Patient stands along the 30-degree line on the overlay and performs a D2 diagonal proprioceptive neuromuscular facilitation pattern.

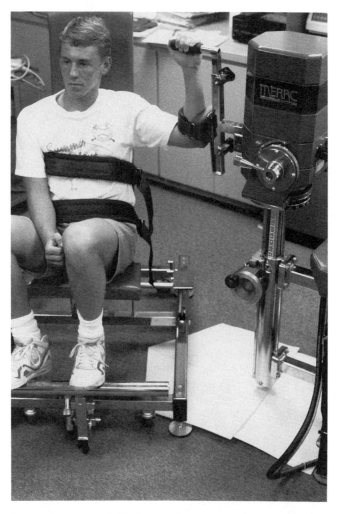

**Fig. 42-8.** Baseball pitcher performing rotational strength training in POS. Technique is described in Fig. 42-7, with MERAC chair positioned along POS line on the plastic overlay. To simulate throwing motion, the chair may be moved perpendicular to the apex of the plastic overlay into the frontal plane. (From Wooden et al,[24] with permission.)

7) is instituted after bilateral testing indicates that rotator cuff muscle peak torque and power are within 20 percent of the involved extremity and that external to internal rotation ratio values are at least greater than 50 percent.

The return-to-function stage represents the final stage for most shoulder rehabilitation programs. The goal for this stage is to prepare the athlete to return to his or her preinjury sport or activity by developing exercises that simulate the motor requirements for optimum performance. Figure 42-8 is an example of training the glenohumeral rotators of baseball pitchers. The POS position is used to enhance the length–tension relationship of the external rotators for optimum force output.

## SUMMARY

The POS represents a positional strategy for shoulder rehabilitation. The author of this chapter has found this position to be experimentally and experientially superior to either the frontal or the sagittal planes for external shoulder rotational strengthening and for stretching the glenohumeral capsule. After satisfactory shoulder strength and range of motion are restored and the patient is pain-free, the clinician has the discretion to position the upper limb to simulate preinjury training. For example, shoulder rotation for baseball pitchers can be performed in 90 degrees abduction in the frontal plane to simulate the throwing motion, whereas swimmers should perform shoulder rotational strengthening prone.

## REFERENCES

1. Jobe FW, Moynes DR: Delineation of diagnostic criteria and a rehabilitation program for rotator cuff injuries. Am J Sports Med 10:336, 1982

2. Townsend H, Jobe FW, Pink M et al: Electromyographic analysis of the glenohumeral muscles during a baseball rehabilitation program. Am J Sports Med 19:264, 1991

3. Blackburn TA: The off-season program for the throwing arm. p. 277. In Zarins B, Andrews JR, Carson WG (eds): Injuries to the Throwing Arm. WB Saunders, Philadelphia, 1985.

4. Jobe FW, Bradley JP: Rotator cuff injuries in baseball: prevention and rehabilitation. Sports Med 6:378, 1980

5. Pappas AM, Zawacki RM, McCarthy CF: Rehabilitation of the pitching shoulder. Am J Sports Med 13:223, 1985

6. Frankel VH, Nordin M: Basic Biomechanics of the Skeletal System. Lea & Febiger, Philadelphia, 1980

7. Inman VT, Saunders M, Abbott LC: Observations on the function of the shoulder joint. J Bone Joint Surg 26A:1, 1944

8. Neer CS: Impingement lesions. Clin Orthop 173:70, 1983

9. Cyriax J: Textbook of Orthopedic Medicine. 7th Ed. Vol. 1. Balliere Tindall, London, 1979

10. Saha AK: Mechanics of elevation of glenohumeral joint. Acta Orthop Scand 44:668, 1973

11. Reid DC, Saboe L, Burnham R: Common shoulder problems in the athlete. In Donatelli R (ed): Physical Therapy of the Shoulder. 2nd Ed. Churchill Livingstone, New York, 1991

12. Cook EE, Gray VL, Savinar-Nogue E et al: Shoulder antagonist strength ratios: a comparison between college-level baseball pitcher and nonpitchers. J Orthop Sports Phys Ther 8:451, 1987

13. Soderberg GJ, Blaschak MJ: Shoulder internal and external rotation peak torque production through a velocity spectrum in differing positions. J Orthop Sports Phys Ther 8:518, 1987

14. Davies G: A Compendium of Isokinetics in Clinical Usage: Workshop and Clinical Notes. S and S Publishers, LaCrosse, WI, 1984

15. Ivey FM, Calhoun JH, Rusche K et al: Isokinetic testing of shoulder strength: normal values. Arch Phys Med Rehabil 66:384, 1985

16. Alderink GJ, Kuck DJ: Isokinetic shoulder strength of high school and college age baseball pitchers. J Orthop Sports Phys Ther 7:163, 1986

17. Hinton RY: Isokinetic evaluation of shoulder rotational strength in high school baseball pitchers. Am J Sports Med 16:274, 1988

18. Connelly-Maddux RE, Kibler WB, Uhl T: Isokinetic peak torque and work values for the shoulder. J Orthop Sports Phys Ther 1:264, 1989

19. Poppen NK, Walker PS: Normal and abnormal motion of the shoulder. J Bone Joint Surg 58A:195, 1976

20. Johnston TB: Movements of the shoulder joint—plea for use of "plane of the scapula" as the plane of reference for movements occurring at hunero-scapula joint. Br J Surg 25:252, 1937

21. Kondo M, Tazoe S, Yamada M: Changes of the tilting angle of the scapula following elevation of the arm. In Bateman JE, Welsh PR (eds): Surgery of the Shoulder. CV Mosby, St Louis, 1984

22. Lucas D: Biomechanics of the shoulder joint. Arch Surg 107:425, 1973

23. Greenfield B, Donatelli R, Wooden M et al: Isokinetic evaluation of shoulder rotational strength between the plane of the scapula and the frontal plane. Am J Sports Med 18:2, 1990

24. Wooden M, Greenfield B, Johanson M et al: Effects of strength training on throwing velocity and shoulder muscle performance in teenage baseball players. J Orthop Sports Phys Ther 15:5, 1992

25. Freedman L, Munro RR: Abduction of the arm in the scapular plane: scapular and glenohumeral movements. A roentgenographic study. J Bone Joint Surg 48A:1503, 1966

26. Albert MS, Wooden MJ: Isokinetic evaluation and treatment of the shoulder. p. 63. In Donatelli RA (ed): Physical Therapy of the Shoulder. 2nd Ed. Churchill Livingstone, New York, 1991

# 43

# Isokinetic Exercise and Testing for the Shoulder

*KEVIN E. WILK*
*CHRISTOPHER A. ARRIGO*

It is a capital mistake to theorize before one has data.
Sir Arthur Conan Doyle

The use of isokinetic exercise and testing appears to be in a period of flux. Since its conception in 1969 by James Perrine, isokinetics became extremely popular during the late 1970s and the 1980s. In the past several years, the clinical trend appears to be favoring a decrease in isokinetic exercise and a greater focus on functional activities. The author believes the use of isokinetics remains most appropriate, because isokinetic exercise provides the clinician with objective reproducible clinical outcome measurements pertaining muscular performance. Thus, isokinetic test results document objective patient progression and/or regression regarding muscular performance. These results are important in the treatment of the shoulder patient.

The glenohumeral joint is an inherently unstable joint.[1–4] The arthrology consists of a large oval humeral head articulating with a small convex glenoid fossa, which represents a ball-and-socket-type joint.[5] This type of joint geometry allows a tremendous amount of movement; however, stability is compromised. The functional stability of the glenohumeral joint is accomplished through the joint's dynamic stabilizing components. The dynamic stabilizers of the shoulder complex are the rotator cuff musculature, the long head of the biceps brachii, the deltoid, and some of the scapulothoracic musculature.

The primary function of the rotator cuff muscles is one of dynamic glenohumeral stability.[1,3] These muscles function to steer the humeral head and control humeral head displacement through a co-contraction of these muscles, which results in increased joint compression forces. Next, the rotator cuff functions as a fine tuner during strenuous activities, especially overhead motions such as throwing, tennis, or elevated work activities. Last, the rotator cuff's secondary function is one of primary movement, such as with external and internal rotation of the shoulder.

It is obvious that the glenohumeral joint must rely extensively on the shoulder musculature and rotator cuff for dynamic stability during different strenuous activities. Therefore, the objective documentation of the strength, power, and endurance of the shoulder musculature is necessary to predict adequately a return to injury-free sporting activities or strenuous activities.

When a clinician refers to the assessment of muscular strength, one often thinks of the manual muscle testing (MMT) techniques. The earliest description of MMT was by Robert Lovett in 1912.[6] Since its conception, there have been several revisions in this technique. Two of the most popular versions of MMT have been developed by Kendall[7] and by Daniels and Worthingham.[8] Several inconsistencies are found in both the application and grading of these two techniques.[9,10] Also, inter-rater reliability is poor,[11,12] and the grading is relatively subjective.[13,14] Wilk et al[15] demonstrated bilateral isokinetic knee extension deficits ranging from 23 to 31 percent in 176 arthroscopic knee patients who exhibited bilaterally equal and normal grade (5/5)

MMT. Last, MMT tells the examiner nothing regarding muscular performance parameters such as work, power, and endurance; rather, it determines the ability of the subject to exert force at one particular point in the range of motion.[10] Thus, the face validity of MMT for the orthopaedic and sports medicine patient may not be completely acceptable in all instances.[9,10]

Therefore, a reasonable clinical addition to MMT is the use of isokinetic testing of the shoulder. Isokinetic testing affords the clinician the ability to document muscular performance objectively in a way that is both safe and reliable using either isolated or combined movement patterns. This objectivity ensures appropriate patient progression or regression, as well as assisting the clinicians with the determination of functional questions such as, When can I hit a golf ball? begin throwing? begin hitting a tennis ball? or return to overhead work activities? Consequently, isokinetics affords the clinician objective criteria and provides reproducible data to monitor patient function and plan patient progression.

## ISOKINETIC TESTING OF THE SHOULDER

To assess the muscular performance characteristics of the shoulder joint that has sustained a repetitive micro- or a macrotraumatic injury, the clinician should consider the daily activities the patient is returning to and the sport activities the patient may be participating in. This type of information provides the clinician with the rationale for which position to test the shoulder in. Most commonly, the shoulder is placed at risk of sustaining a microtraumatic injury when elevation, abduction, and rotation are required while performing a wide variety of activities. Examples of these superimposed activities include throwing, tennis, swimming, volleyball, and a variety of work-related activities such as painting and maintenance work. In these types of patients (the overhead athlete or worker), the authors recommend testing in the 90-degree abducted 90-degree elbow flexed position for shoulder internal and external rotation (Fig. 43-1).

In contrast, for the patient who has sustained a macrotraumatic shoulder injury, involving either the capsule or rotator cuff, and daily activities that do not necessitate repetitive overhead motions, testing is rec-

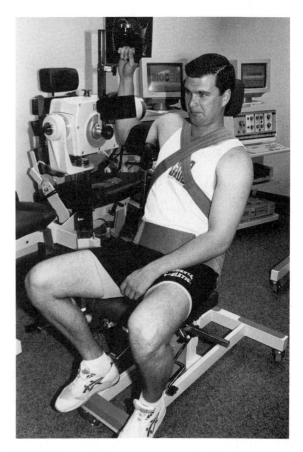

**Fig. 43-1.** The 90-degree abducted position for shoulder external/internal rotation.

ommended in a less-demanding position. This position is referred to as a modified neutral position[16] (Fig. 43-2) or the scapular plane position (Fig. 43-3). We recommend using this testing position in the low-demand shoulder patient or in the patient who is involved in activities most frequently below 90 degrees of abduction.

Wilk et al,[17] recognizing inconsistencies in testing methodology of different published articles, suggested a standardized isokinetic testing protocol for the shoulder. This standardized isokinetic testing protocol is referred to as the thrower's series.[17] The goal of a standardized testing protocol is to improve test–retest reproducibility[18] and to allow the clinician the ability to share test data.[10,17] In this chapter, the authors present an expansion of the "thrower's series" and explain the modifications of this protocol to the general orthopaedic patient. Fourteen "variables" exist that must be

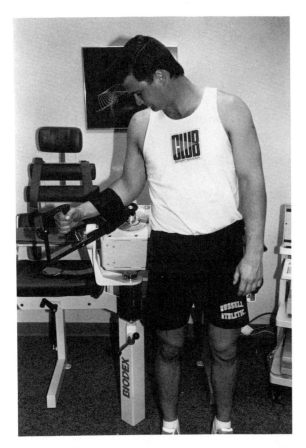

**Fig. 43-2.** Modified neutral position for shoulder external/internal rotation. Dynamometer is tilted 20 to 30 degrees and shoulder is abducted approximately 20 to 30 degrees.

cally injured shoulder. In the low-demand shoulder patient, routine tests recommended include internal/external rotation and shoulder flexion/extension. The testing sequence is specifically standardized, with the internal and external rotators always evaluated first, followed by either shoulder abduction/adduction or flexion/extension.

It is necessary to test the shoulder in a position that closely resembles its position of function during activity, while isolating the specific muscle groups desired. To approximate functional positioning and ensure muscular isolation, most testing is performed in the seated position. This position allows for normal gravitational forces acting on the trunk and upper extremities and enhances glenohumeral joint stabilization. The appropriate stabilization of the trunk, hip, and lower extremities during isokinetic testing of the shoulder is highly recommended (Fig. 43-4).

Testing of the shoulder's external and internal rotators can be performed in several test positions. These positions include the 90/90-degree test position (Fig. 43-1), modified neutral position (Fig. 43-2), scapular plane position (Fig. 43-3), neutral position (Fig. 43-5), and/or the 90/90-degree seated position (Fig. 43-6). Several authors demonstrated significant torque value variations by altering the subjects' test position.[25-31] Greenfield et al[26] tested external/internal rotation in both the scapular and frontal planes, reporting no significant internal rotation peak torque difference but

standardized and controlled to ensure an objective, reliable, and reproducible isokinetic evaluation of the shoulder (Table 43-1).

The first variable is to evaluate the planes of motion to test. In the overhead athlete, it has been reported that the shoulder's external/internal rotators, adductors/abductors, and horizontal abductors/adductors are the most critical to be tested.[17,19-24] Therefore, isokinetic testing in the thrower's series recommends the evaluation of the shoulder's internal and external rotators, as well as the abductors and adductors.[17] Because isokinetic testing of the horizontal abductors and adductors is performed in either the supine and/or prone position, these nonfunctional postures are not recommended in the testing sequence for the microtraumati-

**Table 43-1. Standardized Isokinetic Testing Protocol**

1. Planes of motion to evaluate
2. Testing position/stabilization
3. Axis of joint motion
4. Client education
5. Active warm-up
6. Gravity compensation
7. Rest intervals
8. Test collateral extremity first
9. Testing environment
   a. Standardized verbal commands
   b. Standardized visual feedback
   c. Free from distractions
   d. Tester skill
10. Testing velocities used
11. Test repetitions performed
12. System calibration
13. System level/stabilized
14. Use of windowed data/semihard end stop

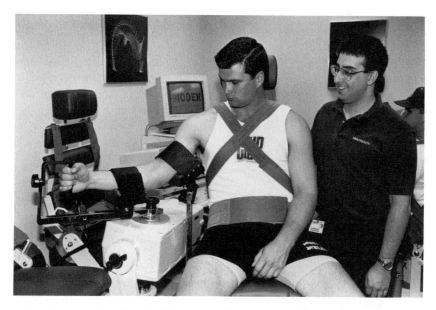

**Fig. 43-3.** Scapular plane position for shoulder external/internal rotation. Shoulder is abducted and flexed to 45 degrees.

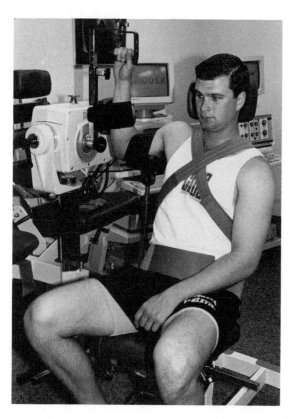

**Fig. 43-4.** Trunk, hip, and lower extremity is stabilized to eliminate muscular substitution during shoulder testing.

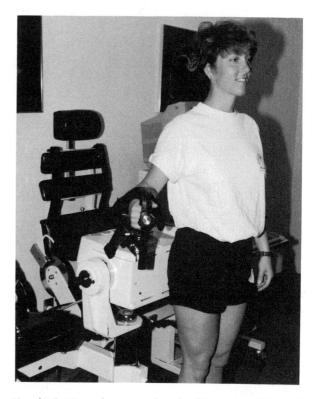

**Fig. 43-5.** Neutral position for shoulder external/internal rotation. Dynamometer is level, and shoulder is abducted slightly.

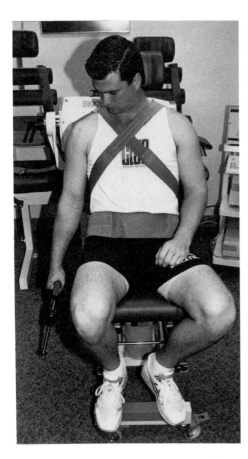

**Fig. 43-6.** Shoulder abduction/adduction in seated position.

increased external rotation torque values in the scapular plane. Walmsley and Szybbo[31] assessed external/internal rotation peak torque values in three test positions: neutral, 90 degree abduction, and 90 degree flexion. They found increased internal rotation torque values in the neutral position, and the highest external rotation values were exhibited in the 90 degree flexion position. Hinton[27] reported increased torque for internal rotation in the neutral position compared with the 90 degree abducted position, and external rotation was found to be equal in both positions.

Soderberg and Blaschek[25] tested external/internal rotation in six different test positions. They concluded that the internal rotation exhibited increased torque production in a neutral position, defined as 0 to 20 degrees of shoulder abduction; and external rotation torque was enhanced in the 90-degree abducted posi-

tion or neutral position.[25] Ellenbecker et al[30] tested external/internal rotation in the plane of scapulae versus the frontal plane and reported no significant differences in torque production in either the supine or seated position. Hellwig and Perrin[29] reported no significant differences in external/internal rotation in the frontal plane compared with the scapular plane during concentric and eccentric muscular contractions.

Considering these investigations, the pathophysiology of rotator cuff injuries, and the function of the shoulder muscles, a continuum of external/internal rotation exercise positions can be developed (Figs. 43-7 and 43-8). The natural progression of this continuum

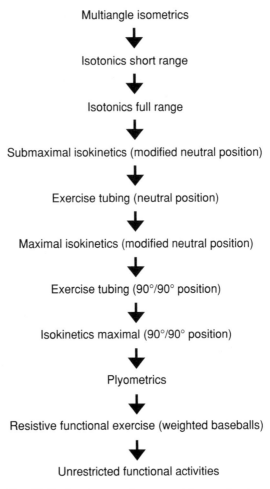

Multiangle isometrics

↓

Isotonics short range

↓

Isotonics full range

↓

Submaximal isokinetics (modified neutral position)

↓

Exercise tubing (neutral position)

↓

Maximal isokinetics (modified neutral position)

↓

Exercise tubing (90°/90° position)

↓

Isokinetics maximal (90°/90° position)

↓

Plyometrics

↓

Resistive functional exercise (weighted baseballs)

↓

Unrestricted functional activities

**Fig. 43-7.** Continuum of rotator cuff strengthening.

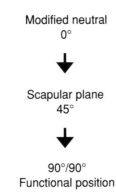

Modified neutral
0°

↓

Scapular plane
45°

↓

90°/90°
Functional position

**Fig. 43-8.** External/internal rotation rehabilitation position continuum.

is from 0 degrees abduction through the scapular plane and up to the functional 90-degree abducted position, which maximizes the external/internal rotation length tension relationship. This position also maximally stresses the dynamic stabilizing function of the rotator cuff musculature. This exercise continuum allows for the progression of static shoulder stability from a position of maximal joint stability to one of minimal stability. As with any form of exercise, if symptoms develop at any stage, the activity is regressed to a asymptomatic level and readvanced only when appropriate. The clinician should be aware that the test results generated in any one specific position cannot be compared with test results obtained in a different test position.

The third parameter that should be addressed is to ensure that the axis of joint motion is aligned with the axis of rotation of the shaft of the dynamometer. This alignment is necessary for accuracy in torque measurement.[10] Although not yet documented for the shoulder, changes in lever arm length of 2.5 in. or greater during knee extension/flexion testing has been shown to significantly alter torque production.[32–34] It is recommended that when testing shoulder abduction/adduction, the axis of the dynamometer be aligned 1 to 2 cm distal to the acromioclavicular joint. In testing the internal/external rotation, the axis of rotation is aligned through the center of the olecranon and the shaft of the humerus.

The next parameter ensures that the subject is informed as to the purpose and the intent of the isokinetic test. The subject should be familiarized with the testing device, how it functions, and what results will be provided. An informed client will be less apprehensive and will produce more consistent, reproducible results. Two investigators[35] demonstrated that subjects allowed previous isokinetic exposures show significantly favorable responses on isokinetic testing. Mawdsley and Knapik[35] reported significant differences between values demonstrated in the first testing session and those of the remaining six test trials. Wilk (unpublished data) has shown that subjects allowed one practice session before testing produced more consistent torque values in 83 to 88 percent of all test trials. Therefore, it is recommended that, whenever possible, clients undergo at least one isokinetic exposure before testing.

The fifth testing guideline is the use of an active warm-up before isokinetic testing. Several studies have shown no direct relationship between a warm-up and increased isokinetic torque production.[36,37] There is definite basic science research that documents the need for an active warm-up from a physiologic basis; however, this has not been found to enhance isokinetic testing.[38–41] Based on these basic exercise physiology principles, a standardized upper extremity warm-up is performed before isokinetic testing of the shoulder. This graded active warm-up activity includes a 5-minute upper body ergometer session at 90 repetitions per minute at a 60 kg/m work load. An isokinetic warm-up or familiarization period before testing includes five submaximal isokinetic repetitions and one maximal repetition at each angular test velocity before testing at that velocity.[35]

The effects of gravity must be addressed, and therefore, the authors recommend gravity compensation of the limb before testing. Significant differences have been demonstrated during isokinetic testing of muscle groups that were gravity-compensated when compared with those that were not.[42,43] Although no specific investigations have shown this fact during shoulder testing, it is generally accepted that, when gravity compensation is not used, the muscles assisted by gravity will show higher torque values, whereas the muscles working against gravity will show significantly smaller torque values. Also, as isokinetic angular velocities increase, so does the relative effect of gravity on torque values.[44,45] Therefore, gravity compensation should be performed before each test on every client.

The seventh parameter, controlling the rest interval during testing, is the next factor that must be addressed to ensure reproducibility. Ariki et al[46] showed that the optimal period of rest between each isokinetic test speed is 90 seconds. In evaluating the shoulder isokinetically, this time period of rest should be used at each test speed.

Testing the uninvolved side first is the next parameter to standardize. This serves three important functions: (1) It establishes a base line of data for the involved side, (2) it evaluates the client's willingness to be tested, and (3) it serves to decrease patient apprehension by allowing exposure to an isokinetic movement in the contralateral extremity first.[10,16]

The testing environment should be one that promotes concentration and assists in eliminating distractions. A designated room for testing is encouraged to isolate the subject from interrruptions, distractions, or additional activities that may impede a consistent test effort.

The verbal commands provided each client should be standardized to improve reproducibility. Johansson et al[47] demonstrated that loud verbal commands resulted in greater isometric torque values compared with softer verbal commands. This has been empirically stated during manual resistance techniques.[48] Thus, it is recommended that verbal commands during isokinetic testing be consistent, encouraging, and moderate in intensity.

The subjects' knowledge of results of torque production during testing is the third component of the testing environment to control. Several investigators reported that knowledge of results during strength testing may enhance some parameters of performance.[49-53] Therefore, visual feedback in the form of knowledge of results can significantly influence testing performance and must be consistently used or not used during isokinetic testing. Because visual feedback has been shown to enhance torque values and promote earlier fatigue, its use is not recommended.[10,53]

The final component of the testing environment is the skill and experience of the examiner. An experienced examiner can greatly allay subject apprehension, improve reproducibility of testing, and maximize the efficiency and efficacy of isokinetic shoulder assessment.

The tenth guideline is the selection of the angular velocities to be used during shoulder testing. Table 43-2 illustrates the current angular velocity classifications for isokinetic testing devices. Because of the extremely high angular velocities the shoulder obtains during throwing, golf, or tennis,[19,20,24,54] testing at slow isokinetic speeds may be inappropriate and, in fact, may impart undue forces on the glenohumeral joint.[55] Therefore, the authors recommend testing the shoulder at angular velocities of 180, 300, and 450 degrees/s.

The number of repetitions performed during isokinetic shoulder testing should be standardized. Davies[16] previously stated that 10 isokinetic repetitions produce an optimal training effect for both peak torque and average power parameters. Based on this observation, isokinetic evaluation of the shoulder is performed using 10 repetitions at 180 degrees/s, 15 repetitions at 300 degrees/s, and 10 repetitions at 450 degrees/s. Although it has been demonstrated that peak torque for both internal and external rotation, as well as the abductors and adductors of the shoulder, is produced during the second or third test repetition in 96 percent of all cases,[56] 10 to 15 test repetitions are used during isokinetic shoulder testing to ensure the optimal assessment of total work, average power parameters, and endurance parameters.

The twelfth parameter to consider is the significance of test system calibration. Although most manufacturers recommend calibration every 30 days to ensure validity in testing measures, the authors recommend calibration of the testing system be performed every 2 weeks.

The next guideline is to ensure that the isokinetic system is level and stabilized to the floor. A level and stable system will minimize artifact, overshoot, and oscillation interference during testing. Each of these aberrant recordings may lead to misinterpretation of test data, especially during shoulder abduction/adduction testing.[17,57,58]

The fourteenth and final parameter concerns data collection during isokinetic testing of the shoulder. During shoulder abduction/adduction testing, there exists the potential for error caused by end-stop oscilla-

**Table 43-2. Isokinetic Angular Velocity Classification**

| 15°–60°/s | 60°–180°/s | 180°–300°/s | 300°–500°/s |
|---|---|---|---|
| Slow velocity | Intermediate velocity | Fast velocity | Functional velocity |

tion and torque curve spiking.[57,58] These torque spikes are produced by combining the long lever arm, high test speeds, and large torque values demonstrated during testing with an abrupt terminal end point. Any abrupt end point results in the spiking of the torque curve graph for beyond the actual values produced.

The author recommends controlling this aberrant data production by using a semihard (firm) end stop and windowing the isokinetic data collection during shoulder abduction/adduction or shoulder flexion/extension testing. An end stop is used to cushion the end range and decelerate the lever arm during testing. A "firm" or semihard end stop results when the end-stop control is turned one-quarter turn from the hard end point. This type of end stop prevents excessive deceleration produced by a soft stop or the abrupt end-stop oscillation that occurs when a hard end stop is used.[57] End-stop oscillation is also prevented by windowing the test results so that any data not obtained at the pre-set isokinetic test speed or at 95 percent of that speed will not be recorded.

The use of a standardized method of isokinetic assessment of the shoulder addresses one of the main pitfalls inherent in the use of isokinetic testing: not using a standardized testing protocol with each evaluation performed. The 14 components addressed in this protocol are discussed to satisfy this limitation by outlining a clinically functional, activity-specific, and consistent means to evaluate the shoulder isokinetically. The authors feel the overhead athlete should be tested in the 90/90-degree seated position, whereas the low-demand shoulder patient may be tested in a more inherently stable, modified neutral or scapular plane position. The tester should use a position that places the client in the most frequent functional position for that particular client.

## ISOKINETIC REHABILITATION PRINCIPLES

The three basic categories of isokinetic exercise for the shoulder complex are: (1) on-axis planes and movements, (2) scapulothoracic patterns, and (3) off-axis planes and movements. On-axis planes or movements are referred to as isolated movement patterns in which the axis of rotation of the dynamometer is aligned with the axis of the joint motion. The scapulo-

thoracic patterns are isolated movements for the scapular muscles, while the off-axis movements are defined as movements in which the axis of the dynamometer is not aligned with the axis of joint motion, which usually results in combined movement patterns.

## On-Axis Planes and Movements

### Shoulder Abduction/Adduction

Shoulder abduction/adduction is a movement that we commonly used in the seated position (Fig. 43-6). This movement pattern attempts to isolate the shoulder abductors (deltoid, supraspinatus) and the adductors (pectoralis major, latissimus dorsi, teres major). Several authors have demonstrated a positive correlation between isokinetic shoulder adduction strength and arm velocity during throwing.[59,60] This correlation makes isokinetic exercise of this movement pattern extremely beneficial in functional strengthening of the shoulder complex in the throwing athlete. The authors also believe that the shoulder adductors serve a vital role in glenohumeral joint stability.

### Shoulder External/Internal Rotation

Shoulder external/internal rotation is a frequently tested movement of the shoulder. Positions to isolate the external/internal rotation of the shoulder include neutral position (Fig. 43-5), modified position (Fig. 43-2), scapular plane (Fig. 43-3), and 90-degree abducted position (Fig. 43-1). These positions are listed from maximal inherent stability to minimal inherent stability. As stated previously, each position will render different torque measurements compared with another position, and the clinician should be aware of these torque results and should employ consistency when comparing data from one test to another.

### Shoulder Flexion/Extension

Shoulder flexion/extension can be accomplished in several positions; seated (Fig. 43-9), prone (Fig. 43-10), supine (Fig. 43-11), and modified supine (Fig. 43-12). The supine position is frequently used to emphasize the shoulder flexors and to provide scapular stability (through the contact of the scapula on chair). Conversely, the prone position is used to emphasize the shoulder extensors and to challenge the scapular stabilizing muscles.

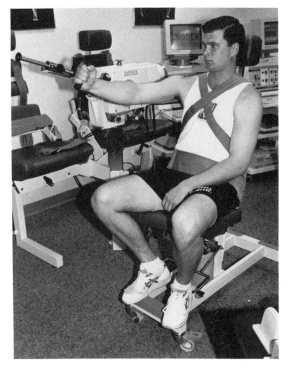

**Fig. 43-9.** Shoulder flexion/extension in seated position.

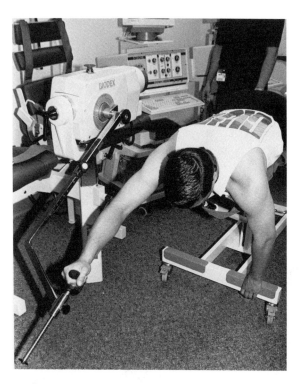

**Fig. 43-10.** Shoulder flexion/extension in prone position.

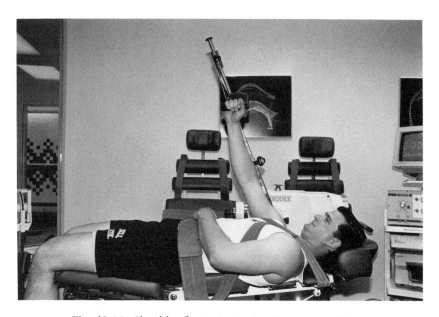

**Fig. 43-11.** Shoulder flexion/extension in supine position.

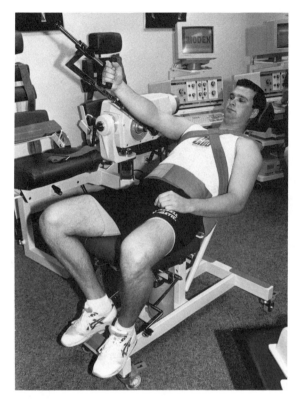

**Fig. 43-12.** Shoulder flexion/extension in modified supine position; chair is tilted approximately 45 degrees.

## Shoulder Horizontal Abduction/Adduction

Shoulder horizontal abduction/adduction can be used in the supine position (Fig. 43-13). This movement is important to the overhead athlete such as the thrower, tennis player, or racquet sport athlete to simulate the follow-through phase. The clinician must proceed with care when using horizontal adduction because this movement may cause impingement syndrome.

## Scapulothoracic Patterns

Adequate scapulothoracic muscular performance is paramount to the symptom-free function of the shoulder complex. A proper exercise regimen to strengthen the scapular muscles ensures the maintenance of the normal length–tension relationship of the glenohumeral joint, a stable base from which the upper extremity can function. These three components ensure that the scapulothoracic musculature provides proximal stability for the scapula to allow distal mobility of

the arm. Two commonly used scapular patterns are (1) scapular protraction and (2) scapular retraction.

### Scapular Protraction

A standing modified unilateral push-up activity performed isokinetically can mimic the function of the serratus anterior performing a wall push-up maneuver (Fig. 43-14). It can be used both concentrically and eccentrically for serratus strengthening. The serratus anterior muscle is an important element to scapular motion and control and must be exercised adequately to improve shoulder function.[61]

### Scapular Retraction

Scapular retraction can be accomplished by shortening the lever arm of motion above the elbow in the sagittal plane; the scapular retractors can be adequately strengthened isokinetically (Fig. 43-15). This motion overloads the rhomboids, middle trapezius, and posterior deltoid during scapular retraction.

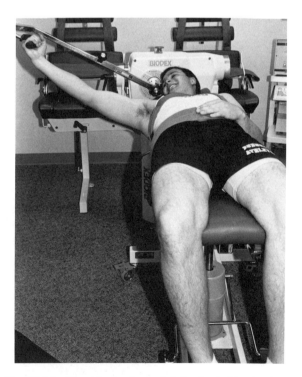

**Fig. 43-13.** Shoulder horizontal abduction/adduction in supine position.

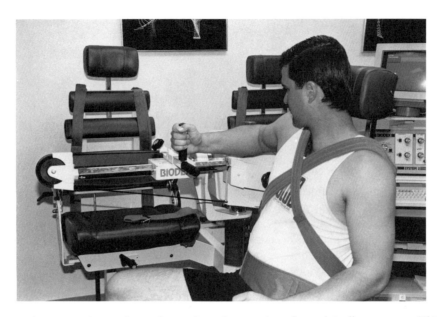

**Fig. 43-14.** Scapular protraction performed seated; motion consists of a push/pull movement. (This movement is employed by utilizing the closed chain attachment by Biodex, Shirley, NY)

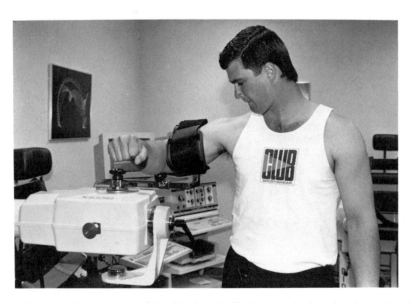

**Fig. 43-15.** Scapular retraction is accomplished isokinetically in sagittal plane by shortening knee lever arm attachment and strapping to arm.

## Off-Axis Patterns

### Supraspinatus/Scaption Exercise

As described by Jobe, this isokinetic exercise position approximates the muscle testing position for the supraspinatus at a 45-degree oblique plane (Fig. 43-16).[62–65] This off-axis pattern for the supraspinatus muscle can be used for isometric or isotonic muscular contraction.

### Diagonal Patterns

Diagonal combined movement patterns are exceptional exercise movements to replicate many dynamic upper extremity work and sport activities. These movements use reciprocal movement patterns and emphasize functional movements for the entire shoulder complex. The D2 flexion pattern (abduction, flexion, external rotation) is used to strengthen the posterior rotator cuff muscles and scapular retractors (Fig. 43-17). The D2 extension pattern (extension, adduction, internal rotation) is used to strengthen the adductor and internal rotators of the shoulder (Fig. 43-18).

The angular velocities (isokinetic speeds) frequently used during the rehabilitation process are described in Figs. 43-19 to 43-21. These pyramids are referred to isokinetic velocity spectrums.[16] The patient performs 10 repetitions at each of the predetermined speeds, followed by 90 seconds of rest and then 10 repetitions at the next isokinetic velocity.[16] This process is continued until all the prescribed speeds have been performed. Figure 43-19 illustrates the intermediate velocity spectrum used for short movement patterns such as shoulder external/internal rotation and scapular patterns. Figure 43-20 illustrates the fast velocity spectrum most often used for larger movement patterns such as shoulder flexion/extension and abduction/adduction. The functional velocity spectrum (Figure 43-21) is used for the upper extremity athletic patient and can be used for any single plane movement or diagonal pattern.

## INTERPRETATION OF TEST DATA

A copious amount of data is generated from an isokinetic evaluation of the shoulder. The data can be subdivided into topics identifying torque parameters, acceleration and deceleration characteristics, and muscular performance parameters. The remainder of this chapter briefly defines and discusses these parameters.

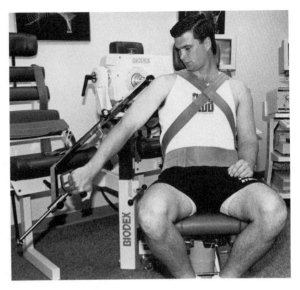

**Fig. 43-16.** Isolation of supraspinatus muscle is performed in plane of scapula. This movement is referred to as scaption.

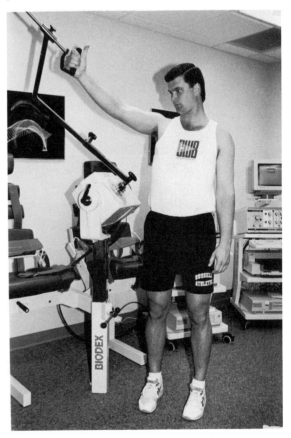

**Fig. 43-17.** Diagonal D₂ flexion pattern for shoulder's abductors, flexors, and external rotators.

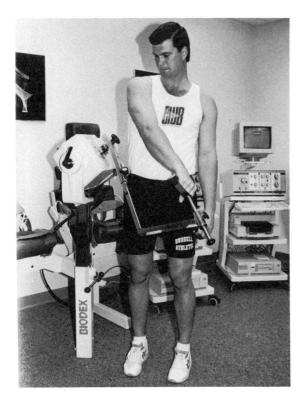

**Fig. 43-18.** Diagonal D$_2$ extension pattern for shoulder. This movement consists of shoulder extension, adduction, and internal rotation.

Torque is defined as force times the perpendicular distance from the axis of rotation. The term *peak torque* expresses a single repetition event that is the highest point on the graph regardless of where it occurs in the range of motion.[16] The average torque of all the test repetitions performed during one set is referred to as the *mean peak torque*. Mean peak torque values may provide more valuable information to the clinician regarding muscular performance than a single repetition peak torque value.

The test parameter referred to as *time rate to torque development* is an example of an acceleration parameter. This test parameter represents how quickly the subject can generate torque. The time rate to torque development can be expressed as a factor of time, such as at 0.2 seconds, or as a factor of joint position, such as at any specific joint angle or pre-determined torque value. This test parameter may prove beneficial to the clinician in determining the acceleration capability of the shoulder's internal rotators.

The next test parameter to consider is the force decay rate of the torque curve or the deceleration of the muscle group. On torque curve observation, it should appear straight or slightly convex. A torque curve whose force decay rate is concave indicates an inability or difficulty in producing force near the end range of motion.

The next area of data interpretation is classified as the muscular performance parameters.[66] These include total work, average power, and muscular endurance characteristics. Total work is defined as torque times an arc of movement. It represents the volume of area contained in the torque curve. The term *maximum work repetition* is the single repetition during which the maximum amount of work occurred. Average power is torque times an arc of movement divided by time, or work divided by time. This parameter is represented in watts. Both work and power can also be expressed in relation to body weight, such as work-to-body weight ratios. Also, work can be expressed as

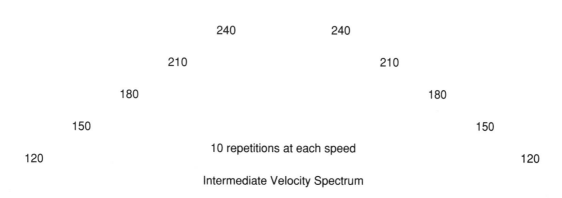

**Fig. 43-19.** Intermediate velocity spectrum.

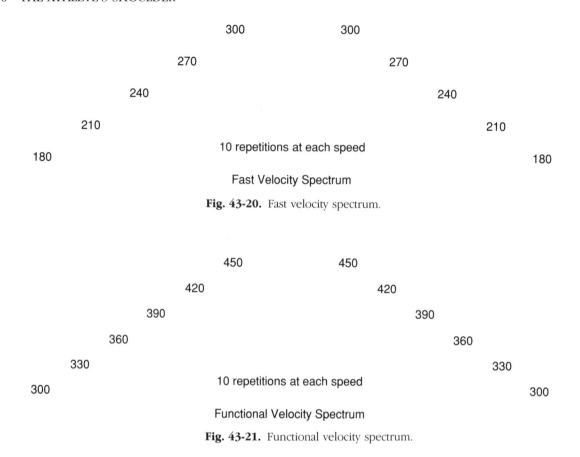

**Fig. 43-20.** Fast velocity spectrum.

**Fig. 43-21.** Functional velocity spectrum.

work in the first third and work in the last third of the repetition set. This represents the total amount of work performed in the first 33.3 percent of the set, and work in the last third is the last 33.3 percent. The work fatigue percentage is the ratio of change between the first third and the last third of any test.

As the reader can see, a tremendous amount of data can be produced by an isokinetic shoulder test. These data may create a paradox for the tester. Three commonly used parameters for data interpretation of the shoulder are (1) bilateral comparison, (2) unilateral data comparison, and (3) torque-to-body ratios. The current literature has produced significant controversy in data comparison. Some of this confusion may be attributed to the inconsistencies in the test positions used and differences in testing apparatus. Several investigators have shown significant differences between results gathered on different testing devices.[67–71] Re-

sults of isokinetic testing cannot be compared from one device or system with results from another device or system.

In regards to bilateral comparison of peak torque of the dominant versus nondominant shoulder, Wilk et al[72] reported their results of isokinetic testing 150 professional baseball pitchers. The results indicate, with regard to bilateral comparison of external/internal rotation testing, that the throwing shoulder is equal to the nonthrowing shoulder (Table 43-3). The bilateral comparison of abduction/adduction indicated no significant differences in peak torque for the shoulder's abductors, whereas the adductors exhibited a significant difference at both test speeds (180 and 300 degrees/s)[58] (Table 43-4). Table 43-5 illustrates the collective work of different investigators who have documented bilateral peak torque comparisons of the shoulder.

Unilateral muscle ratios express the balance between the agonist and antagonist muscle groups. Several investigators have published data regarding external/internal rotation ratios of the shoulder.[16,73–76] Ivey et al[77] reported a ratio of 66 percent at 60, 180, and 300 degrees/s. Cook et al[75] demonstrated an external/internal rotation ratio of 70 percent at 180 degrees/s and 300 degrees/s on the throwing shoulder and a ratio of 83 percent and 87 percent at the respected speeds for the nonthrowing shoulder. Davies[16] reported a ratio of 66.6 percent at 60 and 300 degrees/s. Table 43-6 represents the external/internal rotation unilateral muscle ratios for the shoulder from different investigators.[16,27,72–76] The unilateral muscle ratio for the shoulders abductors/adductors has been reported at 2 to 1 by several authors.[73,76] Wilk et al[58] found the abduction/adduction ratio for the dominant shoulder (throwing shoulder) to be 83 and 94 percent at 180 and 300 degrees/s. The nondominant shoulder abduction/adduction muscular ratio is 66 and 70 percent at the reported speeds.[58] Table 43-7 represents the collective work values of different authors regarding the abduction/adduction muscle ratios of the shoulder.[16,66,73,76]

The last torque parameter expressed in the literature is torque-to-body weight ratios. Table 43-8 represents the torque-to-body weight ratios for the shoulder external/internal rotation and abductors/adductors.[73]

There may exist differences in isokinetic muscular performance among different types of sporting athletes, subject's age and skill, and pathologic condition. For that reason, Tables 43-9 to 43-11 represent descriptive data from several authors regarding tennis players[78–82] and swimmers (TS Murphy, unpublished data).[83] These data are provided to assist the reader in

**Table 43-3. Comparison of Mean Peak Torque ± SD Between Dominant and Nondominant Throwing Arms for Shoulder External/Internal Rotation[a]**

| | External Rotation | | Internal Rotation | |
|---|---|---|---|---|
| Test Speed | Dominant (ft-lb) | Nondominant (ft-lb) | Dominant (ft-lb) | Nondominant (ft-lb) |
| 180°/s | 34.5 ± 6.2 | 36.5 ± 6.8[b] | 53.9 ± 8.8 | 52.4 ± 9.5 |
| 300°/s | 29.3 ± 5.1 | 30.1 ± 6.3 | 49.0 ± 8.5 | 48.0 ± 10.4 |

[a] $n = 150$.
[b] Respective pair showed statistically significant difference ($P < .05$).

**Table 43-4. Mean Peak Torque ± SD Between Dominant and Nondominant Throwing Arms for Shoulder Abduction/Adduction[a]**

| | Abduction | | Adduction | |
|---|---|---|---|---|
| Test Speed | Dominant (ft-lb) | Nondominant (ft-lb) | Dominant (ft-lb) | Nondominant (ft-lb) |
| 180°/s | 56.1 ± 12.5 | 58.6 ± 9.7 | 68.1 ± 12.6 | 62.5 ± 10.5[b] |
| 300°/s | 40.3 ± 15.7 | 38.4 ± 14.7 | 61.0 ± 12.5 | 54.6 ± 13.2[b] |

[a] $n = 131$.
[b] Statistically significant difference ($P < .05$) between respective pairs.

**Table 43-5. Bilateral Comparisons**

| | Dominant Stronger | Nondominant Stronger | Equal Bilateral |
|---|---|---|---|
| External rotation | Brown[74] | Alderink, Hinton | Cook, Ivey,[77] Jobe,[63] Wilk[72] |
| Internal rotation | Brown, Cook,[75] Hinton[27] | — | Alderink, Ivey, Jobe[63] Wilk et al.[72] |
| Abduction | — | — | Alderink,[73] Wilk et al.[72] |
| Adduction | Alderink,[73] Wilk[58] | — | — |
| Flexion | — | — | Alderink,[73] Cook et al.[75] |
| Extension | Alderink | — | Cook et al.[75] |

**Table 43-6. External/Internal Rotation Unilateral Muscle Ratios**

| | | Degrees/second | | | | | | |
|---|---|---|---|---|---|---|---|---|
| | | 60 | 90 | 120 | 180 | 210 | 240 | 300[a] |
| Alderink and Kuck[73] | Dominant | — | 66 | 68 | — | 71 | — | 70 |
| | Nondominant | — | 70 | 72 | — | 76 | — | 76 |
| Brown et al[74] | Dominant | — | — | — | 67 | — | 61 | 65 |
| | Nondominant | — | — | — | 71 | — | 66 | 65 |
| Cook et al[75] | Dominant | — | — | — | 70 | — | — | 70 |
| | Nondominant | — | — | — | 81 | — | — | 81 |
| Davies[16] | | 64 | — | — | — | — | — | 66.6 |
| Hinton[27] | Dominant | — | 69 | — | — | — | 71 | — |
| | Nondominant | — | 76 | — | — | — | 80 | — |
| Ivey et al[77] | | 66 | — | — | 66 | — | — | — |
| Wilk et al[72] | Dominant | — | — | — | 65 | — | — | 61 |
| | Nondominant | — | — | — | 64 | — | — | 70 |

[a] Values expressed in %.

the interpretation of the isokinetic shoulder test data in different overhead athletic populations.

Another parameter worthy of investigation is the load range. The load range refers to the percent of motion spent at the pre-set isokinetic speed. During an isokinetic test, the subject accelerates to speed, engages the speed (load range) and then decelerates near end range. The pre-set range of motion is then divided by the load range to obtain a percentage. Brown et al[84] have used this parameter to study elite junior tennis players. We utilize this parameter to monitor patient progress from test to retest.

When interpreting the results of an isokinetic shoulder test, 10 key parameters have been identified for routine evaluation and interpretation:

1. bilateral peak torque comparison
2. unilateral muscle ratios
3. torque/body weight ratios
4. bilateral work comparison
5. bilateral average power comparisons
6. work/body weight ratios
7. power/body weight ratios

8. torque at 0.2 s for the internal rotation
9. endurance–work fatigue ratios
10. acceleration/deceleration load range parameters

(The values for most of these parameters are listed in Table 43-12.)

Several pitfalls should be avoided when performing an isokinetic shoulder test. First, the test–retest should be performed in the identical position, at the same speeds, and using the same testing protocol.[10,17,18] When the test position or protocol is altered, the test results will be significantly affected. Second is only interpreting bilateral peak torque comparisons to determine patient's progress.[10,66] The review of the literature in this chapter illustrates bilateral comparisons are inconsistent and specifically altered by test position. Next is relying on torque curve shapes to determine different pathologies. The authors have experienced, after several hundred preoperative tests, that torque curves are not consistently generated by any specific shoulder pathologies. Fourth, do not solely rely on peak torque measurements to determine a patient's status. Power, work, and time parameters must be con-

**Table 43-7. Unilateral Muscle Ratios Abduction/Adduction**

| | | Degrees/second | | | | | |
|---|---|---|---|---|---|---|---|
| | | 60 | 90 | 120 | 180 | 210 | 300[a] |
| Alderink and Kunk[73] | Dominant | — | 54 | 54 | — | 50 | 51 |
| | Nondominant | — | 57 | 57 | — | 52 | 50 |
| Davies[16] | | 66 | — | — | 56 | — | 46 |
| Ivey et al[77] | | 50 | — | — | 50 | — | 50 |
| Wilk[66] | Dominant | — | — | — | 83 | — | 94 |
| | Nondominant | — | — | — | 66 | — | 70 |

[a] Values represent %.

## Table 43-8. Torque-to-Body Weight Ratios[a]

| °/sec | Abduction Dominant | Abduction Nondominant | Adduction Dominant | Adduction Nondominant | External Rotation Dominant | External Rotation Nondominant | Internal Rotation Dominant | Internal Rotation Nondominant |
|---|---|---|---|---|---|---|---|---|
| 90 | 27 | 26 | 50 | 46 | 15 | 15 | 22 | 22 |
| 120 | 25 | 25 | 47 | 45 | 14 | 15 | 21 | 21 |
| 210 | 21 | 21 | 43 | 41 | 13 | 14 | 19 | 19 |
| 300 | 18 | 18 | 36 | 36 | 13 | 13 | 18 | 18 |

[a] Values expressed in %.
(Data from Alderink and Kuck.[73])

## Table 43-9. Isokinetic Muscular Performance Data of Collegiate Tennis Players[a]

| | Men 60°/s | Men 180°/s | Men 210°/s | Women 60°/s | Women 180°/s | Women 210°/s |
|---|---|---|---|---|---|---|
| Eccentric peak torque/body weight ratio external rotation | 80 | 80 | 77 | 46 | 47 | 46 |
| Eccentric peak torque/body weight ratio internal rotation | 99 | 91 | 96 | 56 | 56 | 57 |
| Concentric peak torque/body weight ratio external rotation | 43 | 41 | 40 | 25 | 22 | 22 |
| Concentric peak torque/body weight ratio internal rotation | 59 | 49 | 50 | 34 | 27 | 25 |
| External rotation/internal rotation ratio concentric | 59 | 49 | 50 | 80 | 82 | 89 |
| External rotation/internal rotation ratio eccentric | 84 | 92 | 81 | 87 | 93 | 89 |
| Eccentric/concentric ratio external rotation | 202 | 206 | 202 | 103 | 107 | 119 |
| Eccentric/concentric ratio internal rotation | 183 | 202 | 201 | 123 | 143 | 173 |

[a] All values represent %.
(Data from Ellenbecker.[78])

## Table 43-10. Isokinetic Muscular Performance Data of Collegiate Tennis Players

| | Dominant 60°/s | Dominant 300°/s | Nondominant 60°/s | Nondominant 300°/s |
|---|---|---|---|---|
| Internal rotation (peak torque) (ft-lbs) | 30 | 21 | 24 | 16 |
| External rotation (peak torque) (ft-lbs) | 18 | 13 | 17 | 11 |
| Internal rotation torque/body weight % | 20 | 13 | 15 | 10 |
| External rotation torque/body weight % | 12 | 8 | 11 | 7 |
| External rotation/internal rotation % | 61 | 65 | 70 | 69 |

(Data from Chandler et al.[80])

## Table 43-11. Isokinetic Muscular Performance Data of Scholastic Swimmers

| | 120°/s Internal Rotation (ft-lb) | 120°/s External Rotation (ft-lb) | 120°/s External Rotation/Internal Rotation (%) | 180°/s Internal Rotation (ft-lb) | 180°/s External Rotation (ft-lb) | 180°/s External Rotation/Internal Rotation (%) |
|---|---|---|---|---|---|---|
| Pretraining | 36 | 20 | 57 | 32 | 19 | 58 |
| 3-Week post-training program | 42 | 32 | 75 | 41 | 30 | 73 |

(From TS Murphy, unpublished data.)

## Table 43-12. Key Parameters for Routine Evaluation and Interpretation[a]

| | External Rotation (%) | Internal Rotation (%) | Abduction (%) | Adduction (%) |
|---|---|---|---|---|
| Bilateral peak torque comparison | 100–110 | 115–125 | 100–110 | 120–135 |
| Unilateral muscle ratios | 66–70 | 66–70 | 82–88 | 82–88 |
| Torque/body weight ratios | 18–23 | 28–33 | 26–32 | 32–38 |
| Bilateral total work comparison | 105–115 | 118–128 | 110–119 | 115–130 |
| Bilateral total power comparison | 107–118 | 119–139 | 110–120 | 118–128 |
| Torque at 0.2 s for internal rotation | | 80–85 | | |
| Work–endurance ratios | 60–68 | 65–75 | 60–68 | 68–78 |

[a] Data represents values at 180°/s.

sidered to determine muscular performance. Next, realize this is not the only test. Rely on your clinical examination, functional testing, and special tests to assist in determining the condition of the shoulder. Last, the examiner should window all test data to prevent misinterpretation.

# CONCLUSION

The shoulder exhibits tremendous motion with inherently poor stability. The dynamic stabilizers (neuromuscular control) provide the shoulder with much-needed stability during different functional activities. Because of the greatly imposed demands on the shoulder musculature, the clinician must routinely assess the status of the neuromuscular system in an objective, reliable, and reproducible method. Isokinetics provides the clinician with a reproducible, objective, and safe muscular performance testing and exercise tool. The clinician is encouraged to use a standardized testing protocol to improve test–retest reproducibility. Also, a standardized testing protocol will allow clinicians to compare and share data, opening effective communication among sports medicine practitioners. Additionally, when reviewing published data the reader must consider test position and the testing protocol before using that data. Isokinetics should remain a vital tool to the rehabilitation team.

# REFERENCES

1. Inman VT, Saunders M, Abbott LC: Observations on the function of the shoulder joint. J Bone Joint Surg 26:1, 1944
2. Matsen FA, Harryman DT, Sidles JA: Mechanics of shoulder instability. Clin Sports Med 10:783, 1991
3. Saha AK: Dynamic stability of the glenohumeral joint. Acta Orthop Scand 42:491, 1971
4. Silliman JF, Hawkins RJ: Current concepts and recent advances in the athlete's shoulder. In Hawkins RJ (ed): Basic Science and Clinical Application in the Athlete's Shoulder. Clin Sports Med 10:18, 1991
5. Williams PH, Warwick R: Gray's Anatomy. 36th Ed. WB Saunders, Philadelphia, 1980
6. Wright W: Muscle training in the treatment of infantile paralysis. Boston Med Surg 167:567, 1912
7. Kendall FD, McCreary EK: Muscle Testing and Function. 3rd Ed. Williams & Wilkins, Baltimore, 1983
8. Daniels L, Worthingham C: Muscle Testing: Techniques of Manual Examination. 5th Ed. WB Saunders, Philadelphia, 1986
9. Mayhew TP, Rothstein JM: Measurement of muscular performance with instruments. p. 57. In Rothstein JM (ed): Measurement in Physical Therapy. Churchill Livingstone, New York, 1985
10. Wilk KE: Dynamic muscle strength testing. p. 123. In Amundsen LR (ed): Muscle Strength Testing: Instrumented and Noninstrumented Systems, Churchill Livingstone, New York, 1990
11. Iddings D, Smith L, Spencer W: Muscle testing, part 2: Reliability in clinical use. Phys Ther Rev 41:249, 1961
12. Wintz M: Variations in current manual muscle testing. Phys Ther Rev 39:466, 1959
13. Nicholas J, Sapega A, Kraus H, Webb J: Factors influencing manual muscle tests in physical therapy. J Bone Joint Surg 60:186, 1978
14. Nitz M: Variations in current manual muscle testing. Phys Ther Rev 39:466, 1959
15. Wilk KE, Arrigo CA, Andrews JR, Hinger DE: A comparison of manual muscle test results to isokinetic peak torque results in 100 ACL reconstructed knees. Presented at APTA, Denver, CO, 1992
16. Davies GJ: A Compendium of Isokinetics in Clinical Usage. 3rd Ed. S & S Publishers, Onolaska, WI, 1987
17. Wilk KE, Arrigo CA, Andrews JR: Standardized isokinetic testing protocol for the throwing shoulder: the thrower's series. Isokin Exerc Sci 1:63, 1991
18. Byl NN, Wells L, Grady D et al: Consistency of repeated isokinetic testing: effect of different examiners, sites, and protocols. Isokin Exerc Sci 1:122, 1991
19. Dillman CJ: Biomechanics of pitching. Presented at the 1991 Injuries in Baseball Conference, Birmingham, AL, January 25, 1990
20. Dillman CJ, Fleisig GS, Werner SL, Andrews JR: Biomechanics of the Shoulder in Sports: Throwing Activities. Post Graduate Studies in Physical Therapy, Forum Medicum, Pennington, NJ, 1990
21. Jobe FW, Tibone JE, Perry J et al: An EMG analysis of the shoulder in throwing and pitching. A preliminary report. Am J Sports Med 11:3, 1983
22. Jobe FW, Moynes DR, Tibone JE et al: An EMG analysis of the shoulder in pitching. A second report. Am J Sports Med 12:218, 1984
22. Figoni SF, Morris AF: Effects of knowledge of results on reciprocal isokinetic strength and fatigue. J Orthop Sports Phys Ther 6:104, 1984
23. Pappas AM, Zawacki RM, McCarthy CF: Rehabilitation of the pitching shoulder. Am J Sports Med 13:223, 1985
24. Pappas AM, Zawacki RM, Sullivan TJ: Biomechanics of baseball pitching. A preliminary report. Am J Sports Med 13:216, 1985

25. Soderberg GJ, Blaschek MJ: Shoulder internal and external rotation peak torque production through a velocity spectrum in differing positions. J Orthop Sports Phys Ther 8:518, 1987

26. Greenfield BH, Donatelli R, Wooden MJ, Wilken J: Isokinetic evaluation of shoulder rotational strength between plane of the scapula and functional plane. Am J Sports Med 18:124, 1990

27. Hinton RY: Isokinetic evaluation of shoulder rotational strength in high school baseball pitchers. Am J Sports Med 16:274, 1988

28. Hageman PA, Mason DK, Rydlund KW et al: Effects of position and speed on eccentric and concentric isokinetic testing of the shoulder rotators. J Orthop Sports Phys Ther 11:64, 1989

29. Hellwig EV, Perrin DH: A comparison of two positions for assessing shoulder rotator peak torque: the traditional frontal plane versus the plane of the scapula. Isokin Exerc Sci 1:202, 1991

30. Ellenbecker TS, Feiring DC, Dehart RL: Isokinetic shoulder strength: coronal versus scapular plane testing in upper extremity unilaterally dominant athletes. Presented at the annual conference of American Physical Therapy Association, Denver, CO, June 1992

31. Walmsley RP, Szybbo C: A comparative study of the torque generated by the shoulder internal and external rotators in different positions and at varying speeds. J Orthop Sports Phys Ther 9:217, 1987

32. Johnson RJ, Wilk KE: The effect of lever arm pad placement upon the isokinetic torque during knee extension and flexion. Phys Ther 68:779, 1988

33. Siewert MW, Ariki PK, Davies GJ et al: Isokinetic torque changes based on lever arm placement. Phys Ther 65:715, 1985

34. Taylor RC, Casey JJ: Quadriceps torque production on the Cybex II dynamometer as related to changes in lever arm length. J Orthop Sports Phys Ther 8:147, 1986

35. Mawdsley RH, Knapik JJ: Comparison of isokinetic measurements with test repetitions. Phys Ther 62:169, 1982

36. Davies GJ: Cybex II isokinetic dynamometer measurements on the acute effects of direct active warm-ups and direct passive warm-ups on knee extension/flexion and power. Presented at annual conference of American Physical Therapy Association, June 1978

37. Wiktorsson-Moller M, Oberg B, Edstrand V et al: Effects of warming up, massage and strengthening on range of motion and muscle strength in the lower extremity. Am J Sports Med 11:249, 1983

38. Asmussen E, Boje O: Body temperature and capacity for work. Acta Physiol Scand 10:1, 1945

39. Astrand PO, Rodahl K: Textbook of Work Physiology: Physiologic Basis of Exercise. 2nd Ed. McGraw-Hill, New York, 1977

40. Franks DB: Physical warm-up. In Morgan WP (ed): Ergogenic Aids and Muscular Performance. Academic Press, Orlando, FL, 1972

41. Martin BV, Robinson S, Wiogoma DC et al: Effect of warm-up on metabolic responses to strenuous exercise. Med Sci Sports Ex 7:146, 1975

42. Caizzo VJ: Alterations in the in vivo force velocity curve. Med Sci Sports Exerc 12:134, 1980

43. Fillyaw M, Bevins T, Fernandez L: Importance of correcting isokinetic peak torque for the effect of gravity when calculating knee flexor to extensor muscle ratios. Phys Ther 66:23, 1986

44. Nelson SG, Duncan PW: Correction of isokinetic and isometric torque recordings for the effects of gravity. Phys Ther 63:674, 1983

45. Winter DA, Wells RP, Orr GW: Errors in the use of isokinetic dynamometers. Eur J Appl Physiol 46:317, 1981

46. Ariki PK, Davies GJ, Siewert MW et al: Optimum rest interval between isokinetic velocity spectrum rehabilitation speeds (abstract). Phys Ther 65:735, 1985

47. Johansson CA, Kent BE, Shepard KF: Relationship between verbal command volume and magnitude of muscle contraction. Phys Ther 63:1260, 1983

48. Knott M, Voss D: Proprioceptive Neuromuscular Facilitation. Hoeber Medical Division, Harper & Row, New York, 1968

49. Hald RD, Bottken EJ: Effects of visual feedback on maximal and submaximal isokinetic test measurements of normal quadriceps and hamstring. J Orthop Sports Phys Ther 9:86, 1987

50. Manzer CW: The effect of knowledge of output on muscle work. J Exp Psychol 18:80, 1935

51. Pierson WR, Rasch PJ: Effect of knowledge of results on isometric strength scores. Res Q 35:313, 1964

52. Ulrich C, Burke RK: Effect of motivational stress on physical performance. Res Q 28:403, 1957

53. Figoni SF, Christ CB, Massey BH: Effects of speed, hip and knee angle, and gravity on hamstring to quadriceps torque ratios. J Orthop Sports Phys Ther 9:287, 1988

54. Bradley JP, Tibone JE: Electromyographic analysis of muscle action about the shoulder. In Hawkins RJ (ed): Basic Science and Clinical Application in the Athlete's Shoulder. Clin Sports Med 10:789, 1991

55. Elsner RC, Pedegana LR, Lang J: Protocol for strength testing and rehabilitation of the upper extremity. J Orthop Sports Phys Ther 4:229, 1983

56. Arrigo CA, Wilk KE: Peak torque and total work repetition during isokinetic testing of the shoulder. Isokin Exerc Sci (submitted for publication)

57. Wilk KE, Arrigo CA, Keirns MA: Shoulder abduction/adduction isokinetic test results: window vs unwindow data collection. J Orthop Sports Phys Ther 15:107, 1992

58. Wilk KE, Andrews JR, Arrigo CA et al: The isokinetic

abductor and adductor strength characteristics of professional baseball pitchers. Am J Sports Med (submitted for publication)

59. Bartlett LR, Storey MD, Simons BD: Measurement of upper extremity torque production and its relationship to throwing speed in the competitive athlete. Am J Sports Med 17:89, 1989

60. Pedegana LR, Elsner R, Roberts D et al: The relationship of upper extremity strength to throwing speed. Am J Sports Med 10:352, 1982

61. Moseley JB, Jobe FW, Pink M et al: EMG analysis of the scapular muscles during a shoulder rehabilitation program. Am J Sports Med 20:128, 1992

62. Jobe FW, Bradley JP: Rotator cuff injuries in baseball: prevention and rehabilitation. Sports Med 6:378, 1980

63. Jobe FW, Moynes DR: Delineation of diagnostic criteria and a rehabilitation program for rotator cuff injuries. Am J Sports Med 10:336, 1982

64. DeLuca CJ, Forrest WJ: Force analysis of individual muscles acting simultaneously on the shoulder joint during isometric abduction. J Biomechanics 6:385, 1973

65. Townsend H, Jobe FW, Pink M, Perry J: Electromyographic analysis of the glenohumeral muscles during a baseball rehabilitation program. Am J Sports Med 19:264, 1991

66. Wilk KE: Isokinetic testing and exercise for the shoulder complex. Presented at annual conference of Biodex Corporation, Ft. Lauderdale, FL, October 3, 1991

67. Francis K, Hoobler T: Comparison of peak torques of the knee flexor and extensor muscle groups using the Cybex II and Lido 2.0 isokinetic dynamometers. J Orthop Sports Phys Ther 8:480, 1987

68. Wilk KE, Johnson RJ: A comparison of peak torque values of knee extensors and flexor muscle groups using the Biodex, Cybex, Kin-Com isokinetic dynamometer. Phys Ther 67:789, 1987

69. Wilk KE, Johnson RJ: A comparison of peak torque values of knee extensor and flexor muscle groups using the Biodex, Cybex, and Lido isokinetic dynamometer. Phys Ther 68:792, 1988

70. Thompson MC, Shingleton LG, Kegerreis ST: Comparison of values generated during testing of the knee using the Cybex II+ and Biodex mode B-2000 isokinetic dynamometers. J Orthop Sports Phys Ther 11:108, 1989

71. Gross MT, Huffman GM, Phillips CN, Wray JA: Intramachine and intermachine reliability of the Biodex, Cybex for knee flexion and extension peak torque and angular work. J Orthop Sports Phys Ther 13:329, 1991

72. Wilk KE, Andrews JR, Arrigo CA et al: The internal and external rotator strength characteristics of professional baseball pitchers. Am J Sports Med 21:61, 1993

73. Alderink GJ, Kuck DJ: Isokinetic shoulder strength of high school and college aged pitchers. J Orthop Sports Phys Ther 7:163, 1986

74. Brown LP, Niehues SL, Harrah A et al: Upper extremity range of motion and isokinetic strength of the internal and external shoulder rotators in major league baseball players. Am J Sports Med 16:577, 1988

75. Cook EE, Gray VL, Savinor-Nogue E et al: Shoulder antagonistic strength ratios: a comparison between college-level baseball pitchers. J Orthop Sports Phys Ther 8:451, 1987

76. Williams M: Manual muscle testing, development and current use. Phys Ther Rev 36:717, 1956

77. Ivey FM, Calhoun JH, Rusche K et al: Normal values for isokinetic testing of shoulder strength (abstract). Med Sci Sports Exerc 16:274, 1988

78. Ellenbecker TS: Eccentric and concentric isokinetic strength characteristics of the rotator cuff. Presented at annual conference of American Physical Therapy Association, Boston, MA, June 20, 1991

79. Ellenbecker TS: A total arm strength profile of highly skilled tennis players. Isokin Exerc Sci 1:9, 1991

80. Chandler TJ, Kibler WB, Stracener EC et al: Shoulder strength, power, and endurance in college tennis players. Am J Sports Med 20:455, 1992

81. Kibler WB, McQueen C, Uhl T: Fitness evaluations and fitness findings in competitive junior tennis players. Clin Sports Med 7:403, 1988

82. Ng LR, Kramer JS: Shoulder rotator torques in female tennis and non-tennis players. J Orthop Sports Phys Ther 13:40, 1991

83. Falkel JE, Murphy TC, Murray TF: Prone positioning for testing shoulder internal and external rotation on the Cybex II isokinetic dynamometer. J Orthop Sports Phys Ther 8:368, 1987

84. Brown LE, Whitehurst DN, Buchalter M: Isokinetic load range during shoulder external/internal rotation in elite male junior tennis players. Presented at annual conference, American Tennis Professionals, New York, Sept 3, 1992

# 44

# Plyometrics for the Shoulder Complex

*KEVIN E. WILK*
*MICHAEL L. VOIGHT*

The rehabilitation process has changed dramatically in the past several years. A relatively new concept in the rehabilitation of the athletic shoulder is plyometrics. In the rehabilitation of athletic injuries and in sport training, the concept of specificity has emerged as an important parameter in determining the proper choice of an exercise program.[1] The imposed demands during training must mirror those incurred during athletic competition. In many athletic events, these stresses center around a muscle's capacity to exert its maximal force output in a minimal amount of time. Success is dependent on the speed at which muscular force can be generated. A form of exercise training that attempts to combine strength with speed of movement is plyometrics.

Although the term *plyometrics* is relatively new, the basic concepts are old. The roots of plyometric training can be traced to Eastern Europe, where it was simply known as jump training. The actual roots of the word *plyometric* are a little confusing. "Plyo" comes from the Greek word *plythein,* which means to increase. *Plio* is the Greek word for "more," and "metric" literally means to measure. The practical definition of plyometrics is a quick powerful movement involving a prestretching of the muscle, thereby activating the stretch–shortening cycle. As the eastern block countries began to dominate sports requiring power, their training methods became the focus of attention. After the 1972 Olympics, articles began to appear in coaching magazines outlining a strange system of leaps and bounds used to increase speed. As it turns out, the eastern block nations were not the originators of plyo-

metrics, just the organizers. This system of hops and jumps has been used by American coaches for years as a form of conditioning. Rope jumping and bench hops have been used for years as a method to increase reaction time and quickness. The organization of this method of conditioning has been credited to the legendary Soviet jump coach Yuri Verkhoshanski, who, during the late 1960s, began to tie this miscellaneous program of hops and jumps into an organized plan of training.[2] The actual term *plyometrics* was first introduced in 1975 by American track coach Fred Wilt.[3] A literature review shows that since 1969, many authors have used variances of Verkhoshanski's method in an attempt to establish the best plyometric technique and training program.[4–8] Although there is agreement surrounding the benefits of basic plyometric principles, there is controversy regarding an optimal training routine.[9–12] Today, the chief proponents of plyometrics are still in the track and field society, as they continue to use Verkhoshanski's "reactive neuromuscular apparatus" for reproducing and enhancing the reactive properties of the lower extremity musculature.[7,8,13] The main purpose of plyometric training is to increase the excitability of the neurologic receptors for improved reactivity of the neuromuscular system.

Most of the literature to date on plyometric training has been focused on the lower quarter. Adaption of the plyometric principles can be used to enhance the specificity of training in other sports or activities that require a maximum amount of muscular force in a minimal amount of time. All movements in competitive athletics involve a repeated series of stretch–shortening cycles. The musculature surrounding the shoulder girdle possesses the same physiologic characteristics as the lower extremity. Therefore, different forms of plyometric exercises can be applied to the upper quarter to exploit the stretch–shortening cycle. The intensity of the upper-quarter plyometric program is much less due to the small muscle mass as compared with the lower quarter.

Perhaps in no one single athletic endeavor is the use of elastic loading to produce a maximal explosive concentric contraction and the rapid decelerative eccentric contraction seen more than in the violent activity of throwing a baseball. Similar stretch–shortening movements can be seen in such sports as tennis, swimming, and golf. To replicate these forces during rehabilitation is beyond the scope of every traditional exercise tool. For example, the isokinetic dynamometer that reaches maximal velocities of 450 to 500 degrees/s is not specific to the greater than 7,000 degrees/s seen during a baseball pitch.[14] Consequently, to exercise

with the philosophy of specificity, drills such as plyometrics should be an intricate part of every upper extremity training program to facilitate a complete return to athletic participation. This chapter explains the theoretic basis of plyometrics and presents a philosophy for using the stretch reflex to produce an explosive reaction in the upper extremity. Stretch–shortening exercise drills are classified into two categories: (1) sports enhancement training and (2) neuromuscular control. This chapter primarily discusses sports enhancement training for the upper quadrant.

## NEUROPHYSIOLOGIC BASIS OF PLYOMETRICS

Plyometrics is a form of exercise that uses the elastic and reactive properties of a muscle to generate a maximal force production. In normal muscle function, the muscle is stretched before it contracts concentrically.

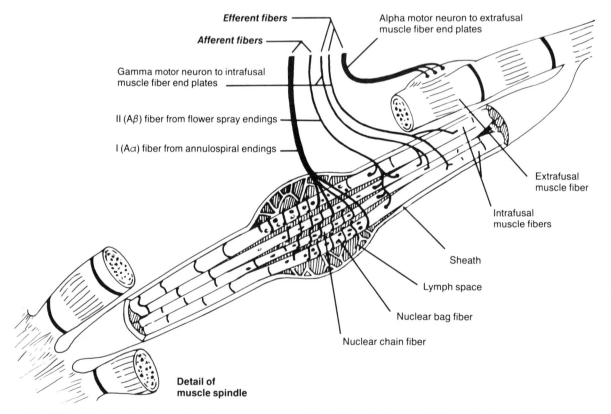

**Fig. 44-1.** Muscle spindle complex is a receptor consisting of intrafusal muscle fibers. Each spindle receives afferent innervation from group Ia (A$\alpha$) fibers and group II (A$\beta$) fibers. Purpose of muscle spindle is to provide information regarding muscular length to central nervous system.

This eccentric–concentric coupling is also referred to as the stretch–shortening cycle. This principle uses the stimulation of the body's proprioceptors to facilitate an increase in muscle recruitment over a minimal amount of time.

The proprioceptors of the body include the muscle spindle, the golgi tendon organ, and the joint capsule/ligamentous receptors.[15,16] Stimulation of these receptors can cause facilitation, inhibition, and modulation of both agonist and antagonist muscles. Both the muscle spindle and golgi tendon organ provide the proprioceptive basis for plyometric training.

The muscle spindle functions mainly as a stretch receptor. The muscle spindle components that are primarily senstitive to changes in velocity are the nuclear bag intrafusal muscle fibers, which are innervated by a type 1a phasic nerve fiber. This response is provoked by a quick stretch, which reflexively produces a quick contraction of the agonistic and synergistic extrafusal muscle fibers (Fig. 44-1). The firing of the type 1a phasic nerve fibers is influenced by the rate of stretch; the faster and greater the stimulus, the greater the effect of the associated extrafusal fibers.[17,18] This cycle occurs in 0.3 to 0.5 ms and is mediated at the spinal cord level in the form of a monosynaptic reflex such as the knee jerk (Fig. 44-2).

The golgi tendon unit is located at the junction between the tendon and muscle both at the origin and insertion and is sensitive to tension.[19] It is arranged in series with the extrafusal muscle fibers and therefore becomes activated with stretch. Unlike the muscle spindle, the golgi tendon organ has an inhibitory effect on the muscle. On activation, impulses are sent to the spinal cord, causing an inhibition of the $\alpha$ motor neurons of the contracting muscle and its synergists and thereby limiting the force produced.

Thus, it has been postulated that the golgi tendon organ is the protective mechanism against overcontraction or stretch of the muscle.[20] Because the golgi tendon organ uses at least one interneuron in its synaptic cycle, inhibition requires more time than the type 1a monosynaptic interneuron excitation.[21]

During concentric muscle contraction, the muscle spindle output is reduced because the muscle fibers are either shortening or attempting to shorten. During eccentric contraction, the muscle stretch reflex serves to generate more tension in the lengthening muscle. When the muscle tension increases to a high or potentially harmful level, the golgi tendon organ fires, thereby generating a neural pattern that reduces the excitation of the muscle. Consequently, the golgi tendon organ receptors may be a protective mechanism,

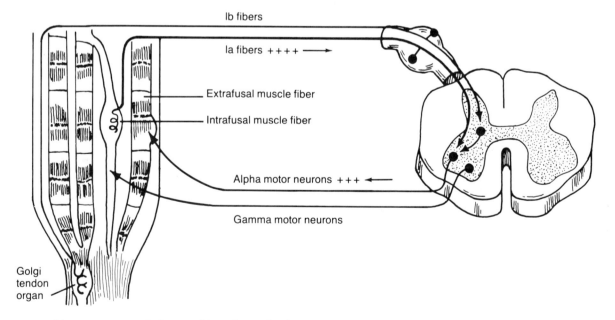

**Fig. 44-2.** Passive stretch (knee jerk). Both intrafusal and extrafusal muscle fibers are stretched; spindle activated. Reflex via group Ia fibers and $\alpha$ motor neurons causes secondary contraction (basis of stretch reflex) stretch too weak to activate golgi tendon organs.

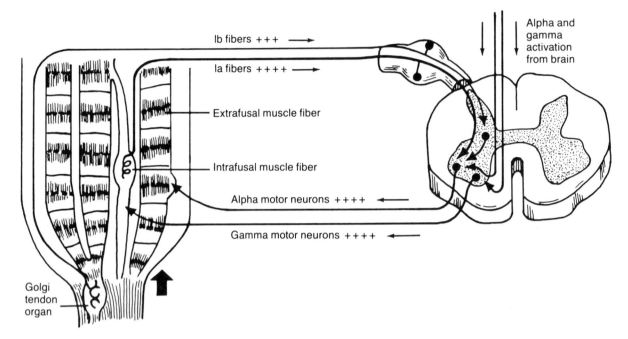

**Fig. 44-3.** Active contraction. Intrafusal as well as extrafusal fibers contract; spindles activated, with increased resistance group Ia fibers activated. Tendon organ activated, if load is too great, causing relaxation.

but in the correctly carried out plyometric exercise, their influences are overshadowed by the reflex arc pathway incorporated with excitation of type 1a nerve fibers (Fig. 44-3).

Another principle to consider when discussing the quick explosion philosophy of plyometrics is which muscles can be best affected. Patten[22] embryologically classified muscles into phasic and tonic groups according to how they arise from the myotomes.[22] Group I muscles (phasic or fast twitch) are innervated by anterior divisions of the plexuses and include the flexors, adductors, and internal rotators. Also included in this category are most two-joint muscles.[20] Group II muscles (tonic or static) include the extensors, external rotators, and abductors. The group I muscles will possess more influence by the type 1a phasic nerve endings, resulting in a greater chance of being facilitated by the plyometric mechanism.

Along with the neurophysiologic stimulus, the positive results of plyometrics also come from the recoil action of elastic tissues.[6,9] Several authors have shown that an eccentric contraction immediately preceding a concentric contraction will significantly increase the force generated concentrically because of the storage of elastic energy.[4,5] The mechanism for this increased concentric force is the ability of the muscle to use the force produced by the elastic component. During the loading of the muscle, when the stretch occurs, the load is transferred to the elastic component and stored as elastic energy. The elastic elements can then deliver increased energy as it is recovered and used for the concentric contraction.[4]

The muscle's ability to use the stored elastic energy is affected by these variables: time, magnitude of stretch, and velocity of stretch. Increased force generation during the concentric contraction is most effective when the preceding eccentric contraction is of short range and performed quickly without delay.[4,5]

The improved or increased muscle performance that occurs with the prestretching of the muscle is the result of the combined effects of both the storage of elastic energy and the myotatic reflex activation of the muscle.[4,5,9] The percentage of contribution from each component is not known at this time.[5] The degree of improvement is dependent on the time frame between the eccentric and concentric contractions.[9]

During plyometric exercise, there are three phases: the setting or eccentric phase, the amortization phase, and the concentric response phase (Table 44-1). The eccentric or setting phase begins when the athlete mentally prepares for the activity and lasts until the stretch stimulus is initiated. Advantages of a correct setting stage include increasing the muscle spindle activity by prestretching the muscle before activation and mentally biasing the $\alpha$ motor neuron for optimal extrafusal muscle contraction.[11,23]

The duration of the setting phase is determined by how much impulse is desired for facilitation of the contraction. With too much or prolonged loading, the elapsed time from eccentric to concentric contraction will prevent exploitation of the stretch–shortening myotatic reflex.[18,24]

The second phase of the plyometric response is the amortization phase. This phase is the amount of time between undergoing the yielding eccentric contraction and initiation of a concentric overcoming force. By definition, it is an electromechanical delay between the eccentric and concentric contractions during which the muscle must switch from overcoming work to imparting the necessary amount of acceleration in the required direction.

The final period of the plyometric exercise is the concentric response phase. It is during this phase that the athlete concentrates on the effect of the exercise and prepares for initiation of the second repetition.

Plyometric exercise helps to improve physiologic muscle performance in several ways. Although increasing the speed of the myotatic stretch–reflex response would increase performance, it has not been documented in the literature. It has been documented that the faster a muscle is loaded eccentrically, the greater the concentric force produced. Eccentric loading places stress on the elastic components, thereby increasing the tension of the resultant rebound force.

A second possible mechanism for the increased force production involves the inhibitory effect of the golgi tendon organs on force production. Because the golgi tendon organ serves as a protective mechanism limiting the amount of force produced within a muscle, its stimulation threshold becomes the limiting factor. It may be possible to desensitize the golgi tendon organ thereby raising the level of inhibition and ultimately allowing increased force production with greater loads applied to the musculoskeletal system.

The last mechanism by which plyometric training may increase muscular performance centers around neuromuscular coordination. Explosive plyometric training may improve neural efficiency and thereby increase neuromuscular performance.

Neural adaptation allows the individual to better coordinate the activities of the muscle groups, thereby affecting a greater net force even in the absence of morphologic change within the muscles themselves. The neurologic system is enhanced to become more automatic.

Successful plyometric training relies heavily on the rate of stretch rather than the length of the stretch. If the amortization phase is slow, elastic energy is wasted as heat and the stretch reflex is not activated. The more quickly the individual is able to switch from yielding

### Table 44-1. Plyometric Phases

| | |
|---|---|
| Phase 1 | Eccentric phase—(setting) preloading period |
| Phase 2 | Amortization phase—time between eccentric and creative phase |
| Phase 3 | Concentric phase—facilitated contraction (pay-off) |

### Table 44-2. Upper Extremity Plyometrics

Warm-up exercises
    Medicine ball rotation
    Medicine ball side bends
    Medicine ball wood chops
    Tubing external rotation/interior rotation
    Tubing diagonal patterns (D2)
    Tubing biceps
    Push-ups
Throwing movements
    Medicine ball soccer throw
    Medicine ball chest pass
    Medicine ball step & pass
    Medicine ball side throw
    Tubing plyos interior rotation/external rotation
    Tubing plyos diagonals
    Tubing plyos biceps
    Plyo push-up (boxes)
    Push-up (clappers)
Trunk extension/flexion movements
    Medicine ball sit-ups
    Medicine ball back extension
Medicine ball wall exercises
    Soccer throw
    Chest pass
    Side-to-side throw
    Backward side-to-side throw
    Forward two hands through legs
    One-hand baseball throw

work to overcoming work, the more powerful the response.

The implementation of the plyometric program begins initially with the development of an adequate strength base. The development of a greater strength base results in greater force generation due to both the increased cross-sectional area and the resultant elastic component. To produce optimal strength gains, a structured plan must be instituted to prevent potential overuse injuries.

Plyometric exercise serves to train the neuromuscular system by teaching it to better accept the increased strength loads. Using the stretch reflex helps to improve the ability of the nervous system to react with maximal speed to the lengthening muscle. This allows the muscle to contract concentrically with maximal force. Because the plyometric program attempts to modify and retrain the neuromuscular system, the exercise program should be designed with sport specificity in mind.

The upper extremity program is organized into four different exercise groupings: (1) warm-up exercises,

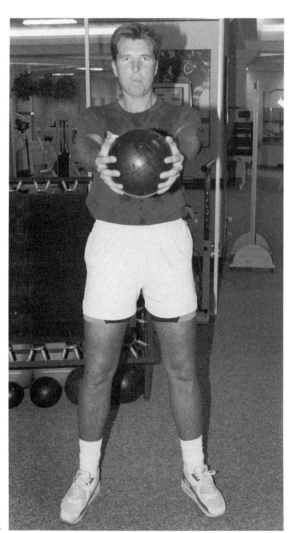

A

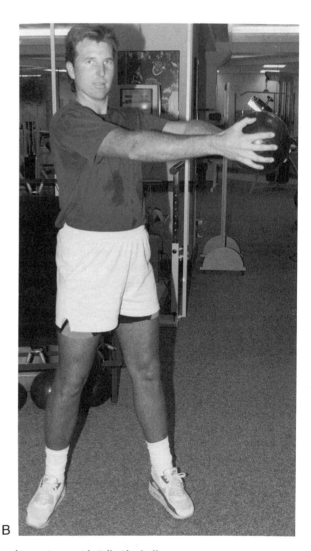

B

**Fig. 44-4.** Warm-up exercise: trunk rotations with 9-lb Plyoball.

(2) throwing movements, (3) trunk extension/flexion exercises, and (4) medicine ball wall exercises (Table 44-2).

## WARM-UP EXERCISES

These exercises are designed to provide the body and especially the shoulder, arm, and trunk an adequate physiologic warm-up before beginning a plyometric program. An active warm-up should facilitate muscular performance by increasing blood flow, muscle/core temperature, speed of contraction, oxygen use, and nervous system transmission.[13,17,19,25,26] The warm-up exercises are listed in Table 44-2. The first three warm-up exercises use a 9 lb medicine ball or a rubber-coated ball called a Plyoball. These warm-up exercises include trunk rotations (Fig. 44-4), trunk side bends (Fig. 44-5), and trunk wood chops (Fig. 44-6). The next two warm-ups are performed with exercise tubing for internal and external rotation movements of the shoulder with the arm in a position of 90 degrees of shoulder

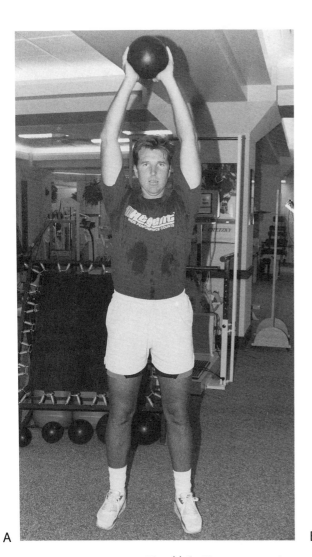

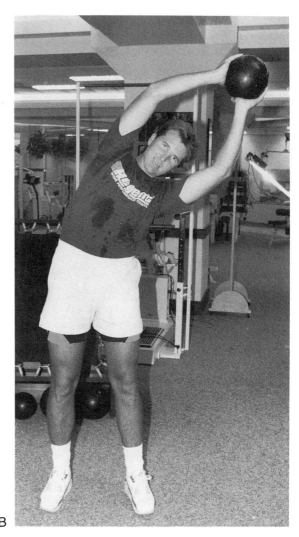

A                                   B

**Fig. 44-5.** Warm-up exercise: trunk side bends with 9-lb Plyoball.

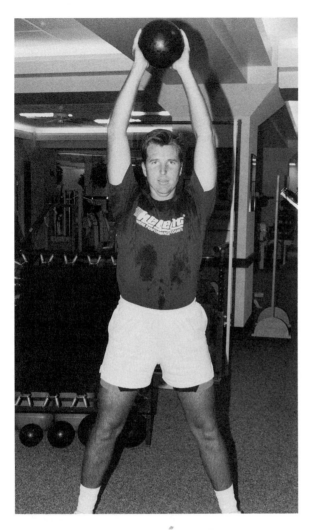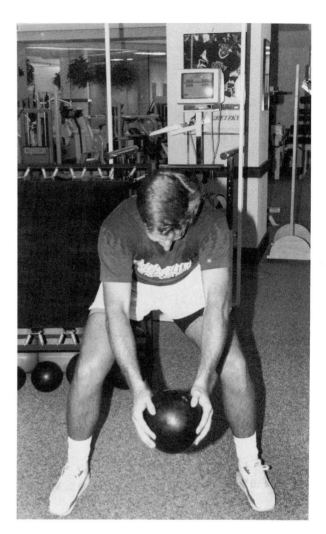

**Fig. 44-6.** Warm-up exercises: wood chop with 9-lb Plyoball.

abduction and 90 degrees of elbow flexion (Fig. 44-7) to stimulate the throwing position. The last warm-up exercise is push-ups with both hands on the ground (Fig. 44-8). Athletes perform two to three sets of 10 repetitions for each of these warm-up exercises.

## THROWING MOVEMENT PLYOMETRICS

The exercises in this group attempt to isolate the muscles and muscle groups necessary for throwing. These exercises are performed in movement patterns similar to the throwing motion. Table 44-2 lists these plyometric exercises. The first four drills are throwing movement plyometrics using a 4 lb Plyoball. The first drill is a two-hand overhead soccer throw (Fig. 44-9), followed by a two-hand chest pass (Fig. 44-10). The next two throws incorporate a step and pass (Fig. 44-11) and a side throw (Fig. 44-12). These exercises can be performed with a partner or with the use of a spring-loaded bounce-back device called the Plyoback (Functionally Integrated Technology, Dublin, Ca.) (see Figs. 44-27 and 44-28).

The next four plyometric drills require exercise tubing. The first movement is plyometrics for the external

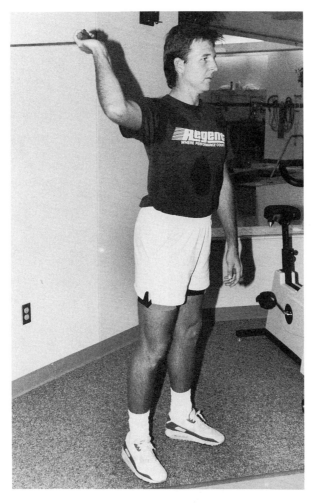

**Fig. 44-7.** Warm-up exercises: internal/external rotation with shoulder abduction of 90 degrees and elbow flexed 90 degrees using exercise tubing.

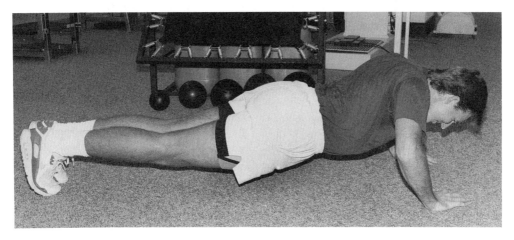

**Fig. 44-8.** Warm-up exercises: push-ups with two hands on the ground.

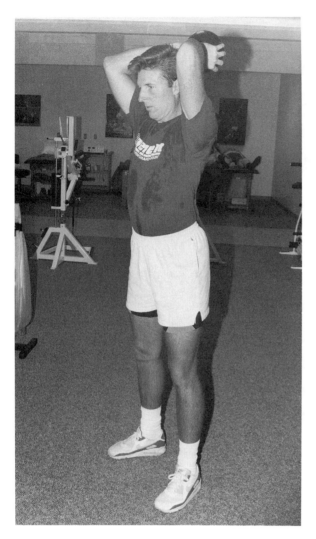

**Fig. 44-9.** Throwing movement exercises: two-hand overhead soccer throw with a 4-lb Plyoball.

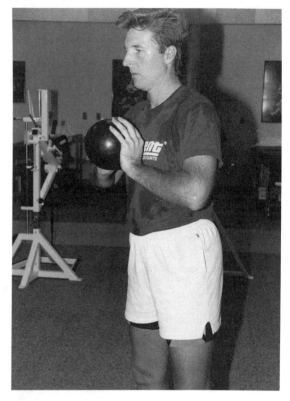

**Fig. 44-10.** Throwing movement exercises: two-hand chest pass throw with a 4-lb Plyoball.

rotators (Fig. 44-13). In this exercise, the athlete stands, bringing the tubing back into external rotation, and holds that position for 2 seconds. Then the athlete allows the external rotation musculature to release this isometric contraction, thus allowing the tubing to pull the arm into internal rotation. Thus, the external rotation are eccentrically controlling this movement. Once the arm reaches horizontal, the external rotations then contract concentrically to bring the tubing back into external rotation. This constitutes one plyometric repe-

tition. This movement is then continued for 6 to 8 repetitions. Similar movements are performed for the internal rotators (Fig. 44-14) and for proprioceptive neuromuscular facilitation diagonal patterns including D2 flexion (Fig. 44-15) and D2 extension of the upper extremities[27-29] (Fig. 44-16). Plyometrics are also performed for the elbow flexors, using exercise tubing (Fig. 44-17). Push-ups to strengthen the serratus anterior, pectoralis major, deltoid, triceps, and biceps musculature are also performed. Plyometric contractions for push-ups are performed using a 6- to 8-in. box or the ground in a depth-jump training manner (Fig. 44-18).

All these exercises are performed for two to four sets of six to eight repetitions two to three times weekly.

The purpose of these exercises is to provide the athlete with advanced strengthening exercises that are more aggressive and at higher exercise levels than

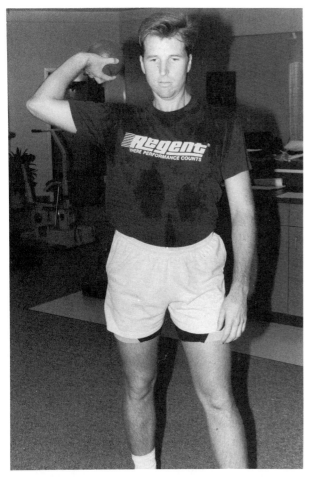

**Fig. 44-11.** Throwing movement exercise: one-hand step and pass throw with a 4-lb Plyoball.

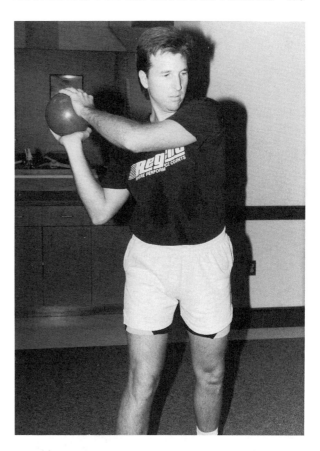

**Fig. 44-12.** Throwing movement exercises: two-hand side throw with a 4-lb Plyoball.

those provided by a simple dumbbell exercise program. These programs can only be used once the athlete has performed a strengthening program for an extended period of time and shows a satisfactory clinical examination.

## TRUNK EXTENSION/ FLEXION PLYOMETRICS

The next two groups of plyometric drills are for trunk strengthening purposes, emphasizing the abdominals and trunk extensors. The exercises in this group are medicine ball sit-ups (Fig. 44-19) and prone back extension (Fig. 44-20).

## PLYOBALL WALL EXERCISES

The last group of exercises or drills uses a 2- and 4-lb medicine ball or Plyoball and a wall, which allows the athlete the opportunity to perform plyometric medicine ball drills without a partner. Also, these exercises of drills can be performed with the Plyoback device. This affords the athlete the luxury to train alone. The first five exercises in this session include a two-handed overhead soccer throw (Fig. 44-21), a two-handed chest pass (Fig. 44-22), a two-handed side-to-side throw (Fig.

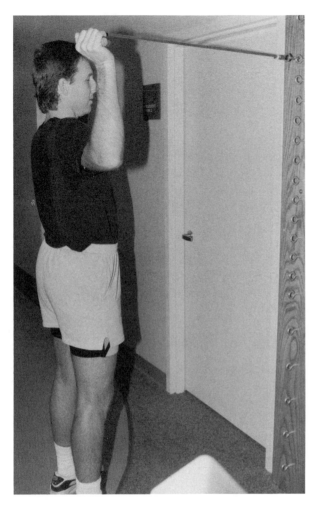

**Fig. 44-13.** Throwing movement exercises: external rotation ploymetrics with exercise tubing.

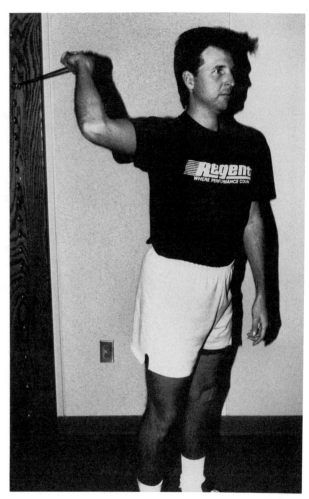

**Fig. 44-14.** Throwing movement exercises: internal rotation plyometrics with exercise tubing.

44-23), a backward two-handed side-to-side throw (Fig. 44-24), and a forward two-handed pass through the legs (Fig. 44-25). Lastly, using a smaller 2 lb medicine ball, the athlete performs a one-handed plyometric baseball throw (Figs. 44-26 and 44-27). These exercises can be performed in the kneeling position to eliminate the use of the lower extremities and to increase the demands on the trunk and upper extremities.

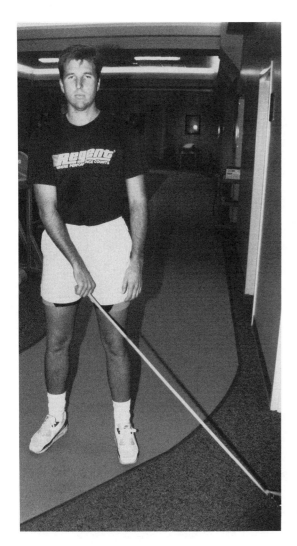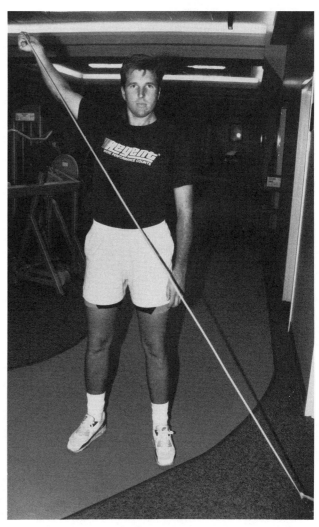

**Fig. 44-15.** Throwing movement exercises: proprioceptive neuromuscular facilitation diagonal pattern D2 flexion plyometrics with exercise tubing.

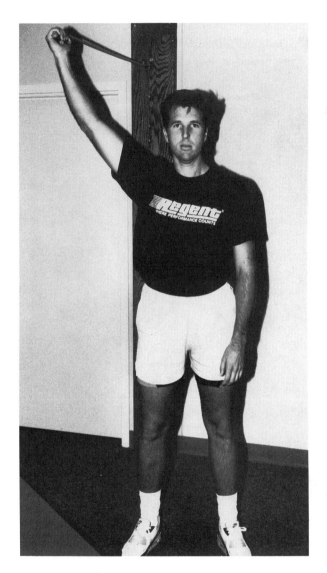 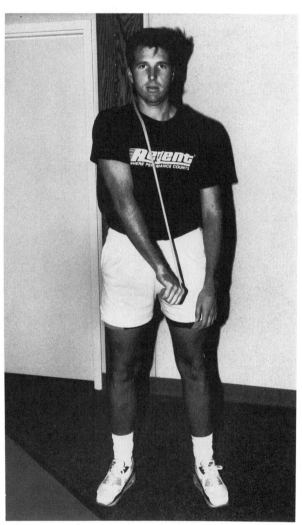

**Fig. 44-16.** Throwing movement exercises: proprioceptive neuromuscular facilitation diagonal pattern D2 extension plyometrics with exercise tubing.

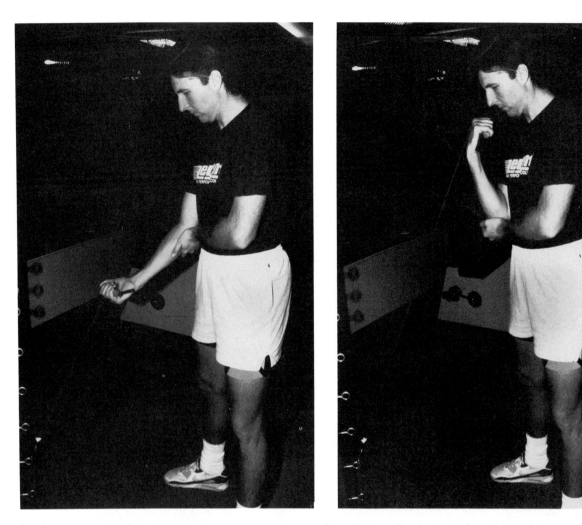

**Fig. 44-17.** Throwing movement exercises: elbow flexion plyometrics with exercise tubing.

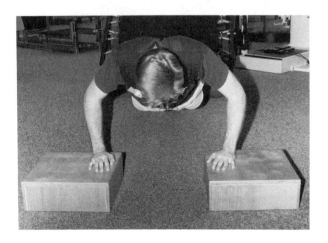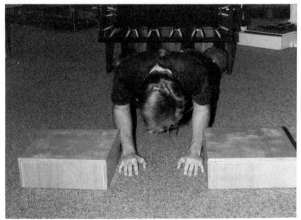

**Fig. 44-18.** Throwing movement exercises: plyometric push-ups using a 6-in. box.

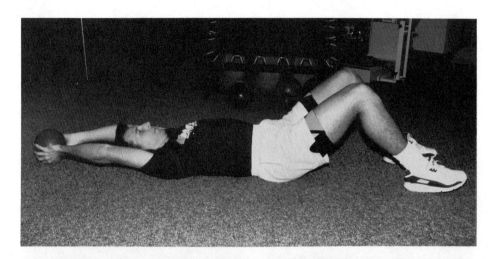

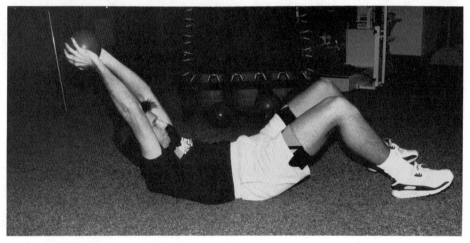

**Fig. 44-19.** Trunk extension/flexion exercises: Plyoball sit-ups (4-lb Plyoball).

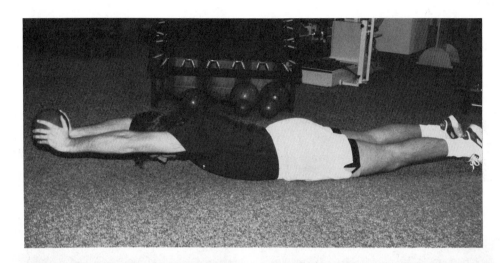

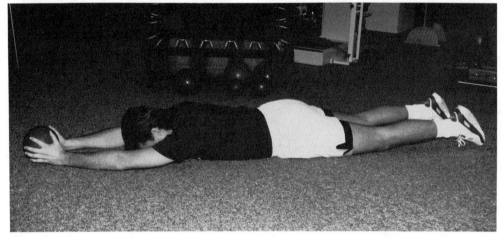

**Fig. 44-20.** Trunk extension/flexion exercises: prone back extensions with a 4-lb Plyoball.

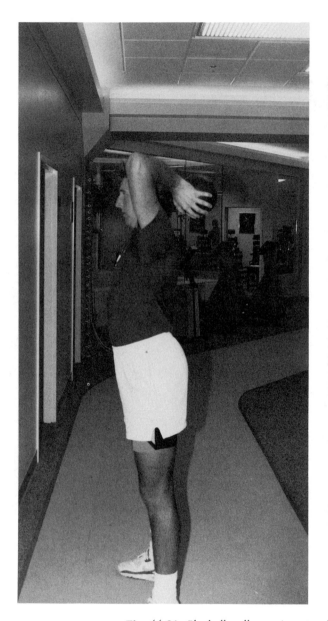
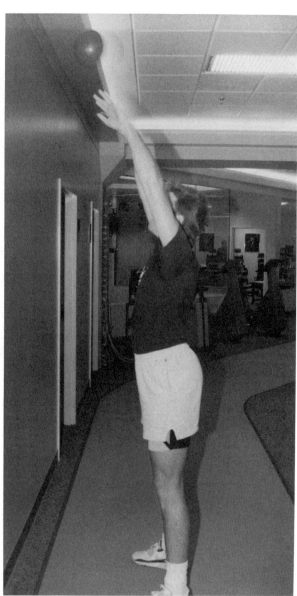

**Fig. 44-21.** Plyoball wall exercises: two-hand soccer throw with 4-lb Plyoball.

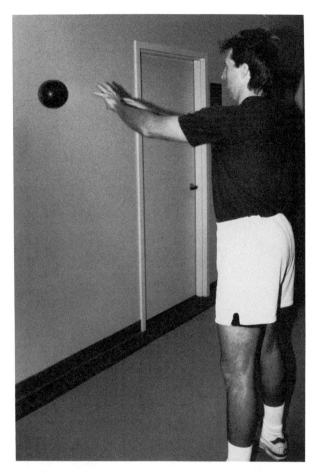

**Fig. 44-22.** Plyoball wall exercises: two-hand chest pass with 4-lb Plyoball.

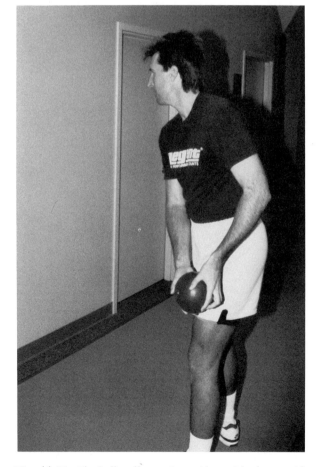

**Fig. 44-23.** Plyoball wall exercises: side-to-side throw with 4-lb Plyoball.

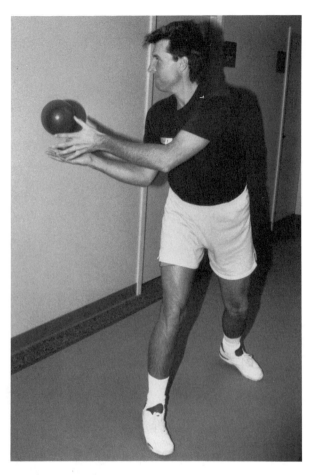

**Fig. 44-24.** Plyoball wall exercises: backward side-to-side throw with 4-lb Plyoball.

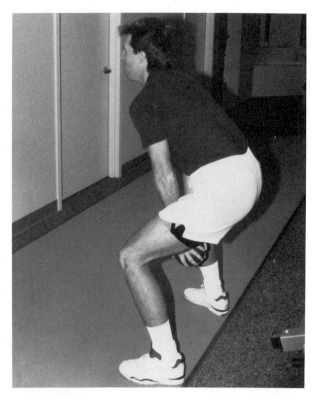

**Fig. 44-25.** Plyoball wall exercises: two-hand pass through the legs with 4-lb Plyoball.

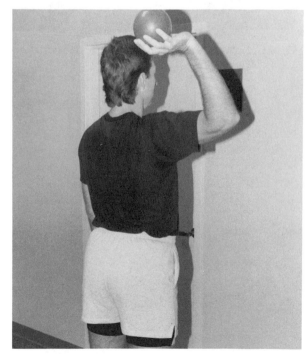

**Fig. 44-26.** Plyoball wall exercises: baseball throw of 2-lb Plyoball into a wall.

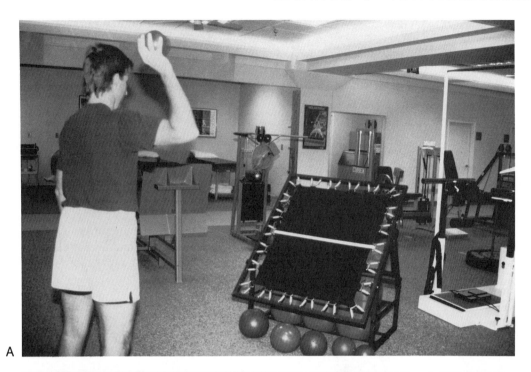

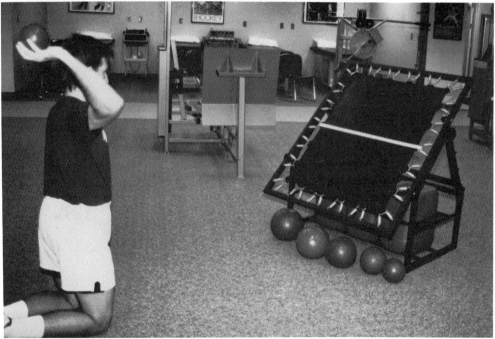

**Fig. 44-27.** Plyometric throwing drill: (**A**) baseball throw of 2-lb Plyoball into the Plyoback (Functionally Integrated Technology, Dublin, CA) device; (**B**) in the kneeling position.

## SUMMARY

Contraindications to performing plyometric upper extremity exercises include individuals exhibiting acute inflammation or pain, immediate postoperative athletes, and individuals with gross shoulder and/or elbow instabilities. The most significant contraindication to implementing a plyometric exercise program is in individuals who have not been involved in any type of weight training program or in those individuals who have not been participating in a training program. This exercise program is intended to be an advanced strengthening program for the competitive athlete. The clinician should be aware of the adverse reactions secondary to this form of exercise, such as postexercise soreness and delayed onset muscular soreness. Also,

this form of exercise should not be performed for an extended period of time because of the large stresses that occur during exercising. Rather, this form of exercise is used during the first and second of preparation phases of training, using the concept of periodization[30] (Fig. 44-28).

This chapter provides the reader with an introduction to the concept of plyometric training, the historical review of the concept, a review of the neurophysiologic response during plyometric training, and a plyometric training program. We encourage the clinician to implement some of these concepts when rehabilitating the competitive athlete. Also, we suggest alterations in this program while using the plyometric concepts. We strongly recommend clinical research to document the efficiency of this training program.

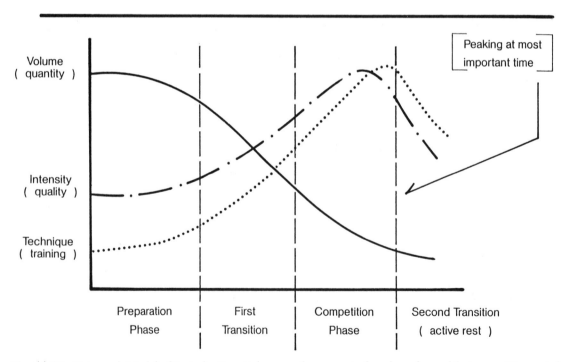

**Fig. 44-28.** Matveyev's Model of Periodization. Volume = the amount of work performed (sets, repetitions, etc.); intensity = the quality of effort; technique = the activity or skill.

# REFERENCES

1. Allman FL: Sports Medicine. Academic Press, Orlando, FL, 1974
2. Verkhoshanski Y: Perspectives in the improvement of speed–strength preparation of jumpers. Yessis Rev Soviet Phys Educ Sports 4:28, 1969
3. Wilt F: Plyometrics, what it is and how it works. Athletic J 55:76, 1975
4. Assmussen E, Bonde-Peterson F: Storage of elastic energy in skeletal muscle in man. Acta Physiol Scand 91:385, 1974
5. Bosco C, Komi P: Potentiation of the mechanical behavior of the human skeletal muscle through pre-stretching. Acta Physiol Scand 106:467, 1979
6. Cavagna G: Elastic bounce of the body. J Appl Physiol 29:29, 1970
7. McGarlane B: Special strength: horizontal and vertical. Track Field Q Rev 83:51, 1983
8. Polhemus R, Burkhardt E: The effects of plyometric training with ankle and vest weights on conventional weight training programs for men. Track Field Q Rev 80:59, 1980
9. Cavagna G, Disman B, Margari R: Positive work done by a previously stretched muscle. J Appl Physiol 24:21, 1968
10. Chu D: Plyometric exercise. Natl Strength Conditioning Assoc J 6:56, 1984
11. Lundin PE: A review of plyometric training. Natl Strength Conditioning Assoc J 7:65, 1985
12. Scoles G: Depth jumping—does it really work? Athletic J 58:48, 1978
13. Adams T: An investigation of selected plyometric training exercises on muscular leg strength and power. Track Field Q Rev 84:36, 1984
14. Pappas AM, Zawacke RM, Sullivan TJ: Biomechanics of baseball pitching: a preliminary report. Am J Sports Med 13:216, 1985
15. Buchwald JS: Exteroceptive reflexes and movement. Am J Phys Med 46:121, 1967
16. Granit R: Receptors and Sensory Perception. Yale University Press, New Haven, CT, 1962
17. Astrand P, Rodahl K: Textbook of Work Physiology. McGraw-Hill, New York, 1970
18. O'Connel A, Gardner E: Understanding the Scientific Bases of Human Movement. Williams & Wilkins, Baltimore, 1972
19. Franks BD: Physical warm-up. In Morgan WP (ed): Ergogenic Aids and Muscular Performance. Academic Press, Orlando, FL, 1972
20. Granit R: The Basis of Motor Control. Academic Press, Orlando, FL, 1970
21. Brodal A: Neurological Anatomy in Relation to Clinical Medicine. Oxford University Press, New York, 1969
22. Patten BM: Human Embryology. McGraw-Hill, New York, 1953
23. Eldred E: Functional implications of dynamic and static components of the spindle response to stretch. Am J Phys Med 46:129, 1967
24. Komi P, Bosco C: Utilization of stored elastic energy in leg extensor muscles by men and women. Med Sci Sports 10:261, 1978
25. DeVries HA: Physiology of Exercise for Physical Education and Athletics. WC Brown, Dubuque, IA, 1974
26. McArdle WD, Katch FI, Katch VL: Exercise Physiology; Energy, Nutrition, and Human Performance. Lea & Febiger, Philadelphia, 1981
27. Knott M, Voss DE: Proprioceptive Neuromuscular Facilitation. 2nd Ed. Harper & Row, New York, 1968
28. Sullivan PE, Markos PD, Minor MD: An Integrated Approach to Therapeutic Exercise; Theory & Clinical Application. Reston Publishing Co., Reston, VA, 1982
29. Voss DE, Knott M, Kabat M: Application of neuromuscular facilitation in the treatment of shoulder disabilities. Phys Ther Rev 33:536, 1953
30. Matveyev L: Fundamentals of Sports Training. Progress Publishers, Moscow, 1977

# 45

# The Decelerator Mechanism: Eccentric Muscular Contraction Applications at the Shoulder

*J. GREGORY BENNETT*
*NORMAN A. MARCUS*

It has long been appreciated that a good "follow-through" demanding a rapid deceleratory rotational component of shoulder motion is essential in sports such as pitching, golf, and tennis. One might question this conventional wisdom by pointing out that the action on the ball has already been accomplished by this time, and hence its trajectory is already determined. This observation clearly misses the point—to excel at such sports one must reproducibly accelerate and then abruptly decelerate the arm in a consistent pattern that does not cause injury. The accomplishment of only one satisfactory golf swing is never enough, although often that is all that may be achieved (Fig. 45-1).

In throwing sports, the shoulder rotates faster than 7,000 degrees/s and then decelerates over a very brief interval.[1] The muscles that accomplish the acceleration are relatively large—the pectorals major and minor, the latissimus dorsi, the triceps, and the anterior deltoid muscles.[2] After release, the rapidly moving extremity has principally the supraspinatus, teres minor, and infraspinatus muscles to rely on, short and relatively small muscles, to slow down a limb with a very large moment of inertia. These muscles are asked to accomplish this task by contracting while they are lengthening (an eccentric muscle action) and to replicate this motion many dozens or even hundreds of times in a single athletic session. It is for this reason that physical therapy paradigms emphasizing eccentric muscle exercise

have potential for the throwing athlete in both the rehabilitation and training setting.

## DECELERATOR (ECCENTRIC) MECHANISM

Errors in deceleration, regardless of the joint or muscle groups involved, have long been identified with orthopaedic injuries, especially sports. Hughston et al[3] first spoke of the bodies' deceleration mechanism relative to the quadriceps femoris musculature in anterior knee pain (Fig. 45-2). Since that time, errors in the deceleration phenomena, or eccentric muscle action, have received increased scrutiny in the scientific literature.[4–6]

Eccentric muscle action, by definition, is muscular lengthening while resisting a load whether it be the weight of a body part or the body part plus a foreign object such as a tennis racket. Negative work is performed and energy is absorbed. Eccentric muscle action functions to decelerate a load and/or body parts and for shock absorption in activities such as walking and running. By comparison, concentric muscle action involves shortening of a muscles' length and functions to accelerate the body part or external load. Positive work is performed.[7]

The third type of muscular action, isometric action, involves active tension of the muscle without changing

567

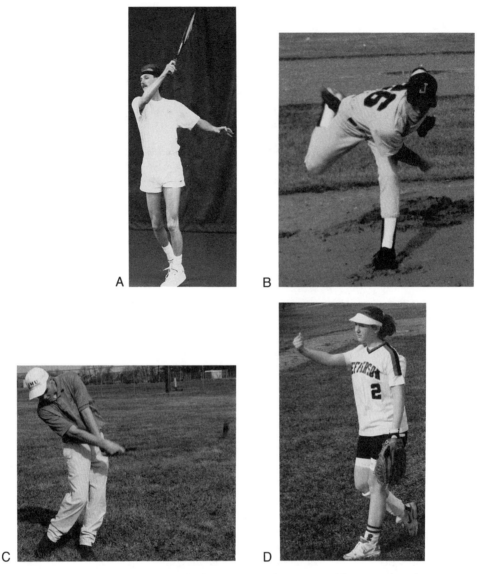

**Fig. 45-1.** Deceleration (eccentric muscle action) plays a major role in most athletic events and activities of daily living. Sports with major deceleration activity at the shoulder include, but are not limited to, tennis, baseball, golf, and fast pitch softball.

the muscle's length. No external work is performed, and isometric muscle action functions to stabilize body parts. Most activities require combinations of concentric, eccentric, and isometric muscle action. For instance, when throwing a baseball, the rotator cuff musculature performs all three muscular actions. The subscapular muscle is involved in acceleration (concentric action), the supraspinatus stabilizes the humerus (isometric action), and the supraspinatus, infra-

spinatus, and teres minor are active in deceleration (eccentric action).

The advent of isokinetic dynamometry in the late 1960s allowed, for the first time, the study of maximal muscle force production in vivo. Research in the area of muscle dynamics has been prolific; however, much of the scientific data reflects only concentric muscle action because of the limitations of early dynamometry. The advent of devices such as the Kin-Com (Chatta-

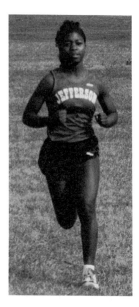

**Fig. 45-2.** Running (and walking) require coordinated deceleration action by the quadriceps femoris, gluteal, and trunk extensor muscles.

nooga Corp., Chattanooga, TN) has allowed further exploration of human muscle action by allowing maximal testing of both the concentric and the eccentric components of muscle action. The importance of this becomes obvious given the instances of eccentric or deceleration variences explained in this text. The importance is further compounded by several physiologic differences between concentric and eccentric muscular action. These differences for the most part preclude inferences regarding eccentric muscle function from data derived from concentric muscle action. An appropriate model using eccentric muscle action is required.

This chapter explores the physical components of concentric and eccentric muscle actions and how they affect motor adaptation. Also, basic applications and implications for injury and rehabilitation are explored, in particular as applied to the shoulder.

## PHYSIOLOGY

Several studies have been conducted comparing energy demand, electromyographic (EMG) output, and force production between concentric and eccentric muscle action. Also, studies have been published comparing relative muscle soreness and the effect of speed

on force output during concentric versus eccentric muscle action (Table 45-1).

The first and most striking difference between concentric and eccentric muscle action is the maximal tension each is capable of producing. The lay person would readily concede it is much easier to go down steps (eccentric muscle action) than it is to go up steps (concentric muscle action). The amount of work performed in both cases is similar (i.e., moving the weight of the body the distance of a flight of steps). Work here is relative and excludes the effect of gravity and potential energy. Yet the perceived exertion is much lower descending stairs. Laboratory research has substantiated this perception. Komi and colleagues, as well as others, demonstrated in several instances that eccentric muscle actions are capable of producing the greatest tensile force[8-12] (Fig. 45-3). A particularly interesting study performed by Komi examined the force–velocity relationship of concentric and eccentric muscle actions.[9] In all instances, eccentric muscle actions produced the greatest amount of tension. Interestingly, as velocity increased, concentric tension decreased, whereas eccentric tension increased. This is critically important to clinicians using isokinetic exercise. Therapists often increase the speed of exercise to diminish force, a method that is only appropriate concentrically. The tension ratio of eccentric to concentric at higher velocities (7 cm/s) became nearly 2:1[13] (Fig. 45-4). Cress et al,[14] in a similar study using isokinetic dynamometry, found that during increases in eccentric velocities, force levels remained consistent; however, increases in concentric speed led to diminished force production.

Because eccentric muscle actions produce greater tension than their concentric counterpart, the meta-

**Table 45-1. Concentric Versus Eccentric Muscle Action**

| | |
|---|---|
| EMG | More concentric fiber activation is required (higher amplitude EMG signal) at the same resistance compared with eccentric fiber activation. |
| Energy | More energy (as reflected by oxygen demand) is used for concentric work compared with the same amount of eccentric work. |
| Muscle soreness | Eccentric exercise is far more likely to create muscle soreness than similar amounts of concentric exercise. |
| Force development | More force can be generated eccentrically than concentrically. |

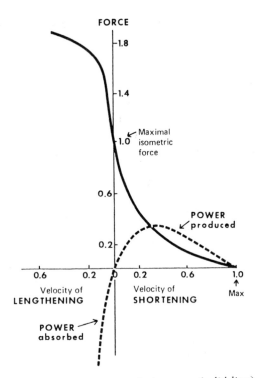

**Fig. 45-3.** The classic force-velocity curve (solid line) obtained on an isolated muscle. It shows the maximal force that can be developed when a muscle is contracting at different speeds. The maximal force in a concentric activity is less than in an isometric contraction. A rapid eccentric contraction produces the highest force. The maximal power (i.e., the force times the velocity of contraction) is represented by the dashed line.

bolic demand during eccentric muscle action would be expected to be greater. However, an extensive amount of research on the subject has shown the opposite to be true.[13,15-17] Knuttgen et al[17] compared oxygen consumption, heart rate, and pulmonary ventilation during concentric and eccentric bicycling. Oxygen consumption increased with intensity for both concentric and eccentric activity but at a far greater rate during concentric exercise. Similar results were found for heart rate and pulmonary reactions. Their study in essence showed that when generating the same tension, eccentric muscle actions caused smaller circulatory and pulmonary reactions and used a much smaller volume of oxygen[17] (Fig. 4-5). Similar results have been substantiated by Newham et al[18] in comparison of ultrastructural changes caused by concentric and eccentric

muscle actions. Not only were metabolic costs less during eccentric exercise, but electromyographic (EMG) activity was diminished at the same tension. EMG activity, which is a reflection of fiber electrical activity and not strength, suggests the conclusion that fewer fibers are producing equal tension to the concentric counterpart. In other words, fewer fibers contract eccentrically than concentrically to produce equal amounts of tension. Given that fewer muscle fibers are activated, it is consistent that eccentric activity creates a lower metabolic demand. This, too, can be exploited clinically. By using primarily eccentrically loaded exercises, patients with poor endurance should be able to tolerate longer workouts. This could be particularly applicable in neurologic cases and in early orthopaedic rehabilitation when emphasis is placed on endurance and not on strength.

Another consideration in a metabolic comparison would be the work performed by Friden and colleagues[19] regarding adaptive responses to eccentric exercise. They found eccentric strength to be remarkably trainable and showed strength gains of 375 percent during their experimental period of 8 weeks. Coinciding with these gains was the confirmation of decreased oxygen consumption during eccentrics, which they expressed as improved nervous coordination.[19]

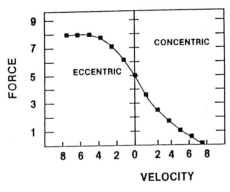

**Fig. 45-4.** Relationship of force attained by an isolated muscle during maximal stimulation at various velocities: for concentric contractions, velocity of shortening; for isometric contractions, zero velocity; and for eccentric contractions, velocity of lengthening. Each point represents the force the muscle generates in a single experiment. The muscle length remains constant. (From Knuttgen and Kraemer,[33] with permission.)

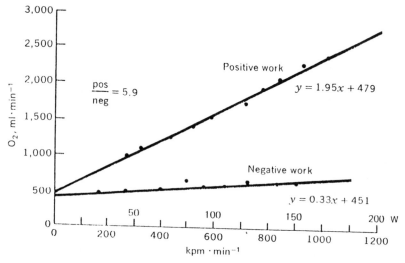

**Fig. 45-5.** Oxygen uptake in positive (upper curve) and negative (lower curve) work. The work consisted of riding a bicycle on a motor-driven treadmill. Uphill was positive work and downhill was negative work (with the movements of the pedals reversed). The work load equals the product of the weight of the subject plus the bicycle times the vertical distance that this weight was lifted or lowered. Oxygen uptake was also measured at zero load (free wheeling). Rate of pedaling = 45 rpm. The average cost of positive work was 5.9 times higher than that of negative work. (From Asmussen,[34] with permission.)

The final physiologic difference found when comparing concentric and eccentric muscle actions is the production of delayed onset muscle soreness (DOMS). The scope of this paper is not to discuss in detail the physiologic factors that cause soreness but rather to provide an overview of the phenomenon of muscle soreness. A study by Newham and co-workers[20] comparing pain and fatigue secondary to concentric and eccentric exercise found that only the eccentrically trained group experienced DOMS. Although many authors believe that only eccentric exercise causes muscle soreness, it is not without controversy.[18,21,22] Tiidus and Ianuzzo[23] found that overall intensity was the primary factor in creating DOMS, especially as compared with duration. Their work, though, also substantiates the previously established premise that eccentric exercise is the primary cause of soreness. Given the previously established information that eccentric muscle action creates the greatest tension, eccentric exercise would create more profound DOMS. It is important to note that DOMS is not necessarily harmful. There is no evidence that DOMS causes any long-term damage or leads to long-term functional impairment.[13,21] In fact, the best way to avoid DOMS is through repetitive

exercise.[21] The ability of eccentric exercise to improve strength is well established and accepted.[9,13,15,19,24]

In summary, it becomes apparent that different forms of exercise have vastly different effects on skeletal muscle. Despite that the same muscle is involved in both eccentric and concentric activity, several important differences occur between concentric and eccentric action. Eccentric action produces significantly greater tension with maximal voluntary effort. At equal tension, eccentrics use less oxygen, place lower demand of the cardiorespiratory system, and show lower EMG activity (see Table 45-1).

The applications and implications of deceleration in sports and rehabilitation are numerous. Increasingly, applications for eccentric rehabilitation are found in the literature.[24,25] The development of dynamometers capable of measuring deceleration capacity promises to further research in this area. The throwing shoulder is an area of particular interest. Because shoulder injuries often involve the deceleration mechanism (the rotator cuff), further exploration is necessary. Specifically, impingement syndromes and rotator cuff injuries require closer analysis. Many authors consider the two intricately linked, particularly in instances of overuse or chronic stress injuries. Unfortunately, no examples were found in the scientific literature showing the efficacy of a particular exercise program in either a prophylactic or rehabilitative sense. To date, only examples of exercises that emphasize particular muscles or muscle groups with empirical support for their application are found.[2,4,8,25]

Patients with rotator cuff tendinitis and an adequate subacromial space may often benefit from rehabilitation of the cuff muscles in their eccentric phase of muscle action. It is important that high-velocity eccentric exercise be restricted until after the acute inflammatory phase subsides; thereafter, eccentric rehabilitation becomes useful at increasingly greater velocities. We have not seen exacerbation of symptoms in this situation from the rehabilitation itself nor rotator cuff inflammation or rupture. Patients with overt subacromial crepitus and type III acromions[26] have been excluded from this type of exercise until the underlying pathology was corrected.

Eccentric muscle action has many unique properties that made it well adapted to the requirements of sport. In the shoulder, relatively small muscle groups with low oxygen demand may function repetitively at high velocities of rotation to result in a smooth, balanced throw. In some disease states, rehabilitation of the eccentric muscles may be useful in restoring improved kinematics of the shoulder, providing the cuff is not inflamed, grossly damaged, or impinging severely. In such cases, rehabilitation alone may be detrimental to treatment.

The optimal paradigm for eccentric exercise has yet to be identified. Present technology partially emulates the throwing motion and does succeed in placing eccentric load on the muscles. Future research may result in even better models such that rehabilitation of the deceleration mechanism more closely approximates its function in sport. As this goal is achieved, it should be possible to obtain better measurements of muscle function during the throwing motion and to analyze patterns of weakness requiring treatment.

# APPLICATIONS AT THE SHOULDER

Symptoms of the rotator cuff muscles are multifactorial and may originate in any one case from factors that are primarily mechanical (i.e., acromial morphology),

vascular, or traumatic. In cases in which impingement is the primary problem, it is unlikely that rehabilitation alone by any technique will solve a problem based on insufficient subacromial space. In the postoperative phase, however, it is precisely these muscles that require retraining to achieve better kinematics. It can therefore be of benefit to obtain preoperative isokinetic tests (including eccentrics) both to establish a baseline and to instruct the patient in appropriate rehabilitation techniques that will be used later. If impingement is a secondary phenomenon in some patients caused by microsubluxation, one might expect rehabilitation to have a more satisfactory effect, as long as capsular tissues maintain their competency.

Several parameters are tested and evaluated in our clinics. Test speeds were arbitrarily chosen to be 50 and 150 degrees/s. Many clinicians choose to test at higher velocities to be more "functional," but because we test the eccentric component, lower velocities were chosen. Motions tested include flexion, abduction, internal rotation, and external rotation. Also, horizontal flexion is often tested from 90 degrees of abduction, especially in those individuals doing a lot of overhead activity (Table 45-2; Fig. 45-6). It is our opinion that the ability to work overhead for sustained periods is frequently overlooked in testing and rehabilitation programs.

## Eccentrics and Shoulder Dysfunction

Eccentric muscle action, as mentioned earlier in this text, plays an important role in shoulder function. EMG studies by Jobe et al[27] and others[28,29] demonstrated the musculature of the rotator cuff functions primarily eccentrically in sports. This phenomena probably extends to activities of daily living as well but is not documented in the literature. It is well documented that the rotator cuff is frequently involved in shoulder pathology,[30–32] making adequate eccentric or deceleration capacity paramount to preventing or relieving shoulder symptoms.

**Table 45-2. Selected Isokinetic Test Parameters for Concentric and Eccentric Evaluation**

| | |
|---|---|
| Velocities | 50 and 150 degrees/s |
| Positions | Abduction |
| | Internal Rotation |
| | Horizontal Flexion |
| | Flexion |
| | External Rotation |

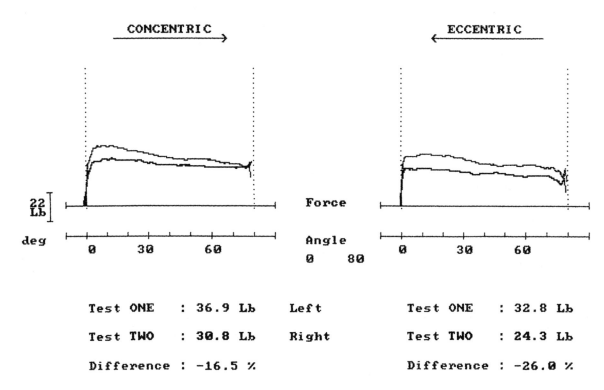

```
Patient   : EXTERNAL ROTATORS
Date      : 03/03/93
Joint     : Shoulder
Physician : THAL
Diagnosis : RTC TENDINITIS
```

```
        Procedures            Test ONE              Test TWO

        Date       :          03/03/93              03/03/93
        Side       :            Left                 Right
        Move. Patt.:           Ext rot              Ext rot
        Lever Arm  :           22 cm.               22 cm
        Angles     :        0 to 80 deg.         0 to 80 deg.
        Velocity   :             60                   60
        File       :          11.CHA               11.CHA
```

**CONCENTRIC** →                     ← **ECCENTRIC**

22 Lb              Force

deg                Angle
                   0    80

0    30    60                          0    30    60

```
Test ONE   : 36.9 Lb    Left      Test ONE   : 32.8 Lb

Test TWO   : 30.8 Lb    Right     Test TWO   : 24.3 Lb

Difference : -16.5 %              Difference : -26.0 %
```

```
Assessment: CONCENTRIC DEFICIT OF 16.5%
            ECCENTRIC DEFICIT OF 26%
```

**Fig. 45-6.** Sample isokinetic test data demonstrating a force output deficit in the shoulder external rotators. Note the increased amplitude of the deficit during eccentric muscle action.

Unfortunately, most existing isokinetic data examine only the concentric component of rotator cuff action and specifically concentric external rotation. Because the supraspinatus is not primarily an external rotator and the rest of the cuff musculature acts primarily eccentrically, concentric analysis of external rotation may be inadequate. Ideally, studies will be forthcoming comparing and analyzing the eccentric action of the rotator cuff.

A novel approach to rehabilitation of rotator cuff tendinitis has been developed in our clinic, especially for throwing athletes. A comprehensive approach to rehabilitation is advocated and undertaken. This chapter focuses only on the unique applications of our program, and a comprehensive approach is discussed elsewhere in this textbook. The unique application of our program is the rapid application of eccentric or deceleration forces to the rotator cuff in external rotation. An outline of this program is presented in Table 45-3. This component is part of a comprehensive program including modalities and concentric exercise as mentioned earlier. All types of exercise including isometric and isotonic muscle actions are thoroughly incorporated.

The purpose of this program is to simulate the rapid reversal from concentric internal rotation to eccentric external rotation to eccentric extenal rotation that occurs at ball release. Isokinetic machines cannot switch muscle action in mid-arc of motion, so a slight modification was made. Patients are positioned in a seated posture with the actuator aligned with the plane of the scapula. In cases of instability, care is taken to protect the patient from recurrence by positioning the humerus in a more stable position, such as 45 degrees of flexion. The patient experiences a concentric external rotation muscle action at a relatively slow speed, which is doubled when the eccentric action begins (see Table 45-3). By doing this, the patients are taught rapid activation of eccentric muscle action, as is required in throwing sports. The results of this type of rehabilitation in addition to traditional intervention has been encouraging.

Eccentric muscle action is routinely incorporated into our spectrum approach to rehabilitation. Our approach is to exercise muscles globally, that is both concentrically and eccentrically for each muscle group. Additional emphasis is then placed on that component in which the muscle most frequently acts. The internal rotators primarily accelerate to receive concentric emphasis and so forth depending on the musculature. As with all rehabilitation programs, exercise must be modified to the involved pathologies with appropriate constraints made for healing tissues.

## SUMMARY

Eccentric muscle action has several unique features compared with its concentric counterpart. At equal external loads, less muscle activation (based on EMG) occurs and less energy is expended during eccentric muscle action. Many sports injuries are identified as occurring during deceleration requiring strong eccentric muscle action.

However, most activities of daily living require both concentric and eccentric muscle action. A cup of coffee must be successfully accelerated and decelerated to drink it. Stairs must be both ascended and descended. It would, therefore, be an error to only exercise the concentric or eccentric component of muscular action. A comprehensive program emphasizing both concentric and eccentric muscle action is advocated. Special emphasis can then be added to that component that is sports-specific or lifestyle-specific.

**Table 45-3. A Novel Protocol to Adjunct Rotator Cuff Rehabilitation Emphasizing Rapid Deceleration**

| Dynamometer mode | Isokinetic concentric/eccentric or passive |
|---|---|
| Motion | External rotation |
| Concentric velocity (degrees/s) | 50 |
| | 75 |
| | 100 |
| Eccentric velocity (degrees/s) | 100 |
| | 150 |
| | 200 |

## REFERENCES

1. Perry J: Anatomy and biomechanics of the shoulder in throwing, swimming, gymnastics, and tennis. Clin Sports Med 2:247, 1973
2. Ryu RKN, McCormick J, Jobe FW, Moynes DR, Antonelli DJ: An EMG analysis of shoulder function in tennis players. Am J Sports Med 16:481, 1988

3. Hughston JC, Walsh WM, Puddu G: Patellar Subluxation and Dislocation. WB Saunders, Philadelphia, 1984

4. Ellenbecker TS, Davies GS, Rowinski MS: Concentric versus eccentric isokinetic strengthening of the rotator cuff: objective data versus functional tests. Am J Sports Med. 16:64, 1988

5. Tomberlin JP, Basford JR: A comparitive study of eccentric and concentric quadriceps strengthening (abstract). Phys Ther 67:790, 1987

6. Highenboten CL, Jackson AW, Meske NB: Concentric and eccentric torque comparisons for knee extension and flexibility in young adult males and females using the kinetic communicator. Am J Sports Med 64:248, 1985

7. Åstrand P, Rodahl K: Textbook of Work Physiology. McGraw-Hill, New York, 1977

8. Kanecki M, Komi PV, Aura O: Mechanical efficiency of concentric and eccentric exercises performed with medium to fast contraction rates. Scand J Sport Sci 6:15, 1984

9. Komi PV: Measurement of the force–velocity relationship in human muscle under concentric and eccentric contraction. Med Sport 8:224, 1973

10. Komi PV, Burkirk ER: Effect of eccentric and concentric muscle conditioning on tension and electrical activity of human muscle. Ergonomics 15:417, 1972

11. Komi PV, Rusko H: Quantitative evaluation of mechanical and electrical changes during fatigue loading of eccentric and concentric work. Scand J Rehabil Med 3:121, 1974

12. Rogers KL, Berger RA: Motor unit involvement and tension during maximum voluntary concentric, eccentric, and isometric contractions of the elbow flexors. Med Sci Sports 6:253, 1974

13. Komi RV: Relationship between muscle tension, EMG and velocity of contraction under concentric and eccentric work. In Desmedt JD (ed): New Developments in Electromyography and Clinical Neurophysiology. Vol. 6. Karger, Basel, 1973

14. Cress NM, Peters KS, Chandler JM: Eccentric and concentric force–velocity relationships of the quadriceps femoris muscles. J Orthop Sports Phys Ther 16:82, 1992

15. Asmussen E: Positive and negative work. Acta Physiol Scand 28:364, 1953

16. Bigland B, Lippold OC: The relation between force, velocity and integrated electrical activity in human muscles. J Physiol 123:214, 1954

17. Knuttgen HG, Nadel ER, Pandolf KB, Patton JF: Effects of training with eccentric muscle contraction on exercise performance, energy expenditure and body temperature. Int J Sports Med 3:13, 1982

18. Newham DJ, McPhail G, Mills KR, Edwards RHT: Ultrastructural changes after concentric and eccentric contractions of human muscle. J Neurol Sci 61:109, 1983

19. Friden J, Seger J, Sjostrom M, Ekblom B: Adaptive response in human skeletal muscle subjected to prolonged eccentric training. Int J Sports Med 4:177, 1983

20. Newham DJ, Mills KR, Quigley BM, Edwards RHT: Pain and fatigue after concentric and eccentric muscle contractions. Clin Sci 6:455, 1983

21. Armstrong RB: Mechanisms of exercise-induced DOMS: a brief review. Med Sci Sports Exerc 16:629, 1984

22. Byrnes WC, Clarkson PM, Katch FI: Muscle soreness following resistance exercises with and without eccentric contraction. Res Q 56:283, 1985

23. Tiidus PM, Ianuzzo ED: Effects of intensity and duration of muscle exercise on delayed soreness and serum enzyme activities. Med Sci Sports Exerc 15:461, 1983

24. Bennett JG, Stauber WT: Evaluation and treatment of anterior knee pain using eccentric exercise. Med Sci Sports Exerc 18:526, 1986

25. Curwin S, Stanish W: Tendinitis: Its Etiology and Treatment. Collamore Press, Toronto, 1984

26. Bigliani LU: Morphology of the acromion and its relationship to rotator cuff tears. Orthop Trans 10:228, 1986

27. Jobe FW, Tibone JE, Perry J et al: An EMG analysis of the shoulder in throwing and pitching. A preliminary report. Am J Sports Med 11:3, 1983

28. Chandler TJ, Kibler WB, Stracener EC et al: Shoulder strength, power, and endurance in college tennis players. Am J Sports Med 20:455, 1992

29. Jobe FW, Moynes DR, Tibone JE et al: An EMG analysis of the shoulder in pitching. A second report. Am J Sports Med 12:218, 1984

30. Hawkins RJ, Kennedy JC: Impingement syndrome in athletes. Am J Sports Med 8:151, 1980

31. Tibone JE, Elrod B, Jobe FW et al: Surgical treatment of tears of the rotator cuff in athletes. J Bone Joint Surg 68A:887, 1986

32. Neer CS II: Impingement lesions. Clin Orthop 173:70, 1983

33. Knuttgen HG, Kraemer WJ: Terminology and measurement in exercise performance. J Applied Sport Sci Res 1:1, 1987

34. Asmussen E: Positive and negative muscular work. Acta Physiol Scand 28:364, 1953

# 46

# Open and Closed Chain Rehabilitation for the Shoulder Complex

*DANIEL CIPRIANI*

Rehabilitation of the shoulder girdle complex is certainly one of the most comprehensive challenges for the health care practitioner. This intricate network of force couples, muscle synergies, deceleration mechanisms, and soft tissue guide wires operates to provide the athlete with an incredible means of functional adaptability.[1-5] And because the shoulder girdle complex is capable of greater mobility than any other joint complex, a sound understanding of the biomechanics of movement involving the shoulder is imperative. Unfortunately, the shoulder girdle complex presents a further complication to the practitioner—the upper extremity functions well in both open kinematic chain activities as well as closed kinematic chain activities. Normal shoulder girdle biomechanics and the approaches to rehabilitation are greatly affected by these two variables.

## CLOSED CHAIN VERSUS OPEN CHAIN

Identifying the differences between the open chain segment and the closed chain segment can be made more effective by evaluating the concepts of function, gravity, muscle action, and proprioception as they relate to the mechanics of movement. By definition alone, it is generally accepted that closed chain activity involves movement of the proximal segments in relation to a fixed distal segment, such as occurs during the stance phase of gait. In this instance, the distal segment (the foot) is fixed while the proximal knee and hip move as the body passes over the fixed foot. Open chain activity, however, involves movement of the distal segment in relation to a fixed proximal segment. Again using the example of gait, the swing phase illustrates the distal foot and leg moving in relation to the fixed hip.

### Function

Thus in terms of function and the kinetic chain concept of activity, the lower extremities tend to function predominantly in a closed chain environment, with the foot in contact with the ground more so than moving through the air. Walking, running, and standing all involve closed chain function of the lower extremity. And although the lower extremity does perform some open chain activity (swing phase of gait), most injuries and difficulties with rehabilitation will center around the closed chain functions of the lower extremity.

The upper extremity, however, tends to function predominantly in an open chain environment. Most activities of daily living, as well as most athletic events, require freely moveable hands to manipulate our environment. Feeding and grooming, as well as throwing and swinging a racquet, all require open chain function of the upper extremity. And just as the lower extremity must function in an open chain environment, the upper extremity must be able to function in a closed chain

577

environment. Athletes fall and push and swing from bars, all of which necessitates movement of the shoulder and arm around a fixed distal hand. From a rehabilitation standpoint, this dual role of the upper extremities complicates our mission for returned function after injury. Not only must we attempt to create a shoulder joint that is stable and mobile, we need to create an upper extremity that can function well in an unstable environment as well as a mobile environment.[6]

## Gravity

When assessing the effects of gravity on human function, the concepts of open and closed chain environments become more important. In the closed chain environment, such as with gait or falling on an outstretched arm, gravity is creating an acceleration of movement—specifically toward the ground. Gravity assists in closing the chain.[6] Thus the action of muscles will predominantly focus on decelerating this motion with eccentric contractions. Closed chain gait is a sequence of gravity acceleration controlled by eccentric muscle decelerations. In the open chain, however, gravity creates a challenge to any imposing load by providing us with an invisible force that resists our movements. Thus, to initiate an open chain movement requires a concentric muscle force against gravity. Eventually, an eccentric contraction must occur to return us to our normal starting point.

Based on function and muscle action, it appears that most closed chain function would require predominantly an eccentric contraction to slow down the effects of gravity, whereas open chain function would require predominantly concentric contractions to initiate movement. However, any health care professional evaluating human movement and injury pathology will argue that open chain activity actually requires a fine balance between concentric and eccentric muscle contractions; this fact alone complicates our rehabilitation and training methods for the upper extremity.

## Muscle Action

An additional area of complication relates to the speed of muscle function and the differences between open chain and closed chain activities. Evaluating gait, a closed chain activity, shows a fairly consistent pattern of joint accelerations and decelerations, all relatively reproducible in the rehabilitation setting. Evaluating a volleyball serve, however, reveals a full spectrum of angular accelerations at the shoulder joint and upper extremity. The toss hand may go through a limited range of movement at a set speed. However, the sending arm may first wind up slowly in the early stage, accelerate quickly into full flexion to create an opportunity for an elastic recoil, followed by an extremely high-velocity angular acceleration into diagonal extension of the shoulder. Or in the case of lifting a heavy crate, the shoulder muscles may be functioning isometrically, with no speed at the shoulder. Open and closed chain function creates for us multiple speeds, quite variable and often very difficult to reproduce in the rehabilitation setting.

Finally, in reference to the upper extremity and the differences between open and closed chain activities, we need to look more closely at the actual type of muscle action occurring. For instance, the latissimus dorsi is well accepted as an extensor and internal rotator of the shoulder. However, based on recent observations, the latissimus dorsi, when functioning in a closed chain, actually functions as a trunk extensor by way of its attachment into the thoracolumbar fascia.[7] A more simplistic example of the changing muscle functions in relation to the type of kinetic chain activity is seen with the biceps, which creates elbow flexion of the

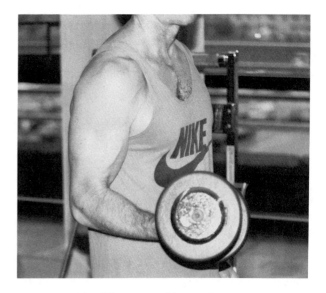

**Fig. 46-1.** Normal biceps function.

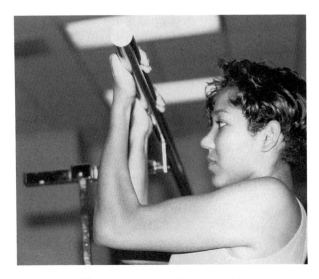

**Fig. 46-2.** Reverse muscle action of biceps.

forearm moving on the humerus in the open chain and elbow flexion with the humerus moving on the fixed forearm in the closed chain (Figs. 46-1 and 46-2).

## Proprioception

When discussing the differences between open chain and closed chain function, it is always necessary to discuss the concepts of proprioception, as they are affected by these two types of activity. From an advantage standpoint, the lower extremities benefit greatly from the closed chain environment they function in. This environment provides a unique perception tool for the moving athlete, namely, the ground. Ground reaction forces provide the athlete with a key proprioceptive feedback system, queuing the joints with information regarding spacial relationships, forces of muscle contractions, and the speed of movement. Open chain function is rather void of this important assistance for proprioception and must function based on the feedback of gravity and rotational activities within the joints. The upper extremity, as well as the lower extremity, must rely solely on the feedback from the joint mechanoreceptors, muscle spindles, golgi tendon organs, and visual cues to assist in controlled, focused movement in the open chain. This is not to say that these receptor systems are not sufficient for normal

function; unfortunately, injury to the musculoskeletal system has been shown to affect these proprioceptive devices, and thus any additional support is appreciated and must be taken advantage of.[8–13]

## SHOULDER REHABILITATION AND THE KINETIC CHAIN CONCEPT

### Review of Literature: Current Concepts

A great deal has been written dealing with proper shoulder rehabilitation exercises.[1,6,14,15–21] Some of the more typical and well-accepted exercises are described by Anderson[14] in his review of shoulder exercises. This review consists of both open and closed chain strengthening and stretching. Warner et al[20] supported the need for these exercises in a review of the instability patterns and impingement potentiators of the shoulder girdle, with specific recommendations regarding muscle imbalances between the internal and external rotators of the shoulder. Wagner[21] described the typical rotator cuff exercises, which generally include internal and external rotation against resistance in different arm positions using free weights. A recent electromyographic analysis of these rehabilitation exercises showed strong support for varying the positions of the arm during exercise. These investigators were able to outline specific exercises to isolate different components of the rotator cuff and shoulder girdle musculature.[5]

The greatest common denominator of these rehabilitation exercises is the influence of open chain strengthening approaches. The upper extremity is primarily an open chain tool, and most overuse sports injuries occur during open chain function—especially during decelerations. Traumatic falls on the outstretched arm in a closed chain position also contribute to the rehabilitation setting. However, it is not the fall itself that poses the problem down the road for the athlete; the unstable or dysfunctional shoulder caused by the closed chain injury can become a chronic problem for open chain function. This makes it more important than ever to provide the athlete with not only a comprehensive open chain rehabilitation environment but also an innovative closed chain training period. As reported by Nash[18] in his review of rotator cuff problems, shoulder

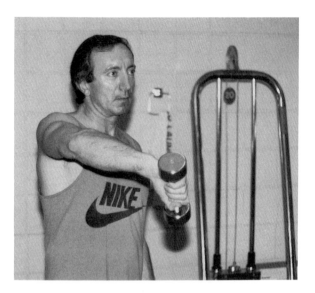

**Fig. 46-3.** "Empty can" exercise.

rehabilitation programs fail most often because they are not "extensive enough."

The design of a shoulder rehabilitation program must therefore consider multiple factors: the goal of the athlete and the type of functional environment to which they plan to return. Will this environment re-quire primarily open chain activities at set speeds, or will they need to be able to function in a closed chain environment with multiple speeds? Also the influences of posture and overall trunk and leg strength must be considered. Are the rehabilitation approaches the same for an athlete with a thoracic kyphosis and rounded shoulders predisposed to impingement problems? How much influence do the lower extremities have on the ability to throw a baseball any distance or speed? Thus, the series of events surrounding upper extremity function are very much based on a "chain reaction" of activities surrounding the entire moving system.[6]

## Traditional Kinetic Chain Exercises

Current shoulder rehabilitation exercises incorporate both free weights and mechanical forms of resistance. The more traditional free-weight exercises include sidelying external rotation, the "empty can" (Fig. 46-3), bench pressing, and overhead presses. Also, emphasis is being placed on the posterior shoulder to include exercises such as the bent-over row, bent-over flies (Figs. 46-4 and 46-5), and the lateral pull-down. These same exercises with free weights can be easily repro-duced using rubber tubing, manual resistance, soup cans, or other forms of external resistance.

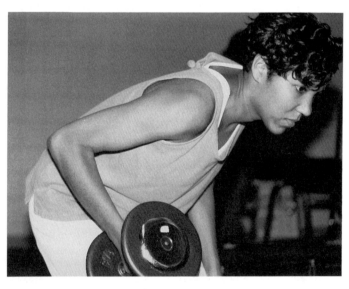

**Fig. 46-4.** Bent-over row.

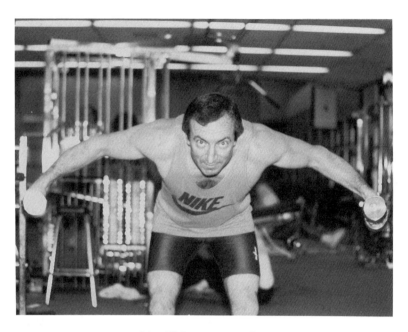

**Fig. 46-5.** Bent-over flies.

Mechanical resistance to the shoulder is much more specific. While the free-weight exercises require ongoing muscle input from the postural and trunk muscles to stabilize, many mechanical apparatus fix the trunk and postural muscles to facilitate total isolation of the particular muscles to be addressed. The advantage to this approach is especially effective in the early stages of rehabilitation, when the clinician needs to isolate, re-educate, and protect the athlete from extraneous movements. However, as the athlete improves, a shift must occur to a more free-standing, total body functional training approach. The appropriate biomechanics of the shoulder is very much influenced by the entire system.

## Traditional Open Kinetic Chain Rehabilitation

### Return to Function

The greatest advantages of the free-weight, open chain approach to shoulder strengthening are found in the exact nature of the exercises.[3,15] Free-weight exercises provide an environment that is not only functional but also traditional in the sense that open chain activities

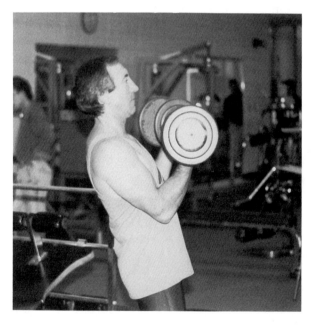

**Fig. 46-6.** Involvement of trunk.

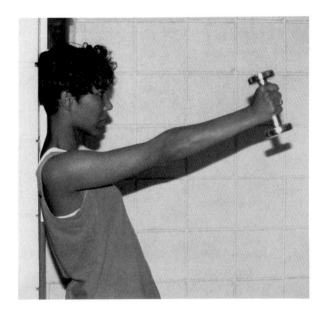

**Fig. 46-7.** Isolated shoulder flexion.

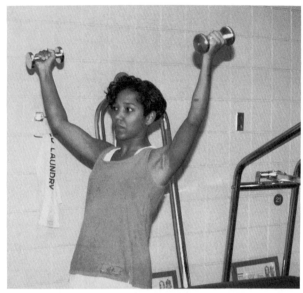

**Fig. 46-8.** Diagonal patterns.

against gravity-enhanced forces are familiar to the shoulder girdle muscles. Free-weight exercises require that not only do the prime movers take part in the action but that the stabilizing muscles and the synergists must also assist in the movement pattern (Fig. 46-6). Because free weights require active participation of the entire trunk and lower extremities, greater muscle involvement is facilitated. However, if the goal is to isolate a particular shoulder muscle, free weights can allow fairly precise isolation of a movement. The preacher curl, sidelying external rotation, and front raises with the back stabilized are just a few examples (Fig. 46-7).

### Position Awareness

From a neuromuscular standpoint, free-weight open chain exercises are extremely effective for reproducing resistance throughout a proprioceptive neuromuscular facilitation diagonal pattern, either unilaterally or bilaterally (Fig. 46-8). And because free-weight exercises are generally performed standing, balance and coordination against a dynamic external load can be challenged. Thus the athlete's position awareness can be enhanced as a moving extrinsic load is applied to the body. Eliminating visual cues by performing these

same exercises with eyes closed is an additional method to challenge the rehabilitating athlete further (Fig. 46-9). Finally, the neuromuscular challenge imposed by open chain free weights provides effective feedback to the muscles of static posture, creating a situation that requires alert and facilitated muscle spindles to maintain a static posture in conjunction with a moving shoulder girdle.

### Substitution

In the early phases of shoulder rehabilitation, the benefits of open chain exercises can also be used to focus on identifying pathologic weak links in the muscular system. After injury and during rebuilding, a tendency exists for surrounding muscles to substitute function for the weaker, injured, or involved muscle. This form of substitution is usually deemed inappropriate, as the normal or effective biomechanics of the shoulder girdle are altered. For instance, the elevating of the shoulder girdle to compensate for a weak rotator cuff could be detrimental to the rehabilitation process. Open chain exercises allow us to observe these abnormal patterns of substitution, patterns that may not be as readily available in a fixed motion system.

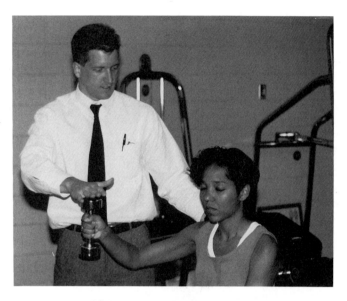

**Fig. 46-9.** Position awareness: eyes closed.

## Legal Cheating

In the same terms, as rehabilitation progresses and an athlete improves in strength of the involved muscle, it becomes even more important to recognize the avenues an athlete may take to compensate for fatigue and weakness that may occur with additional activity. Strengthening exercises appear to be most beneficial when the exercise is taken to the point of muscular failure. The method in which the athlete compensates for this failure may clue the clinician as to the patterns an athlete may use to substitute (Fig. 46-10). This legal cheating is as important as abnormal substitution from the standpoint that substitution is certainly going to occur and therefore we need to be aware of how it will occur and if we can improve the strength and function of these substitutors.[15]

The tendency to substitute is readily recognized during open chain exercises, as the weaker muscles fail and additional support is recruited from the stabilizers and synergists. And although substitution is natural, in the early stages of rehabilitation it is important that it be recognized and trained appropriately. Once an appropriate foundation is built within the prime muscle, legal cheating can then take the place of substitution, and normal function substitution can be allowed to occur.

## Variance of Position

One additional benefit of open chain exercise, especially with free-weight-type equipment, is the ability to vary the position of the athlete during an exercise. The clinician is thus able to provide the athlete with a controlled environment of varied positions for the

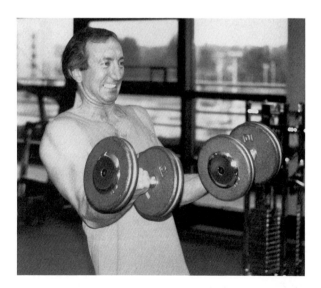

**Fig. 46-10.** Substitution during biceps curls.

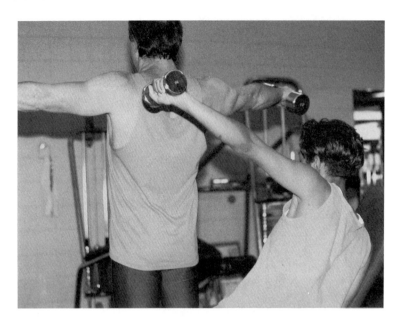

**Fig. 46-11.** Variance of position: lateral fly.

same exercise. This allows us to recreate some of the "real world" forces that an athlete will face at a level that is safe and sufficient. Figures 46-11 and 46-12 show some of the different clinically controlled variations of common free-weight exercises. During these exercises, the perceived forces of gravity and extrinsic load change dramatically.

## Nontraditional Open Chain Exercises

The addition of plyometrics to the rehabilitation environment has been an exciting and worthy adjunct to traditional functional retraining. The upper extremities experience these plyometric forces daily, from activities as simple as taking milk out of the refrigerator to more complicated tasks such as shrugging off a would-be tackler in football. A load is experienced, with a brief eccentric contraction, followed by an explosive, controlled concentric contraction of the effected muscle groups. Traditional plyometrics include a myriad of weighted balls (Plyoballs) and elastic tubing exercises aimed at challenging the forceful phase shift of a plyometric contraction.

Also, it is possible to take advantage of the athlete's own body weight for dynamic exercise, challenging the plyometric phase shift. Exercises initially described

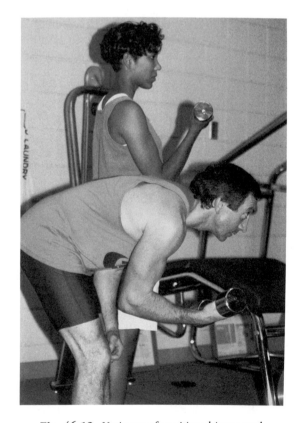

**Fig. 46-12.** Variance of position: biceps curl.

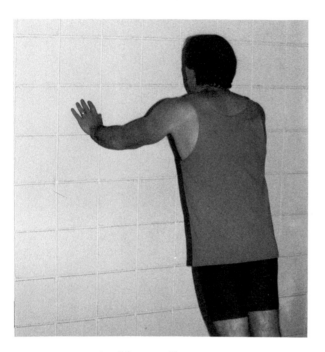

**Fig. 46-13.** Wall reactions.

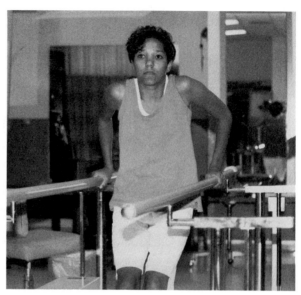

**Fig. 46-14.** Basic dips.

by Gray termed *wall reactions* require that an athlete fall toward a wall, forcefully decelerate their motion, and then quickly accelerate away from the wall.[6,15] This form of plyometrics is ideal for challenging the athlete with controlled falls—until the athlete is prepared to actually fall to the ground. And although this form of exercise looks like a closed chain exercise, controlling the hand to catch the body's falling weight is an effective open chain proprioceptive challenge (Fig. 46-13). Also, wall reactions can be performed at increasing distances from the wall, thereby increasing the magnitude of muscle contraction necessary to arrest motion and then accelerate motion.

## Traditional Closed Chain Exercises

Mechanical resistance, provided by an external fixed motion apparatus, provides the clinician with the opportunity to isolate and emphasize a particular muscle group or movement pattern. Greater objectivity regarding progression, overall strength, and isolated function are certainly advantages to mechanical apparatus. Additional traditional closed chain exercises would include those that use the athlete's body as the external resis-

tance. For instance, chin-ups take advantage of the reverse muscle action of the biceps as the humerus is moved on a fixed forearm. Dips provide an environment requiring proximal stabilization with motion of the shoulders as the distal hands are fixed (Fig. 46-14). Although chin-ups and dips are considered closed chain because of the fixed distal segments, that the trunk is now moving freely through space provides a certain reverse open chain challenge to the upper extremity. And, in fact, wall reactions (described earlier) can be performed in both an open and closed chain format.

## Nontraditional Closed Chain Exercises

To provide additional creative and challenging exercises in a closed chain to the rehabilitation program, clinicians only need to look in their clinic at some of their traditional lower extremity exercise devices. These lower extremity exercises can in some ways be modified and adapted to provide for an unusual upper extremity challenge. After all, with the body's ability to respond and adapt to changing stresses, it becomes vital to continue providing changing stresses for the athlete to adapt to. Figures 46-15 to 46-19 illustrate some of the less traditional upper extremity exercises

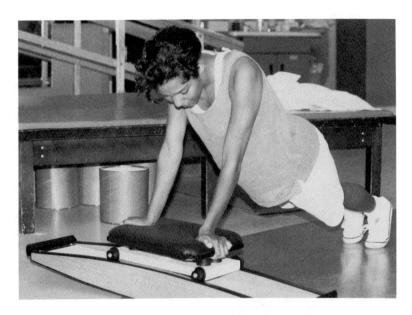

**Fig. 46-15.** Upper extremity profitter: dynamic push-up.

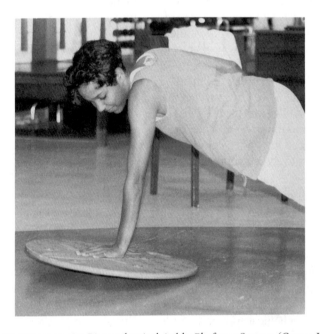

**Fig. 46-16.** Upper extremity Biomechanical Ankle Platform System (Camp, Jackson, MI).

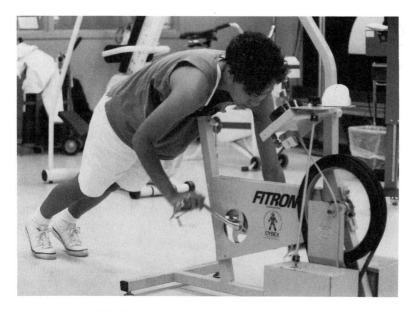

**Fig. 46-17.** Stationary bike dynamic stability.

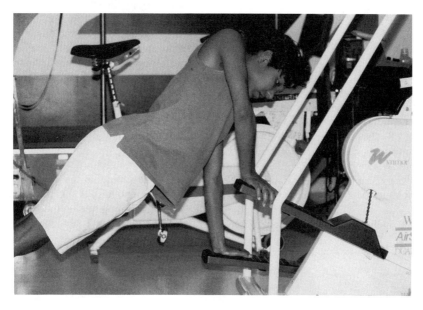

**Fig. 46-18.** Hand stair climber.

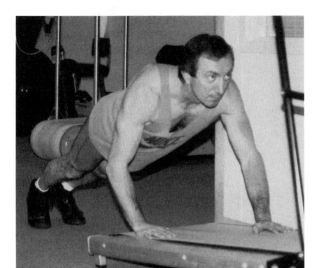

**Fig. 46-19.** Treadmill: hand gait.

available. These exercises require that the shoulder girdle complex function not only with great stability but also with great mobility on a dynamically fixed distal segment.

# REFERENCES

1. Jobe FW, Moynes DR, Brewster CE: Rehabilitation of shoulder joint instabilities. Orthop Clin North Am 18:473, 1987

2. Frame MK: Anatomy and biomechanics of the shoulder. p. 1. In Donatelli R (ed): Physical Therapy of the Shoulder. 2nd Ed. Churchill Livingstone, New York, 1991

3. Norkin CC, Levangie PK: The shoulder complex. p. 207. In: Joint Structure and Function: A Comprehensive Analysis. 2nd Ed. FA Davis, Philadelphia, 1992

4. Soderberg GL: The shoulder. p. 109. In: Kinesiology: Applications to Pathological Motion. Williams & Wilkins, Baltimore, 1986

5. Townsend H, Jobe FW, Pink M, Perry J: Electomyographic analysis of the glenohumeral muscles during a baseball rehabilitation program. Am J Sports Med 19:264, 1991

6. Gray GW: Chain Reaction: Successful Strategies for Closed Chain Testing and Rehabilitation. Wynn Marketing, Adrian, MI, 1990

7. Porterfield J, DeRosa C: Mechanical Low Back Pain: Perspectives in Functional Anatomy. WB Saunders, Philadelphia, 1991

8. Dvir Z, Koren E, Halperin N: Knee joint position sense following reconstruction of the anterior cruciate ligament. J Orthop Sports Phys Ther 10:117, 1988

9. Garn SN, Newton RA: Kinesthetic awareness in subjects with multiple ankle sprains. Phys Ther 68:1667, 1988

10. Gray GW: Rehabilitation of running injuries: biomechanical and proprioceptive considerations. Top Acute Care Trauma Rehabil 1:67, 1986

11. Ingersoll CD, Knight KL: Patellar location changes following EMG biofeedback or progressive resistive exercises. Med Sci Sports Exer 23:1122, 1991

12. Keshner EA: Controlling stability of a complex movement system. Phys Ther 70:844, 1990

13. Lentell GL, Katzman LL, Walters MR: The relationship between muscle function and ankle stability. J Orthop Sports Phys Ther 11:605, 1990

14. Anderson TE: Rehabilitation of common shoulder injuries in athletes. J Musculskeletal Med 5:15, 1988

15. Cipriani DJ, Gray GW: Open and closed chain rehabilitation of the shoulder. In: The Challenge of Shoulder Rehabilitation: A Multidisciplinary Approach. Meeting Planners, Virginia Beach, VA, 1990

16. Glousman RE, Jobe FW: How to detect and manage the unstable shoulder. J Musculoskeletal Med 7:93, 1989

17. Mulligan E: Conservative management of shoulder impingement syndrome. Athl Training 23:348, 1988

18. Nash HL: Rotator cuff damage: re-examining the causes and treatments. Phys Sports Med 16:129, 1988

19. O'Connell PW, Nuber GW, Mileski RA, Lautenschlager E: The contribution of the glenohumeral ligaments to anterior stability of the shoulder joint. Am J Sports Med 18:579, 1990

20. Warner JP et al: Patterns of flexibility, laxity, and strength in normal shoulders and shoulders with instability and impingement. Am J Sports Med 18:366, 1990

21. Wagner L: Strengthening the rotator cuff. Natl Strength Condit J 12:54, 1990

# 47

# Conservative Treatment of Shoulder Instability

## JOSEPH S. SUTTER

Instability of the glenohumeral joint is a common yet complex problem that challenges all members of the rehabilitation team. This chapter presents current concepts and techniques regarding conservative management and rehabilitation for shoulder instability.

Several classifications for glenohumeral instability are described in the literature. The degree of instability (subluxation or dislocation), the chronology (acute, chronic, recurrent), and the nature (voluntary or involuntary) are all important parameters that need to be identified and addressed in the rehabilitation program.[1] For organizational purposes, this chapter is presented from the perspective of etiology (trauma, microtrauma, or atraumatic). The rehabilitation program is initially focused on anterior instability, and modifications for posterior and multidirectional instability are discussed at the end of the chapter.

No single rehabilitation program is absolute or correct. Therefore, the "cookbook" approach is a disservice both to the patient and to the practitioner. This text serves as a guideline to be modified as indicated by individual considerations and treatment responses. References are cited when available, but much of this rather clinical approach is based on clinical experience.

## REHABILITATION AFTER TRAUMATIC ANTERIOR GLENOHUMERAL DISLOCATION

Anterior dislocation represents more than 90 percent of all glenohumeral dislocations, and trauma is the most common cause.[2,3] The injury usually occurs when the arm is forced beyond its available range of motion into the combined position of external rotation, extension, and abduction.[1,4] Several investigators have reported a high recurrence rate of dislocation, ranging from 60 to 90 percent in the young and active population.[3,5,6] Other studies reveal that these percentages have been greatly reduced after a short period of immobilization and a supervised rehabilitation program.[7,8] Newer arthroscopic stabilization procedures have shortened rehabilitation times and allowed greater recovery of motion, which makes surgery a more favorable option after traumatic dislocation.[9-12] If surgery is declined, it seems reasonable to propose a rehabilitation period of approximately 12 weeks after the first-time dislocation. However, patients who have had multiple dislocations and are experiencing daily symptoms caused by instability are not usually benefited by conservative measures. A course of surgical stabilization and supervised postoperative rehabilitation is indicated for this patient.

Conservative treatment after dislocation is 3 weeks of immobilization in a sling or immobilizer followed by an approximate 12-week rehabilitation program to regain range of motion, strength, and neuromuscular control of the arm. The immobilization period is age-dependent, as the older patient is mobilized sooner to avoid potential complications of adhesive capsulitis. However, it is imperative to rule out possible fractures and associated rotator cuff tears, which would dictate a different course of rehabilitation.

All patients can benefit from early physical therapy intervention involving instruction in isometric exercises to the glenohumeral musculature and dynamic

589

exercise of the distal limb joints and the scapulothoracic region. The exercises are intended to reduce muscle atrophy and to improve circulatory and metabolic processes to help maintain a more "physiologic limb" during immobilization. The exercises are performed in a protected position of glenohumeral internal rotation at a frequency of three-five times per day and five-ten repetitions of each exercise. The patient can also be instructed in cervical range of motion exercises, massage, positioning, and the home application of heat and ice in attempts to reduce pain and expedite the healing process. These simple techniques are often quite helpful early on. Patients older than 40 years are also started on gentle and controlled pendulum exercises at 7 to 10 days that are performed in the sling.

After the immobilization period, a general recovery of motion is encouraged from 120 to 150 degrees of active flexion at 4 to 6 weeks, with full flexion attained at 6 to 8 weeks postinjury (Table 47-1). External rotation is limited to 30 degrees for the first 6 weeks and is progressed to full range of motion at 8 to 10 weeks. The combined position of external rotation and abduction is approached last. Although the time schedule for older patients is more aggressive, healing tissues are not stressed for the first 6 weeks.

Range of motion is best recovered in an active assisted manner initially. Pulley and L-bar (Breg Corp; Vista, CA) exercises are useful for the patient at home. The patient is instructed to work in desired ranges and to move gradually into tightness or stiffness but to stop short of any significant pain. Exercises are performed for 5 to 10 minutes twice per day. In the clinic, the therapist can work effectively with the patient in the supine position. One can use active assisted and active exercises in a very controlled fashion by providing

### Table 47-1. General Rehabilitation Timeframe After Initial Anterior Dislocation

Phase 1. Immobilization—3 weeks
   *Exercises:* distal joints of arm and hand to tolerance, glenohumeral isometrics, dynamic resistive scapular exercise

Phase 2. Motion recovery—3–8 weeks
   *Exercises:* an overlapping sequence of active assisted–active resistive exercise. External rotation with abduction is approached last

Phase 3. Strengthening and neuromuscular training—6–12 weeks
   *Exercises:* scapular and rotator cuff musculature emphasis, weight-bearing exercises

Phase 4. Functional progression—12–20 weeks

Phase 5. Return to activity—20–26 weeks

manual assistance and/or resistance. The therapist can stabilize the shoulder and control the range of motion and forces such that undue stress is not applied to the involved structures. Elevation is first regained in the sagittal and scapular planes, while external rotation is initiated with the arm by the side. One gradually progresses to the apprehension position of combined external rotation and abduction from each direction with an appreciation of the type of end feel present. Significant force is rarely necessary to regain full motion, and many younger patients must be restricted from regaining motion too quickly.

Strengthening exercises are initially performed in a high-repetition low-load mode, progressing to sets of 20 to 30 repetitions. This is well tolerated and quite functional, as most use of the shoulder, except with certain athletes, is submaximal and repetitive in nature. Attention is focused on scapular and rotator cuff musculature.

Muscles are strengthened in isolation and with synergistic patterns, and most safely exercised in a midrange that renders the joint in a less vulnerable position. Strengthening exercises are limited to shoulder height and below initially and not progressed above this height unless required by functional demands. The use of long lever arms with resistive exercises is discouraged, as this may produce undesired shear forces at the glenohumeral joint. Accordingly, contact points (hand placement, weight cuffs, machine attachments) during resistive exercise are made at the mid-upper arm rather than at the hand with the elbow extended (Fig. 47-1). As the strengthening program progresses, the resistance is progressively increased and repetitions may be decreased if further muscle hypertrophy and "strength" are desired goals. The rigor of the endurance exercises can also be adjusted as indicated, and upper body ergometers, rowing machines, and pulley systems are all useful. Additionally, the specificity regarding concentric/eccentric muscle function, aerobic/anaerobic energy pathways, and the velocity of movement should be addressed in the final aspects of the strengthening program.

Scapular muscles have been emphasized of late where they were largely disregarded in the past. The concept of proximal stability to allow proper distal mobility and function is a basic concept in normal human movement.[13] Studies involving electromyographic recordings of scapular muscles reveal very high activation during many athletic activities, especially the serratus anterior.[14,15] Thus, the scapular stabi-

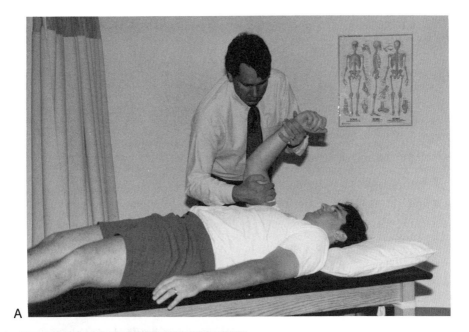

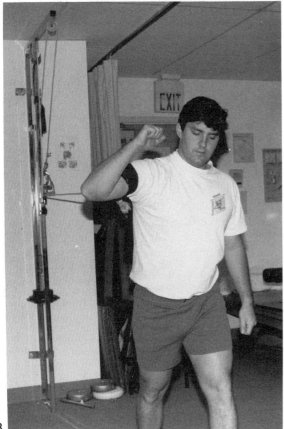

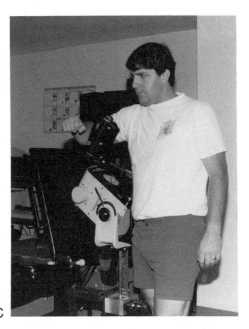

**Fig. 47-1.** Contact points are made at upper arm to maximize joint stability during resistive exercise. (**A**) Manual contact; (**B**) pulley cuff; (**C**) isokinetic pad.

lization program can be considered the cornerstone of the strengthening program. Additional electromyographic investigation has identified exercises with specific scapular muscle activation, which has helped therapists to design more effective exercise programs.[16] Scapular strengthening exercises, including push-ups, shrugs, dips, upright rows, and elevation in the scapular plane, are emphasized in the rehabilitation program. Resistive forms are combinations of manual resistance, body weight, elastic devises, isokinetics, and isotonic equipment.

Clinically, the rotator cuff (specifically the supraspinatus) is adversely affected by the required immobilization. This can present as inadequate humeral head depression with active shoulder elevation. It can be visualized as superior humeral head migration and is often accompanied by excessive scapular shrugging. Different exercises have been described to enhance the performance of the rotator cuff. These include the "empty can" position (elevation with thumb down), isotonic internal and external rotation in sidelying positions, proprioceptive neuromuscular facilitation diagonal patterns, and resisted internal and external rotation in the upright position with the arm at the side using manual, elastic, or isokinetic resistance.[13,17] The prone rotator cuff exercises described by Blackburn et al[18] are beneficial and may enhance the recruitment of scapular muscles. A modification of some of these prone exercises can be made to avoid the extreme apprehension position by simply lowering the arm below the horizontal plane to reduce stress on noncontractile anterior restraints.

Additional exercises that can produce undesired forces on noncontractile restraints must be modified to be performed safely. Push-ups, pull-downs, and the bench press are performed with hands in close and avoiding the last 10 to 20 degrees of shoulder extension (more midrange). Pull-downs and military press performed with widebars and machines are kept in front rather than behind head. Supine fly exercises and the butterfly machines are limited to −30 degrees of the coronal plane while maintaining glenohumeral internal rotation (Fig. 47-2; Table 47-2).

Range of motion and strength are not usually difficult to recover after traumatic dislocation. Perhaps the key parameter of rehabilitation becomes the neuromuscular control of the limb as there is a kinesthetic deficit present after anterior glenohumeral dislocation.[19] The

### Table 47-2. Exercise Modifications per Direction of Instability

| Direction of Instability | Position to Avoid | Exercises to Be Modified or Avoided |
|---|---|---|
| Anterior | Combined position of external rotation and abduction | Fly, pull-down, push-up, bench press, military press |
| Posterior | Combined position of internal rotation, horizontal adduction, and flexion | Fly, push-up, bench press, weight-bearing exercises |
| Inferior | Full elevation, dependent arm | Shrugs, elbow curls, military press |

potential inadequacy of the damaged "static" stabilizers (capsulolabrum complex) also emphasizes the importance of proper neuromuscular control.[1] The required dynamic stabilization is provided by the complex interaction of scapular, rotator cuff, and trunk musculature, which occurs with simultaneous movements at the scapulothoracic, glenohumeral, acromioclavicular, sternoclavicular, and intervertebral joints.[20] Movement must be synchronized such that normal kinematics and biomechanics occur without overstressing any particular structure(s) selectively. The difficulty of this task is clear.

Neuromuscular techniques used early in the program to help establish proper scapulothoracic rhythms and to avoid superior humeral head migration and shoulder shrugging would be the following: Supraspinatus sets at 30 degrees of elevation in the scapular plane held for 5 seconds isometrically, manually resisting excessive scapular movement, and facilitating rotator cuff recruitment with quick stretches, muscle belly "tapping," and electromyographic biofeedback. The use of mirrors or video cameras for visual feedback to the patient with their active assisted and active elevation exercises is also helpful.

Techniques to elicit muscular co-contractions at the shoulder girdle are very useful to help provide dynamic stability. Proprioceptive neuromuscular facilitation techniques include controlled diagonal patterns and rhythmic stabilization, especially with weight-bearing activities.[13] The patient may begin weight-bearing exercises at 6 to 8 weeks if there are no contraindications such as fractures, rotator cuff tears, or posterior instability. One can start in a modified plantigrade position with hands on a table and perform gen-

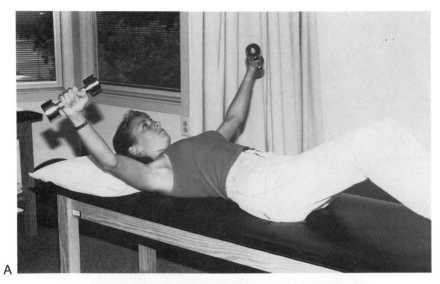

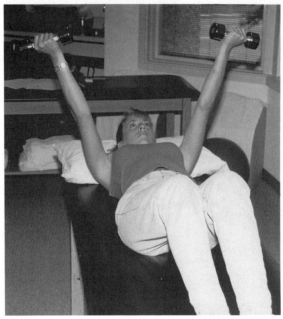

**Fig. 47-2.** Supine fly exercise is modified to avoid undesired joint forces. (**A**) Shoulder is in internal rotation and stopped 30 degrees from the coronal plane with anterior instability; (**B**) shoulder is in external rotation and stopped 30 degrees from the sagittal plane with posterior instability.

tle weight shifts to provide compression into the glenohumeral joint and facilitate co-contractions. With younger patients, this can be progressed to more difficult quadruped and triped positions using different dynamic balance equipment such as large gym balls and wobble boards (Fig. 47-3 and 47-4). The therapist can manually apply resistance in different directions while the patient attempts to maintain balance through the involved upper limb in these quadruped and triped positions. This facilitates the patient to "react" rather than to "act" and is a very challenging and worthwhile activity.

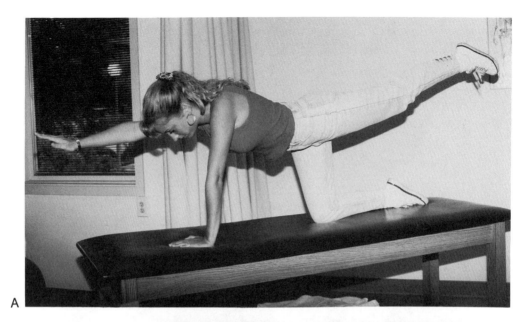

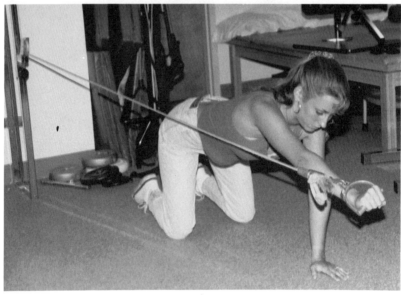

**Fig. 47-3.** Examples of weight-bearing (closed chain) shoulder exercises to facilitate co-contractions and enhance neuromuscular control. (**A**) Two-point balance with outstretched uninvolved arm and contralateral leg. (**B**) Using a pulley system with the involved arm down and stabilizing the body while the uninvolved arm is moving against resistance. (*Figure continues.*)

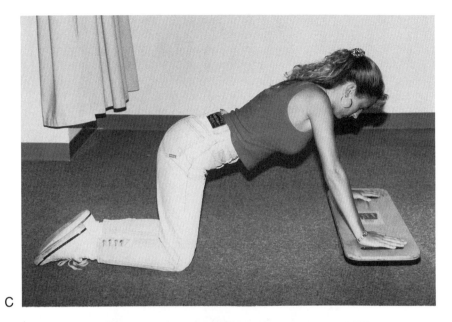

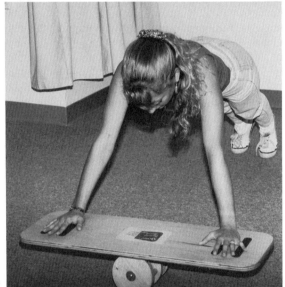

**Fig. 47-3.** (*Continued*). (**C**) Using a balance board with body weight on hands and knees. (**D**) Progressing to balance board with body weight on hands and toes.

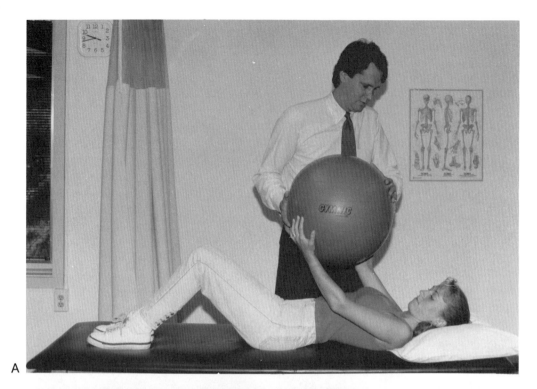

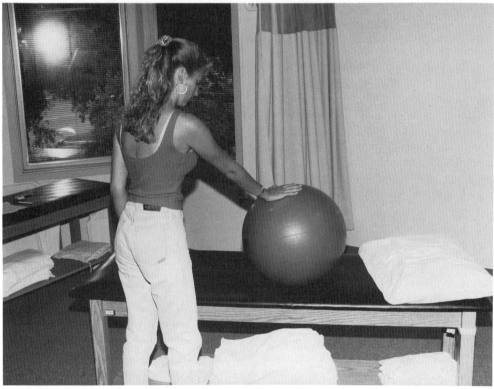

**Fig. 47-4.** Use of balls is an inexpensive and effective tool in many shoulder stabilization programs. (**A**) Resisting diagonal patterns while patient holds ball to elicit co-contractions. (**B**) Patient bears weight through ball to activate scapular musculature and promote neuromuscular control of arm. (*Figure continues.*)

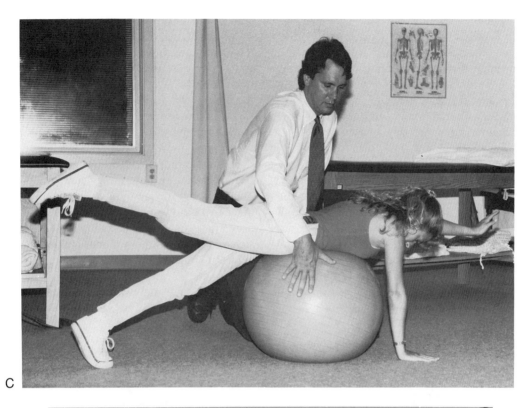

C

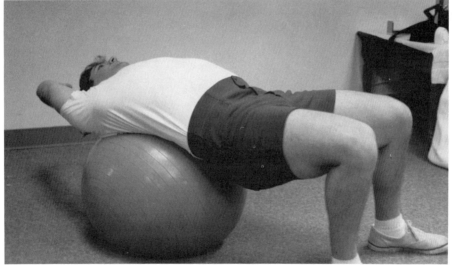

D

**Fig. 47-4.** (*Continued*). (**C**) Advanced closed chain exercise as patient maintains balance through involved arm and resists therapist's attempts to move ball. (**D**) Patient performs self-mobilization of thoracic spine into extension and rotation, which may be hypomobile with anterior shoulder subluxation.

Another similar technique to elicit isometric co-contractions is placing the patient supine with the arm at 90 degrees of elevation (hand toward ceiling). The therapist can apply manual resistance in different directions, varying the timing and intensity, while the patient tries to keep the arm from moving. This can be performed with the arm in different positions depending on deficits and functional needs.

Patients can also be taught to perform isometric co-contractions at home. One example is to have the patient stand with his or her back to the wall and a pillow between the arm and body. The patient squeezes the pillow while pushing the back of the arm into the wall and simultaneously resists internal rotation with the uninvolved arm. This allows co-contractions of the shoulder adductors, extensors, and internal rotators.

Another technique to help improve kinesthetic awareness with shoulder instability is to place the uninvolved arm in a position and ask the patient to close his or her eyes and attempt to match that position with the involved limb (Fig. 47-5). Patients seem to do quite well if the joint is in an invulnerable position. If the shoulder is brought toward the apprehension position, the deficits often become quite apparent. Patients have shown improvement with practice, but no data document a training effect regarding recovery of kinesthetic ability after dislocation of the glenohumeral joint.

The final component of the rehabilitation program deals with task simulation and functional progression. This part of the program must be designed individually but is commonly started around 12 weeks after dislocation. The progression is criteria-based, as dictated by signs and symptoms, but most patients refrain from vigorous overhead activities for at least 4 months. Before discharge, the patient needs to fully understand that the ultimate goal of the rehabilitation is not only to

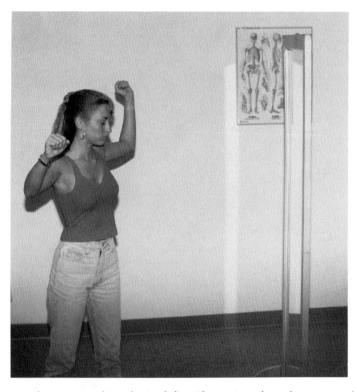

**Fig. 47-5.** A mirror is used to increase kinesthetic ability. The patient closes her eyes and the uninvolved arm is placed in position. The patient is asked to match the contralateral position with the involved arm. As the patient opens her eyes, she can use the visual feedback to help make any necessary correction. Deficits are greater as the shoulder approaches the apprehension position.

restore range of motion, strength, and neuromuscular control but to avoid recurrence of dislocation. The patient must be well educated to avoid the apprehension position with activities of daily living, exercise machines, and other events to avoid placing undesired forces on the restraining structures (see atraumatic anterior instability).

## REHABILITATION FOR ANTERIOR GLENOHUMERAL SUBLUXATION FROM MICROTRAUMA

Repetitive microtrauma leading to anterior instability is most commonly seen in the younger than 35-year-old athlete and worker who are required to use their arms overhead or at extremes of motion.[21] These conditions are generally classified as transient subluxations rather than dislocations and are associated with rotator cuff pathology, muscle imbalances, overuse, faulty biomechanics, and lack of flexibility.[4,21,22]

Successful conservative treatment for anterior subluxation is highly dependent on correctly identifying the causative factors and the involved pathology. Positive findings include a history of using the arm overhead or in the apprehension position with a subjective feeling of the arm slipping, going "dead," or producing an audible cracking or popping.[21,23-25] This can be accompanied by sharp pain with sports involving throwing or similar motions during the late cocking or acceleration phase of the activity. Objectively, the apprehension test[1] performed in the supine position augmented with a posterior fulcrum is a sensitive provocative test in this author's experience. Careful examination of the rotator cuff also must be performed to assess its possible involvement. Other findings on physical examination may reveal general hypermobility throughout the body or a concomitant hypomobility in the upper and midthoracic spine regions. Different imaging tests can be ordered at the discretion of the physician to aid in making a diagnosis.

One key assessment based on the examination is the determination of the amount of inflammation and pain present such that appropriate types of treatment are initiated. If this is a significant problem, no exercise program is started for 1 to 2 weeks. Rather, treatment is initiated with rest, anti-inflammatory medication, and appropriate modality use. A combination of ice massage and electrical stimulation is beneficial in reducing pain and inflammation with this type of patient. A restriction from aggravating factors for 2 to 4 weeks or longer is advised in some cases.

The strengthening and neuromuscular concepts presented after traumatic dislocation are valid with subluxation. These exercises emphasize scapular muscles to provide a stable base for the glenohumeral joint in different positions of elevation. Special attention is also given to rotator cuff endurance to help provide necessary dynamic stabilization. The progression of strengthening exercises should not be rushed. This may require a great deal of patience from both the therapist and the patient, but advancing these programs too quickly or returning to throwing or overhead activities too soon can result in problems. The involved structures are often still vulnerable and irritable, even after a period of rest and initial treatment.

Treatment programs also include joint and soft tissue mobilization as necessary. Examples are posterior capsular mobilization of the glenohumeral joint and extension and rotation of the upper thoracic spine, as hypomobility in these regions may contribute to anterior glenohumeral instability (Fig. 47-4).

After pain has subsided and adequate strength and mobility are attained, a formal functional progression is necessary to incrementally induce stress to the involved tissue and to maximize chances of full recovery. An ergonomic or biomechanical assessment of related activities must first be performed to help avoid continuation of repeated microtrauma to the shoulder.

## REHABILITATION FOR ATRAUMATIC ANTERIOR GLENOHUMERAL INSTABILITY

Atraumatic dislocation and subluxation can present in a volitional or nonvolitional manner and may be due to structural congenital anomalies of the glenohumeral joint or to systemic disorders such as Ehlers-Danlos syndrome, which results in inadequate connective tissue.[1] The condition may present as unidirectional, but it is often associated with multidirectional instability to be discussed later.[1,4]

Conservative care for this type of anterior instability is directed toward patient education and motivation, postural corrections, and stabilization exercises. Many of these patients have a painful and frustrating history associated with their condition. It is of the utmost importance to establish good rapport and communication with these patients if one expects long-term patient compliance and an ultimate decrease in symptoms.

Education consists of explaining the nature of the problem to the patient and then identifying activities of daily living that aggravate symptoms. Unrecognized repetitive microtrauma is often experienced in simple tasks of dressing, sleeping, carrying, and reaching. Simple examples of activities of daily living that produce stress on the anterior restraints of the shoulder include sleeping on the back with an arm under the pillow, fixing hair with the shoulder in the apprehension position, reaching into the backseat of a car while the body faces straight ahead, placing a backpack on with the arm abducted, and leaning back on outstretched arms behind the back while in the long sitting position.

Posture can also affect shoulder function. One example is proper lumbar support while sitting. This improves the positioning of the head and scapulothoracic region and allows the glenohumeral joint to operate from a safer and more efficient position. Regardless of the sophistication of an exercise program, modifications must be made in these simple daily activities to reduce symptoms effectively.

Exercise programs are initiated at very submaximal levels, designed to be performed in a pain-free manner so that the patient does not become discouraged. Attention is again concentrated on scapular and rotator cuff musculature, as they are often found to be weak, and scapular winging is not uncommon. Isometrics for glenohumeral muscles with the arm by the side in a neutral position are used early and are well tolerated if the patient controls the amount of tension properly. Each exercise is performed 5 to 10 repetitions and 2 to 3 times daily. Dynamic resistive exercises for the scapular musculature can be introduced early in the program, while this is delayed for a few weeks for the glenohumeral joint. Many of the dynamic glenohumeral exercises are performed in limited arcs of motion, and the shoulder is not "loaded" in the apprehension position. Elbow curls and glenohumeral rotation exercises are performed with the arm by the side using isotonic, isokinetic, or elastic resistance. The exercise program usually includes weight-bearing exercises previously described. The application of heat 2 to 3 times daily is often more effective than ice in reducing soreness from the onset of the exercise. Formal supervised rehabilitation usually consists of two to three weekly visits for 1 to 2 months, after which the patient is placed on a home exercise program. Ongoing periodic monitoring helps to ensure patient compliance and allows for modifications of the home program.

## REHABILITATION FOR POSTERIOR GLENOHUMERAL INSTABILITY

Posterior instability is much less common than anterior instability but may be unrecognized in many cases.[24] Axial loading of the glenohumeral joint in the position of adduction, flexion, and internal rotation such as falling on outstretched arms is a common method of posterior dislocation.[1,26] Automobile accidents and seizures can also produce posterior dislocations.[1,27] Patients with posterior subluxation may complain of pain with a follow-through type of motion involving internal rotation and flexion or horizontal adduction. Provocative tests include the posterior draw, the jerk test, and the push–pull test.[1] Many of the concepts and guidelines presented for anterior instability remain valid, although some of the techniques used are quite different or "reversed" in some cases. The differences rather than the similarities will be emphasized.

In general, the rehabilitation program is more conservative with a timeframe 2 to 4 weeks slower than with anterior instability because of decreased familiarity and success. If immobilization is required, the arm is maintained in slight external rotation and abduction as with an abduction pillow. The position of internal rotation, flexion, and horizontal adduction is clinically unstable and can be considered the apprehension position with posterior instability.[28] Accordingly, this position is approached last and the arm is not loaded at the end range. Most weight-bearing exercises must be modified or avoided. Push-ups are replaced with isotonic scapular protraction exercises performed supine in the plane of the scapular, maintaining glenohumeral external rotation. Adequate humeral support is provided posteriorly using towels or bolsters to prevent posterior translation of the humerus with supine exercises. Scapular protraction can also be resisted manually in sidelying or using elastic or pulleys in the upright position. The bench press is performed in an inclined position with posterior humeral support. Efforts are submaximal, a wide grip is used, and the elbows are not locked-out in extension. Supine flies are stopped approximately 30 degrees short of the sagittal plane, maintaining glenohumeral external rotation. With daily activities, the patient is cautioned to avoid reaching across the body and bearing weight through the arms, which may occur with pushing activities or in kneeling or prone positions.

# REHABILITATION FOR MULTIDIRECTIONAL GLENOHUMERAL INSTABILITY

Multidirectional instability is a diagnosis that is experiencing an increasing recognition. By definition, multidirectional instability will have an inferior component in addition to either anterior or posterior instability or both.[29] Multidirectional instability is most often atraumatic and may be associated with general ligamentous laxity. Surgery is not indicated with most atraumatic conditions. In all cases, it is essential to establish the direction and the degree of instability to implement proper treatment plans. Therefore, a careful examination with special attention to provocative tests is once again essential. A positive sulcus sign is consistent with inferior instability.[1,29]

Most of the concepts already presented regarding shoulder stabilization are valid (see atraumatic anterior instability). Considerations not yet presented would relate to the inferior component of the instability. Modifications of posture, daily activities, and exercises are directed at avoiding stress to the inferior restraints. This would include proper support of the arms in a sitting position and avoidance of the arms in the dependent position or overhead with any significant amount of weight in the hands. Exercises to avoid are dead lifts, military presses, and shrugs with weights in the hands. Resistance can be applied with weights or manually to the suprascapular area to allow shrugs to be performed safely. Elbow curls are performed with support beneath the elbow or upper arm. The use of long lever arms or weights in the hands with the elbows extended is avoided and replaced with more proximal resistance points about the upper arm as with pulley

cuffs or manual contact. Isometrics, scapular stabilization, and midrange dynamic exercises are emphasized. Significant attention is devoted to different motor/sensory techniques to enhance neuromuscular control and kinesthetic awareness as described previously.

Patient motivation and compliance are again of the utmost importance as many of these patients also have had a most frustrating experience with their shoulders. There is no single magic answer, but all aspects of the program must be used as indicated to help reduce symptoms and improve functional capabilities. The multidirectional instability is often a most difficult condition that requires activity modification and avoidance of many sports involving the shoulder. It may be helpful for the patient to think in terms of improving rather than becoming entirely asymptomatic.

# REFERENCES

1. Matson FA, Thomas SC, Rockwood CA: Glenohumeral instability. p. 526. In Rockwood CA, Matson FA (eds): The Shoulder. WB Saunders, Philadelphia, 1990
2. Cave EF, Burke JF, Boyd RJ: Trauma management. p. 437. Yearbook Book of Medical Publishers, Chicago, 1974
3. Rowe CR: Prognosis in dislocations of the shoulder. J Bone Joint Surg 38A:957, 1956
4. O'Brien SJ, Warren RF, Schwartz E: Anterior shoulder instability. Orthop Clin North Am 18:395, 1987
5. McLaughlin HL, Cavallaro WU: Primary anterior dislocation of the shoulder. Am J Surg 80:615, 1950
6. Henry JH, Gening JA: Natural history of glenohumeral dislocation revisited. Am J Sports Med 10:135, 1982
7. Aronen JG, Regan K: Decreasing the incidence of recurrence of first time anterior shoulder dislocations with rehabilitation. Am J Sports Med 12:283, 1984
8. Yoneda B, Welsh RP, MacIntosh DL: Conservative treatment of shoulder dislocation in young males (proceedings). J Bone Joint Surg 64:254, 1982
9. Grana WA, Buckley PD, Yates CK: Arthroscopic Bankart suture repair. Am J Sports Med 21:348, 1993
10. Caspari RB, Savoie FH: Arthroscopic shoulder reconstruction: Bankhart repair. p. 514. In McGinty JB (ed): Operative Arthroscopy. Raven Press, New York, 1990
11. Morgan CD, Bordenstab AB: Arthroscopic Bankart suture repair: technique and early results. Arthroscopy 3:111, 1987
12. Altchek DW, Warren RF, Skyhar MJ: Shoulder arthroscopy. p. 276. In Rockwood CA, Matson FA (eds): The Shoulder. WB Saunders, Philadelphia, 1990

13. Knott M, Voss DE: Proprioceptive Neuromuscular Facilitation. Harper & Row, New York, 1968

14. Jobe FW, Tibone JE, Perry J: An EMG analysis of the shoulder in throwing and pitching. A second report. Am J Sports Med 12:218, 1984

15. Ryu RK, McCormick J, Jobe FW: An electromyographic analysis of shoulder function in tennis players. Am J Sports Med 16:481, 1988

16. Mosely JB, Jobe FW, Pink M: EMG analysis of the scapular muscles during a shoulder rehabilitation program. Am J Sports Med 20:128, 1992

17. Jobe FW, Moynes DR: Delineation of diagnostic criteria and a rehabilitation program for rotator cuff injuries. Am J Sports Med 10:336, 1982

18. Blackburn TA, McCleod WD, White B: EMG analysis of posterior rotator cuff exercises. Athletic Training 25:40, 1990

19. Smith RL, Brunolli J: Shoulder kinesthesia after anterior glenohumeral joint dislocation. Phys Ther 69:106, 1989

20. Glousman RE, Jobe FW, Tibone JE: Dynamic EMG analysis of the throwing shoulder with glenohumeral instability. J Bone J Surg 70A:220, 1988

21. Jobe FW, Tibone JE, Jobe CM: The shoulder in sports. p. 961. In Rockwood CA, Matsen FA (eds): The Shoulder. WB Saunders, Philadelphia, 1990

22. Warner JJ, Mianelli LJ, Arslanian LE: Patterns of flexibility, laxity, and strength in normal shoulders and shoulders with instability and impingement. Am J Sports Med 18:366, 1990

23. Rockwood CA Jr: Subluxation of the shoulder—the classification, diagnosis, and treatment. Orthop Trans 4:306, 1979

24. Rowe CR, Zarin B: Chronic unreduced dislocations of the shoulder. J Bone Joint Surg 64A:494, 1982

25. Simonet WT, Cofield RH: Prognosis in anterior shoulder dislocation. Am J Sports Med 12:19, 1984

26. Moeller JC: Compound posterior dislocation of the shoulder. J Bone Joint Surg 57A:1006, 1975

27. Hawkins RH, Neer CS II, Pianta RM: Locked posterior dislocation of the shoulder. J Bone Joint Surg 69A:9, 1987

28. Rockwood CA: Posterior dislocation of the shoulder. p. 806. In Rockwood CA, Green DP (eds): Fractures in Adults. JB Lippincott, Philadelphia, 1984

29. Neer CS II: Shoulder Reconstruction. WB Saunders, Philadelphia, 1990

# Editors' Preferred Method

In this chapter the author presents a thorough, logical, and traditional conservative treatment program for the patient with a traumatic or atraumatic unstable shoulder. We classify shoulder instability as traumatic, atraumatic, or acquired. Matsen[1] has provided us with a useful acronym to remember this classification. Traumatic patients exhibit *u*nilateral/*u*nidirectional instability, caused by a *B*ankart lesion, and usually these patients require *s*urgery to stabilize the shoulder joint (TUBS). We might add that these patients are the most difficult to rehabilitate conservatively, especially if they desire overhead movements. The next type of patient is the *a*traumatic, *m*ultidirectional unstable patient, usually *b*ilaterally involved, in whom *r*ehabilitation is the first line of defense; if conservative treatment fails then an *i*nferior capsular shift procedure is performed (AMBRI). Burkhead et al[2] reported only 15 percent

good to excellent result with conservative treatment in patients with traumatic shoulder dislocation, while obtaining a success rate of 85 percent with the atraumatic patient. The acquired instability patient is the overhead athlete (thrower, tennis player, swimmer) who, because of repetitive microtraumatic stresses applied to the glenohumeral capsule, has developed significant laxity to allow the tremendous movement necessary for these sports.

The most common complication following traumatic anterior shoulder dislocation is recurrent dislocation. The patient's age has been shown to have the most significant effect on subsequent dislocations. In patients under the age of 20 years, the incidence of recurrent dislocations is greater than 85 percent,[3,4] and over 40 years of age, the incidence reduces to 10 to 15 percent. Most recurrences occur within the first two years of the initial traumatic dislocation[5,6,7] and are most common in males.[8] Therefore, it appears that traumatic shoulder dislocation sustained by a relatively young individual is likely to lead to recurrent dislocations. This is probably due to traumatic injury causing an avulsion of the glenohumeral ligament from the anterior glenoid lip and neck of the scapula (Bankart lesion). In the older individual, injuries usually cause a stretch of the capsule or an avulsion of the greater tuberosity, and either may heal to produce adequate stability.[9] Reeves[10] has reported the force required to dislocate a cadaveric specimen is about 70 N; less force is required in subjects under 20 or over 40 years of age.

The editors' treatment for traumatic shoulder dislocations has changed dramatically in the past several years. If the patient is not a surgical candidate, for whatever reason, and a conservative treatment is attempted, our program is based on immediate motion and strengthening. Several investigators have documented that the incidence of recurrent instability is not affected by the type or length of glenohumeral immobilization.[11,12,13] The editors' preferred method is based on four critical components: (1) immediate motion/strengthening; (2) preventing rotator cuff "shutdown" (i.e., muscular atrophy or neuromuscular dissociation); (3) re-establishing dynamic stability through the force couples of the glenohumeral joint, and (4) adequate retention of proprioception.

We use a program in which the patient begins active assisted motion exercises immediately after the initial dislocation. The motion is gradually increased in a non-painful fashion. A sling may be used, and exercising is avoided for the first two days to diminish pain. Additionally mid-range isometrics are performed to prevent muscular atrophy and dissociation owing to pain inhibition. We believe that immobilization may result in increased laxity because of a decrease in dynamic stability through rotator cuff muscular inhibition, atrophy, and increased pain owing to a lack of movement. Thus, motion and strengthening exercises that are pain-free stimulate collagen synthesis and collagen fiber organization and neuromodulate pain.[14,15,16] After motion has been restored, the patient can perform rhythmic stabilization drills in the mid range of motion, diagonal proprioceptive neuromuscular facilitation patterns, external/internal rotation, and shoulder flexion. Additionally, weight-bearing exercises may be performed to initiate co-contractions about the glenohumeral joint; often these drills can be performed immediately after the injury. Strengthening exercises should emphasize the muscles on each side of the joint and re-establishing dynamic stability through the force couples of the glenohumeral joint. The patient is then progressed to neuromuscular control exercise drills that are performed at the end range of motion and in the apprehensive position. The patient's arm is placed in abduction and external rotation. The patient is asked to hold that position while the therapist applies a force to rotate the shoulder externally and internally. Similar drills can be used during PNF $D_2$ flex patterns at end range in the supine, sidelying, and seated positions. Additional exercises such as isokinetics, isotonics, and scapular strengthening should be performed.

The purpose of this program is to re-establish full motion within two weeks and then progress to exercise drills to enhance neuromuscular control of the glenohumeral joint to provide dynamic functional stability. Programs that emphasize dynamic shoulder stability appear to be successful in selected patients. Aronen[17] and Yoneda[18] have reported 75 to 83 percent satisfactory results, whereas Burkhead[2] reported 15 percent good to excellent results in trauma-induced instability. This program has proven beneficial for the patient who does not require overhead movements.

The editor's preferred treatment for the multidirectional atraumatic unstable shoulder patient is similar to the program previously described. The success of this program is often determined by the patient's tissue status and program compliance. Hawkins[19] has reported that patients with multidirectional instability (MDI) often exhibit a collagen deficiency, whereas the patient's collagen regenerates at a quicker rate. We emphasize dynamic stability exercises for all the muscles that surround the shoulder joint (the circle dynamic stability concept, Ch. 30). The circle dynamic stability concept describes the dynamic stabilizers of the glenohumeral joint, which are the muscular structures on both sides of the joint (anteriorly and posteriorly). These muscles are referred to as the force couples, and we believe they are the essential stabilizers. They can be effectively exercised with PNF, which uses rhythmic stabilization techniques, neuromuscular control drills, and isometric contractions. If the instability is severe, traditional exercises are often unsuccessful, and the therapist must use manual techniques to stabilize the humeral head within the glenoid, or have the patient use the sidelying position to promote gravitational stability to the shoulder while performing various exercises.

We have found that compliance is an extremely important factor. The patient must continue to exercise to enhance dynamic stability; if the exercises are discontinued, subluxation frequently reoccurs.[20,21] Also, when the MDI patient starts the conservative program, we emphasize performing the strengthening exercises 4 to 5 times per day for 5 to 10 minutes to enhance the resting tone of the shoulder muscles. The success rate of conservative treatment for the atraumatic shoulder is dramatically enhanced compared with the traumatic unstable shoulder; in general the success rate is 80 percent or better.[2,22,23] If this conservative treatment plan is unsuccessful, an inferior capsular shift procedure has proven extremely successful in reestablishing joint stability.[23]

# REFERENCES

1. Matsen FA, Harrgmon DT, Sidles JA: Mechanics of glenohumeral instability. Clin Sports Med 10(4):783, 1991
2. Burkhead WZ, Rockwood CA: Treatment of instability of the shoulder with an exercise program. J Bone Joint Surg 74A:890, 1992
3. McLoughlin HL, Cavallaro WV: Primary anterior dislocation of the shoulder. Am J Surg 80:615, 1950
4. Watson-Jones R: Dislocation of the shoulder joint. Proc R Soc Med 29:1060, 1936
5. DePalma AF: Surgery of the Shoulder. 3rd Ed. JB Lippincott, Philadelphia, 1973
6. Bankart ASB: The pathology and treatment of recurrent dislocation of the shoulder joint. Br J Surg 26:23, 1939
7. Rowe CR: Prognosis in dislocations of the shoulder. J Bone Joint Surg 38A:957, 1956
8. Moseley HF: The basic lesions of recurrent anterior dislocations. Surg Clin North Am 43:1631, 1963
9. Matsen FA, Thomas SC, Rockwood CA: Glenohumeral Instability. p. 526. In Rockwood CA, Matsen FA (eds): The Shoulder. WB Saunders, Philadelphia, 1990
10. Reeves B: Experiments on the tensile strength of the anterior capsular structures of the shoulder region. J Bone Joint Surg 50B:838, 1968
11. Ehgartner K: Does the duration of cast fixation after shoulder dislocations have an influence on the frequency of recurrent dislocations? Arch Orthop Trauma Surg 89:187, 1977
12. Hovelius L: Recurrences after initial dislocation of the shoulder. J Bone Joint Surg 65A:343, 1983
13. Rowe CR, Sakellarides HT: Factors related to recurrences of anterior dislocations of the shoulder. Clin Orthop 20:40, 1961
14. Akeson WH, Woo SLY, Ariel D: The connective tissue response to immobility: biochemical changes in periarticular connective tissue of the immobilized rabbit knee. Clin Orthop 93:356, 1973
15. Woo SLY, Mathews SV, Akeson WH: Connective tissue response to immobility. Arthritis Rheum 18:257, 1973
16. Wyke BD: The neurology of joints. Ann R Coll Surg Engl 41:25, 1966
17. Aronen JC, Regan K: Decreasing the incidence of recurrence of first time anterior shoulder dislocations with rehabilitation. Am J Sports Med 12:283, 1984
18. Yoneda B, Welsh RP, MacIntosh DL: Conservative treatment of shoulder dislocation in young males. J Bone Joint Surg 64B:254, 1982
19. Hawkins RJ, Bell R: Collagen analysis in patients with multidirectional instability. American Shoulder and Elbow Surgeons Specialty Day. Anaheim, CA, March, 1991
20. Wilk KE, Andrews JR: Current concepts in the treatment of shoulder instability. Orthopaedic Phys Ther Home Study Course LaCrosse, WI, July, 1993
21. Wilk KE, Arrigo CA: Current concepts in the rehabilitation of the athletic shoulder. J Orthop Sports Phys Ther (submitted for publication, 1993)
22. Rowe CR, Pierce DS, Clark JG: Voluntary dislocation of the shoulder. A preliminary report on a clinical, electromyographic and psychiatric study of twenty-six patients. J Bone Joint Surg 55A:445, 1973
23. Neer CS, Foster CR: Inferior capsular shift for involuntary inferior and multidirectional instability of the shoulder. A preliminary report. J Bone Joint Surg 62A:897, 1980

# 48

# Conservative Management of Shoulder Impingement

*MICHAEL A. KEIRNS*

## DEFINITION

Using the arm in a repetitive overhead activity may compromise the structures in the subacromial space, thus causing injury to the rotator cuff and subsequent shoulder dysfunction.[1,2] Several authors recognized this subacromial entrapment; however, we are indebted to Charles Neer for popularizing this pathologic mechanism of injury and classifying it as "impingement syndrome."[3-8] The impingement syndrome is characterized as a continuum beginning with an inflammatory process and progressing to fibrosis and ending in rotator cuff rupture.[9]

The subacromial space normally measures 7 to 12 mm and is bordered superiorly by the acromion, acromioclavicular joint, and the coracoacromial ligament.[10,11] Inferiorly this space is bound by the head of the humerus (Fig. 48-1). As the acromiohumeral distance becomes narrowed with elevation of the arm, especially when the movement involves internal rotation, the structures within become "pinched" against the anterior edge of the acromion and the coracoacromial ligament.[12-14]

The structures in the subacromial space that become compromised during the impingement process include the supraspinatus tendon, the long head of the biceps tendon, the subacromial bursa, and to a lesser extent, the infraspinatus tendon.[9] The greatest encroachment occurs near the attachment of the supraspinatus to the greater tuberosity, the "critical zone."[6,15] The possibility of diminished blood flow to the critical zone emphasizes its significance as a precursor for pathology.

## CAUSES OF IMPINGEMENT

As with any pathologic condition, it is important for the rehabilitation team to determine and treat the cause and not just eliminate the symptoms. Once the diagnosis of impingement is made, there is the need to distinguish whether the mechanical impingement is occurring secondary to structural or functional causes.

The structural causes of impingement encompass congenital abnormalities and/or degenerative alterations in the subacromial arch. Whether these transformations are the cause or consequence of impingement is difficult to determine. Bigliani and Morrison[16,17] described a high correlation (.95) between the types of acromion processes and impingement diagnosis with rotary cuff involvement. In their morphologic study, type III anterior hooked acromion processes (Fig. 48-2) were found to be associated with rotator cuff tears in 70 percent of the cases; however, a causal relationship could not be determined. In other words, did the rotator cuff tear, with subsequent humeral head elevation, cause the proliferation of the acromion process, or did the hooked acromion process cause the rotator cuff tear? Or finally, did both elevation of the humerus and rubbing of the acromion cause the resultant findings of impingement?

Uhthoff et al[18] showed that most rotator cuff tears are degenerative in nature and are present on the articular side (i.e., on the side facing the humeral head). Ozaki et al[19] presented a cadaver study indicating that these tears on the articular side were not associated with degeneration of the acromion undersurface. In contrast, they found complete and bursal rotator cuff

605

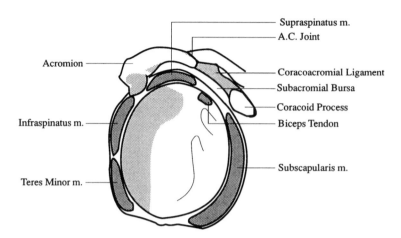

**Fig. 48-1.** Anatomic predispositions of impingement. (*A.C.,* acromioclavicular)

tears were associated with pathologic changes of the acromion. They postulated that a vicious cycle develops, beginning with a tear of the rotator cuff on the bursal side; followed by pathologic changes of the undersurface acromion; and ending with the subsequent acromion lesion abrading the cuff facilitating the degenerative process. Consequently, it is important to break this cycle by restoring the humeral head depression and minimizing this degenerative cycle. Should clients with structural changes in the arch not respond to conservative care or alterations in activity, surgical intervention may be the appropriate treatment of choice.[7,20–23]

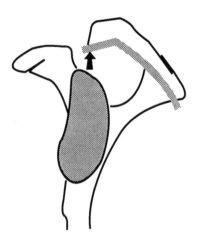

**Fig. 48-2.** Type III hooked acromion, which predisposes impingement of structures in the subacromial space.

Functional causes of impingement include (1) glenohumeral capsular laxity or tightness, (2) cervical spine dysfunction with radiculopathy, (3) postural deviations, and (4) inadequate rotary cuff function with diminished humeral head depression. Capsular laxity, which is prevalent with an athletic population, can alter normal humeral head translations during overhead activity. During athletic endeavors, such as the acceleration phase of a baseball pitch, the glenohumeral joint's static stabilizers must withstand tremendous torques (upwards of 71 Nm) as the arm accelerates 7,000 degrees/s[2.24,25]

Anterior capsular tension and/or the articular congruencies, not the contraction of the muscles, mediate a 10-mm humeral posterior translation during the late cocking and early acceleration of this pitch.[26–29] With capsule laxity, this accessory movement cannot be controlled by the static constraints, thereby allowing the humeral head to ride forward and thus cause shoulder impingement.[30] If a diagnosis of impingement syndrome is made secondary to hypermobility, treatment should focus on the primary diagnoses of subluxating shoulder.[31,32]

Just as hypermobility can be a precursor for impingement, so too can the hypomobility of the glenohumeral joint. Cofield and Simonet[33] described how the patient with adhesive capsulitis may be predisposed to having the shoulder entrapment in the subacromial space. Stiffness involving the posterior capsule can cause the humeral head to roll up on the posterior capsule like

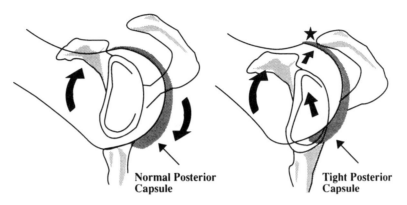

**Fig. 48-3.** Influences of posterior capsule on forcing humeral head elevation causing impingement. Normal posterior capsule allowing normal humeral head translation; tight posterior capsule causing humeral head elevation.

a yo-yo (Fig. 48-3). Subsequent humeral pressure is placed upward against the anteroinferior acromion. Treatment of this client should focus on increasing the mobility of the static constraints, especially the posterior capsule.[34,35]

Differential diagnoses need to be made with respect to the possibility of cervical dysfunction causing functional entrapment of the subacromial space. Nerve root entrapment at the C5-C6 level can facilitate weakness of the rotary cuff with subsequent diminished humeral head depression.[36,37]

There may also be nerve root entrapment for the scapula stabilizers.[38] Poor scapula stabilization can diminish scapula humeral rhythm and hinder the correct spacing of the subacromial opening. Moreover, posture can influence both the cervical dysfunction and correct scapula positioning. The client with postural deviation and/or cervical dysfunction should respond favorably to conservative physical therapy management.

The final and most important component in understanding the causation of the impingement syndrome is the influence of the rotator cuff tendons in maintaining humeral head location in the glenoid fossa. The rotator cuff is the prime mover in the depressor mechanism of the humeral head.[39–42] McMasters[43] has shown normal tendons to be exceedingly strong and resistant to pathology. However, in the case of the rotator cuff, light and scanning electron microscopes have confirmed rotator cuff microtears and hyalinization.[44] The pathogenesis of the rotator cuff tendon failure comes from a combination of adverse effects: (1) repeated mechani-

cal trauma from pinching, (2) ischemia causing predisposition for injury, and (3) diminished healing secondary to compromised vascularity.[7,45,46] Deficiency of the rotator cuff will allow the upward pull of the deltoid to force elevation of the humeral head (Fig. 48-4).[47–51]

When not corrected, the functional causes of impingement listed above can cause elevation of the humeral head with associated rotator cuff trauma. This is a self-perpetuating process with facilitation of an

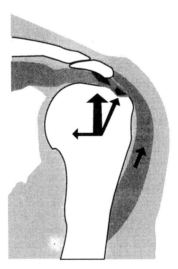

**Fig. 48-4.** Force vector diagram showing how the influences of the deltoid resultant vector can cause humeral elevation. Impingement can be magnified with diminished rotator cuff influences.

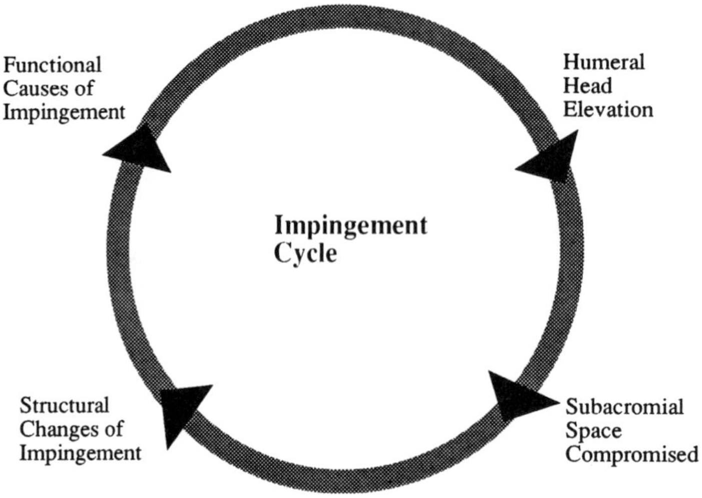

**Fig. 48-5.** Impingement cycle is a continuum that can begin anywhere in the sequence and can formulate a vicious succession.

impingement cycle (Fig. 48-5). As the subacromial structures become compromised, structural changes are forthcoming.

## IMPORTANCE OF SUBACROMIAL SPACE VASCULARITY

Lindbloom[52] in 1939 suggested that the Codman's critical zone of the supraspinatus tendon was avascular. Iannotti et al[53] and Moseley and Goldie[6] found later through laser doppler evaluations that there actually is adequate blood supply to this area; however, it is a zone of anastomoses between the osseous vessels (the anterior and posterior humeral circumflex) and tendinous vessels (the suprascapular and subscapular) (Fig. 48-6).

The classical study of Rathbun and MacNab[46] showed attenuation of this blood supply during certain activities. There is a diminished filling of the blood quantity when the arm is held in adduction and neutral position. It was then proposed that the tendon failure is eminent when the humerus is allowed to "wring out" the underdeveloped blood supply to the critical zone. With diminished vascularity to the arm, there is a decreased blood supply for nutrition and oxidation necessary to the healing process.

Another important finding in vascularity with respect to rehabilitation was the study performed by Sigholm et al,[54] in which the subacromial pressure was measured during shoulder elevation. By using micropipette infusion technique, it was found that the pressure in the subacromial space was raised from 8 mmHg to 56 mmHg with 45 degrees of arm flexion with 1 kg weight. This elevation is sufficient to compromise the microvascularity of the arm held in an elevated position.[55]

## NONOPERATIVE MANAGEMENT

Conservative treatment has proven to be very effective and is the treatment of choice in rehabilitation of the impingement patient.[7,9,23,56] Many rehabilitation programs have been outlined for treatment of the impingement with the common denominator of allowing adequate rest and promoting rotator cuff strengthening.[22,57–63] The goal of this rehabilitation program is to present a physiologically based program that is scientifically backed and goal-oriented with criteria established for progression. The main emphasis is placed on the vascularity influences and outlined progression. A basic rationale in developing a rehabilitation protocol is that compromised circulation diminishes the

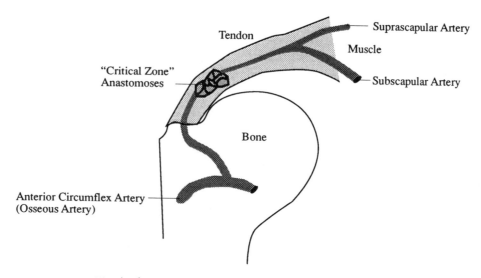

**Fig. 48-6.** Vascularity of critical zone is a period of transition.

healing capabilities of the shoulder. This reduction in vascularity is particularly important with respect to accelerating rotator cuff healing, chiefly because the rotator cuff communicates with the joint fluid and bursal fluid that remove any hematoma, contributing to cuff healing.

The program proposed in this chapter places the primary focus of rehabilitation needs on facilitating subacromial tissue healing and diminishing humeral head elevation. Attention is centered on humeral head depression and vascularity to the subacromial space, both to facilitate healing and to minimize continued ischemic pathology. This program establishes four stages through which the client must pass before completion of the rehabilitation program. Each stage has goals that are established and criteria that must be met before moving on to the next stage.[63b] When initiating the rehabilitation program, it is first important to ensure differential diagnosis has been made. Then, one must assess at what stage in the rehabilitation program the person is and how far the impingement pathology has progressed according to Neer's[9] classification. Although not a cookbook, this rehabilitation protocol will, through systematic re-evaluations, progress the surgical and nonsurgical clients quickly and safely through their rehabilitation program.

## Stage I: Acute Inflammatory Stage

During this stage, an acute inflammatory process exists in the shoulder. There is bleeding into the tissue with subsequent impaired healing, secondary to increased capillary pressure on the damaged tissue.[64] Stage I inflammatory process is characterized by (1) inability to sleep on the affected extremity, (2) discomfort at rest, (3) warmth felt with palpation of the joint, (4) pain and weakness with isolated muscle evaluation, (5) diffuse tenderness with palpation, (6) positive impingement signs, and (7) pain with overhead activity.[36,65-70] The rehabilitation goals in order of importance during this stage include (1) decreasing the inflammatory process, (2) educating the patient, (3) maintaining joint mobility, and (4) preventing atrophy. It needs to be thoroughly emphasized during this stage that the impingement symptoms not be exasperated.

### Decreasing the Inflammatory Process

Proven adjuncts in diminishing the chemical reaction of the inflammatory process are rest, therapeutic modalities, and nonsteroidal anti-inflammatory agents. By alleviating the inflammatory mechanism, there will be an associated decrease in pain and swelling. Success in achieving these goals has been accomplished through an array of modalities to include microcurrent, pulsed electromagnetic field therapy, iontophoresis, and phonophoresis.[71] The author's choice of modalities to treat the acute inflamed shoulder include cryotherapy and low-frequency transcutaneous electrical nerve stimulation (TENS).

Cold applications diminish the inflammatory condition by acting as vasoconstrictors and reducing metabolic activity.[72,73] Cooling also diminishes discomfort associated with the acute shoulder injury by increasing the threshold of pain in nerve fibers stimulation.[74,75] Through this cold-induced analgesia, normal shoulder motion can be facilitated.[76] Application of the shoulder cold therapy can be effective with ice massage for 15 to 20 minutes with the arm position in abduction (Fig. 48-7).

Classically, TENS has been used for the purpose of pain alleviation. Low-frequency TENS has also been found effective to increase microcirculation and facilitate the absorption of calcific deposits in the shoulder tendons.[77,78] The most effective treatment points are thought to be associated with stimulation of the acupuncture points.[79] Figure 48-8 displays an effective inferential pad setup using acupuncture sites successful in treating shoulder dysfunction. The points used in this arrangement include Jianjing (G.B. 21), Binao (L.I.

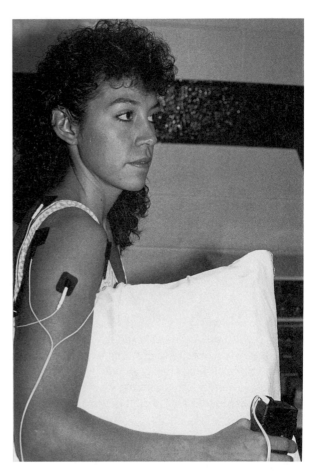

**Fig. 48-8.** Successful method of TENS setup.

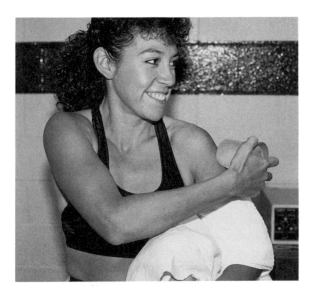

**Fig. 48-7.** Ice massage performed with shoulder abduction.

14), Juga (L.I. 16), and Jianya (L.I. 15).[80] Any modality is only an adjunct in a physical therapy clinic and should be used with prudence.

Although injections can be a useful tool in diminishing the inflammatory process and differentiating the impingement diagnoses, caution must be exercised in recommending steroid injections. Steroid injection in or near the cuff and biceps tendons may produce tendon atrophy or may reduce the capability of damaged tendon to repair itself.[81-83] Moreover, Kennedy and Willis[84] concluded collagen necrosis occurred with steroid injection. Finally, control studies have been performed showing minimal effectiveness alone with the use of steroid injections.[85,86]

## Patient Education

Patient education begins with instruction as to the pathogenesis of the injury. Understanding the problem may enlighten the client as to the therapeutic rationale for avoiding activities that can cause persisting shoulder pathology. The rehabilitation program should be outlined with the short-term and long-term goals emphasized; the criteria for the stage advancement should be highlighted. Educating the client will also promote compliance throughout the rehabilitation program.

When outlining motions to refrain from, it is particularly important to advise avoiding shoulder activities where the humerus is 10 degrees higher than the scapular spine. Higher angles approximate the humerus

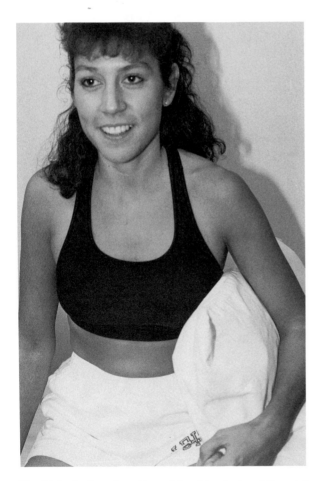

**Fig. 48-9.** Preferred position of shoulder during daily activities of living.

with the acromion and can impede the microvascularity of the subacromial space.[22] If symptoms persist at the waist level, the overhead limitation is set at that height. Avoidance of reaching and lifting activities should be emphasized so not to traumatize the associated structures.[87,88] The inflammatory process needs rest and protection to heal, and any activity causing pain should be avoided.[89]

Besides emphasizing the don'ts, it is also equally important to inform clients of how they should protect the arm. A critical part of the home care is to advise the patient of the following: (1) Minimize the time that the arm rests at the side; (2) when sitting, have the arm propped and supported approximately 45 degrees away from the side (Fig. 48-9); and (3) when sleeping, lie on the contralateral side with a pillow under the arm for maintenance of the desired position (Fig. 48-10). These recommendations facilitate circulation to the hypovascular zone of the subacromial space.[46,63]

Active rest is important in the rehabilitation of the individual with impingement symptoms, although activities that may be engaged in should be outlined. Aerobic non-weight-bearing arm activities, such as running in the pool, stationary bike riding, and stairmaster exercises, are indicated. The vascularity improvement in the nonexercising extremity may promote the healing process and facilitate progression in the rehabilitation process.[90] It is important for the therapist to observe and modify the exercise program and activity to guarantee no shoulder stress occurs.

### Maintenance of Joint Mobility

Immobility and the inflammatory process associated with stage I can result in increased scar tissue formation and eventual joint capsule contracture.[91] Therefore, during the early stages of rehabilitation, it is critical to maintain the mobility of the associated joints.[92-95] These are to include the glenohumeral, scapulothoracic, acromioclavicular, and sternoclavicular joints. The glenohumeral joint should be influenced by grades I and II cephald-caudal glides in the scapular plane to diminish the discomfort associated with the inflammatory process of the joint.[95-97] Maintenance of the humeral depression and evaluation of capsular tightness can also be addressed, with ensuing treatments as indicated and tolerated.

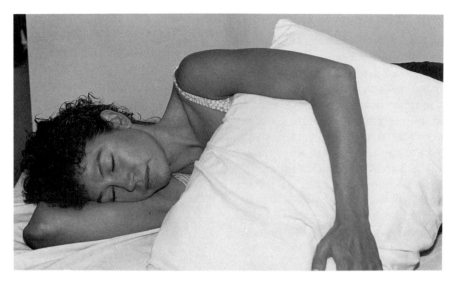

**Fig. 48-10.** Preferred position of shoulder during sleeping; affected shoulder is resting on the pillow.

Adequate scapulothoracic, acromioclavicular, and sternoclavicular joint mobility are essential for assurance of normal joint play and movement.[94] Grades I, II, and III joint mobilization are indicated to allow normal arthrokinematics during range of motion exercises.[94,95,98] Through joint mobilization, a skilled manual therapist can prevent complications of abnormal shoulder rhythms and ensuing diminished shoulder mechanics. While performing the joint mobilization, it is critical not to facilitate the inflammatory process.

Along with joint mobilization, active assisted range of motion exercises should be introduced to facilitate maintenance and increases in soft tissue flexibility. The motion should begin with pendulum activity with progression to rope and pulley motion. The rope and pulley exercise should begin with the flexion motion, performed with the palm supinated and the humerus externally rotated (Fig. 48-11). This allows the greater tuberosity to glide laterally of the anterior acromion, thereby lessening the chance of subacromial impingement.

The pulley maneuver is an advantageous way to perform range of motion because it allows gravity to assist with humeral depression. The goal of the active assisted range of motion is not to accomplish soft tissue remodeling and therefore performance of these exercises requires only a pause at the extremes of motion. The purpose of the range of motion exercises is to accom-

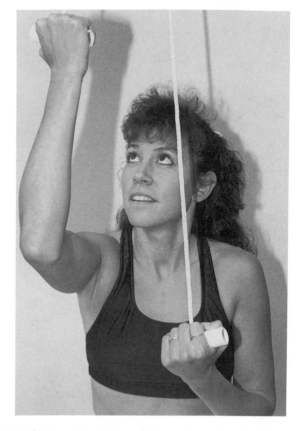

**Fig. 48-11.** Arm position during active assisted pulley exercise.

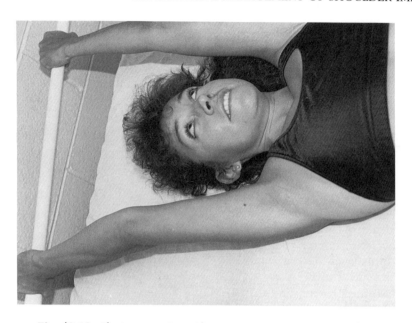

**Fig. 48-12.** Flexion exercise with correct arm position using T bar.

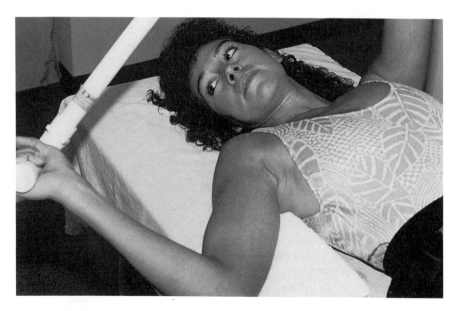

**Fig. 48-13.** External rotation with arm in scapular plane using T bar.

**Table 48-1. Stage I: Modified Isometrics Exercises**

| Position | Activity | Limitation |
| --- | --- | --- |
| Standing | External rotation | Submax |
| Standing | Internal rotation | Submax |
| Standing | Abduction | Submax |
| Standing | Flexion | Submax |
| Standing | Extension | Submax |
| Sidelying | Scapular motions | Submax |

plish a pumping action with redistribution of the waste products and neuromodeling of the associated musculature. Full flexion is the aspiration; however, as with any activity, it is crucial to avoid any discomfort associated with the movement.

After the pulley exercise, the T bar, or cane, maneuver should be performed in flexion and scapular-plane external rotation. Just as in the pulley flexion motion, the contralateral extremity should assist with the flexion action and the arm should maintain external rotation and supination (Fig. 48-12). External rotation is then performed with the T bar by placing the shoulder in the scapular plane with 45 degrees of abduction[99-101] (Fig. 48-13).

### Prevent Muscular Atrophy

The next goal of stage I is to retard muscular atrophy. When shoulder injury occurs, muscle atrophy occurrences happen secondary to reflexive retardation and disuse.[102-106] Costill et al[107] have shown the physiologic characteristics of this atrophy to be a decrease in muscle oxidative enzyme system with a predilection for effects on volume and diameter of type I slow-twitch fiber. The shoulder muscles that are affected most substantially are the tonic rotary cuff musculature.[108] Consequently, when addressing beginning shoulder rehabilitation, it is important to emphasize the preservation of rotator cuff strength and endurance. Because recruitment order begins with the type I fibers, submaximal modified isometrics are indicated to facilitate the rotator cuff musculature. Modified isometrics are illustrated as standing motions of 10 degrees or less in a slow rhythmic action with submaximal effort. The modified isometrics are performed with the arm supported at 45 degrees of abduction and are preferable

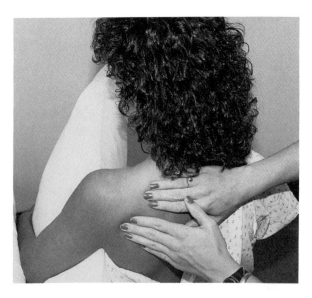

**Fig. 48-14.** Massage to supraspinatus and infraspinatus fossa.

because they facilitate a concentric contraction that will exercise the contraction component of the muscle.[109] This in turn facilitates an increase in vascularity and minimizes the stress at the tendinous junction, which needs protection at this point in rehabilitation.

Three sets of 12 to 20 repetitions are recommended to facilitate a pumping action and enhance recruitment of the mitrocondria and vascular energy system. The motions performed are listed in Table 48-1. Active rest and using the arm below 90 degrees in a pain-free motion during the normal activities of daily living will assist in minimizing atrophy by recruiting the rotary cuff for stabilization and promoting facilitation of vascularity of the rotary cuff.

## Stage II: Subacute Stage

The criteria for progress into stage II of the rehabilitation program are decreased inflammatory signs characterized by (1) no discomfort at rest, (2) no warmth felt with palpation of joint, and (3) good tolerance of above program. Although the individual may still present the other characteristics mentioned in stage I, the progression to stage II may be within a week. (Be careful not

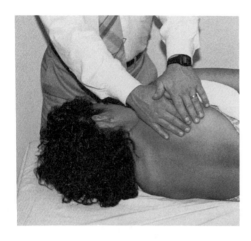

**Fig. 48-15.** Scapula proprioceptive neuromuscular facilitation technique.

to progress according to strict time-based protocol, as the author has observed 70 percernt of the patients will fit the program while 15 percent will need to speed up and another 15 percent will need to be slowed down.) The goals of stage II are the same as stage I, with the primary difference being an emphasis on circulatory advancement.

Circulation enhancement to the subacromial space, the primary focus of this stage, is accomplished by (1) ultrasound to supraspinatus fossa,[110–114] (2) effleurage massage proximal-to-distal to the supraspinatus and infraspinatus muscles while the client's arm is in an abducted position (Fig. 48-14),[115,116] and (3) ice to the supraspinatus and infraspinatus fossa and insertions with the patient's arm in the abducted position.[117,118] Transverse friction massage may be indicated in the case in which the lesion is superficial at the tenoperiosteal junction[36] (i.e., the scenario in which a painful arc is present and the pinching occurs between the greater tuberosity and the acromion). Rationale for use of transverse friction massage centers around causing tissue hyperemia and assisting with remodeling of the lesion.[116,119]

Joint mobility is advanced as tolerated with (1) abduction movement with the rope and pulley, (2) T bar external rotation at 90 degrees of abduction, (3) self-stretch for anterior, posterior, and inferior capsule, and (4) progressive joint mobilization. The prevention

of atrophy exercise program is the same as outlined in stage I with addition of total arm strengthening. This includes (1) scapular stabilization with submaximal proprioceptor neuromuscular facilitation in mid range of motion (Fig. 48-15), (2) submaximal biceps with dumbbell, (3) submaximal triceps performed with a dumbbell as a "kickback," and (4) dumbbell forearm exercises. A light resistance should be used for all isotonic exercises, beginning with three sets of 10 repetitions with progression to 20 repetitions.

## Stage III: Progressive Exercise Stage

The criteria for advancement into this stage is that the patient must present (1) normalized range of motion, (2) symptom-free during activities of daily living, and (3) improved muscular performance. Disappearance of pain and disability does not mean the lesion has healed.[9,89] Rapid progression into this stage is the largest factor in dissatisfied rehabilitation. It is more beneficial to delay progression into this stage, especially with the older population who may have diminished healing capabilities. Brewer[120] and Meyer[121] have shown age-related changes in the rotator cuff to include diminution of vascularity and loss of normal organizational characteristics of tendon.

The goals during this stage include (1) normalize arthrokinematics of shoulder complex, (2) regain and improve strength, and (3) improve neuromuscular control of shoulder.

### Range of Motion Normalized

The range of motion and arthrokinematics are normalized through aggressive joint mobilization, self-capsule stretching, and T bar active assisted range of motion in all planes. The joint mobilization is performed to address limitations found with clinical evaluation. The keys for the joint mobilization include (1) oscillations in caudal motion to treat abduction, (2) ventral accessory glides to increase external rotation, (3) dorsal accessory glides to increase internal rotation, and (4) lateral distraction to increase general motions. Self-capsule stretches are performed to specifically address limitations found in clinical evaluation with inferior, anterior, and posterior regions outlined (Figs. 48-16 and 48-17). The range of motion exercises are per-

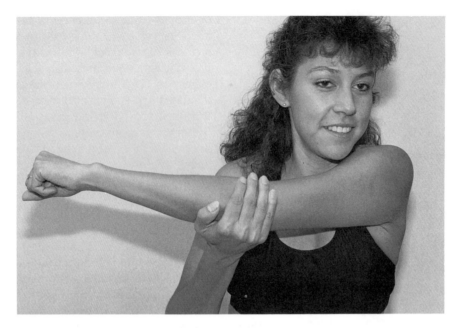

**Fig. 48-16.** Posterior capsule self-stretch.

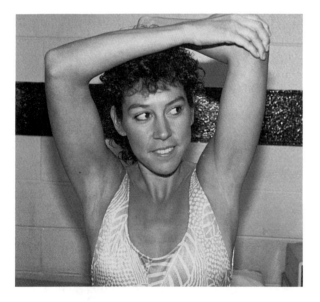

**Fig. 48-17.** Inferior capsule self-stretch.

formed before and after an arm ergometer warm-up.[122,123]

### Regain and Improve Strength

The main emphasis of stage III is restoration of the rotator cuff effectiveness and total arm strength. In the early stages of the progressive exercise program, endurance of the rotator cuff is emphasized. This is accomplished by arm ergometry and initiation of an isotonic dumbbell program for the shoulder musculature (Table 48-2). If available, a cable system is effective in progressing the shoulder strengthening program by adjusting the lever arm and minimizing the stress on the humeral depressors (Fig. 48-18).

**Table 48-2. Stage III: Isotonic Shoulder Exercise Program**

| Position | Motion | Limitation |
|----------|--------|------------|
| Prone | Extension | Pain |
| Prone | Horizontal abduction | Pain |
| Standing | Flexion | 90 Degrees |
| Standing | Abduction | 90 Degrees |
| Standing | Supraspinatus | 80 Degrees |
| Sidelying | Rotations | Arm abducted |

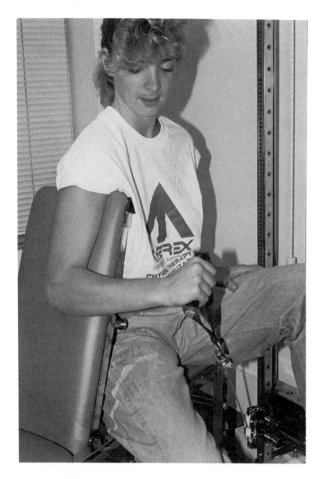

**Fig. 48-18.**  Cable used with external rotation.

**Table 48-3. Variables for Strength Training Program**

Repetitions
Weight
Sets
Concentric versus eccentric
Rest between exercises and sets?
Type of exercise (e.g., dumbbell versus isokinetic versus tubing)
Level of intensity
Order of exercises
Frequency of workouts
Isolation of muscle or muscle groups

the choices of exercise. Ten variables should be focused on to organize the appropriate strength training program (Table 48-3). Understanding the needs of the shoulder will dictate the optimal manipulation of these 10 parameters. The needs of the shoulder might include (1) type of muscle involved—phasic versus tonic,[129] (2) energy system used,[130,131] (3) demands to be placed on the shoulder with return to individual activities of daily living to include manual labor or athletic participation,[24,132,133] and (4) prevention of exercises or activities that preempt the impingement cycle.

In the advanced stages of the progressive exercise program, strength and power of the shoulder musculature should be centered on. Exercises should focus on duplicating the stresses that will be placed on the shoulder when the client returns to their normal upper extremity activities.

The concept of specialization is used during this latter part of stage III.[134] Plyometrics as outlined in Chapter 44 can be used to duplicate the explosive dynamics of overhead athletic participation.[135–137]

## Stage IV: Return to Activity

The guidelines for progression into this stage include (1) full nonpainful range of motion, (2) no pain or tenderness, (3) satisfactory strength evaluation (isokinetic test), and (4) satisfactory clinical examination. The goal of unrestricted symptom-free activity is accomplished by a functional interval program progressing back to full activity. It is important to adapt the activity and make appropriate changes in the movement so not to predispose reoccurrence of impinge-

Surgical tubing can also be an important adjunct in designing an adaptable exercise program; however, caution must be made not to perform full range of motion initially for the length–tension curve is combated with undue stress on the musculotendinous junctures.[124–126]

Proximal stability with scapula stabilization is also emphasized early on in the exercise plan. The concept of proximal stability for distal mobility is important to allow total arm strengthening without exasperation of the impingement syndrome.[127] This may be accomplished with scapular proprioceptive neuromuscular facilitation patterns and wall push-ups[128] (Fig. 48-19).

As the progressive exercise program is accelerated, the concept of specificity of training should dominate

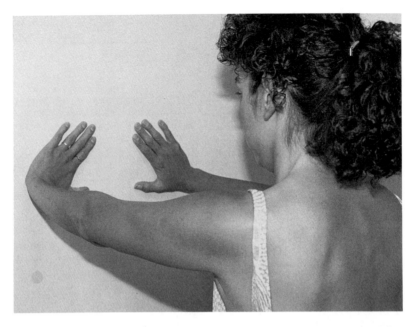

**Fig. 48-19.** Wall push-up for serratus anterior and facilitation of rotary cuff stabilization.

ment.[138,139] During the return to activity, a maintenance program should be instituted to include flexibility exercises, rotator cuff strengthening, and total arm strengthening exercises.

## SUMMARY

The purpose of this chapter has been to outline the conservative treatment of the client presenting with the diagnosis of impingement syndrome. The program emphasizes treating the cause and not just the symptoms. In accomplishing this goal, a progressive stage protocol was presented using goal orientation and criteria progression format. The individualization of every rehabilitation program cannot be compromised during the progression back to normal activity.

## REFERENCES

1. Clancy WG: Symposium: shoulder problems in overhead overuse sports. Am J Sports Med 7:138, 1979
2. Ha'ere GH, Wiley AM: Shoulder impingement syndrome. Clin Orthop 168:128, 1982
3. Armstrong JR: Excision of the acromion in treatment of the supraspinatus syndrome: report of ninety-five excisions. J Bone Joint Surg 31B:436, 1949
4. Codman EA: Rupture of the supraspinatus tendon. p. 123. In: The Shoulder: Rupture of the Supraspinatus Tendon and Other Lesions in or About the Subacromial Bursa. Robert E Krieger, Melbourne, FL, 1984
5. Hammond G: Complete acromionectomy in the treatment of chronic tendinitis of the shoulder. J Bone Joint Surg 44A:494, 1962
6. Moseley HF, Goldie I: The arterial pattern of the rotator cuff of the shoulder. J Bone Joint Surg 45B:780, 1963
7. Neer CS: Anterior acromioplasty for the chronic impingement syndrome in the shoulder. J Bone Joint Surg 54A:41, 1972
8. Neer CS, Welsh RP: The shoulder in sports. Orthop Clin North Am 8:585, 1977
9. Neer CS: Impingement lesions. Clin Orthop 173:70, 1983
10. Cone RO, Resnick D, Danzig L: Shoulder impingement syndrome: radiographic evaluation. Radiology 150:29, 1984
11. Ellman H, Hanker G, Bayer M: Repair of the rotator cuff. J Bone Joint Surg 68A:1136, 1986
12. Peterson CJ, Gentz CF: Ruptures of the supraspinatus tendon—the significance of distally pointing acromioclavicular osteophyte. Clin Orthop 174:143, 1983

13. Neviaser RJ, Neviaser TJ: Reconstruction of chronic tears of the rotator cuff. p. 172. In Bateman JE, Welsh RP (eds): Surgery of the Shoulder. BC Decker, Philadelphia, 1984

14. Craig EV: The geyser sign and torn rotator cuff: clinical significance and pathomechanics. Clin Orthop 191:213, 1984

15. Codman EA: Rupture of the supraspinatus—1834–1934. J Bone Joint Surg 19:643, 1937

16. Bigliani LU, Morrison D, April EW: The morphology of the acromion and its relationship to rotator cuff tears. Orthop Trans 10:228, 1986

17. Morrison DS, Bigliani LU: Variations in acromial shape and its effect on rotator cuff tears. p. 213. In Takagishi N (ed): The Shoulder. Professional Postgraduate Services, Philadelphia, 1987

18. Uhthoff HK, Loehr J, Sarkar K: p. 211. In Takagishi N (ed): The Shoulder. Professional Postgraduate Services, Philadelphia, 1987

19. Ozaki J, Fujimoto S, Yoshiyuki N et al: Tears of the rotator cuff of the shoulder associated with pathological changes in the acromion. J Bone Joint Surg 70A:1224, 1988

20. Apoil A, Dautry P, Koechlin P, Hardy J: The surgical treatment of rotator cuff impingement. p. 22. In Bayley I, Kessel L (eds): Shoulder Surgery. Springer-Verlag, Berlin, 1982

21. DePalma AF: Surgery of the Shoulder. 3rd Ed. JB Lippincott, Philadelphia, 1983

22. Matsen FA, Arntz CT: Subacromial impingement. p. 623. In Rockwood CA, Matsen FA III (eds): The Shoulder. WB Saunders, Philadelphia, 1990

23. Hammond G: Complete acromionectomy in the treatment of chronic tendinitis of the shoulder. A follow-up of ninety operations of eighty-seven patients. J Bone Joint Surg 53A:173, 1971

24. Pappas AM, Zawacki RM, Sullivan TJ: Biomechanics of baseball pitching: a preliminary report. Am J Sports Med 13:216, 1985

25. Poppen NK, Walker PS: Forces at the glenohumeral joint in abduction. Clin Orthop 135:165, 1978

26. Schwartz RE, O'Brien SJ, Warren RF et al: Capsular restraints to anterior-posterior motion of the abducted shoulder: a biomechanical study. Orthop Trans 12:727, 1988

27. Turkel SJ, Panio MW, Marshall JL, Girgis FG: Stabilizing mechanisms preventing anterior dislocation of the glenohumeral joint. J Bone Joint Surg 63A:1208, 1981

28. Poppen NK, Walker PS: Normal and abnormal motion of the shoulder. J Bone Joint Surg 58A:195, 1976

29. Ovesen J, Nielsen S: Stability of the shoulder joint: cadaver study of stabilizing structures. Acta Orthop Scand 56:149, 1985

30. Harryman DT, Sidles JA, Clark JM et al: Translation of the humeral head on the glenoid with passive glenohumeral motion. J Bone Joint Surg 72A:1334, 1990

31. Jobe FW, Tibone JE, Jobe CM, Kuitne RS: The shoulder in sports. p. 961. In Rockwood CA, Matsen FA III (eds): The Shoulder. WB Saunders, Philadelphia, 1990

32. Jobe FS, Moynes D: Delineation of diagnostic criteria and rehabilitation program for rotator cuff injuries. Am J Sports Med 10:336, 1982

33. Cofield RH, Simonet WT: Symposium on sports medicine: Part 2, The shoulder in sports. Mayo Clin Proc 59:157, 1984

34. Bulgen DY, Binder AI, Hazleman BL et al: Frozen shoulder: prospective clinical study with an evaluation of three treatment regimes. Ann Rheum Dis 43:353, 1984

35. Connolly J, Regen E, Evans OB: The management of the painful, stiff shoulder. Clin Orthop 84:97, 1972

36. Cryiax J: Textbook of Orthopaedic Medicine: Diagnosis of Soft Tissue Lesions. Vol. 1. 8th Ed. Bailliere Tindall, London, 1982

37. Thompson RC Jr, Schneider W, Kennedy T: Entrapment neuropathy of the inferior branch of the suprascapular nerve by ganglia. Clin Orthop 166:185, 1982

38. Maigne R: Orthopedic Medicine: A New Approach to Vertebral Manipulations. Charles C Thomas, Springfield, IL, 1984

39. Saha AK: Dynamic stability of the glenohumeral joint. Acta Orthop Scand 42:491, 1971

40. Basmajian JV, Bazant FJ: Factors preventing downward dislocation of the adducted shoulder joint. J Bone Joint Surg 41A:1182, 1959

41. Kapandji IA: The Physiology of the Joints: Upper Limb. Churchill Livingstone, New York, 1982

42. Dempster WT: Mechanisms of shoulder movement. Arch Phys Med Rehabil 46:49, 1965

43. McMasters PE: Tendon and muscle ruptures: clinical and experimental studies on the causes and location of subcutaneous ruptures. J Bone Joint Surg 15A:705, 1933

44. Uhthoff HK, Loehr J, Sarkar K: The pathogenesis of rotator cuff tears. In: Proceedings of the Third International Conference on Surgery of the Shoulder, Fukuora, Japan, 1986

45. Matsen FA, Arntz CT: Rotator cuff tendon failure. p. 647. In Rockwood CA (ed): The Shoulder. WB Saunders, Philadelphia, 1990

46. Rathbun JB, MacNab I: The microvascular pattern of the rotator cuff. J Bone Joint Surg 52B:540, 1970

47. Atwater AE: Biomechanics of overarm throwing movements and of throwing injuries. Exerc Sport Sci Rev 7:43, 1979

48. Inman VT, Saunders JB de CM, Abbott LC: Observations on the function of the shoulder joint. J Bone Joint Surg 26A:1, 1944

49. Saha AK: Dynamic stability of the glenohumeral joint. Acta Orthop Scand 42:491, 1971

50. Weaver HL: Isolated suprascapular nerve lesions. Injury: Br J Accident Surg 15:117, 1983

51. Weiner DS, Macnab I: Superior migration of the humeral head: a radiological aid in the diagnosis of tears of the rotator cuff. J Bone Joint Surg 52B:524, 1970

52. Lindblom K: On pathogenesis of ruptures of the tendon aponeurosis of the shoulder joint. Acta Radiol 20:563, 1939

53. Iannotti JP, Swiontkowski M, Esterhafi J, Boulas HJ: Intraoperative assessment of rotator cuff vascularity using laser Doppler flowmetry. Abstract presented to AAOS Meeting, Las Vegas, NV, 1989

54. Sigholm G, Styf J, Korner L, Herberts P: Pressure recording in the subacromial bursa. J Orthop Res 6:123, 1988

55. Matsen FA III: Compartmental Syndromes. Grune & Stratton, Orlando, FL, 1980

56. Cofield RH: Current concepts review rotator cuff disease of the shoulder. J Bone Joint Surg 67A:974, 1985

57. Hawkins RJ, Kennedy JC: Impingement syndrome in athletes. Am J Sports Med 8:151, 1980

58. Nitz AJ: Physical therapy management of the shoulder. Phys Ther 66:1912, 1986

59. Fowler P: Swimmer problems. Am J Sports Med 7:141, 1979

60. Moynes D: Prevention of injury to the shoulder through exercise and therapy. Clin Sport Med 2:413, 1983

61. Penny JN, Smith C: The prevention and treatment of swimmer's shoulder. Can J Appl Sport Sci 5:195, 1980

62. Richardson AB, Jobe FW, Collins HR: The shoulder in competitive swimming. Am J Sports Med 8:159, 1980

63. Brookes RB: Physiotherapy of supraspinatus tendinitis. Physiotherapy 57:21, 1971

63b. Wilk KE, Arrigo CA, Coursur RE et al: Preventive and Rehabilitative Exercises for the Shoulder and Elbow. American Sports Medicine Institute, Birmingham, AL, p. 4, 1991

64. Peterson L, Renstrom P: Sports Injuries: Their Prevention and Treatment. Year Book Medical Publishers, Chicago, 1986

65. Jackson DW, Reiman RE: Diagnosis of the painful athletic shoulder. In Jackson DW (ed): Shoulder Surgery in the Athlete. Aspen Systems, Rockville, MD, 1985

66. Yocum LA: Assessing the shoulder: history, physical examination, differential diagnosis, and special tests used. Clin Sports Med 2:281, 1983

67. Daniels L, Worthingham C: Muscle Testing Techniques of Manual Examination. WB Saunders, Philadelphia, 1985

68. Kendall HO, Kendall FP: Muscle Testing and Function. Williams & Wilkins, Baltimore, 1985

69. Andrews JR, Gillogly S: Physical examination of the shoulder in throwing athletes. In Zarins B, Andrews JR, Carson WG (eds): Injuries to the Throwing Arm. WB Saunders, Philadelphia, 1985

70. Hawkins RJ, Kennedy JC: Impingement syndrome in athletes. Am J Sports Med 8:151, 1980

71. Binder A, Parr G, Hazelman B: Pulsed electromagnetic field therapy of persistent rotator cuff tendinitis: a double-blind controlled assessment. Lancet 1:695, 1984

72. Clarke R, Mellon R, Lind A: Vascular reactions of the human forearm to cold. Clin Sci 17:165, 1958

73. Janssen CW Jr, Wasleer E: Body temperature, antibody formation and inflammatory response. Acta Pathol Microbiol Scand (C) 69:555, 1967

74. Lee JM, Warren MP, Mason SM: Effects of iced on nerve conduction velocity. Physiotherapy 64:2, 1978

75. Stangle L: The value of cryotherapy and thermotherapy in the relief of pain. Physiother Can 27:135, 1975

76. Knight KL: Cryotherapy: Theory, Technique and Physiology. Chattanooga Corp., Tennessee, 1985

77. Kaada B: Treatment of peritendinitis calcaria of the shoulder by transcutaneous nerve stimulation. Acupunct Electrother Res 9:115, 1984

78. Kaada B: Vasodilation induced by transcutaneous nerve stimulation in peripheral ischemia. Eur Heart J 3:303, 1983

79. Santiesteban AJ: Physical agents and musculoskeletal injuries. p. 201. In Gould JA, Davies GJ (eds): Orthopedic and Sports Physical Therapy. CV Mosby Co, St. Louis, 1985

80. Yao JH: Acutherapy; Acupuncture T.N.S. and Acupressure. Acutherapy Postgraduate Seminars, Libertyville, IL, 1984

81. Lund IM, Donde R, Knudsen EA: Persistent local cutaneous atrophy following corticosteroid injection for tendinitis. Rheumatol Rehabil 18:91, 1979

82. Rostron PK, Orth MCH, Wigan FRCS, Calver RF: Subcutaneous atrophy following methylprednisolone injection in Osgood-Schlatter epiphysitis. J Bone Joint Surg 61A:627, 1979

83. Uitto J, Teir H, Mustakellio KK: Corticosteroid induced inhibition of the biosynthesis of human skin collagen. Biochem Pharm 2:2161, 1972

84. Kennedy JC, Willis RB: The effects of local steroid injections on tendons: a biomechanical and microscopic correlative study. Am J Sports Med 4:11, 1976

85. Wirthington RH, Girgis, FL, Seifert MH: A placebo controlled trial of steroid injections in the treatment

of supraspinatus tendinitis. Scand J Rheumatol 14:76, 1985

86. Valtonen EJ: Double acting betamethasone in the treatment of supraspinatus tendinitis: a comparison of subacromial and gluteal single injections with placebo. J Int Med Res 6:643, 1978

87. Herberts P, Kadefors R, Hogfors C, Sigolm G: Shoulder pain and heavy manual labor. Clin Orthop 191:166, 1984

88. Rowe CR: Ruptures of the rotator cuff. Surg Am 43:1531, 1963

89. Peacock EE: Wound Repair. WB Saunders, Philadelphia, 1981

90. Falkel JE, Angle DD, Chleboun GS: Blood flow in the nonexercising limb during cycle and arm crank ergometry. Unpublished data.

91. Evans P: The healing process at cellular level: a review. Physiotherapy 66:256, 1980

92. Cookson JC, Kent BE: Orthopedic manual therapy: an overview. Part 1: The extremities. Phys Ther 59:136, 1979

93. Barak T, Rosen ER, Sofa R: Mobility: passive orthopedic manual therapy. p. 212. In Gould FA, Davies GJ (eds): CV Mosby, St. Louis, 1985

94. Paris SV: Extremity Dysfunction and Mobilization: Prepublication Manual. Institute Press, Atlanta, 1980

95. Maitland GD: Peripheral Manipulation. 4th Ed. Butterworth, London, 1977

96. Paris SV: Spinal manipulative therapy. Clin Orthop 179:55, 1983

97. Wyke B: Articular neurology: a review. Physiotherapy 58:94, 1972

98. Kaltenborn FM: Mobilization of the Extremity Joints. 3rd Ed. Olaf Bokhandel, Oslo, 1980

99. Saha AK: Mechanism of shoulder movements and a plea for the recognition of "zero position" of glenohumeral joint. Indian J Surg 12:153, 1950

100. Freedman L, Monroe RR: Abduction of the arm in the scapular plane: scapular and glenohumeral movements. J Bone Joint Surg 48A:1503, 1966

101. Das SP, Roy GS, Saha AK: Observations on the tilt of the glenoid cavity of scapula. J Anat Soc India 15:114, 1966

102. Cardenas DD, Stolov WC, Hardy R: Muscle fiber number in immobilization atrophy. Arch Phys Med Rehabil 58:423, 1977

103. Cooper R: Alterations during immobilization and regeneration of skeletal muscle in cats. J Bone Joint Surg 54A:919, 1972

104. Currier DP, Petrille CR, Threlkeld AJ: Effect of graded electrical stimulation of blood flow to healthy muscle. Phys Ther 66:937, 1986

105. Gould N, Donnermeyer D, Pope M et al: Transcutaneous muscle stimulation as a method to retard disuse atrophy. Clin Orthop 164:215, 1982

106. Wolf E, Magora A, Goen B: Disuse atrophy of the quadriceps muscle. Electromyography 11:479, 1971

107. Costill DL, Fink WJ, Habansly AJ: Muscle rehabilitation after knee surgery. Physician Sportsmed 5:71, 1977

108. Granit R: The Basis of Motor Control. Academic Press, New York, 1970

109. Curin S, Stanish WD: Tendinitis: its etiology and treatment. DC Heath, Toronto, 1984

110. Abramson KI, Burnett C, Bell Y et al: Changes in blood flow, oxygen uptake and tissue temperatures produced by therapeutic physical agents. Am J Phys Med 39:51, 1960

111. Griffin JE, Karselis TC: Physical Agents for Physical Therapists. Charles C Thomas, Springfield, IL, 1978

112. Griffin JE: Physiological effects of ultrasonic energy as it is used clinically. J Am Phys Ther Assoc 46:18, 1966

113. Lehmann JF, DeLateur BJ, Stonebridge FB, Warren CG: Therapeutic temperature distribution produced by ultrasound as modified by dosage and volume of tissue exposed. Arch Phys Med Rehabil 48:662, 1967

114. Lota MJ: Electronic plethysmographic and tissue temperature studies of effect of ultrasound on blood flow. Arch Phys Med Rehabil 46:315, 1965

115. Beard G, Wood EC: Massage: Principles and Techniques. WB Saunders, Philadelphia, 1974

116. Hovind H, Nielson SL: Effect of massage on blood flow in skeletal muscle. Scand J Rehabil Med 6:74, 1974

117. Kowal MA: Review of physiological effects of cryotherapy. J Orthop Sports Phys Ther 5:66, 1983

118. Lehmann JF, Waren CG, Scham SM: Therapeutic heat and cold. Clin Orthop 99:207, 1974

119. Cyriax J: Textbook of Orthopaedic Medicine: Treatment by Manipulation Massage and Injection. Vol. 2. 10th Ed. Bailliere Tindall, London, 1980

120. Brewer BJ: Aging of the rotary cuff. Am J Sports Med 7:102, 1979

121. Meyer AW: The minute anatomy of attrition lesions. J Bone Joint Surg 13A:341, 1931

122. Moore MA, Hutton RS: Electromyographic investigation of muscle stretching techniques. Med Sci Sports Exerc 12:322, 1980

123. De Vries HA: Physiology of Exercise for Physical Education and Athletics. Brown, Dubuque, IA, 1980

124. Frankel BH, Nordin M: Basic Biomechanics of the Skeletal System. Lea & Febiger, Philadelphia, 1980

125. Kulwig K, Andrews JG, Hay JG: Human strength curves. Exerc Sports Sci Rev 12:417, 1984

126. Komi PV: Training of muscle strength and power: interaction of neuromotoric, hypertrophic and mechanical factors. Int J Sports Med 7:10, 1986

127. Stockmeyer SA: An interpretation of the approach of Rood to the treatment of neuromuscular dysfunction. Am J Phys Med, 46:900, 1967

128. Knott B, Voss DE: Proprioceptive Neuromuscular Facilitation. 2nd Ed. Harper & Row, New York, 1968

129. Patten BM: Human Embryology. McGraw-Hill, New York, 1953

130. Brodal A: Neurological Anatomy in Relation to Clinical Medicine. Oxford University Press, New York, 1969

131. Astrand P, Rodahl K: Textbook of Work Physiology. McGraw-Hill, New York, 1970

132. Herbert P, Kadefors R, Hogfors C, Sigholm G: Shoulder pain and heavy manual labor. Clin Orthop 191:166, 1984

133. King JW, Brelsford HJ, Tullos HS: Analysis of the pitching arm of the professional baseball pitcher. Clin Orthop 67:116, 1970

134. Fleck SJ, Kraemer WJ: Designing Resistance Training Programs. Human Kinetics, Champaign, IL, 1987

135. Komi P, Bosco C: Utilization of stored elastic energy in leg extensor muscles by men and women. Med Sci Sports 10:261, 1978

136. Lundin PE: A review of plyometric training. Nat Strength Conditioning Assoc J 7:65, 1985

137. Eldred E: Functional implications of dynamic and static components of the spindle response to stretch. Am J Phys Med 46:129, 1967

138. Barnes OA, Tullos HS: An analysis of 100 symptomatic baseball players. Am J Sports Med 6:62, 1978

139. Perry J: Anatomy and biomechanics of the shoulder in throwing, swimming, gymnastics and tennis. Clin Sports Med 2:247, 1983

140. Wilk KE, Arrigo CA: An integrated approach to upper extremity exercises. Orthop Phys Ther Clin North Am 1(2) 337, 1992

# 49

# Rehabilitation after Total Shoulder Surgery

*JOHN W. BRAUTIGAM*
*DENISE L. MASSIE*

Total shoulder replacement is an orthopaedic surgical procedure that is most appropriately referred to as a "replacement reconstruction."[1] This term indicates that the prosthetic implant is only part of the surgery. Emphasis is also placed on soft tissue reconstruction and balance. As mentioned in Chapter 29, the goals in total shoulder replacement arthroplasty are dependent on specific pathology and disease state. For complete rehabilitation to occur, it is imperative for the physical therapist to have a thorough understanding of the different pathologies and an understanding of how the rehabilitation goals may vary accordingly.

Although the total shoulder replacement was the first joint arthroplasty procedure completed, it is currently a less commonly performed joint replacement procedure compared with the hip and knee. As a result, many physical therapists working in an orthopaedic setting have a greater knowledge base and feel more confident in their ability to work with total hip and total knee patients. This is a paradoxical situation when considering the importance of rehabilitation for surgical success at the hip, knee, and shoulder. Callaghan (orthopaedic surgeon, Duke University, personal communication, 1988) stated that the surgical success of total hip replacement arthroplasty is 90 percent surgery and 10 percent rehabilitation, and the success of total knee replacement arthroplasty is 50 percent surgery and 50 percent rehabilitation. Meanwhile, he contended that the success of total shoulder replacement arthroplasty is 10 percent surgery and 90 percent rehabilitation.

Throughout the evolution of the total shoulder re-placement procedure, different implant categories for prosthetic design were developed. Currently, orthopaedic surgeons most commonly use two implant categories. The term *hemiarthroplasty* refers to replacement of the humeral head only. The term *nonconstrained total shoulder replacement* refers to the replacement of the humeral head and glenoid. Because both of these categories use nonconstrained glenoid components, soft tissue reconstruction and rehabilitation is paramount in achieving maximal stability and function.

## PATHOLOGY IN DISEASED STATES

As mentioned in Chapter 29, different pathologic and disease states cause degeneration and destruction of the glenohumeral joint.[2,3] These include glenohumeral arthritis, avascular necrosis of the humeral head, collagen vascular diseases (i.e., rheumatoid arthritis), traumatic arthritis, acute fractures, neoplasms, and rotator cuff arthropathy.

Several factors that may cause modifications in the rehabilitation protocol include the integrity of the rotator cuff and deltoid musculature, soft tissue contractures, and simulation of normal shoulder bony anatomy. Optimal surgical results are based on preservation of the deltoid and rotator cuff, preservation of humeral length, prosthetic simulation of normal anatomy, and rehabilitation of soft tissues.[1–4]

Communication between the surgeon and physical therapist is a necessity to ensure complete and safe rehabilitation. A review of medical records, patient history, and physician referral may not provide adequate information, especially for rotator cuff integrity and viability.

## NORMAL SHOULDER ANATOMY AND BIOMECHANICS

The shoulder joint allows for the greatest range of motion of all joints in the body. Because the shoulder girdle's only attachment to the axial skeleton comes at the sternoclavicular joint, the soft tissue structures play an important role for both stability and mobility. Anatomic comparisons of the shoulder, knee, and hip joints outline the structural support of each articulation. The hip provides strong skeletal support, strong ligamentous support, and strong muscular support. The knee provides weak skeletal support, moderate ligamentous support, and strong muscular support. The shoulder provides weak skeletal support, moderate ligamentous support, and moderate muscular support.[5,6] It is evident from these comparisons why the reconstruction and rehabilitation of the soft tissue structures are regarded as significant in the success of the total shoulder replacement arthroplasty.

Another factor leading to the difficulty in the rehabilitation of the shoulder is the need to mobilize the subacromial space. Soft tissue contractures including shortening of the pectoralis minor and major, coracobrachialis, anterior deltoid, and biceps musculature, besides adhesions and contractures of the anterior capsule, contribute to the compromise of this space.[1,3,4] The function of the rotator cuff musculature acting as a humeral head depressor for movements involving glenohumeral elevation is important in maintaining the mobility of the subacromial space.

As described in the literature, shoulder movements are possible by the use of force couples at both the glenohumeral and scapulothoracic joints.[7] Force couples enable the shoulder to be the most mobile joint in the body. The surrounding shoulder musculature provides for proximal and distal glenohumeral stability and mobility. The shoulder musculature and its relationship to the force couples are summarized in Table 49-1.

It is important to remember that the shoulder musculature is weakened by two factors: the acute or chronic trauma (i.e., rotator cuff pathology, adhesive capsulitis, soft tissue shortening, and contractures) and the induced trauma of surgery. To achieve maximal function, the force couples involved in attaining shoulder movements must be addressed on an individual basis.

### Table 49-1. Shoulder Musculature and Its Relationship to Joint Force Coupler

| Motion | Glenohumeral Joint | Scapulothoracic Joint |
|---|---|---|
| Abduction | Rotator cuff (primarily supraspinatus) Deltoid | Upper trapezius Lower trapezius Serratus anterior |
| Flexion | Anterior deltoid Coracorbrachialis Pectoralis major (clavicular portion) Rotator cuff | Upper trapezius Lower trapezius Serratus anterior |
| Adduction | Rhomboids Teres major | Triceps (long head) Latissimus dorsi |
| Extension | Teres major Teres minor Posterior deltoid Latissimus dorsi | Rhomboids Middle trapezius Latissimus dorsi |
| Internal rotation | Latissimus dorsi Teres major Subscapularis Pectoralis major | Serratus anterior Pectoralis minor |
| External rotation | Infraspinatus Teres minor | Rhomboids Trapezius |

## GENERAL PRINCIPLES OF REHABILITATION

A goal-oriented approach based on specific pathology is the foundation for total shoulder replacement arthroplasty rehabilitation. The general goals of the rehabilitation program include pain relief, increased passive and active range of motion, increased strength, and increased shoulder function. Hopkinson (orthopaedic surgeon, Walter Reed Army Medical Center, personal communication, 1989) stated that timely surgical intervention is often a key to attaining these goals. Often times, the degeneration and weakening of the rotator cuff musculature, as well as associated soft tissue shortening and/or contractures, are limiting factors in achieving maximal function. The presence of significant soft tissue pathology will dictate the need for limited goals to be established. Because the emphasis of rehabilitation is on the soft tissue structures, surgery before soft tissue deterioration allows for optimal success.

Before the implementation of a specific exercise regime, the physical therapist must have a knowledge of the factors affecting the biomechanical stability and mobility of the total shoulder replacement. Communication with the surgeon is necessary regarding humeral shortening and/or tuberosity repair, glenoid erosion, rotator cuff integrity, and joint contractions and/or capsular adhesions.[1-4] These factors will dictate the specific plan of care and establishment of goals.

Knowledge of these factors is also important with regard to time constraints for healing. Rotator cuff and deltoid musculature healing requires approximately 6 weeks. Reformation of the subacromial bursa requires approximately 3 months.

In general, the rehabilitation program can be divided into three phases. The first phase, from weeks 1 to 6, is termed the *recovery of motion* phase. The second phase, from the sixth week to the third month, is termed the *recovery of strength or neuromuscular control* phase. The third phase, beginning the third month, addresses the increase in activities of daily living and neuromuscular coordination. The breakdown of the rehabilitation program into phases regarding range of motion, strength, and function does not imply that the exercises should focus only on these specific components. In phase I, the recovery of motion phase, specific exercises to increase neuromuscular control are initiated. In phase 3, range of motion and shoulder strengthening exercises are continued. The program is divided into phases only to focus on the activities of primary importance during this time.

A preoperative evaluation by the physical therapist is beneficial in establishing postsurgical goals. This evaluation should include measures for active and passive range of motion, strength, pain, and function. Preoperative exercises including range of motion and isometrics will stretch and strengthen soft tissue components and aid the postoperative program. Instruction in the entire postoperative exercise regime is also performed at this time.

The acute phase of total shoulder replacement arthroplasty rehabilitation should focus on passive and active assistive range of motion exercises. Multiple daily exercise bouts in short duration are preferred. Neer[1,3,4] recommended five exercise bouts daily of at least 5 minutes in duration. The use of local ice application during the acute phase of the rehabilitation process is indicated for control of the local inflammatory response and pain relief. Moist heat applications before exercise for analgesia are most appropriately used after the first 4 to 6 weeks. Some discomfort in the performance of the specific exercises is expected; however, performance of the exercises to the point of excruciating pain will increase the local inflammatory response and is detrimental to the program. Obviously, tolerance to pain varies with each patient and requires subjective evaluation by the therapist. Also, pool therapy after adequate wound healing may be used at different points in the rehabilitation program. The water may serve as an assistive or resistive medium.

The issue of scapular mobility versus scapular stability and whether the specific shoulder motion occurs at the glenohumeral joint or scapulothoracic joint are most appropriately addressed after at least the initial 6 weeks of rehabilitation.

## SPECIFIC PROGRAM FOR ASEPTIC NECROSIS OR INCONGRUITY OF THE HUMERAL HEAD WITH INTACT TUBEROSITIES, ROTATOR CUFF, AND GLENOID

This program is a modification of the original Neer protocol.[1,4] Neer based his original protocol on a hospital stay of approximately 21 days. This program has been modified to be consistent with the current length of hospitalization. As mentioned in Chapter 29, this is not a "cookbook" approach. The need for daily evaluation and progression on an individual basis is emphasized during hospitalization. The exercise program is dependent on the patient's compliance and overall motivation level. At least biweekly follow-ups are recommended. At 6 weeks, progressive resistance exercises with light weights and proprioceptive neuromuscular facilitation patterns are incorporated. Six months of vigorous physical therapy is recommended both at home and with periodic monitoring. Consider the scapular mobility versus stability issue after 6 to 8 weeks of rehabilitation. The specific program, with regard to initiation of postoperative day exercises and program instruction is shown in Appendix 49-1.

## TECHNIQUE FOR ACUTE FRACTURES AND FRACTURE DISLOCATIONS

The rehabilitation protocol for actue fractures and fracture dislocations is modified to allow sufficient time for fracture healing.[1,3] The patient is placed in a shoulder immobilizer and instructed not to attempt to raise or lean on the affected arm for 6 weeks. Tanner and Cofield[8] advocated initiation of physical therapy before 2 weeks after the operation. Passive and active assisted range of motion exercises including external rotation, flexion, and extension and passive pendulum exercises are the only exercises to be performed during the initial 6 weeks. The patient may progress to a more aggressive exercise regime after 6 weeks as indicated by the surgeon. It is important for the physical therapist to communicate with the surgeon regarding the status of bony repair and possible contraindications and/or indications in the rehabilitation program.

## SHOULDER CONTINUOUS PASSIVE RANGE OF MOTION

A shoulder continuous passive motion machine is used with different techniques as indicated by the orthopaedic surgeon.[9] The shoulder continuous passive motion may be administered in either a supine or standing position. The initial setup should be conducted by the physical therapist, and the limits of motion should be set to the patient's tolerance. The rate of motion may be set from 2 to 5 degrees/s. Specific limitations to the range of motion should be in accordance with the pathology and prescribed by the surgeon. The continuous passive motion is a useful adjunct to therapy; however, it may not be indicated in all conditions.

## SUMMARY

Rehabilitation based on sound physiologic principles, surgical technique regarding involved structures, and communication among the surgeon, physical therapist, and patient is imperative for optimal surgical results. Program modification and appropriate progression must be performed on an individual basis. The primary goals of total shoulder replacement arthroplasty are decreased pain and increased function of the affected shoulder. Individual goals are based on the patient's desires and functional needs. Limited goals for range of motion, restricted function, and limitations must be identified for specific individuals. Patient education regarding the continued improvement in strength and function over months and years through continuation of an independent home program must be emphasized. Improvements in prosthetic design, timely patient selection, and emphasis on complete rehabilitation will no doubt lead to increased function and better quality of life for the entire total shoulder replacement arthroplasty patient population in the future.

## REFERENCES

1. Neer CS II: Surgical Protocol. Neer II Proximal Humerus. Arthroplasty of the Shoulder: Neer Technique. Minnesota Mining and Manufacturing Company, St Paul, MN, 1982
2. Neer CS II: Articular replacement for the humeral head. J Bone Joint Surg 37A:215, 1955
3. Neer CS II, Watson KC, Stanton FJ: Recent experience in total shoulder replacement. J Bone Joint Surg 64A:319, 1982
4. Hughes M, Neer CS II: Glenohumeral joint replacement and postoperative rehabilitation. Phys Ther 55:850, 1975

5. Klafs CE, Arnheim DD: Modern Principles of Athletic Training. CV Mosby, St Louis, 1981

6. Warwick R, Williams P: Gray's Anatomy. 36th Ed. WB Saunders, Philadelphia, 1980

7. Kapandji IA: The Physiology of the Joints. Vol. 1. 5th Ed. Churchill Livingstone, New York, 1982

8. Tanner NW, Cofield RH: Prosthetic arthroplasty for fractures and fracture-dislocations of the proximal humerus. Clin Orthop 179:116, 1983

9. Craig EV: Continuous passive motion in the rehabilitation of the surgically reconstructed shoulder. A preliminary report. Orthop Transactions 10:233, 1986

# Appendix 49-1

1. Patient is cautioned not to attempt to raise or lean on arm for the first 10 days after surgery.
2. Immobilization: Shoulder immobilizer is used for the first 10 days after surgery at night (Fig. 49-1). A sling may be used during awake hours on postoperative day 4. A surgeon should be consulted before discontinuing the use of the sling during awake hours. This is greatly influenced by the bony repair of the glenoid and humerus.
3. Postoperative day 1:
   A. Ice bags for 20 minutes in duration applied four to five times daily
   B. Hand, wrist, forearm, and elbow active range of motion exercises (Figs. 49-2 to 49-4)
   C. Shoulder sets (isometrics) with submaximal contraction performed by squeezing the hand and "setting" the musculature of the upper extremity (Fig. 49-5). This should be performed to patient's tolerance
   D. Pendulum exercises may be performed in a sling (Fig. 49-6)
   E. Patient may ambulate with assistance
4. Postoperative day 2:
   A. Gravity-assisted pendulum exercises (Figs. 49-7 and 49-8)
   B. External rotation exercises with assistance provided by the opposite hand (Fig. 49-9) or wand (Fig. 49-10) in a supine position. External rotation may be limited because of the status of the subscapularis repair noted by the surgeon at the time of surgery
5. Postoperative day 3:
   A. Standing assisted shoulder extension with wand (Fig. 49-11)
   B. Standing or sitting assisted flexion manually (Fig. 49-12) or with a pulley (Fig. 49-13)
   C. Supine gravity-assisted flexion with wand (Fig. 49-14) or with opposite hand (Fig. 49-15)
   D. Shoulder isometrics in neutral position for external rotation, extension, and abduction (Figs. 49-16 to 49-18). Emphasis should be placed on submaximal contractions

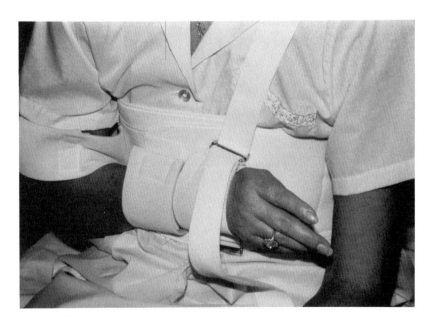

**Fig. 49-1.**

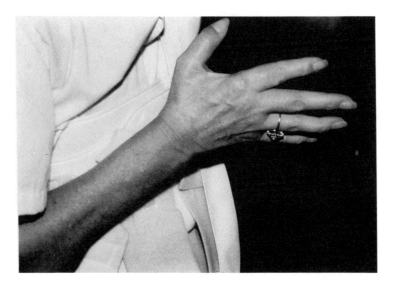

**Fig. 49-2.**

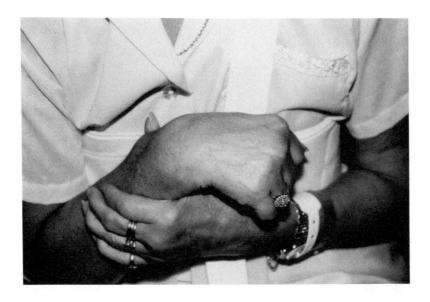

**Fig. 49-3.**

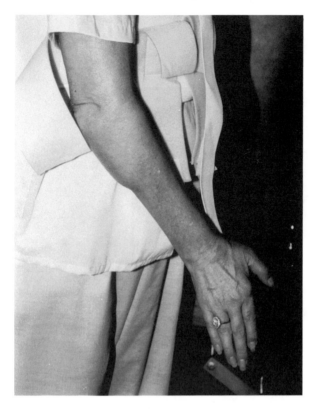

Fig. 49-4.

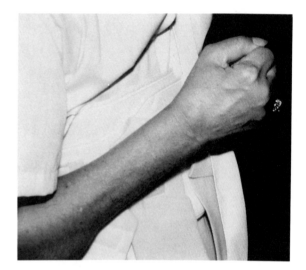

Fig. 49-5.

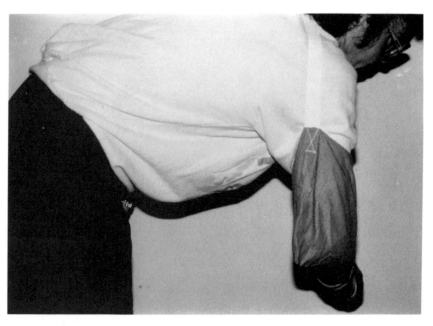

Fig. 49-6.

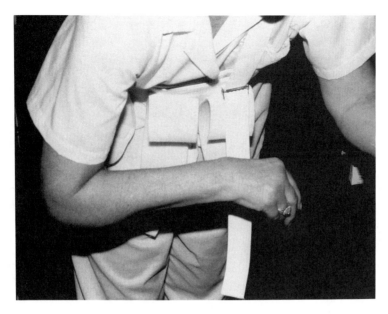

Fig. 49-7.

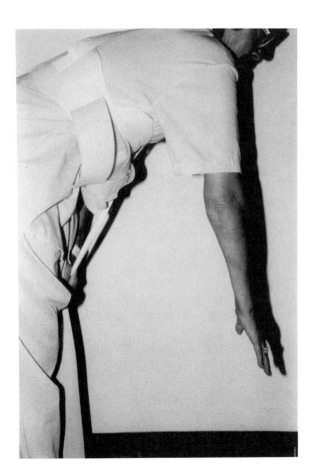

Fig. 49-8.

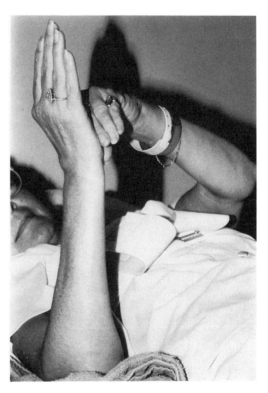

Fig. 49-9.

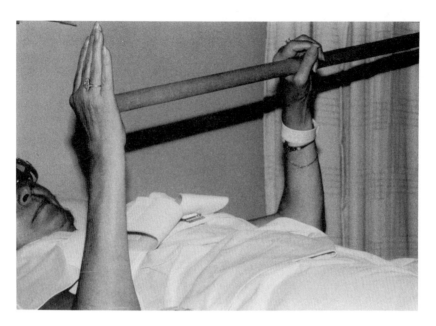

**Fig. 49-10.**

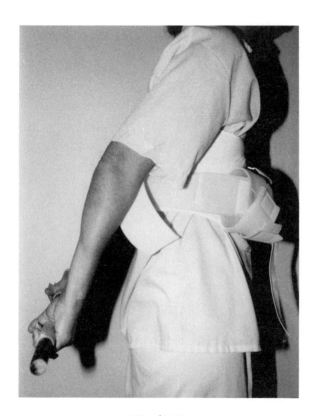

**Fig. 49-11.**

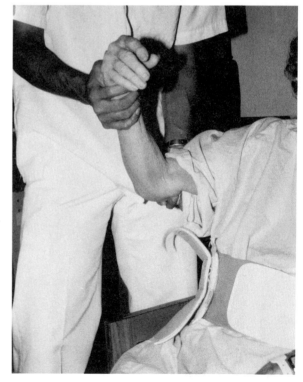

**Fig. 49-12.**

6. Postoperative days 5 to 7:
   A. Sitting assisted flexion using a table (Figs. 49-19 and Fig. 49-20)
   B. Standing assisted external rotation using door frame (Fig. 49-21). Caution should be taken, and extreme external rotation should be avoided secondary to the subscapularis incision
   C. Standing assisted flexion with wand (Fig. 49-22) or door (Fig. 49-23)
   D. Standing active range of motion for shoulder flexion, extension, and internal and external rotation. This should be performed through a limited, pain-free arc

7. Hospital discharge criteria (postoperative days 7 to 10):
   A. Passive range of motion for shoulder flexion of 120 to 140 degrees
   B. Passive range of motion for shoulder external rotation of 20 to 30 degrees
   C. A thorough understanding of the exercise home program
   D. Occupational therapy training in activities of daily living
   E. Independent transfer and ambulation

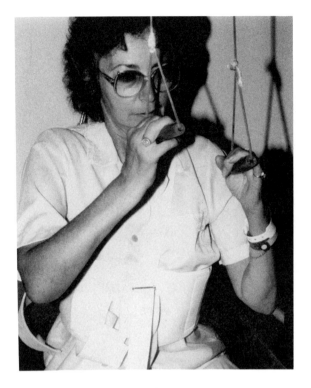

**Fig. 49-13.**

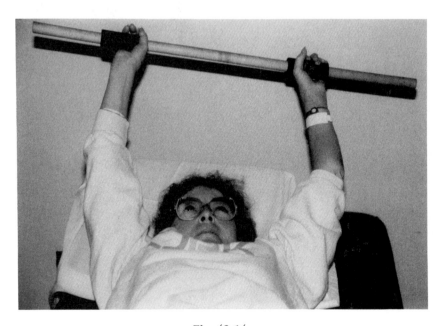

**Fig. 49-14.**

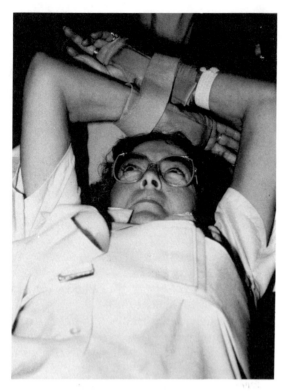

Fig. 49-15.

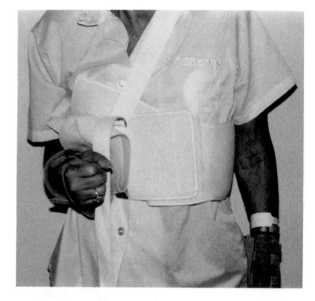

Fig. 49-17.

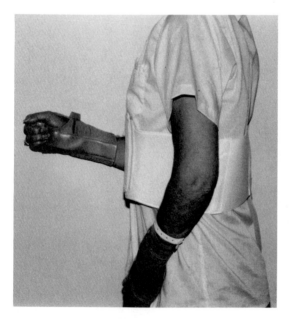

Fig. 49-16.

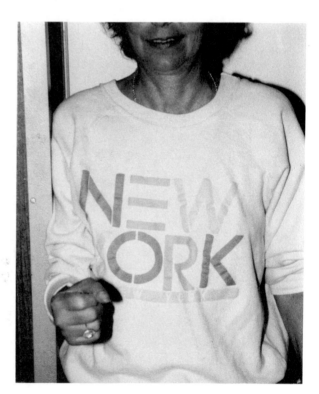

Fig. 49-18.

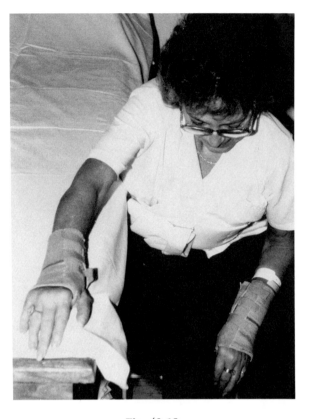

**Fig. 49-19.**

8. Postoperative days 12 to 14:
   A. Supine eccentric flexion from 90 to 0 degrees (Fig. 49-24)
   B. Spaghetti tubing exercises for extension (Fig. 49-25), flexion (Fig. 49-26), external rotation (to neutral only) (Fig. 49-27) through limited arc
9. Postoperative day 30:
   A. Begin active range of motion exercises through entire range as tolerated. Progress from supine to standing as needed
   B. Internal rotation with spaghetti tubing
   C. Pool therapy is initiated using the water as both an assistive and resistive medium. No swimming
   D. Passive range of motion continues with stretching to the end point in the range
10. Follow-up:
   A. Check progress every 3 months
   B. Continue daily home program of exercise
   C. Emphasize to the patient that function continues over months or years

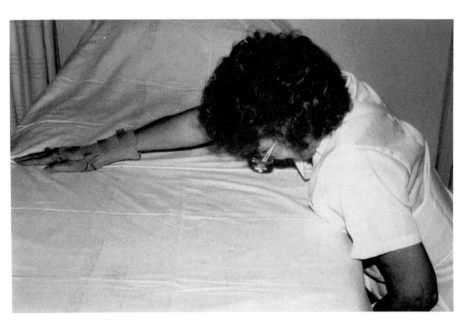

**Fig. 49-20.**

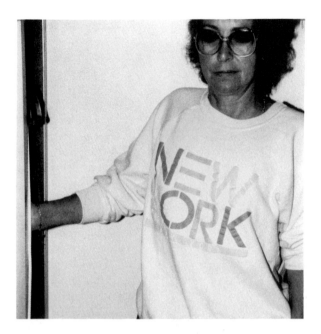

**Fig. 49-21.**

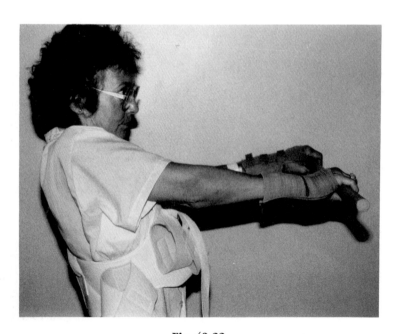

**Fig. 49-22.**

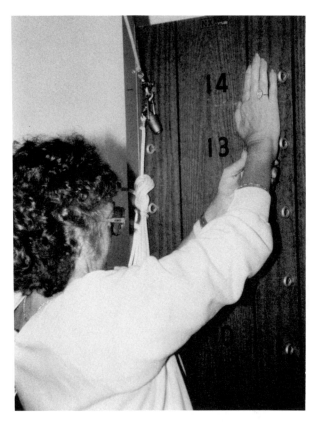

**Fig. 49-23.**

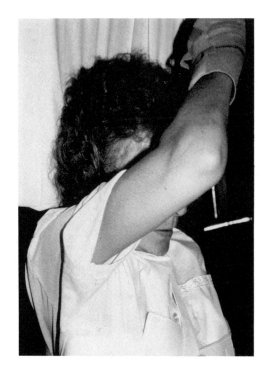

**Fig. 49-24.**

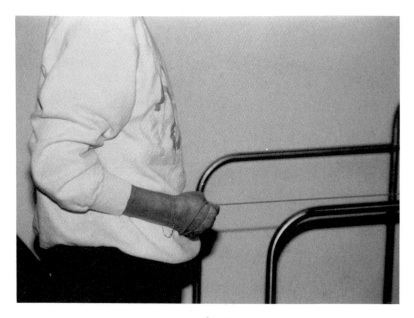

**Fig. 49-25.**

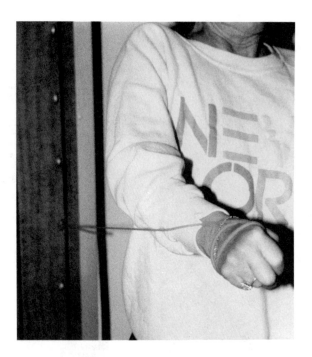

**Fig. 49-26.**

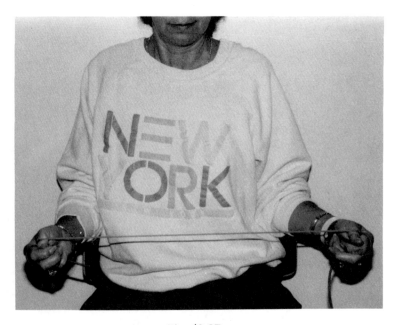

**Fig. 49-27.**

# Editors' Preferred Method

The rehabilitation program after shoulder replacement reconstruction surgery can be difficult, challenging, and frustrating to both the health care providers and the patient. It usually represents a long term process. From the articles of Neer et al.,[1,2,3] Cofield,[4] Post,[5] and others[6,7,8] we believe we have learned to approach this patient population in a different manner.

As reported by the authors of this chapter, Neer[1] cited the most common diagnostic indications for total shoulder replacement surgery as (cited order of occurrence) rheumatoid arthritis, osteoarthritis, previous trauma, prosthetic revisions, arthrosis secondary to primary dislocations, and rotator cuff arthropathy. These diagnoses represent a wide spectrum of patients, from systemic disorders to traumatic injuries.

We have determined that at least six critical factors affect the rehabilitation of these patients:

1. Underlying predisposing condition
2. Patient age
3. Activity level desired
4. Type of surgery and prosthesis
5. Patient variables (health, other pathologies, strength, etc.)
6. Tissue status of patient

Based on these factors, and particularly the first and last factors listed above, we have established two very different treatment programs for the total shoulder patient. The first patient group is considered the normal tissue rehabilitation group. These patients process good muscle tissue and bone quantity, and the causative factor for surgery is often trauma. This patient group is generally younger and wants an active lifestyle. The goal of this normal tissue rehabilitation group is more joint mobility and less inherent joint stability. In contrast, the second patient group we consider the tissue deficiency group. These patients exhibit poor or inadequate bone and muscular tissue because of systemic disorders, congenital dysplasia, surgical revisions, repeated trauma, or inadequate tissues. The ultimate goal for this patient group is joint stability, pain-free function, and less but adequate mobility. In this second group, motion is slowed to allow capsular scar formation to enhance glenohumeral joint stability. These patients exhibit poor tissue, thus process inadequate dynamic stability for the glenohumeral joint. Neer referred to this type of patient as the "limited goals" category.[9,10] The glenohumeral joint, owing to its inherent joint geometry, depends significantly on the dynamic stabilizers for functional stability. Therefore the tissue-deficient group must compensate for this insufficiency. The following tables list treatment approaches for the normal-tissue and the tissue-deficient groups of total shoulder replacement patients.

## POSTOPERATIVE REHABILITATION PROGRAM, NORMAL TISSUE GROUP

### Phase One—Immediate Motion Phase (Week 0–4)

**Goals:** Increase passive range of motion
Decrease shoulder pain
Retard muscular atrophy and prevent rotator cuff shutdown

**Exercises:** Continuous passive motion
Passive range of motion exercises
    Flexion (0-90°)
    External rotation (at 30° abduction) 0–30°
    Internal rotation (at 30° abduction) 0–35°
Pendulum exercises
Elbow wrist range of motion
Grasping exercises for hand
Ice and modalities for pain control

Isometrics (external and internal rotation, abduction) Day 10
Electrical muscle stimulation (if needed)
Rope and pulley (2nd week)

## Phase Two—Active Motion Phase (Week 4–10)

**Goals:**    Improve shoulder strength
Improve range of motion
Increase functional activities
Decrease pain

**Exercises:**    Active assisted range of motion with T-bar
Flexion, external and internal rotation (begin week 2)
Rope and pulley (flexion)
Pendulum exercises
Active range of motion (supine flexion)
Seated flexion (short arc 45–90°)
Seated abduction
Exercise tubing internal/external rotation (week 4)
Dumbbell bicep/tricep
Scapulothoracic strengthening
Joint mobilization

## Phase Three—Strengthening Phase

Initiation of this phase begins when patient exhibits

Passive range of motion
Flexion 0–160°
External rotation 0–75°
Internal rotation 0–80°
Strength ³/₅ of external rotation/abduction/internal rotation

**Goals:**    Improve strength of shoulder musculature
Neuromuscular control of shoulder complex
Improve functional activities

**Exercises:**    Exercise tubing—internal/external rotation
Dumbbell strengthening
Abduction
Supraspinatus
Scapulothoracic
Stretching exercise
T-bar
Rope and pulley

## POSTOPERATIVE REHABILITATION PROGRAM, TISSUE-DEFICIENT GROUP

### Phase One—Immediate Motion Phase (Week 0–4)

**Goals:**    Increase passive range of motion
Decrease shoulder pain
Retard muscular atrophy

**Exercises:**    Continuous passive motion
Passive range of motion
Flexion (0–90°)
External rotation (at 30° abduction) 0–20°
Internal rotation (at 30° abduction) 0–30°
Pendulum exercises
Elbow/wrist range of motion
Gripping exercises
Isometrics external/internal rotation, abduction
Rope and pulley (2nd week)
Active assisted motion exercises (when able)

### Phase Two—Active Motion Phase (Week 4–12)

**Goals:**    Improve shoulder strength
Improve range of motion
Decrease pain/inflammation
Increase functional activities

**Exercises:**  Active assisted range of motion exercises with T-bar

> Flexion, external rotation, internal rotation (Begin week 2–3, or when tolerable)
>
> Rope and pulley flexion
>
> Pendulum exercises
>
> Active range of motion exercises
>> Seated flexion (short arc 45–90°)
>> Supine flexion (full available range)
>> Seated abduction (0–90°)
>> Exercise tubing internal/external rotation (week 4–6)
>> Dumbbell bicep/triceps
>
> Joint Mobilization (week 6–8)

## Phase Three—Strengthening Phase

\* Initiation of this phase begins when patient exhibits

Passive range of motion
> Flexion 0–120°
> External rotation (at 90° abduction ) 30–40°
> Internal rotation (at 90° abduction) 45–55°

Strength level $^4/_5$ for external/internal rotation, abduction

**Goals:**  Improve strength of shoulder musculature

> Improve and gradually increase functional activities

**Exercises:**  Exercise tubing—external/internal rotation

---

\* Note: Some patients will never enter this phase.

Dumbbell strengthening
> Abduction
> Supraspinatus
> Flexion

Stretching exercises

T-bar stretches
> Flexion
> External rotation
> Internal rotation

## REFERENCES

1. Neer CS, Watson KC, Stanton FJ: Recent experience in total shoulder replacement. J Bone Joint Surg 64A:319, 1982
2. Neer CS, McCann PD, Macfarlone EA, Padilla N: Earlier passive motion following shoulder arthroplasty and rotator cuff repair. A prospective study. Orthop Trans 2:231, 1987
3. Hughes M, Neer CS: Glenohumeral joint replacement and postoperative rehabilitation. Phys Ther 55:850, 1975
4. Cofield RH: Degenerative and arthritic problems of the glenohumeral joint. p. 678. In Rockwood CA, Matsen FA (eds): The Shoulder. WB Saunders, Philadelphia, 1990
5. Post M: Shoulder arthroplasty and total shoulder replacement. p. 221. In Post M (ed): The Shoulder. Lea & Febiger, Philadelphia, 1988
6. Craig EV: Continuous passive motion in the rehabilitation of the surgically reconstructed shoulder. Orthrop Trans 10:233, 1986
7. Engelhardt E: Ten years of experience with unconstrained shoulder replacement. p. 234. In Bateman VE, Welsh RP (eds): Surgery of the Shoulder. CV Mosby, St. Louis, 1984
8. Hawkins RJ, Bell RH, Jallay B: Experience with the Neer total shoulder arthroplasty: a review of 70 cases. Orthop Trans 10:232, 1986
9. Neer CS, Craig EV, Fukuda H: Cuff tear arthropathy. J Bone Joint Surg 65A:1232, 1983
10. Neer CS, Morrison DS: Glenoid bone-grafting in total shoulder arthroplasty. J Bone Joint Surg 70A:1154, 1988

# 50

# Conditioning of the Shoulder Complex

## VERN GAMBETTA

In overhead movements in sports (throwing, tennis, swimming, etc.), the upper extremity represents the last link in the kinetic chain. Therefore, conditioning the upper extremity should represent the culmination of the total conditioning process designed to prepare the entire body for the competitive demands. Because of their position in the kinetic chain, these structures are asked to produce, transfer, and reduce tremendous amounts of force in very short periods of time. These high force demands dictate the means and methods of conditioning the upper extremity, which are discussed in this chapter.

## OBJECTIVES

The two primary objectives in conditioning the upper extremity are injury prevention and performance enhancement. The two are not mutually exclusive, but closely related. A sound conditioning program will help prevent injuries. A healthy athlete with sound skill patterns cannot help but improve performance given a basic level of ability.

## BASIC PRINCIPLES
### Synergy

The whole is greater than the sum of its parts. No one aspect of a conditioning program can stand alone and be effective. All aspects must operate together to achieve optimum performance levels. An effective con-

ditioning program consists of all aspects of the program working together. Each part of the program is incumbent on the others. If any aspect of the program is not functioning, the whole program is compromised.

## Train for Performance, Not Work Capacity

Emphasize quality of effort, intensity, and correct execution of the exercises to obtain optimum return from training. Just doing a series of exercises to get tired is not conditioning. Training should simulate the muscle action of the activity being prepared for as much as possible.

## Train for Muscular Balance

For coordinated efficient movement, it is necessary to have muscular balance. Muscular balance entails balance bilaterally, antagonist to prime mover, and within the muscle proximal to distal. The inherent structure of the shoulder with three external rotators and five internal rotators causes a muscular imbalance before any activity occurs. This must be addressed in designing a program. It is also common to see the muscles on the dominant side overdeveloped in the throwing athlete. This factor can also predispose the athlete to injury. Therefore, overdevelopment of the dominant side must be addressed in an upper extremity conditioning program. This is achieved by throwing with the opposite arm and using unilateral exercises in the strength conditioning program.

## Train Movements, Not Muscles

Rather than training muscles in isolation, it is sport-specific and functional training to involve the different muscle groups in patterns similar to the activity. Individual muscles can change their function within a single movement or may change functions from one movement to another.[1] There are three functions of muscle action:

1. Move a body segment
2. Resist movement of a body segment
3. Stabilize or fixate a body segment

To apply this principle fully, it is necessary to train all muscle actions concentrically, eccentrically, and isometrically in a similar manner and sequence as they are used in the sport skill.

## Structural (Core) Strength Before Extremity Strength

All movement starts from the stronger slower muscles surrounding the athletes center of gravity and moves out to the extremities. The waist and abdominal area connects the upper body to the lower extremities. A weak core will cause improper postural alignment. Poor postural alignment will predispose the athlete to injury by causing compensatory movements that place even greater stress on the upper extremity. Even though this is not addressed directly in this chapter, it must be constantly considered as an underlying factor in performance enhancement and conditioning.

## Body Weight Before External Resistance

In all strength activities involving the upper extremity, it is first necessary to handle the athlete's own body weight as resistance before attempting external loading. This allows for better development of joint proprioception and allows the ligaments and tendons to adapt more gradually to the stress of training.

## Strength Before Strength Endurance

A base level of strength must be developed before attempting to add endurance to that quality. This is violated in most upper extremity conditioning programs, which begin with strength endurance and work toward strength. This hinders the ultimate development level, because the quality that you are attempting to endure, strength, has not been developed to a sufficient level to operate in a climate of fatigue. This causes technique to deteriorate, which does not allow the athlete to derive full benefit from the exercise. There is also some thought that excessive long-duration low-resistance work may interfere with strength development, which eventually leads to a decrease of maximal force production per unit cross-sectional area of the muscle.

## Synergists Before Prime Movers

Often it is the synergistic muscles that are the limiting factors in performance. In the beginning stages of a conditioning program, the weak smaller stabilizing muscles prevent the athlete from increasing the load on the exercises involving the prime movers in multijoint movements. The rotator cuff group of muscles is an example. Therefore, it is important to develop those muscles within the context of the joint movements so that this will not be a limiting factor in the latter stages of conditioning. Exercises with weights facilitate the activity of the synergistic and stabilizing muscles as well as the prime movers. This is also a good argument against undue reliance on machines for strengthening. Machines provide guided resistance, which does not allow full activation of the synergistic and stabilizing muscles.

## Joint Integrity Before Joint Mobility

Inherently the shoulder joint has sacrificed stability for mobility, resulting in the most mobile joint in the entire body.[2] The issue then is to provide joint stability without a loss of optimum joint range of motion. A well-designed program that stresses muscle balance around the joint will accomplish this purpose.

## Fundamental Movement Skill Before Specific Sport Skill

Without a sound foundation of fundamental movement skills, specific sport skills will not be able to be optimally developed. These movement skills must encompass locomotion, manipulation, and stability. The average athlete that grows up specializing in one sport has a tendency to be very limited in other movement skills not directly involved in the actual sport. This eventually limits higher-level skill development and predisposes the athlete to injury. If this is the case, fundamental movement skills must be addressed as part of the conditioning program.

# TRAINING COMPONENTS

Each of the following components is a factor in performance. They are developed in different manners and with varying degrees of emphasis depending on the sport, position, and physical qualities of the individual relative to the demands of the sport. Each component is a dependent variable and cannot be considered as an isolated independent variable. None of the qualities can be significantly altered without effective the quality of the others. This underscores the significance of a balanced program.

*Work capacity (endurance)* is the ability to tolerate a large workload and to recover adequately to perform the next training session or competition. It is the capacity to resist fatigue. This is a cumulative process that encompasses the sum total of all aspects of training. The key in work capacity is the recovery process to allow for more work of higher quality to be performed in training.

*Strength* is the ability to exert force in a maximum voluntary contraction. Strength is increased either by increasing the cross-sectional area of the muscle or by enhancing neuromuscular recruitment. In conditioning the upper extremity, excessive hypertrophy or "bulk" can be counterproductive to proper skill development. Therefore the emphasis is on enhancement of the recruitment pattern, which dictates the modes and methods of training.

*Power* is the ability to exert the highest amount of force in the shortest amount of time. It is dependent on neural drive from the central nervous system to ensure a high frequency of firing through the motoneurons and a high degree of motor unit recruitment to cause fast high-tension contractions. This quality is highly dependent on the stretch shortening cycle of muscular contraction. The popular term in coaching literature for this phenomenon is *plyometrics*. It is based on the fact that a muscle on a stretch can exert significantly more force. In throwing, the stretch shortening cycle is an important factor in performance because of the production of high joint torques. This is very trainable and is the cornerstone of a conditioning program for throwing.

Plyometrics are specific work for the enhancement of explosive power. It improves the relationship between maximum strength and explosive power. In most athletic events, there is seldom enough time to develop maximum strength. It takes 0.5 to 0.7 seconds to develop maximum strength. There are few explosive/ballistic movements in athletics that take that long. For example, the delivery phase of a pitch takes 0.143 seconds.[3] Therefore, the premium in performance is on generating the highest possible force in a short time.

Plyometric training enhances the muscles ability to tolerate high stretch loads. This increased tolerance develops efficiency of the stretch shortening cycle of muscle contraction. During the stretching (eccentric lengthening) phase of muscle action, a greater amount of elastic energy is stored in the muscle. This elastic energy is then used in the following concentric action, making that movement stronger and faster. The key to the energy transfer is a short coupling time. Coupling time refers to the time it takes for the muscle to change from the lengthening/yielding phase to the shortening phase. This leads us to the key principle of plyometric training: The rate, not the magnitude of the stretch, is what determines the use of elastic energy and the transfer of chemical energy into mechanical work.

The ballistic nature of throwing dictates that the naturally occurring phenomenon of the stretch shortening cycle can be trained. To be most effective, plyometric training should exhibit similar patterns of (1) motor unit recruitment, (2) temporal sequence, and (3) firing frequency to movements in the events.[4] Medicine ball is an excellent means to train this for the upper extremity.

*Speed* is the ability to move the body or parts of the body through a range of motion in the least amount of time. The primary concern with the upper extremity is the speed of the arm resulting in velocity imparted to the ball or the implement being projected.

*Flexibility/mobility* is the ability to move a joint through a great range of motion while still maintaining the integrity of the joint.

*Coordination and skill* are the abilities to perform movements of varying degrees of difficulty with precision and accuracy in accordance with specific objectives. The ultimate goal of a conditioning program is to raise conditioning to the highest possible level to enhance skill.

# GUIDELINES FOR RESISTANCE TRAINING METHODS

## Selection of Exercise Mode

There are many modes of exercise available to choose from; some are more appropriate than others. In selecting the exercise mode, consider the following criteria: (1) facilities available, (2) space and time available, (3) safety, (4) developmental level of the athlete, and (5) goals of the program.

Body weight exercises are a very effective method of exercise for use in beginning a program. The weight-bearing nature of these exercises facilitates joint proprioception. This method is very adaptable to the plyometric method of training. It is necessary to allow a 1 day recovery between bouts of body weight exercises.

Proprioceptive neuromuscular facilitation is diagonal rotational movements designed to strengthen the muscles of the upper extremity in patterns that are similar to the stress imposed in the throwing motion. The quality of this type of training is highly dependent on the person offering the resistance because it is performed manually. It is very effective, and the patterns of contraction can be adapted for use with rubber tubing.

Weight training is perhaps the most popular mode of training and the most misunderstood mode of training for the upper extremity. There are two general categories of weight training: (1) machines, which offer guided resistance; and (2) free weights, which are ballistic and dynamic in nature.

In my opinion there has been an over-reliance on machines. The principal reason is the safety factor and ease of use. I feel that this does not take into account the dynamic ballistic nature of the demands placed on the upper extremity in throwing. Consequently, strength has been developed that is not functional strength, so there is little transfer to performance enhancement or injury prevention. The guided resistance offered by machines does not allow the involvement of the synergistic and stabilizing muscles, nor does it allow the full development of the eccentric action, which is an important factor in throwing.

Free weights are a preferable mode for conditioning the upper extremity. The free weight mode takes two forms: barbells or dumbbells. Dumbbells are preferred because they allow the upper extremities to be used unilaterally as well as allowing for a full range of motion.

Tubing and rubber bands are very effective methods for training the upper extremity. They allow for full range of motion and can accommodate all muscle actions. They are adaptable for use in the plyometric method. This mode can be used daily as long as the volume and intensity is varied. It is also very effective as a warm-up and a cool-down activity.

Medicine ball exercise is one of the most specific modes of training the upper extremity because it is the most dynamic and ballistic. This mode makes full use of the plyometric method. It is highly adaptable. It is possible to perform medicine ball training on consecutive days with proper sequencing of the exercises alternating torso and legs and upper extremity work. It can be adapted for use as a warm-up and cool-down activity.

## Selection of Exercises

Multijoint exercises are preferable over isolated single-joint movements. Unilateral work is preferable over bilateral work. For maximal strength or power development, the optimum number of exercises is two to seven. For strength endurance, the optimum number of exercises is 10 to 12.

## Sequence of Exercises

In setting the sequence of exercises, the prime consideration is the interdependency of muscle groups. It is necessary to consider the role of the prime mover, synergist, and stabilizing muscle in the exercises. "As a general rule, if a muscle is going to be called on to function as a synergist at some point in your workout, you shouldn't work it as a prime mover first."[5] An example would be a latissimus dorsi pull-down. The prime movers are the latissimus dorsi and trapezius muscles with the synergists the biceps. Therefore, the biceps should not be worked first. Another consideration in sequence is to always work the antagonist muscle group. This is necessary for balance.

## Rhythm and Speed of Exercise

It is possible to take the same exercise and have it have a very different training effect by changing the rhythm and speed of exercise. The following are the possibilities: (1) very slow, (2) slow, (3) moderate, (4) fast, (5) varied, and (6) explosive.

## Frequency

Frequency refers to the number of training sessions per training cycle, usually a week. This is dependent on the age and training level of the athlete. The younger the athlete, the smaller number of sessions per week. The older, more mature the athlete, the greater the number of training sessions and the longer the workout session.

## Progression of Exercise

Training should progress in the following manner: (1) simple to complex, (2) easy to hard, (3) volume to intensity, and (4) general to specific.

## MEANS OF TRAINING

The following means of training represent several examples of methods for conditioning the upper extremity. There are literally hundreds of means of training. Space does not permit a detailed discussion of all possibilities. The following were chosen as examples of the application of the previously discussed principles.

## Remedial Shoulder Exercises

Remedial shoulder exercises (Table 50-1) are designed to focus on the rotator cuff and allied structures to develop joint stability and strength in the muscles that decelerate the arm. Not only can these exercises be used for strengthening but they can also be adapted for use in rehabilitation, warm-up, and cool-down.

Prone horizontal abduction
Prone extension

**Table 50-1. Remedial Shoulder Exercise Progression**

| Week | Monday | Wednesday | Friday |
|---|---|---|---|
| | **PHASE 1: BASIC STRENGTH** | | |
| 1 | $1 \times 10$ | $1 \times 10$ | $1 \times 10$ |
| 2 | $2 \times 10$ | $2 \times 10$ | $2 \times 10$ |
| 3 | $3 \times 8$ | $3 \times 8$ | $3 \times 8$ |
| 4 | $4 \times 6$ | $4 \times 6$ | $4 \times 6$ |
| | **PHASE 2: STRENGTH ENDURANCE** | | |
| 1 | $1 \times 20$ | $2 \times 20$ | $3 \times 20$ |
| 2 | $1 \times 30$ | $2 \times 30$ | $3 \times 30$ |
| 3 | $1 \times 40$ | $2 \times 40$ | $3 \times 40$ |
| 4 | $3 \times 20$ | $3 \times 20$ | $3 \times 20$ |
| | **PHASE 3: COMBINATION** | | |
| 1 | $3 \times 6$ | $3 \times 10$ | $3 \times 20$ |
| 2 | $4 \times 6$ | $4 \times 10$ | $4 \times 20$ |
| 3 | $5 \times 6$ | $5 \times 10$ | $5 \times 20$ |
| 4 | $3 \times 20$ | $3 \times 20$ | $3 \times 20$ |
| | **PHASE 4: CONVERSION** | | |
| 1 | $3 \times 6$ | $3 \times 10$ | $3 \times 6$ |
| 2 | $4 \times 6$ | $4 \times 10$ | $4 \times 6$ |
| 3 | $3 \times 6$ | $3 \times 10$ | $3 \times 10$ |
| 4 | $4 \times 6$ | $4 \times 10$ | $4 \times 6$ |

Internal rotation (after phase $2_2$ strength endurance, is completed, only do one set of internal exercises during each workout)
    supine or sidelying
External rotation
    prone or sidelying
Supraspinatus raise (empty can)
Shoulder shrugs
Scapular protraction and retraction

## Arm Strength Throwing Program

The purpose of the arm strength throwing program is to prepare progressively for throwing. It will also serve to increase arm strength. This is performed by gradually using more body parts and increasing the distance and velocity of the throw.

### Warm-up

Arm swings and arm circles and arm stretches to enhance circulation.

### Pattern Throws

1. Kneeling facing the direction of the throw with throwing arm already in up position. *Distance:* 20 ft—effort: easy—number: 10—*emphasis:* proper grip.

2. Kneeling on one knee facing the direction of the throw with throwing arm already in up position (Right-handed thrower on right knee; left-handed thrower on left knee). *Distance:* 30 ft—effort: easy—number: 10—*emphasis:* hitting a target and proper follow-through.

3. Standing—feet in a straddle position facing the direction of the throw with the shoulders turned and the ball in the glove. *Distance:* 40 ft—effort: medium—number: 10—*emphasis:* follow-through.

4. Regular throwing position from a stand. *Distance:* 40 ft—effort: medium—number:10—*emphasis:* staying closed, front shoulder pointing to target.

**Arm Strength Throwing Program
(Table 50-2).**

## Medicine Ball Drills

Medicine ball drills are a plyometric form of training that is highly specific to the patterns of muscle action in throwing. These exercises maximally stress the stretch shortening component of muscle action. By adjusting the volume, intensity, and amplitude, they can be adapted for use in rehabilitation, warm-up, and cooldown.

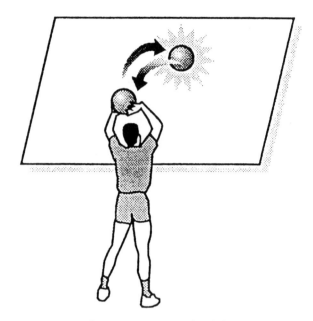

**Fig. 50-1.** Two-arm overhead throw.

### Two-Arm Overhead Throw (Fig. 50-1)

Extend the legs and the back and throw the ball forward to a partner or against a wall. When catching, allow the weight of the ball to stretch you back into the starting position and immediately repeat the action.

**Table 50-2. Arm Strength Throwing Program**

| Number of Throws[a] | Distance (ft) | Short Hop Throws to a Target | Distance (ft) |
|---|---|---|---|
| **PHASE 1** | | | |
| 20 | 45 | 20 | 45 |
| 20 | 60 | | |
| Days per week | 2 | 2 | |
| **PHASE 2** | | | |
| 40 | 60 | 15 | 60 |
| 20 | 90 | | |
| Days per week | 3 | 3 | |
| **PHASE 3** | | | |
| 50 | 90 | 15 | 90 |
| 25 | 120 | | |
| Days per week | 3 | 3 | |
| **PHASE 4** | | | |
| 20 | 150 | 15 | 90 |
| 20 | 180 | | |
| Days per week | 4 | 4 | |
| **PHASE 5** | | | |
| 25 | 180 | 15 | 90 |
| 15 | 240 or longer | | |
| Days per week | 4 | 4 | |

[a] All throws should be performed with a crow hop.

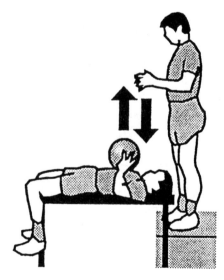

**Fig. 50-2.** Plyometric bench press throw.

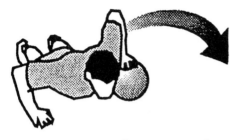

**Fig. 50-3.** Medicine ball cross-over push-ups.

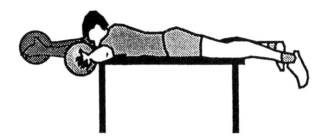

**Fig. 50-5.** Reach-outs.

## Plyometric Bench Press Throw (Fig. 50-2)

Catch the ball over the chest and bend the arms, absorbing the weight of the ball. Quickly throw the ball back to a partner standing above.

## Medicine Ball Cross-over Push-ups (Fig. 50-3)

Move the ground hand to the top of the ball, so that both hands are on the ball. Remove the opposite hand from the ball to the ground and perform a single-arm push-up. Repeat in the opposite direction.

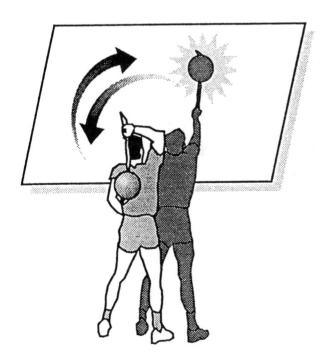

**Fig. 50-4.** One-arm chops against the wall.

## One-Arm Chops Against the Wall (Fig. 50-4)

Straddle stand, knees slightly flexed, upper body erect with a firm center and the ball held by the rope behind the body. Extend the legs, torso, and arms simultaneously, and execute a chopping action overhead.

## Reach-Outs (Fig. 50-5)

Reach out until the arms are completely extended. Hold one count and slowly return to starting position under control.

## Double-Arm Drops (Fig. 50-6)

Partner drops ball in the hands of the exerciser who decelerates the ball and throws it back to the partner.

## Single-Arm Catch and Stretch (Fig. 50-7)

Partner throws ball into the hand of the exerciser who catches the ball and throws it back to the partner with the opposite hand. The purpose of this drill is to emphasize the eccentric component by catching the ball and putting the muscles on a stretch.

## PERIODIZATION AND PROGRAM DESIGN

The ultimate success of a conditioning program depends on the timing of the application of the different training stimuli. This is achieved by manipulating the variables of volume, intensity, and recovery to force a training adaptation.

A sound program must contain a period of preparation, adaptation, and application. Preparation consists of general work. Adaptation is specialized type of work

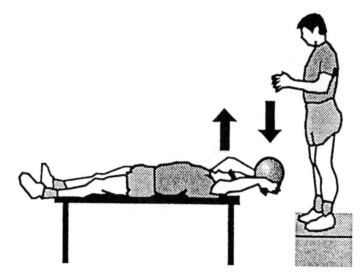

**Fig. 50-6.** Double-arm drops.

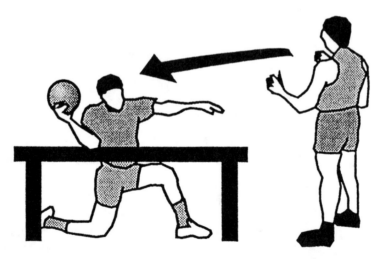

**Fig. 50-7.** Single-arm catch and stretch.

that incorporates the joint dynamics of the sport. Application is specific work that incorporates the joint actions of the sport and the specific movements of the sport.

It is also necessary to keep in mind the immediate, residual, and cumulative effects of training. All too often, the focus is on the immediate and residual training effects. In actuality, the focus must be on the long-term or cumulative training effects. The process of adaptation takes time.

The law of reversibility should receive strong consideration in designing a training program. In coaching language, reversibility means "use it or lose it." If a physical quality is not trained, that quality will decline proportionally to the time it is not emphasized. Therefore, it is unwise to train any physical quality in isolation.

Age dependency is a key aspect in planning a training program. Usually when age is considered as a factor in training, it is chronologic age. In fact, the biologic age of the athlete is a greater variable in the ability to handle a training program. Training age or the number of years that an athlete has been training for a particular activity is a major determining factor in increasing the volume and intensity of training.

The key in designing a program is separating the need-to-do from the nice-to-do activities and focusing in on those methods that will give specific results. This is performed by a thorough evaluation of all physical qualities, posture, and skill level of the individual before designing a program.

## REFERENCES

1. Kreighbaum E, Barthels KM: Biomechanics—A Qualitative Approach For Studying Human Movement. Burgess Publishing, Minneapolis, 1981
2. Cailliet R: *Shoulder Pain.* FA Davis, Philadelphia, 1981
3. Dillman CJ et al: Biomechanics of the shoulder. *In* Sports: Throwing Activities. (in press)
4. Bosco C: Stretch-shortening cycle in skeletal muscle function and physiological considerations on explosive power in man. Athleticstudi 1:7, 1985
5. Robinson J: The Secrets of Advanced Bodybuilders. Health for Life, Los Angeles, CA, 1985

## SUGGESTED READINGS

Curwin S, Stanish WD, *Tendonitis: Its Etiology and Treatment.* Collamore Press, Lexington, MA, 1984

Dominguez RH, Gajda RS: Total Body Training. Warner Books, New York, 1982

Gambetta V, Odgers S: The Complete Guide To Medicine Ball Training. Optimum Sports Training, Sarasota, FL, 1991

Gustavsen R: Training Therapy—Prophylaxis and Rehabilitation. Thieme Inc., New York, 1985

Jones NL, McCartney N, McComas AJ: Human Muscle Power. Human Kinetics Publishing, Champaign, IL, 1986

Stone M, O'Bryant H: Weight Training: A Scientific Approach. Burgess Publishing, Minneapolis, MN, 1987

Wilk KE, Courson R, Dehard R et al: Preventive & Rehabilitative Exercises for the Shoulder & Elbow. American Sports Medicine Institute, Birmingham, AL, 1990

# 51

# Arm Care for the Throwing Athlete

*CHRISTOPHER A. ARRIGO*

Preventing injuries in the throwing athlete is a major responsibility of the sports medicine practitioner. This is particularly true for those individuals involved in the day-to-day management of these athletes. The inherent instability of the shoulder and the huge dynamic muscular contributions required from the rotator cuff and flexor/pronator muscle groups, coupled with the repetitive high-velocity loads placed on the shoulder and elbow, combine to place the throwing arm at risk of sustaining a significant injury. This is particularly true when the demands of an entire competitive season are considered. Although injury prevention includes a year-round program of conditioning and training, the in-season management of the throwing arm provides one of the greatest challenges to the sports medicine team. These challenges include (1) minimizing the effects of microtrauma, (2) controlling the acute inflammatory process, (3) maintaining total arm flexibility, (4) improving total arm strength and power, (5) maintaining cardiovascular/lower extremity conditioning, and (6) communication between the athlete, athletic trainer, coaching staff, physician, and physical therapist. Assisting in the successful maintenance of symptom-free competition or in returning an injured thrower to participation requires a combination of each of these factors. To properly meet these six challenges to in-season management of the throwing arm, sports medicine professionals must possess a thorough knowledge of throwing biomechanics, functional anatomy, physiology, and the exercise tools available to them.

This chapter outlines a functional, physiologic, biomechanical, and practical approach to the in-season management and rehabilitation of the throwing arm as it relates to baseball. This approach is best described as a preventive–rehabilitative process, which combines the use of conditioning to maintain/improve functional performance, flexibility to ensure complete unrestricted range of motion, sport-specific strengthening activities designed to improve total arm strength, and modality interventions to control and minimize the microtraumatic inflammatory events related to throwing.

Microtraumatic injury events are best minimized by combining proper warm-up and stretching with the maintenance of whole body conditioning. The inflammatory process is best controlled with local modalities and the use of an organized postactivity cooldown. Total arm flexibility must be maintained to prepare the surrounding tissues for this type of repetitive, stressful activity. Total arm strength and power must be emphasized to minimize the stresses placed on the throwing shoulder and elbow, thus maximizing symptom-free function through an entire competitive season. Cardiovascular and lower extremity conditioning must also be maintained to ensure whole body functional performance. Communication is the key to successful prevention–rehabilitation. By ensuring all involved parties are aware of the status, activity level, demands, expectations, and time frames involved with every athlete, a planned approach can be carried out to coordinate this process in an extremely effective manner.

# PREVENTION–REHABILITATION

A preventive–rehabilitative approach to managing the throwing arm is grounded in the principle that the throwing arm in particular is constantly in a state of microinjury and repair. Through a competitive season, these demands become greater, and recovery time is increased, resulting in an increased risk of injury. It has been observed that isokinetic values can drop by as much as 15 percent from the beginning to the end of the season for the throwing shoulder.[1] This type of management approach allows for the contributions of both preventive and rehabilitative measures that are not mutually exclusive of one another to minimize, control, and potentially eliminate the harmful side effects of inflammatory microtraumatic injury episodes about the throwing shoulder. The key to prevention–rehabilitation of the throwing arm is flexibility and a balance of power between the opposing muscle groups of the shoulder.

# SPECIAL CONSIDERATIONS

In implementing any form of in-season management program for baseball athletes, several important considerations must be addressed. First and foremost, no program should be dictatorial. Each athlete develops his or her own pregame, postgame, and between game routines. These routines should not necessarily be altered unless they are detrimental to the athlete or the athlete is having problems with his or her arm. Such problems can be manifested as uncontrollable pitches, velocity losses, ineffective outings, increasing time length between outings, stiffness, and/or pain.[1] At this juncture, the determination must be made between the healthy and the injured athlete. Athletes who are healthy but exhibiting some periodic difficulty or those who have a history of arm trouble are the group of athletes that this type of preventive–rehabilitative program is directed toward. Those athletes with overt injuries must be appropriately dealt with outside the confines of a competitive schedule for maximal results.

In the author's experience, the best approach with any group of baseball players is to present formally a summary of all treatments and rehabilitative interventions available in this type of program. This discussion should also include how the program is implemented and what the athlete's responsibilities are within it. This type of a meeting will allow the player's expectations to be blended with the sports medicine team's philosophy to aid in the successful implementation of this type of preventive–rehabilitative program.

# LOCAL MANAGEMENT OF THE SHOULDER AND ELBOW

Implementation strategies for the prevention–rehabilitation of shoulder and elbow conditions related to throwing includes the use of a dynamic treatment plan. This type of approach includes an appropriate evaluation of the dysfunction to determine the exact etiology and pathophysiology of the injury. After the identification of the causative factors, appropriate therapeutic interventions are implemented to maximize symptomatic relief and minimize the effects of inflammation and delayed onset muscle soreness. A continuous process of evaluation and treatment modification must be used to advance these athletes appropriately through the rehabilitation process.

The goal of this local management is to normalize the dysfunction as quickly as possible by combining the use of therapeutic modalities, exercise, and proper training techniques. The involved arm must be conditioned progressively in a controlled environment to ensure that it can accommodate the stress required by the athlete to perform symptom-free throwing activities.[2]

Four key components comprise the local management of the throwing arm: (1) therapeutic modalities, (2) flexibility, (3) therapeutic exercise, and (4) conditioning.

Therapeutic modalities can often be incorporated into the treatment program to assist in the appropriate management of acute, subacute, and chronic conditions of the shoulder and elbow. Many different modalities are available to aid in preparing an athlete for competition, facilitating "cool-down" after activity, or simply as an adjunct to flexibility and strengthening exercises. These interventions can serve to minimize the inflammatory reaction and enhance tissue healing about the throwing shoulder and elbow.[2]

Flexibility exercises are paramount to a successful preventive–rehabilitative program for the throwing arm. Their benefits include (1) increased power through a greater range of motion, (2) decreased chance of muscular and joint injury, (3) increased fluidity of motion, (4) decreased postactivity soreness, (5) increased blood flow before activity, and (6) decreased anxiety.[3] Although this chapter focuses on flexibility exercises for the shoulder and elbow, whole body flexibility activities for the hip flexors, quadriceps, hamstring, groin, and trunk should also be performed before activity.

Rotator cuff and elbow strengthening activities are also critical to maintaining total arm strength and a balance between the shoulder accelerator and decelerator muscle groups. The external rotators and biceps must be able to decelerate the throwing aim, whereas the internal rotators and triceps must accelerate it. Maintaining rotator cuff and elbow strength during the competitive season with a light-weight, controlled strengthening program will minimize the risk of injury occurrence by maximizing muscular balance, coordination, and power during throwing activities.

Conditioning, the final concept, is largely beyond the scope of this chapter. However, a program of lower extremity and cardiovascular activities performed between outings to address endurance, sport-specific training, and strengthening activities is a must for any preventive–rehabilitative program.

To present this material most effectively, in a logical and sequential manner, the concepts briefly discussed above will be incorporated as they directly relate to specific areas of the in-season management for the throwing arm. The following discussions will be directed toward starting pitchers initially with specific adaptations for relief pitchers presented separately later in the chapter.

## PREPARTICIPATION ACTIVITIES

### Therapeutic Modalities

The use of a limited number of therapeutic modalities before competition may be beneficial in certain situations to increase soft tissue extensibility, promote increased blood flow, create a tissue temperature rise, and facilitate the preparation of the throwing arm for athletic competition. In the author's experience, the modalities that are most effective in this category include superficial thermotherapy, ultrasound, and phonophoresis. In selected conditions, iontophoresis and

high-voltage pulsed galvanic stimulation may also be of benefit before participation.

Moist hydrocollator packs are beneficial for superficial heating of the shoulder/elbow before warm-up activities and throwing. One megahertz ultrasound can also be selectively applied to the shoulder and/or elbow to (1) decrease pain, (2) promote tissue healing, (3) decrease muscle spasm, (4) increase soft tissue extensibility, and (5) decrease inflammation.[2] Ultrasound can produce the deepest tissue temperature rise of all the heating modalities.[2] This, along with its mechanical effects of cavitation, make it an ideal preparatory modality before physical activity. Appropriately used, these heating modalities can be beneficial in the management of many overuse pathologies, including tendinitis, bursitis, joint sprains, and musculotendinous strains.

Phonophoresis, the use of ultrasound with a 10 percent hydrocortisone, anti-inflammatory cream, is often beneficial in the local management of minimally painful inflammatory conditions before participation. The combination of effects between the ultrasound and the hydrocortisone cream serves to minimize the symptoms and maximize symptom-free performance related to mild overuse inflammatory reactions about the throwing shoulder and elbow.

The application of ultrasound to the throwing arm is best accomplished in one of three manners: (1) to the anterior shoulder with the athlete supine and the involved arm slightly internally rotated, hand resting comfortably on the hip to expose the greater tuberosity (Fig. 51-1), (2) to the posterior shoulder with the athlete prone and the affected arm supported off the side of the treatment table to facilitate access to the posterior rotator cuff underneath the deltoid, and (3) to the elbow via underwater ultrasound except in the application of phonophorosis.

### Stretching

Throwing athletes who are stiff and have difficulty loosening up or those with a history of arm trouble may benefit from the use of a specialized arm stretching routine just before full body warm-up activities. This type of stretching can be performed by the pitchers themselves or with the assistance of a T bar (see Appendix at end of book). It is imperative to stretch the inferior, anterior, and posterior aspects of the shoulder

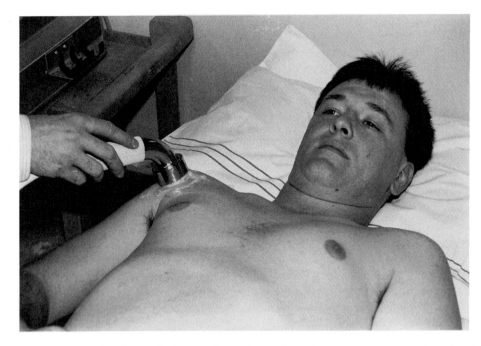

**Fig. 51-1.** Anterior glenohumeral ultrasound with internal rotation to expose the greater tuberosity.

by performing shoulder flexion, external rotation, and internal rotation stretches in a static progressive fashion. The author prefers the use of a passive stretching routine before activity for this purpose.

Fauls[1] originated a stretching routine that has enjoyed great success over the years and has empirically been shown to facilitate the warm-up process, saving a pitcher as many as 25 pitches. The stretching routine presented here is a variation of Fauls' shoulder stretching routine originally taught this author by Fauls.[1]

Five general principles of stretching should be followed when using this routine[1]:

1. Stretching should be performed before throwing, preferably within 15 minutes of the normal warm-up.
2. Stretching is performed passively with the athlete completely relaxed.
3. All stretching should be performed to the limit of available motion without pain.
4. It is imperative that the stretches be performed in their presented order, one after another for continuity. Continuity ensures that each stretch will flow readily to the next.

5. The number of stretches performed should be varied to fit the needs of the athlete being stretched

Table 51-1 outlines the 12 stretches used in this passive stretching routine.[1] Beginning in position 1, the athlete lies on the nonthrowing side, facing the athletic trainer. The athlete's head is supported on a pillow or with the nonthrowing arm, and the athlete is asked to relax completely. All the explanations pro-

**Table 51-1. Fauls Shoulder Stretch**

| | |
|---|---|
| Position 1: Sidelying | |
| Stretch 1: | Shoulder roll |
| Stretch 2: | Pectoral stretch |
| Stretch 3: | Shoulder extension |
| Stretch 4: | Shoulder flexion |
| Stretch 5: | Shoulder circles |
| Position 2: Supine | |
| Stretch 6: | "The pump" stretch |
| Stretch 7: | Shoulder flexion |
| Stretch 8: | Internal rotation |
| Stretch 9: | External rotation |
| Stretch 10: | Elbow circles |
| Stretch 11: | Wrist circles |
| Stretch 12: | Arm waves |

vided are intended for proper application of this program with a right-handed pitcher. The reverse would be true in applying these activities to a left-handed thrower.

### Stretch 1: Shoulder Roll

The pitcher's arm is placed on the athletic trainer's left shoulder. The athletic trainer cups the pitcher's shoulder with both hands and rotates the entire shoulder girdle complex 10 times in both a clockwise and counterclockwise fashion (Fig. 51-2). These rotations are performed in small circles. The object is to move the scapulothoracic and clavicular articulations and not the glenohumeral joint.

For continuity from stretch 1 to stretch 2, the pitcher's arm is moved from the trainer's left shoulder to the trainer's right forearm at the crease of the elbow.

### Stretch 2: Pectoral Stretch

The athletic trainer places the right hand on the superior aspect of the athlete's scapula. The athlete's arm is then bent at the elbow across the trainer's right forearm to place the humerus parallel to the treatment table above the athlete's head. The trainer blocks the left elbow against the athlete's hip for stability and places the left hand on the inferior aspect of the scapula (Fig. 51-3). The athletic trainer then "pulls" the scapula toward him- or herself while "pushing" the arm over the athlete's head with the right elbow. The stretch is held for 5 to 7 seconds and released. Usually this stretch is reapplied three to five times in this fashion.

For continuity from stretch 2 to stretch 3, the athlete's arm is "flipped" from the trainer's right forearm to the left hand.

### Stretch 3: Shoulder Extension

The athletic trainer places the right hand on the superior lateral aspect of the scapula over the acromioclavicular joint. The trainer then grasps the athlete's right wrist with the left hand. The athlete's arm is then moved into extension as far as possible while keeping the elbow straight and the arm parallel to the treatment surface (Fig. 51-4). As the arm is stretched back, firm pressure should be applied to the scapula in a compressive fashion. This stretch is held for 3 to 5 seconds

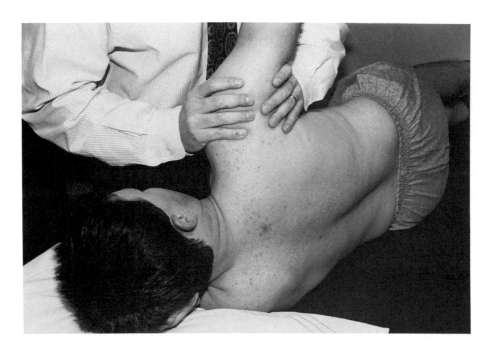

**Fig. 51-2.** Sidelying shoulder roll.

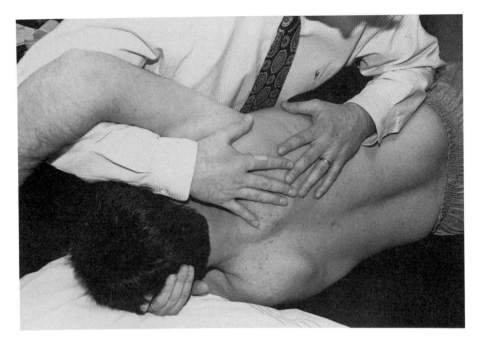

**Fig. 51-3.** Sidelying pectoral stretch.

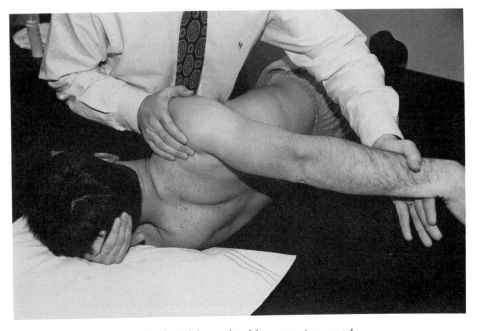

**Fig. 51-4.** Sidelying shoulder extension stretch.

in the end range and then released slightly. This pattern is repeated between three to five times to complete the stretch.

For continuity from stretch 3 to stretch 4, the athlete's arm is moved from the athletic trainer's left hand into the right hand and brought into full overhead elevation over the athlete's ear.

## Stretch 4: Shoulder Flexion

The athletic trainer cups the left hand over the top of the athlete's shoulder while grasping the right wrist with the right hand. The athlete's arm is then extended parallel to the table, directly over the right ear. Firm pressure is applied to the posterolateral aspect of the shoulder using the left hand as a fulcrum to extend the arm downward toward the table as far as possible (Fig. 51-5). This position is held for 3 to 5 seconds, released, and then the stretch is reapplied from three to five repetitions.

For continuity from stretch 4 to stretch 5, the athlete's arm is brought out of full elevation to approximately 90 degrees of abduction and elbow flexion. The athletic trainer grasps the athlete's right wrist with the right hand, and the elbow is cupped with the left hand for support.

## Stretch 5: Shoulder Circles

From this starting position, the upper arm is rotated in as big a circle as possible while keeping the forearm parallel to the treatment table (Fig. 51-6). The rotation movement is initiated with the trainer's left hand pushing the athlete's elbow first in a clockwise and then in a counterclockwise direction. Each direction is repeated five to eight times to complete this stretch.

The next seven stretches are performed in the supine position. The body is positioned so that the shoulder and arm are just slightly off the outside edge of the treatment table.

## Stretch 6: "The Pump Stretch"

From a crouched position, the athletic trainer slides the left hand under the athlete's arm at the level of the axilla and places it on the athlete's chest. At the same time, the trainer grasps the athlete's arm just above the wrist with the right arm. In this position, the athlete's arm should be supported by the trainer's anterior el-

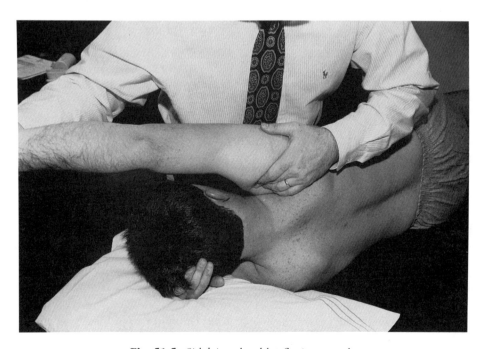

**Fig. 51-5.** Sidelying shoulder flexion stretch.

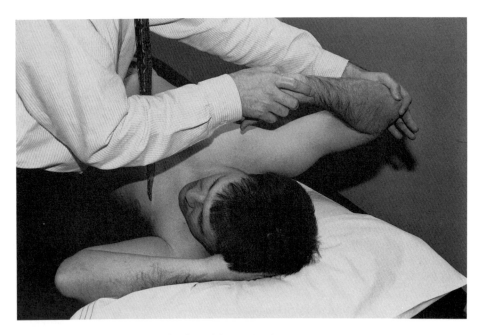

**Fig. 51-6.** Sidelying shoulder circles.

bow. Using the left arm as a fulcrum, the athletic trainer pushes the athlete's arm back in an attempt to move it perpendicular with the body while the elbow remains fully extended (Fig. 51-7). The stretch is held for 5 to 7 seconds, relaxed, and then repeated from three to five repetitions.

For continuity from stretch 6 to stretch 7, the trainer stands up bringing the athlete's arm into forward flexion to grasp the right wrist with the left hand.

### Stretch 7: Shoulder Flexion

The athletic trainer first stabilizes the lateral scapula with the right hand. Then, with mild traction applied to the long axis of the arm, the trainer's left hand moves the athlete's arm into extreme forward flexion (Fig. 51-8). This stretch is held for 5 to 7 seconds, released, and repeated from three to five times.

For continuity from stretch 7 to stretch 8, the athletic trainer continues to grasp the dorsal aspect of the athlete's wrist with the left hand. The right hand is then moved from the scapula to the posterior surface of the elbow to cup it for support. The athlete's arm is allowed to relax completely into a 90 degree elbow flexed position while the shoulder is maintained

in 90 degrees of abduction parallel to the treatment table.

### Stretch 8: Internal Rotation

While maintaining the athlete's arm in this 90 degree abducted, 90 degree elbow flexed position, the athletic trainer moves the shoulder into extreme internal rotation with the left hand while stabilizing the elbow with the right (Fig. 51-9). This position is held for a 5- to 7-second stretch, relaxed, and then as previously described, three to five repetitions are repeated.

For continuity from stretch 8 to stretch 9, the athletic trainer simply slides the right hand up the anterior forearm to grasp the volar portion of the athlete's wrist while the left hand slides down the forearm to support the flexed elbow.

### Stretch 9: External Rotation

The athletic trainer now moves the shoulder into extreme external rotation with the right hand. The left hand continues to stabilize the elbow in 90 degrees of flexion and 90 degrees of shoulder abduction (Fig. 51-10). Again, this position is held for 5 to 7 seconds,

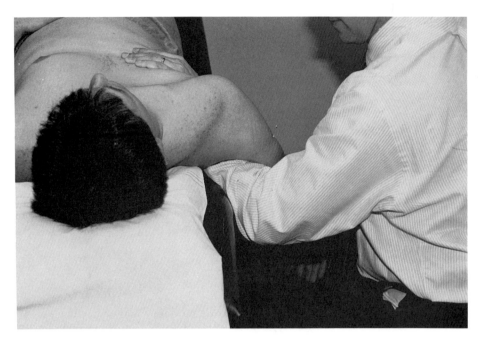

**Fig. 51-7.** Supine "pump stretch."

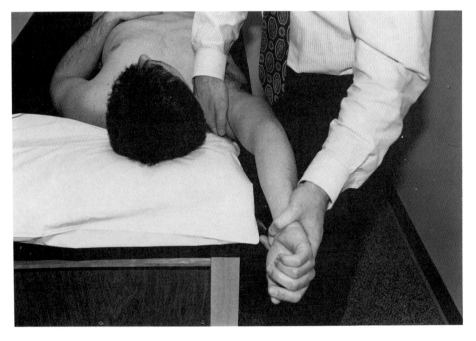

**Fig. 51-8.** Supine shoulder flexion stretch.

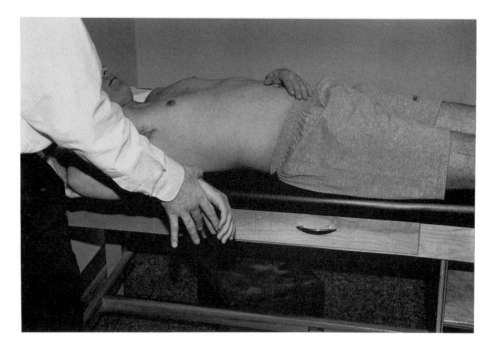

**Fig. 51-9.** Supine internal rotation stretch.

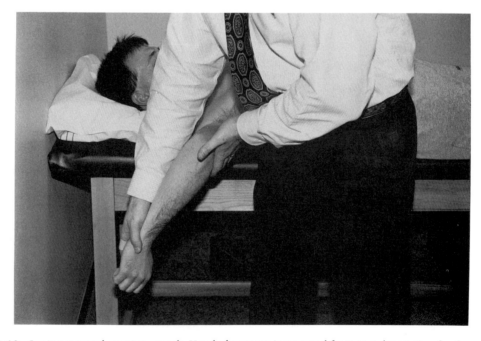

**Fig. 51-10.** Supine external rotation stretch. Hand placement is reversed from text description for figure clarity.

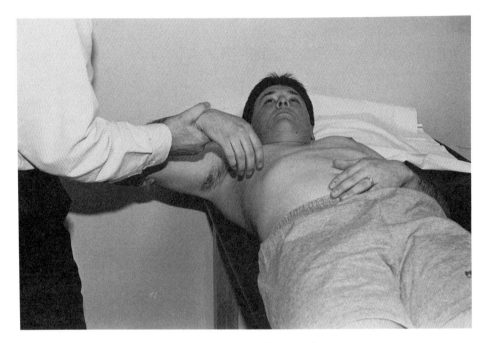

**Fig. 51-11.** Supine elbow circles.

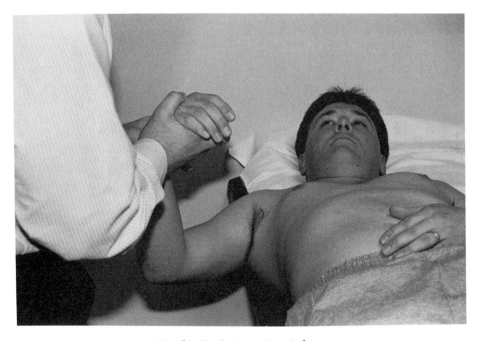

**Fig. 51-12.** Supine wrist circles.

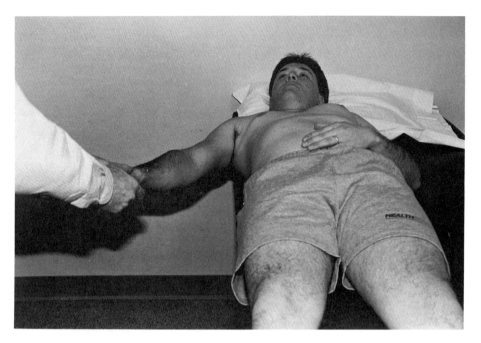

**Fig. 51-13.** Supine arm waves.

relaxed, and repeated from three to five times to complete the stretch.

### Stretch 10: Elbow Circles

While maintaining the same head positioning as described for external rotation above, the elbow is gently rotated in as large an arc as possible in both clockwise and counterclockwise directions (Fig. 51-11). Five to six rotations are performed in each direction.

For continuity from stretch 10 to stretch 11, the athletic trainer's right hand is slid from the athlete's wrist to their palm and the trainer's left hand from the elbow to grasp and support the wrist.

### Stretch 11: Wrist Circles

From this hand positioning, the athletic trainer simply rotates the wrist in both clockwise and counterclockwise directions four to five times (Fig. 51-12).

### Stretch 12: Arm Waves

The trainer grasps the athlete's hand with both hands, holding it in a palm-down position. With the athlete's arm relaxed and limp, the athletic trainer uses both hands to lift up and down evenly, causing the athlete's arm to move in a wave-like manner (Fig. 51-13). After 10 to 15 waves, the athletic trainer should toss the athlete's relaxed arm onto the chest to finish the stretch.

After this stretch, pitchers should immediately begin warming up. The use of this type of stretching routine with an organized warm-up before pitching follows one of the most important concepts in arm care purported by Fauls—"Pitchers should warm up to throw; not throw to warm up."[1]

This type of warm-up activity should include (1) jogging to "break a sweat," (2) different lower extremity and trunk flexibility exercises, (3) beginning tossing from 30 ft progressing to a comfortable long-toss distance, and (4) finally, to a bull pen warm-up as needed before competition.

## ARM CARE BETWEEN INNINGS

There are several avenues to consider in the appropriate care of the pitching arm between innings: (1) Pitchers should use at least two long-sleeved undershirts and change them as needed to facilitate heat exchange and the sweating mechanism; (2) plenty of fluids should be encouraged between innings to avoid dehydration during activity; (3) the throwing arm, back, and neck should remain warm and covered with a jacket to minimize inactivity stiffness between innings; (4) during long offensive innings, pitchers should get up, stretch, and toss on the side as necessary to prevent stiffness from occurring; and (5) during hot and humid weather, towels soaked in a mixture of ice water and aromatic spirits of ammonia may be beneficial to cool and refresh players between innings.

## POSTPARTICIPATION ACTIVITIES

Immediately after pitching or throwing activities, the cooling-down process begins. Depending on the amount of throwing performed, some pitchers may need to add additional aerobic activities before the cooling-down process. This is usually accomplished with low-intensity distance running or stationary cycling for 15 to 30 minutes. The use of this type of postpitching aerobic activity is encouraged to assist in the mobilization of inflammatory infiltrates and microtraumatic waste products from the muscle groups most strenuously exerted during pitching. Ideally, this type of activity should be performed before initiating any organized cool-down activities to maximize the effectiveness of these interventions. This cool-down process has historically been the domain of "icing-down" a player's arm. Although icing may be beneficial in many instances, the author does not believe that it is mandatory; icing should be used if a pitcher requests it, has a history of arm trouble, or if experiencing intermittent symptoms related to overuse.

The key to all postparticipation activities is that aggressive interventions initiated immediately after throwing will facilitate the healing and recovery process. Proper activities to minimize secondary tissue hypoxia, control effusion, mobilize lactic acid, and control noxious stimuli all combine to facilitate recovery between throwing activities by decreasing the acute inflammatory reaction and delayed onset muscle soreness. One of the most effective measures to accomplish these goals with the throwing arm, as with most injuries, is the combination of cryotherapy and elevation. The use of cryotherapy serves to limit the formation

of tissue debris by minimizing the increase in tissue oncotic pressure, inducing vascular spasm, increasing endothelial adhesiveness, and decreasing tissue metabolism.[4] Together these factors serve to decrease the secondary hypoxic injury and, thus, facilitate healing and recovery. The use of cryotherapy serves to decrease tissue damage, swelling, muscle spasm, and pain, all of which allows for a quicker resolution of postpitching trauma and decreased disability time.[4] The use of elevation during cryotherapy application also decreases capillary hydrostatic pressure to aid in limiting edema formation in the usually dependent upper extremity.[4] The most effective use of this technique requires the application of several ice bags applied to the throwing arm from the shoulder girdle to the wrist and held in place with elastic bandages. The

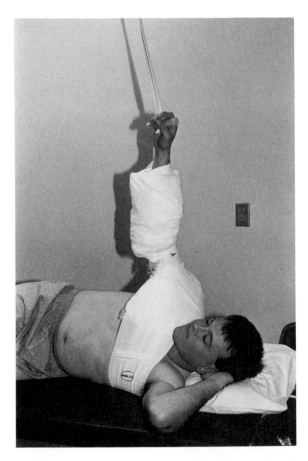

**Fig. 51-14.** Throwing arm cryotherapy with suspension elevation.

athlete is then positioned sidelying with the throwing arm elevated by grasping a rope connected to the ceiling[1] (Fig. 51-14). Cryotherapy is used for 20 to 25 minutes after activity to attain a complete numbing effect of the upper extremity.

Cryotherapy application is then followed by a postgame "milking massage" to flush by-products from the throwing arm and minimize metabolic waste and effusion accumulation. This type of compressive massage increases external pressure, decreases underlying blood flow, helps to control edema formation, and promotes the reabsorption of edema systemically.[4] During the application of this technique, the athlete remains in a sidelying position, grasping a rope suspended from the ceiling as described above. The arm is then massaged with a combination of cooled lotion

and alcohol. The massage is performed using effleurage strokes beginning at the wrist and moving gradually to the forearm, elbow, upper arm, and shoulder girdle (Fig. 51-15). The stroking action of the massage is always directed toward the heart. The total time of this milking massage ranges from 5 to 10 minutes as tolerated by the athlete.[1]

## REHABILITATIVE MANAGEMENT

Rehabilitative exercises should play an integral part of the between-outing training and conditioning program for any throwing athlete. These exercises must isolate the rotator cuff, biceps, and elbow musculature in a fashion that replicates the demands placed on the throwing arm during competition. The performance of this type of exercise program is directed toward maintaining or improving total arm strength power and endurance through an entire baseball season. The thrower's 10 exercise program, as detailed in Chapter 32 of this book, provides an effective exercise program designed to isolate and emphasize the musculature most important to the throwing athlete. Table 51-2 outlines these specific rotator cuff and arm exercises. Between outings, these exercises should be performed using 3 to 5 lbs of weight for three to five sets of 10 repetitions as tolerated by stiffness, soreness, and the amount of pitching performed. The elastic tubing exercises outlined in this exercise program should be performed from two to four sets of 10 to 15 repetitions each. The intensity, duration, and load of this rehabilitative program will fluctuate and should most appropriately be determined by the athlete for each successive

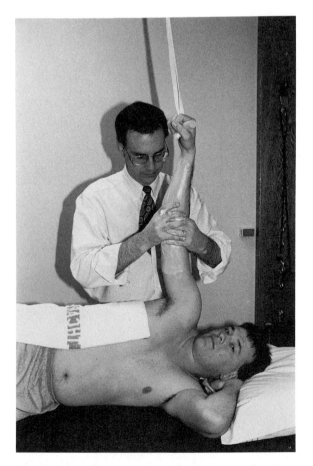

**Fig. 51-15.** Milking massage with suspension elevation.

**Table 51-2. Thrower's 10 Exercise Program**

Dumbbell Exercises
    Shoulder abduction
    Shoulder scaption (elevation with internal rotation in scapular plane)
    Prone horizontal abduction
    Prone extension
    Prone rowing
    Wrist flexion/extension; forearm supination/pronation
Elastic Tubing Exercises
    Internal rotation in 90-degree abduction
    External rotation in 90-degree abduction
    Diagonal $D_2$ flexion pattern
    Biceps curl/triceps extension

session. Recommendations regarding the frequency and intensity of this program during a competitive season are outlined in the next section of this chapter.

## ARM CARE BETWEEN STARTS

The activities performed between starts are the most essential to keeping a pitcher in the rotation, effective, and symptom-free. A 5-day pitching rotation is currently used most often in competitive baseball. Maximizing the available therapeutic, rehabilitative, and conditioning interventions during the 4 days between starts is a prerequisite to successful in-season arm care. Although this type of program will vary greatly from pitcher to pitcher and organization to organization, some general guidelines and comments follow. The reader is reminded that an in-depth discussion of conditioning principles and practices is discussed in Chapter 50.

The first day after a start should combine several types of training and rehabilitative activities, including (1) self, active assisted, and/or passive stretching as previously described, (2) heavy weight work for both the upper and lower extremities (machines and free weights), (3) thrower's 10 exercise program at 3 lbs, three sets of 10 repetitions and light tubing resistance, (4) 10 to 14 40- to 50-yd sprints, (5) abdominal strengthening exercises, (6) 20 to 30 minutes of aerobic activity, and (7) local modalities to minimize soft tissue inflammation and microtrauma as needed.

An aggressive stretching program including shoulder flexion, external rotation, and internal rotation at a minimum should be performed daily between stints. Stretching activities should be performed two to three times a day to ensure adequate arm flexibility is maintained. The passive stretching routine previously described is an excellent adjunct to decrease postpitching soreness during this first day time frame.

The local modalities of greatest benefit during this interim time frame include (1) ultrasound, (2) high-voltage pulsed galvanic stimulation, and (3) iontophoresis. Low-dose pulsed ultrasound may be extremely beneficial in the management of acute inflammatory reactions and in the mobilization of tissue exudates. The use of ultrasound in conjunction with a controlled rehabilitative exercise program can serve to minimize symptoms between starts and maximize pitching effectiveness without risking severe shoulder or elbow injury.

Also, phonophoresis, as previously described, is often used to minimize acute microtraumatic symptoms and facilitate continued training. The use of ultrasound in the presence of these acute to subacute conditions serves to warm up the affected area before activity. This is particularly effective before stretching muscular and connective tissue, as well as serving to decrease the risk of further injury.[2] High-voltage pulsed galvanic stimulation is an effective pain control modality that may be beneficial in the presence of acute symptoms between starts. Its use to break a pain–spasm–pain cycle can be most beneficial during these brief 4-day active rest periods. Iontophoresis has limited benefits as a local modality. It is most beneficial when pain/symptoms can be localized to one point-specific area to be treated. The use of iontophoresis in diffuse conditions is not as effective in the throwing athlete. Although marked pain and inflammatory symptom reductions can be achieved with the use of iontophoresis, its application is limited to persistent, unresponsive, and isolated musculotendinous inflammatory conditions.

The second postpitching day's activity should include (1) aggressive stretching, (2) abdominal strengthening exercises, (3) thrower's 10 exercise program, (4) distance running program, and (5) 10 to 15 minutes of long toss.

The third day uses a combination of activities including (1) stretching activities, (2) heavy weight training activities, (3) distance running program, (4) 10 to 14 40-yd sprints, and (5) 10 to 15 minutes of full-speed bull pen work.

The fourth and final between-activity day combines stretching and gentle long tossing with a light thrower's 10 exercise program and running activities as needed in preparation for competition the next day.

## SPECIAL CONSIDERATIONS FOR RELIEF PITCHERS

Managing the arm care needs of the relief pitcher poses several particular difficulties for the sports medicine team. The relief pitcher can throw more frequently, on successive days, with short notice and with fluctuating regularity compared with the starting pitchers. Although none of the principles, specific interventions, or conditioning requirements are significantly altered for the relief pitcher, their application is greatly changed to match the constantly varying level of pitching participation.

Relief pitchers must maximize their time and effort to maintain an adequate level of conditioning and arm strength to minimize their risk to overuse throwing-related injuries. In general, alterations are small in nature and follow the guideline of more frequent activities at lesser intensities and loads than those used by starting pitchers.

A regular daily pregame routine should be used for the relief pitcher, including a proper warm-up and light running activities. All stretching and/or local modalities incorporated into the relief pitcher's routine can be implemented at appropriate stages of the game based on the pitcher's specific role (short or long relief). Postgame treatment activities depend greatly on the amount of pitching performed. Brief outings often respond favorably to a milking massage only, whereas more extensive relief efforts may require more aggressive treatment measures. The use of these interventions varies greatly in relief pitchers, and each specific situation and individual must be evaluated for proper use.

The conditioning and rehabilitative portions of a relief pitcher's program do not vary greatly from that of the starting pitcher with one key difference. The reliever always performs the activity after a game and varies the amount of the activity based on the amount thrown that day and a prediction of the amount the reliever may throw the next day.

## SUMMARY

A combination of interventions involving conditioning, rehabilitative, and preventive measures are necessary to maximize the level of symptom-free pitching activity in the competitive athlete. An aggressive, preventive–rehabilitative approach can serve to minimize the microtraumatic inflammatory results of pitching while improving the flexibility, total arm strength, and conditioning of the throwing athlete. Developing a complete in-season management program based on the guidelines presented in this chapter can serve to minimize a pitcher's risk of injury and maximize the competitive effectiveness by addressing all the challenges the in-season management of the throwing arm presents to the sports medicine team. Additionally, a thorough off-season conditioning program must also be followed by the throwing athlete to prepare for the tremendous demands placed on the body during the long competitive baseball season.

## REFERENCES

1. Fauls D: General training techniques to warm up and cool down the throwing arm. p. 266. In Zarins B, Andrews JR, Carson WG (eds): Injuries to the Throwing Arm. WB Saunders, Philadelphia, 1985
2. Giek JH, Saliba EN: Application of modalities in overuse syndromes. Clin Sports Med 6:427, 1987
3. Medich G: Interval throwing programs for baseball players. Sports Med Update 2:9, 1987
4. Knight KL: Cryotherapy: theory, technique, and physiology. Chattanooga Corp., Chattanooga, TN, 1985

# 52

# Interval Sport Programs for the Shoulder

*KEVIN E. WILK*
*CHRISTOPHER A. ARRIGO*

Returning an athlete to unrestricted, symptom-free function requires the integration of continued high level rehabilitative exercises with progressive and graduated sport-specific activities. Adequately incorporating these types of activities during the latter phases of the rehabilitation process serves to minimize this often difficult transitional period for both the athletic patient and the clinician. The last phase of rehabilitation, often called "the return to activity phase," is characterized by a gradual return to sporting activities in an athletic population. During this period patients are instructed to continue performing their established rehabilitation program to facilitate the progression of strength, power, endurance, and flexibility of the shoulder complex. Also, comprehensive total body flexibility and conditioning exercises are accelerated to ensure competitive sport-specific readiness.

Before initiating a gradual progressive return to sporting activities, the athletic patient must exhibit specific criteria: (1) full non-painful range of motion; (2) no pain or tenderness; (3) satisfactory muscular performance based on functional sporting demands (see Ch. 43); (4) satisfactory clinical examination.

The authors have adapted several programs to promote this gradual return to injury-free sporting activities, referred to as "interval programs".[2] The purpose of these interval programs is to increase progressively and systematically the demands placed on the shoulder complex while the patient is performing sport-specific activities. Using this type of gradual return to sporting activities minimizes the risk of re-injury and allows progressive adaptation of the shoulder and other body parts to the repetitive stresses of throwing, tennis, golf, swimming, or other athletic activities. In addition, the interval programs are used to allow athletic patients the opportunity to re-establish their timing, coordination, movement patterns, and synchondrocity of muscle firing before returning to competition. These interval programs can be employed for the competitive athlete as well as the recreational athlete. The patient is encouraged to perform the prescribed exercise program before throwing. These exercises include strengthening, flexibility, and neuromuscular control drills.

## INTERVAL THROWING

For the throwing athlete, the number of throws, distance, intensity, and types of throws are monitored and progressed to facilitate a successful return to competition. The throwing program is organized into two phases: phase I, a long-toss program, and phase II, an off-the-mound program (for pitchers only).

### Long-Toss

The interval long-toss program is performed by all baseball players, positional or pitchers. The throwing mechanics performed in the long-toss program rise a "crow-hop" technique similar to throwing from the outfield. This technique uses a hop, skip, and throw to accentuate lower body and trunk involvement in the throwing motion. The crow-hop method stimulates the throwing act, allowing an emphasis on proper body mechanics. Throwing flat-footed encourages improper body mechanics and places increased stresses on the throwing shoulder. Appendix 52-1 illustrates the interval long-toss program. The thrower progresses through each step with the ultimate goal of throwing 75 repetitions at 180 feet without pain (step 13) for positional players and 150 feet without pain (step 9) for pitchers. The thrower is instructed to throw every other day, or three times per week. The patient progresses from one stage to the next stage, once the number of throws have been achieved without pain while throwing or residual pain. If pain or difficulty occurs the athlete regresses to the previous level or attempts the same step during the next throwing drill.

## Off-the-Mound Throwing

For the pitcher, once 75 throws from 150 feet can be performed without pain, throwing from the mound is initiated. In the phase II throwing program from the mound, the number of throws, intensity (speed), and type of pitches are monitored and systematically progressed (Appendix 52-2). This phase II program is subdivided into three progressive components designed to enable the pitcher to return to symptom-free athletic participation. In stage one, mechanics and velocity are emphasized during fast ball pitching only. In stage two, mechanics, ball location, and confidence are emphasized as the pitcher begins throwing to a hitter. Lastly, in stage three, breaking balls (curve balls, sliders) are initiated as the final progression before competitive return. If a patient complains of pain or an inability to throw at a particular stage, we encourage a light toss program. When the pitcher regresses the program to a light toss (70 percent intensity) from 60 to 75 feet, this allows the pitcher to continue to throw while allowing the arm to calm down.

## Little League

The adolescent baseball player creates a different challenge for the clinician. The little league interval throwing program (Appendix 52-3) is similar to the previously discussed throwing program, with two distinct differences: the throwing distances are shorter and the number of throws less. The young thrower is encour-

aged to progress slowly through these steps and re-establish good throwing mechanics before any return to competitive activity. The adolescent thrower is encouraged to master control and change of velocity instead of throwing breaking balls, which may cause deleterious stress on the elbow and shoulder complex.

## Tennis

The same principles of the interval program can be followed by the tennis player as well (Appendix 52-4). The program for the tennis player progresses from a limited number of forehand and backhand ground strokes, gradually increasing the number of these strokes over a period of 2 to 3 weeks. During this time frame the player gradually initiates overhead and service strokes in combination with his ground strokes. The tennis player begins playing games during the fourth week of this interval program. Occasionally, this type of activity is delayed because of the patient's rehabilitation progression and underlying pathology. The clinician is encouraged to monitor the tennis players' signs and symptoms as they progress through the stages of functional rehabilitation.

## Golf

One of the most commonly utilized programs is the interval golf program (Appendix 52-5). This program begins with the golfer chipping and putting only. This is followed by a gradual progression to short and medium iron strokes. Once a confident, pain-free swing has been re-established, long irons and woods are initiated. The purpose of the interval golf program is to allow golfers time to re-establish their swing pace, weight transfer, and proper mechanics before play is resumed. Once play is resumed the golfer is encouraged to progress 9 holes twice per week, to 9 holes four to five times per week, to 18 holes several times per week. This allows a gradual improvement of endurance and strength as well as an increase in the players tolerance to the microtraumatic stresses.

## CONCLUSIONS

The purpose of these interval programs is to provide the athletic patient with established time frames for a gradual, progressive return to sporting activities. Patients are encouraged to progress at their own rate and to regress or stay at the same phase if pain or dysfunction occurs. In addition, the athletic patient is instructed to perform specific flexibility and strengthening exercises before the interval program, as a warm-up, and afterwards, as part of a cool down. Initially, cryotherapy may be used after the interval program if pain or soreness develop. The use of these interval sport programs is encouraged for the competitive and the recreational athlete.

The athletic patient must be encouraged to continue strengthening and flexibility exercises during this return-to-activity phase of rehabilitation. The interval sport programs are not used to rehabilitate or to "get the athlete in shape" for competition. The athletic patient must and should be in good physical condition to participate in this type of program. The interval program is used for sport-specific training. Therefore, a basic principle supported by the use of these programs is that an athlete must rehabilitate to train for a sport and then perform sport-specific training to participate in sporting activities.

## REFERENCES

1. Wilk KE, Arrigo CA: An integrated approach to upper extremity exercises. Orthop Phys Ther Clin North Am 1(2) 337, 1992
2. Blackburn TA: The off season program for the throwing arm. p. 277. In Andrews JR, Carson WG, Zarins B (eds): Injuries to the throwing arm. WB Saunders, Philadelphia, 1985

# Appendix 52-1

# Interval Throwing Program*
# Phase I: Long-Toss Program

**45-ft Stage**

Step 1: a. Warm-up throwing
     b. 45 ft (25 throws)
     c. Rest 15 min
     d. Warm-up throwing
     e. 45 ft (25 throws)

Step 2: a. Warm-up throwing
     b. 45 ft (25 throws)
     c. Rest 10 min
     d. Warm-up throwing
     e. 45 ft (25 throws)
     f. Rest 10 min
     g. Warm-up throwing
     h. 45 ft (25 throws)

**60-ft Stage**

Step 3: a. Warm-up throwing
     b. 60 ft (25 throws)
     c. Rest 15 min
     d. Warm-up throwing
     e. 60 ft (25 throws)

Step 4: a. Warm-up throwing
     b. 60 ft (25 throws)
     c. Rest 10 min
     d. Warm-up throwing
     e. 60 ft (25 throws)

     f. Rest 10 min
     g. Warm-up throwing
     h. 60 ft (25 throws)

**90-ft Stage**

Step 5: a. Warm-up throwing
     b. 90 ft (25 throws)
     c. Rest 15 min
     d. Warm-up throwing
     e. 90 ft (25 throws)

Step 6: a. Warm-up throwing
     b. 90 ft (25 throws)
     c. Rest 10 min
     d. Warm-up throwing
     e. 90 ft (25 throws)
     f. Rest 10 min
     g. Warm-up throwing
     h. 90 ft (25 throws)

**120-ft Stage**

Step 7: a. Warm-up throwing
     b. 120 ft (25 throws)
     c. Rest 15 min
     d. Warm-up throwing
     e. 120 ft (25 throws)

Step 8: a. Warm-up throwing
     b. 120 ft (25 throws)
     c. Rest 10 min

---

* Throwing is performed every other day. Pre-throwing and post-throwing exercises must be performed.

d. Warm-up throwing
e. 120 ft (25 throws)
f. Rest 10 min
g. Warm-up throwing
h. 120 ft (25 throws)

## 150-ft Stage

Step 9: a. Warm-up throwing
b. 150 ft (25 throws)
c. Rest 15 min
d. Warm-up throwing
e. 150 ft (25 throws)

Step 10: a. Warm-up throwing
b. 150 ft (25 throws)
c. Rest 10 min
d. Warm-up throwing
e. 150 ft (25 throws)
f. Rest 10 min
g. Warm-up throwing
h. 150 ft (25 throws)

## 180-ft Stage

Step 11: a. Warm-up throwing
b. 180 ft (25 throws)
c. Rest 15 min
d. Warm-up throwing
e. 180 ft (25 throws)

Step 12: a. Warm-up throwing
b. 180 ft (25 throws)
c. Rest 10 min
d. Warm-up throwing
e. 180 ft (25 throws)
f. Rest 10 min
g. Warm-up throwing
h. 180 ft (25 throws)

Step 13: a. Warm-up throwing
b. 180 ft (25 throws)
c. Rest 10 min
d. Warm-up throwing
e. 180 ft (25 throws)
f. Rest 10 min
g. Warm-up throwing
h. 180 ft (25 throws)

Step 14: Begin throwing off the mound or return to respective position.

# Appendix 52-2

# Interval Throwing Program
# Phase II: Starting Off The Mound

**Stage I: Fastball Only**

Step 1: a. Interval throwing
 b. 15 throws off mound 50%

Step 2: a. Interval throwing
 b. 30 throws off mound 50%

Step 3: a. Interval throwing
 b. 45 throws off mound 50%

Step 4: a. Interval throwing
 b. 60 throws off mound 50%

Step 5: a. Interval throwing
 b. 30 throws off mound 75%

Step 6: a. 30 throws off mound 75%
 b. 45 throws off mound 50%

Step 7: a. 45 throws off mound 75%
 b. 15 throws off mound 50%

Step 8: a. 60 throws off mound 75%

**Stage II: Fastball Only**

Step 9: a. 45 throws off mound 75%
 b. 15 throws in Batting Practice

Step 10: a. 45 throws off mound 75%
 b. 30 throws in Batting Practice

Step 11: a. 45 throws off mound 75%
 b. 45 throws in batting practice

**Stage III**

Step 12: a. 30 throws off mound 75% warm-up
 b. 15 throws off mound 50% breaking balls
 c. 45-60 throws in batting practice (fastball only)

Step 13: a. 30 throws off mound 75%
 b. 30 breaking balls 75%
 c. 30 throws in batting practice

Step 14: a. 30 throws off mound 75%
 b. 60–90 throws in batting practice 25% breaking balls

Step 15: Simulated game progressing by 15 throws per work-out. Use interval throwing to 120-ft phase (see Appendix 52-1) as warm-up. All throwing off the mound should be done in the presence of the pitching coach to stress proper throwing mechanics. A speed gun should be used to aid in effort control.

# Appendix 52-3

# Little League Interval Throwing Program

The Little League interval throwing program parallels the interval throwing program in returning the Little Leaguer to a graduated progression of throwing distances. Warm-up and stretching should be performed before throwing.

**30-ft. Stage**

Step 1: a. Warm-up throwing
     b. 30 ft (25 throws)
     c. Rest 15 min
     d. Warm-up throwing
     e. 30 ft (25 throws)

Step 2: a. Warm-up throwing
     b. 30 ft (25 throws)
     c. Rest 10 min
     d. Warm-up throwing
     e. 30 ft (25 throws)
     f. Rest 10 min
     g. Warm-up throwing
     h. 30 ft (25 throws)

**45-ft Stage**

Step 3: a. Warm-up throwing
     b. 45 ft (25 throws)
     c. Rest 15 min
     d. Warm-up throwing
     e. 45 ft (25 throws)

Step 4: a. Warm-up throwing
     b. 45 ft (25 throws)
     c. Rest 10 minutes
     d. Warm-up throwing
     e. 45 ft (25 throws)
     f. Rest 10 minutes
     g. Warm-up throwing
     h. 45 ft (25 throws)

**60-ft Stage**

Step 5: a. Warm-up throwing
     b. 60 ft (25 throws)
     c. Rest 15 min
     d. Warm-up throwing
     e. 60 ft (25 throws)

Step 6: a. Warm-up throwing
     b. 60 ft (25 throws)
     c. Rest 10 min
     d. Warm-up throwing
     e. 60 ft (25 throws)
     f. Rest 10 min
     g. Warm-up throwing
     h. 60 ft (25 throws)

**90-ft Stage**

Step 7: a. Warm-up throwing
     b. 90 ft (25 throws)

        c. Rest 15 min

        d. Warm-up throwing

        e. 90 ft (25 throws)

Step 8: a. Warm-up throwing

        b. 90 ft (25 throws)

        c. Rest 10 min

        d. Warm-up throwing

        e. 90 ft (25 throws)

        f. Rest 10 min

        g. Warm-up throwing

        h. 90 ft (25 throws)

# Appendix 52-4

# Interval Tennis Program

Use ice after each day of play.

|  | Monday | Wednesday | Friday |
|---|---|---|---|
| 1st week | 12 FH<br>8 BH<br>Rest 10 min<br>13 FH<br>7 BH | 15 FH<br>8 BH<br>Rest 10 min<br>15 FH<br>7 BH | 15 FH<br>10 BH<br>Rest 10 min<br>15 FH<br>10 BH |
| 2nd week | 25FH<br>15 BH<br>Rest 10 min<br>25 FH<br>15 BH | 30 FH<br>20 BH<br>Rest 10 min<br>30 FH<br>20 BH | 30 FH<br>25 BH<br>Rest 10 min<br>30 FH<br>15 BH<br>10 OH |
| 3rd week | 30 FH<br>25 BH<br>10 OH<br>Rest 10 min<br>30 FH<br>25 BH<br>10 OH | 30 FH<br>25 BH<br>15 OH<br>Rest 10 min<br>30 FH<br>25 BH<br>15 OH | 30 FH<br>30 BH<br>15 OH<br>Rest 10 min<br>30 FH<br>15 OH<br>Rest 10 min<br>30 FH<br>30 BH<br>15 OH |
| 4th week | 30 FH<br>30 BH<br>10 OH<br>Rest 10 min<br>Play 3 games<br>10 FH<br>10 BH<br>5 OH | 30 FH<br>30 BH<br>10 OH<br>Rest 10 min<br>Play set<br>10 FH<br>10 BH<br>5 OH | 30 FH<br>30 BH<br>10 OH<br>Rest 10 min<br>Play 1½ sets<br>10 FH<br>10 BH<br>3 OH |

OH, overhead shots; FH, forehand ground stroke; BH, backhand ground strokes

# Appendix 52-5

# Interval Golf Program

Flexing exercises should be performed before hitting.
Ice should be used after play.

| | Monday | Wednesday | Friday |
|---|---|---|---|
| 1st week | 10 putts<br>10 chips<br>Rest 5 min<br>15 chips | 15 putts<br>15 chips<br>Rest 5 min<br>25 chipping | 20 putts<br>20 chips<br>Rest 5 min<br>20 putts<br>20 chips<br>Rest 5 min<br>10 chips<br>10 short irons |
| 2nd week | 20 chips<br>10 short irons<br>Rest 5 min<br>10 short irons | 20 chips<br>15 short irons<br>Rest 10 min<br>15 short irons<br>15 chips<br>putting | 15 short irons<br>10 medium irons<br>Rest 10 min<br>20 short irons<br>15 chips |
| 3rd week | 15 short irons<br>15 medium irons<br>Rest 10 min<br>5 long irons<br>15 short irons<br>15 medium irons<br>Rest 10 min<br>20 chips | 15 short irons<br>10 medium irons<br>10 long irons<br>Rest 10 min<br>10 short irons<br>10 medium irons<br>5 long irons<br>5 wood | 15 short irons<br>10 medium irons<br>10 long irons<br>Rest 10 min<br>10 short irons<br>10 medium irons<br>10 long irons<br>10 wood |
| 4th week | 15 short irons<br>10 medium irons<br>10 long irons<br>10 drives<br>Rest 15 min<br>repeat | play 9 holes | play 9 holes |
| 5th week | 9 holes | 9 holes | 18 holes |

Chips, pitching wedge; short irons, W, 9, 8; medium irons, 7, 6, 5; long irons, 4, 3, 2; woods, 3, 5; drives, driver.

# 53

# Taping, Strapping, and Bracing of the Shoulder Complex

*JEFF G. KONIN*
*FRANK C. McCUE III*

## HISTORY OF PROTECTIVE EQUIPMENT

Protective equipment, strapping, and taping are commonly performed treatment adjuncts in athletics. The lack of documentation makes it unclear as to when protective equipment was first used. As described by Plutarch, it is believed that the first form of the use of protective equipment took place in ancient times when Termerus would destroy his enemies by running into them head first. The first use of adhesive substances as external devices can be dated back to ancient times as well. The Greeks have been credited with formulating a healing paste that was composed of lead oxide, olive oil, and water, which was used for many different skin conditions.[1]

Today, the difficulty lies not in finding protective equipment or padding but instead in choosing an appropriate, cost-effective brand that will specifically individualize and protect an athlete from injury. Manufacturers have progressed in technology, and several variously designed forms of athletic tapes, pads, and equipment are commercially available. Many organizations and committees have also been formed to provide rules and regulations for the use and conditions of these products.

## PURPOSE OF PROTECTIVE EQUIPMENT

The primary purpose of protective padding and equipment is to dispose and absorb forces of a blow by spreading them over a larger area than the initial point of contact, thus reducing the number and severity of injuries. For many sports, particularly those involving high levels of contact (e.g., football, lacrosse, hockey), protective equipment is part of the uniform. The idea behind this concept is to protect those body parts prone to repeated blows or traumatic contact by the nature of the sport.

## TAPING

Taping of the shoulder can be used as a valuable adjunct to properly supervised therapeutic exercise for an injury. The art of taping is a skill that one can master only with extensive practice.

Although presently there is minimal research on the effectiveness of taping of the shoulder complex, there are some important functions of tape that have been purported in the literature. These functions include (1) increasing joint stability, (2) limiting joint range of motion, (3) improving kinesthetic awareness, (4) stabilizing compressive-type bandages or padding, and (5) preventing further insult to injury.[1,2]

### Taping Materials

#### Elastic

Elastic tape comes in many forms, with names such as Conform (Bike), Elastikon (Johnson & Johnson), Lightplast (Beiersdorf Inc.), and Coban (3M) (Fig. 53-1). This type of tape is made to stretch, so it is highly

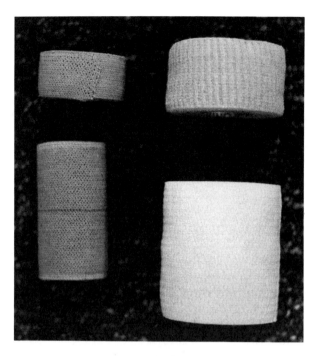

**Fig. 53-1.** Elastic tape is available in many different sizes and materials.

conforming to the affected area of concern. Elastic tape is recommended to be used when attempting to provide a gentle compressive force on tissues. For the shoulder complex, a rugged yet conforming tape should be used. Also, these types of tapes can be used to secure protective padding around the areas of the shoulder that are noncooperative with the application of adhesive tape.

### Adhesive

The primary use for adhesive (linen) tape is to prevent excessive motion of the joints and to aid in the stability of the functioning ligaments. This type of tape is much stronger than elastic tape and is better able to withstand vigorous athletic competition.

Like most other types of tape, adhesive tape comes in many colors, sizes, and strengths. Tape width can vary anywhere from 1/2 to 3 in. The most commonly used adhesive tape in athletic training is of the cloth-backed nature and comes in tubes or speed packs. Speed packs are wound more loosely than tubes and therefore may damage easier.

Three factors should be considered when purchas-

ing adhesive tape; tape grade, adhesive mass, and winding tension. The strength of linen or cloth-backed tape is graded by the number of longitudinal and vertical threads per inch. A stronger grade of tape backing will contain in excess of 85 longitudinal fibers and 65 vertical fibers. In comparison, weaker cloth-backed tape contains 65 or less longitudinal and 45 vertical fibers. Tape grade is always considered in the manufacturer's expenses.[3]

Adhesive mass is simply the tape's ability to adhere to skin surface despite circumstances such as perspiration and physical activity. It is important that the materials comprising this mass contain as few irritants as possible and do not damage superficial layers of skin on removal.

Possibly one of the most important concepts often overlooked when purchasing adhesive tape is the winding tension of each brand. Basically, adhesive tape must contain an even and constant unwinding tension. All principles of taping applications to joints encompass anatomy, biomechanics, and tensile strength of the supporting structures. These techniques are designed with the simple fact that external supportive structures such as tape are of equal tension throughout, therefore not altering any mechanical characteristics of application.

## Principles of Taping

No chapter discussing taping techniques would be complete without including the basic principles of taping. A complete tape job for any structure involving the shoulder complex should be effective and comfortable while affording consistent, compressive tension. The most important aspect of taping is to have a thorough understanding of why a certain technique is being used.

Similar to the taping of any joint, the athlete should be placed in a comfortable position, yet the shoulder should be easily accessible for taping. As long as no open wounds are present, the area may be cleansed and prepared with a skin adherent. If skin irritation is caused by the adherent or from direct taping onto the athlete's skin, a form of underwrap may be used before applying the tape. This is usually made up of a thin, porous, polyurethane foam wrap. However, the effectiveness of the supporting tape is maximized when applied directly to the surface of the skin. All tape should be applied when the skin is at normal body temperature.

Just as important as applying tape correctly is the art of removing tape. Tape can be removed with the aid of bandage scissors or by manual methods and should always be pulled off from the skin in a linear fashion. This is performed in a slow, controlled manner. After removal of the tape, the skin should be cleansed with soap and water to rid the surface of tape residue. A moisturizing cream or antibiotic ointment may then be applied to avoid skin abrasions.

In general, the following guidelines should be followed:

1. *Positioning and preparation:* The area to be taped should be adequately prepared and positioned for easy access.
2. *Removal:* Removal of tape should be slow and controlled, being careful not to damage superficial layers of skin.
3. *Effectiveness:* The effectiveness of any tape job lies within the understanding of why it is being performed and the art of its completeness.
4. *Vision:* Always observe the skin before application and after removal of tape for any irritations.
5. *Equality:* The tension of application should be performed in a smooth, equal, and firm manner.
6. *Natural:* Tape should be applied by following the natural contours of one's anatomy.
7. *Temperature:* Only apply tape and adhesive products when the area of concern is at normal skin temperature.
8. *Individualize:* Not only is each athlete taped individually according to his or her anatomy, so is each strip of tape. Continuous strips of tape may be constricting and lead to circulatory problems.
9. *Overlap:* Each strip of tape applied in sequence should overlap the previous strip by one-half.
10. *Neatness:* Follow each strip of tape by smoothing it down, being careful to avoid any wrinkles or gaps.

# PROTECTIVE PADDING TYPES OF MATERIAL

The athletic trainer must only be skilled at recognizing the indications for using protective padding but must also be aware of the types of materials available. Pads can be designed to absorb shock by constructing them with closed-cell foamy air or water cells, or a semiliquid high-viscous material. Materials can also be combined for functional purposes. For example, a pad can be constructed with a rigid outer layer and a softer inner natural layer.

## Rigid Materials

Many rigid materials are being used for the fabrication of custom padding. Often times, a plastic material is used because of its chemical composition and reaction to heat. Three common types are thermoforming plastics, thermosetting plastics, and thermoplastic foams.[3]

The most popular plastics in athletic training are thermoforming. This plastic can be molded to the body part when heated to between 140° and 180°F. The most common brands are orthoplast (synthetic rubber thermoplast) and aquaplast (a polyester sheet).

A more rigid and difficult to form plaster is the thermosetting type. This usually requires a mold rather than being formed directly on the body part. Thermosetting plasters require higher temperatures to alter the material for fabrication. Examples of this type of plastic are polyvinyl chloride (high-impact vinyl), polyvinyl chloride acrylic (kydex), and thermoplaster acrylic (myoplex).

Plastics containing additional liquids, gases, or crystals that alter their density are called thermoplastic foams. Polyethylene foams such as aloplast and plastazate are two of the most common types of thermoplastic foams.

Other products often used as rigid outer layers of padding are lightcast (Merck Sharpe Dohne Co., Inc., West Point, PA), Hexcelite (Hexcel, Dublin, CA), and RTV-11 (Genulastic Silicone Products, Waterford, NY).

## Soft Materials

Soft materials are equally as important for preventive measures. These can vary in shapes and sizes and are easy to mold to the contours of the body (Fig. 53-2).

Foam rubber is particularly effective because of its variety of thicknesses. It protects the body area from forces while it is resilient and nonabsorbent. Thero-foam (Cramer Products, Gardner, KS) and Ensolite (Whiroyal, Mishawka, IN) are two of the most common types of foams used today.

Felt is another popular soft material. Felt produces a firmer pressure than most foam rubbers because of its comfortable, semiresilient surface. This type of

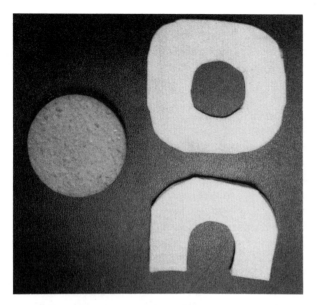

**Fig. 53-2.** Two common forms of soft material are substances derived from felt or foam.

material is composed of matted wool fibers pressed into varying thicknesses. Felt may absorb perspiration and therefore must be replaced daily to enable it to achieve its full effectiveness. However, its ability to absorb moisture allows it to keep better skin contact, thus allowing for a lesser tendency of migration.

Other soft materials such as adhesive felt (mole skin), gauze, cotton, and lamb wools can also be used as an adjunct to fabrication of protective devices.

## PREVENTIVE AND PROTECTIVE EQUIPMENT

Injuries may not be caused only by inadequate protection from equipment but also by improper fitting of the equipment. An example of this takes place at many secondary school levels where coaches, managers, and student trainers are responsible for adequately fitting equipment, yet they may not have been thoroughly trained with the proper knowledge and correct techniques of accomplishing the given task at hand. It is imperative that a qualified professional administer any type of preventive equipment and that each athlete is fitted individually according to the anatomic placement of the desired piece of equipment.

As previously stated, protective equipment can be manufactured commercially or it can be self-fabricated. Regardless of the nature of production, there are five basic concepts that should be addressed with each piece of material or equipment:[4]

1. Does the equipment protect the area of concern appropriately?
2. Can the athlete perform the skills required for his or her sport and position while wearing the device?
3. Will the device maintain a proper anatomic position?
4. Is the device potentially hazardous or injurious to other participants?
5. Is the device legal by the rules and regulations of the athlete's particular sport?

### Fitting Football Shoulder Pads

Shoulder pads are designed to provide four main functions: (1) absorb shock, (2) protect the shoulders, (3) protect the chest, and (4) fit the midcervical spine to the trunk.[2,3,5-8] Proper fit to the chest is important in distributing the shock to the shoulders evenly. Better shoulder protection should allow one to de-emphasize the use of the head as a blocking and tackling instrument. Improperly fit equipment may cause injury or increase the severity of an injury. Like all other fittings, those who fit the shoulder pads must be extremely knowledgeable about fitting techniques.

There are two basic types of shoulder pads: flat pads and cantilever pads[5] (Fig. 53-3). Quarterbacks and receivers use flat pads because they allow greater glenohumeral motion. The cantilever pads are named for the bridge that extends over the superior portion of the shoulder and are worn by players who are in constant contact. There are two components of cantilever pads, the inside and the outside. The inside cantilever is the most common, yet the outside cantilever provides more protection with a larger blocking surface, and thus are used by linemen. Some pads are specifically designed with larger anterior surfaces that are slanted slightly forward for those players receiving blows in a standing position.

In some cases, a pair of anthropometric calipers may be used to help properly fit shoulder pads. With this device, a measurement is taken from the edge of the shoulder across to the opposite shoulder. A similar

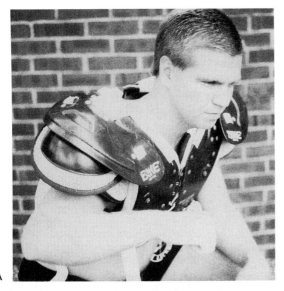
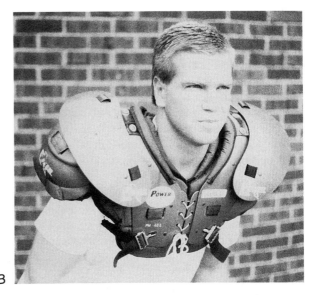

**Fig. 53-3.** (**A**) Flat pads allow for greater glenohumeral motion used by quarterbacks and receivers. (**B**) Cantilever pads used by linemen provide for greater protection of the shoulder girdle.

measurement is then made on the undersurface of the pad and etched on the anterior surface of the pad. These measurements are then used to derive a correct size. Calipers are primarily used to speed the process of fitting. However, all principles of fitting should still be followed for a complete and proper fit. When applying shoulder pads for a fitting evaluation, the following points should be addressed:[1–3]

1. The tip of the shoulder pad should fit just to the lateral edge of the shoulder.
2. The neck opening should be large enough for a player to extend his arm overhead without impinging the neck while not allowing any excessive sliding about the shoulder. Neck openings that are too small may lead to compression of the cervical or deltoid regions. Pads with excessively large neck openings may cause cervical or acromioclavicular injuries.
3. Elastic straps holding the pads to the chest and back must be tight yet comfortable, allowing for equal distribution of forces.
4. The flaps, or epaulets, on the lateral aspect of the pads should completely cover the deltoid region. Additional epaulets may be attached to cover the deltoids adequately.
5. Pay special attention to make sure the anterior por-

tion of the pads adequately cover the sternum and clavicle and that the posterior aspect of the pads completely cover the scapula.

## Maintenance of Equipment

All shoulder pads should be inspected with documentation at the beginning and end of each season. Also, pads should be constantly observed for damaged parts such as cracks, missing or loose rivets, and nonelastic or fraying straps. All defective equipment should be properly repaired by the manufacturer. Taking time to inspect and recondition faulty equipment adequately is significantly worthwhile as it will allow for the equipment to provide the optimal protection for which it was designed.

## PROTECTION OF THE ACROMIOCLAVICULAR JOINT

In many contact sports such as football, lacrosse, and ice hockey, the acromioclavicular joint is susceptible to frequent injury.[9] Athletes with acromioclavicular joint sprains can return to competition with satisfactory functional testing and with the approval of the team physician. However, adequate protection should be provided to the acromioclavicular joint to prevent further injury.

One form of protection is by using a foam pad insert called a shoulder injury pad or a "spider pad" (Adams, Plastics, Inc., Cookeville, TN) (Fig. 53-4). This type of pad is lightweight in nature yet directs the attention of a blow to the acromioclavicular joint toward the elevated foam pad.[10] This is commercially available and should be properly fitted according to the individual athlete.

A specialized pad for the acromioclavicular joint can also be made.[10–12] This is done to provide for a more custom-type fitting for the athlete. Many types of material have been recommended for construction of the pad. The pad basically takes on an elevated donut or dome shape with both a rigid and soft material. The rigid material is molded to the athlete's acromioclavicular joint region. When doing this, a dome of 1 1/2 in. should be constructed, so the acromioclavicular joint itself is not directly in contact with the pad (Fig.

53-5A). A softer material made of foam is then used as a dispersive medium between the athlete's shoulder and the rigid material. This pad can be held in place by taping it to the skin with adhesive tape or by creating a strap or belt system (Fig. 53-5). The key to making a successful acromioclavicular pad is to make sure that the pad is raised off the injured area to distribute the force of a blow around that area, allowing it to be absorbed by the pad itself.

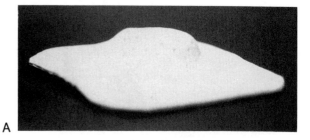
A

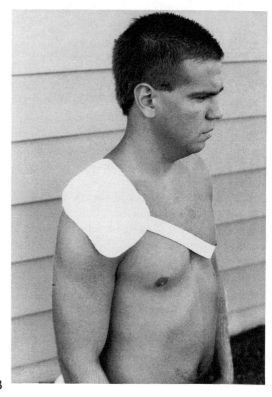
B

**Fig. 53-5.** (**A**) Custom-made acromioclavicular joint pad from rigid material, showing an elevated area where acromioclavicular joint would lie beneath. (**B**) Acromioclavicular pad used with a belt system.

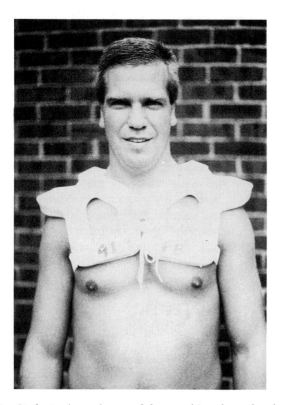

**Fig. 53-4.** Spider pads are soft foam pads used to aid in the dispersing of forces around shoulder region.

## Taping the Acromioclavicular Joint

Taping of the acromioclavicular joint has been used for first- or second-degree sprains, as it may provide some external support while not limiting the athlete's range of motion.

The area of involvement should be cleansed and shaved to allow good contact surfaces. The nipple can be protected with a Bandaid or a small piece of felt or gauze. Initially, two anchors are applied. The first is placed from the chest as its midline, over the shoulder to the back, and ending just below the tip of the scapula. A second anchor is applied from the anterior to the posterior aspect of the thorax (Fig. 53-6A). A series of nonelastic support strips are then placed in an upward manner from the arm to the anchor strips on the shoulder (Fig. 53-6B). Also, more support strips are applied in a diagonal fashion from the arm to the shoulder anchors. This is performed in a fanning pattern, both anterior to posterior and posterior to anterior (Fig. 53-6C). Anchor strips can then be applied from the chest to the back, attaching to the initial anchor. These should be overlapped half-way, allowing for a more stable product (Fig. 53-6D). Similarly, these strips are then applied completely around the chest and arm to "close off" the taping procedure[12] (Fig. 53-6E & F).[13]

# PROTECTING THE GLENOHUMERAL JOINT

## Contusions

Direct blows to the glenohumeral joint are common in contact sports. Complications such as tackler's exostosis and myositis ossificans can be prevented with proper protection to the glenohumeral region.[1,14] Often times the area of concern is just distal to the glenohumeral joint, near the insertion of the deltoid muscle and the origin of the brachialis muscle. This is an area that may not be adequately protected with football shoulder pads. Protective donut-shaped pads can be designed to cover the lateral humerus in a similar manner to the contusion of the acromioclavicular joint (Fig. 53-7). Also, pads can be attached to the epaulets of the athlete's shoulder pads.

## Anterior Stability

One of the most difficult problems that a medical team faces is how to adequately prevent an athlete from recurrent anterior instability of the glenohumeral joint. Because of the complexity of the ligamentous structures involved, there is no true device or taping procedure guaranteed to protect the unstable shoulder. Because the mechanism of injury for anterior subluxation or dislocation is external rotation and abduction of the shoulder, braces have been designed to limit these motions while allowing an athlete to return to competition.[15] However, an athlete who must compete by bringing his or her shoulder into external rotation and abduction is a viable candidate for a reinjury regardless of the type of brace being worn. Many sports, such as skiing, are somewhat style-conscious, and the likelihood of gaining acceptance for any type of brace may be impractical.[16]

Gieck[17] designed a shoulder strap that attaches to the shoulder pad by using a 1.5 in. elastic belt. The buckle of the belt is riveted to the shoulder pad on the opposite side of the injury, allowing for the tension to be adjusted. This shoulder strap will also allow for forward flexion while limiting external rotation from a horizontal, extended, and abducted position. The athlete's positional requirements, his or her functional ability in the strap, and the experience of the athletic trainer who is constructing this device should all be considered when designing a shoulder strap of this nature.

There are many different types of shoulder braces on the market designed to prevent recurrent episodes of anterior subluxation/dislocation. The Shoulder Subluxation Inhibitor (SSI, Physical Support Systems, Inc., Windham, NH)[18] is custom-fitted and made of low- and high-density polyethylene. It is designed with a hyperextension strap used to restrict excessive external rotation about the shoulder (Fig. 53-8). The C.D. Denison-Duke Wyre Shoulder Vest (C.D. Denison Orthopaedic Appliance Co., Baltimore, MD)[19] is constructed of sturdy canvas and is chrome leather stitched with nylon. This harness contains a biceps cuff, with lacer attachment to the chest vest used to limit abduction and extension of the shoulder. Also, laces can be threaded to limit horizontal adduction and shoulder elevation The SAWA Shoulder Orthosis (BRACE International, Scottsdale, AZ)[20] is an off-the-shelf brace made

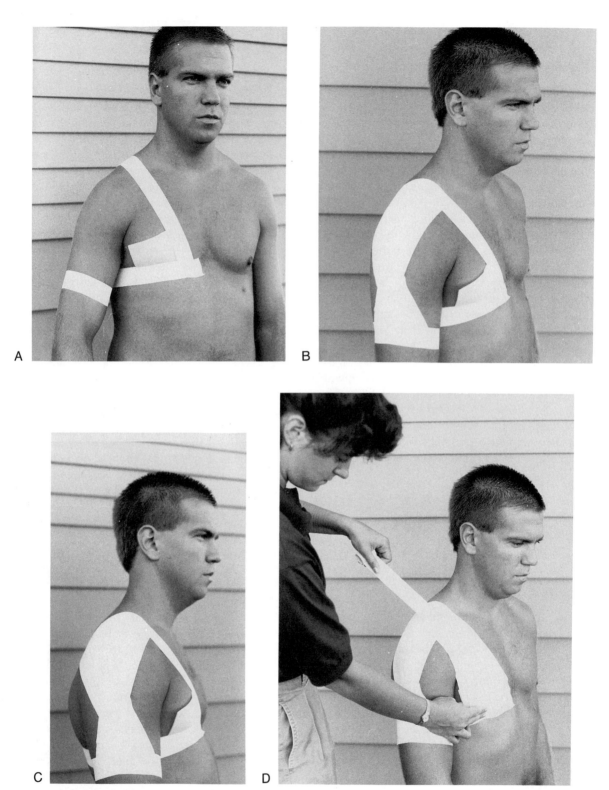

**Fig. 53-6.** Taping of acromioclavicular joint. (**A**) Application of anchors; (**B**) nonelastic support strips applied in an upward manner; (**C**) support strips applied in a fanning manner; (**D**) Anchor strips being applied from the chest to the back overlapping halfway. (*Figure continues.*)

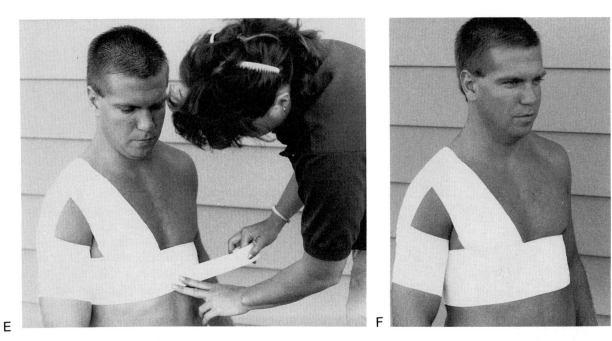

**Fig. 53-6** (*Continued*). (**E**) Anchor strips applied completely around chest and arm to "close off" the taping procedure; (**F**) completed taping of acromioclavicular joint.

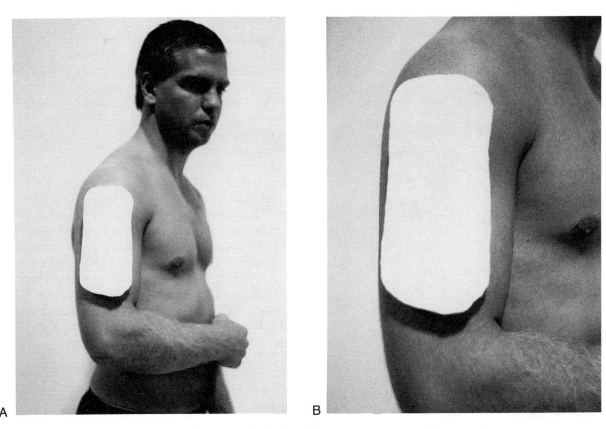

**Fig. 53-7.** (**A & B**) Donut pads for lateral humerus to protect against contusions.

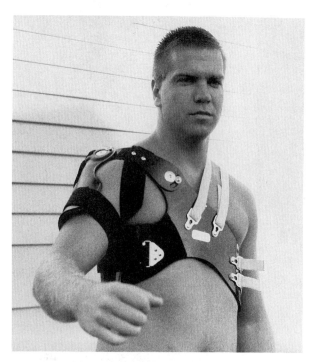

**Fig. 53-8.** Shoulder Subluxation Inhibitor designed to restrict abduction and external rotation.

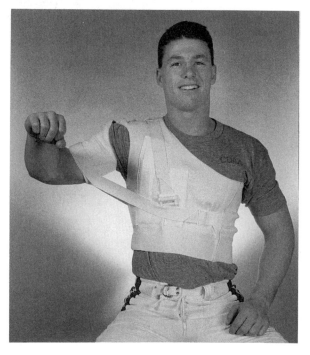

**Fig. 53-9.** SAWA Shoulder Orthosis.

of a hypoallergenic blend of cotton and rubber material. It is reinforced for strength, shape, and form with Velcro-type front closures and fasteners. A glenohumeral Velcro strap attached to a humeral cuff is used to limit adduction, abduction, flexion, and extension (Fig. 53-9).

The ultimate preventive brace for recurrent anterior instability would be one that will allow enough motion for the athlete to be as functional as possible in his or her particular sport, yet be able to provide restricting support to stabilize the glenohumeral joint. Because no surgery or rehabilitative protocol can ever replace the original anatomic and biomechanical functions of the shoulder, more research is needed to help create an individualized shoulder restrictor that is lightweight, comfortable, functional, and effective.

## LEGAL AND ETHICAL CONSIDERSATIONS AND PRINCIPLES

A substantial amount of controversy exists regarding the effectiveness of externally aided devices used for protection of the athletic shoulder. When considering the use of any protective equipment, one should always be aware of the concerns in both the individual sport that the person is participating in and any ethical ramifications that may arise in regards to the design and application of the equipment itself.

Liability is defined as the legal responsibility of a person in a certain situation to do a particular task in a reasonable and prudent manner.[3] Failure to perform such action in a prudent and reasonable manner makes the person legally liable for the results of said action. A tort concept of negligence is held by the courts when it is shown that an individual does something that a reasonably prudent person would not do.[3] More specifically, knowingly using dangerous or faulty equipment is a type of negligence that a trainer, therapist, coach, or team physician can be held accountable for should an accident result from such case.

All athletes and medical personnel should be aware that no single piece of equipment can be 100 percent preventable in terms of injury or reinjury. Therefore, the statement that a piece of equipment can totally prevent a certain injury should be completely avoided in all discussion. The implication of such a statement can lead to implied liability should an injury occur in this situation.

Special interest should be addressed to any self-fabricated device made by the medical staff. In its attempt to prevent reinjury, no piece of equipment should predispose an athlete to further insult. Of primary concern are those devices constructed to limit an athlete's range of motion. The following is a list of suggestions to help maintain safety parameters with the usage of protective equipment:[3]

1. Maintain accurate records of each athlete's injuries, both present and past.
2. Establish qualified and adequate supervision of all equipment.
3. Properly instruct the medical staff, the coaches, and the athletes themselves on correct procedures for equipment fitting.
4. Thoroughly inspect equipment on a regular basis, looking for faulty or hazardous parts.
5. Inform all athletes that no piece of equipment is 100 percent injury preventable.
6. Use sound, logical judgment when applying any type of externally aided device.
7. Have a thorough understanding of the rules of the sport that your athlete is participating in.

It is the ultimate responsibility of the medical staff to ensure that each and every athlete is treated in a reasonable and prudent manner, whereas any person deviating from this principle is subject to ethical and legal complications.

## SUMMARY

The complexity of the shoulder joint has caused many of us to use different methods of prevention and protection through the use of externally aided devices. Taping, strapping, and bracing of the shoulder complex has become a skill in which all of us involved in sports medicine are attempting to become more proficient. An externally aided device will never replace the importance of a thorough rehabilitation program, nor will it restore normal biomechanics of the injured shoulder. However, performed within the guidelines of one's qualifications and legal considerations, externally aided devices for the shoulder can be used as a valuable adjunct for returning an athlete to competition.

## REFERENCES

1. Kuland D: The Injured Athlete. JB Lippincott, Philadelphia, 1988
2. Fahey TD: Athletic Training: Principles and Practice. Mayfield Publishing Co., Palo Alto, CA, 1986
3. Arnheim DD: Modern Principles of Athletic Training. Times Mirror/Mosby College Publishing, St. Louis, 1985
4. Miller R: Presentation on protective padding. NATA National Convention and Symposium, Columbus, OH, 1987
5. Gieck J, McCue FC III: Fitting of protective football equipment. Am J Sports Med 8:3, 1980
6. Malacrea R: Protective equipment fit. Proceedings of the NATA Professional Preparation Conference, NATA Professional Education Committee, Nashville, TN, 1978
7. Roy S, Irvin R: Sports Medicine: Prevention, Evaluation, Management and Rehabilitation. Prentice-Hall, Englewood Cliffs, NJ, 1983
8. Watkins RG: Neck Injuries in Football Players. Clinics in Sports Medicine. WB Saunders, Philadelphia, 1986
9. Silloway KA, McLaughlin RE, Edlich RC, Edlich RF: Clavicular fractures and acromioclavicular joint dislocations in lacrosse: preventable injuries. J Emerg Med 3:2, 1985
10. Biron SA: Acromioclavicular protection of ice hockey players. Athletic Training 18:2, 1983
11. Deitsch MA, Fashover T: Football hip pad protection for hip pointers and AC sprains on ice hockey players. Athletic Training 16:2, 1981
12. Wershing CE: A specialized pad for the acromioclavicular joint. Athletic Training 15:2, 1980
13. Athletic Uses of Adhesive Tape. Johnson & Johnson Consumer Products, Inc., New Brunswick, NJ, 1989
14. Booher JM, Thibodeau GA: Athletic Injury Assessment. Times Mirror/Mosby College Publishing, St. Louis, 1985
15. Rovere GD, Curl WW, Brownig DG: Bracing and taping in an office sports medicine practice. In Collins HR (ed): Clinics in Sports Medicine: Office Practice of Sports Medicine. WB Saunders, Philadelphia, 1989
16. Weaver JK: Skiing-related injuries to the shoulder. Clin Orthop No. 216, March, 1987
17. Gieck J: Shoulder strap to prevent anterior glenohumeral dislocations. Athletic Training 11:1, 1976
18. Shoulder Subluxation Inhibitor: Informative Literature. Physical Supports Systems, Inc., Windham, NH, 1989
19. CD Denison-Duke Wyre Shoulder Vest: Information Packet. CD Denison Orthopedic Appliance Corp., Baltimore
20. SAWA Shoulder Orthosis: Informative Packet. Brace International, Scottsdale, AZ

# Appendix

## Shoulder Rehabilitation Program *To be performed 3 times daily.

### Range of Motion Exercises

1. **Pendulum**
   Lean over table, supporting body with uninvolved arm. Let involved arm hang straight down in a relaxed position. Move your hips to cause the shoulder to move first side-to-side and then in circles, forward, and backward. Begin with small movements and gradually increase. Shoulder should move passively. Repeat _____ sets of _____, _____ daily, _____ weekly.

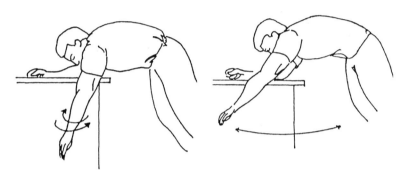

2. **Rope and Pulley**
   The overhead rope and pulley should be positioned in doorway. Sit in chair with back against door, directly underneath pulley.
   A. Shoulder Flexion:
   With elbow straight and thumb facing upward, raise involved arm out to the front of body as high as possible. Assist as needed by pulling down with uninvolved arm. Hold overhead 5 seconds and repeat.
   B. Shoulder Abduction:
   With elbow straight and palm against side, raise involved arm to the side of body as high as possible, turning the palm up as you approach 90°. Assist as needed by pulling down with the uninvolved arm to control lowering and repeat.

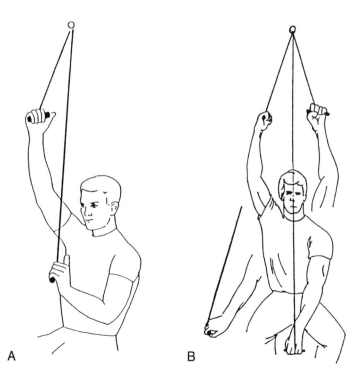

A          B

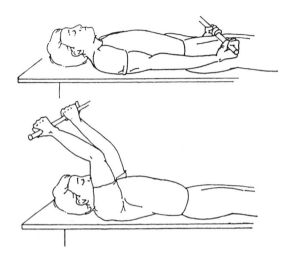

3. **T-Bar Exercises**
   A. Shoulder Flexion:
      Lie on back and grip T-bar between index finger and thumb, elbows straight. Raise both arms overhead as far as possible keeping thumbs up. Hold for 5 seconds and repeat.

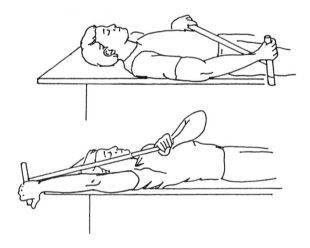

   B. Shoulder Abduction:
      Lie on back with involved arm at side of body, elbow straight and palm against leg. With other hand, push arm overhead, keeping the arm parallel to your side. As the arm reaches 90°, turn palm upwards. Twisting the uninvolved hand up can help. Continue overhead with palm up. Hold at end position 5 seconds and repeat.

## 4. External Rotation

A. Lie on back with involved arm against body and elbow bent at 90°. Grip T-bar handle and with uninvolved arm, push involved shoulder into external rotation. Hold for 5 seconds. Return to starting position and repeat.

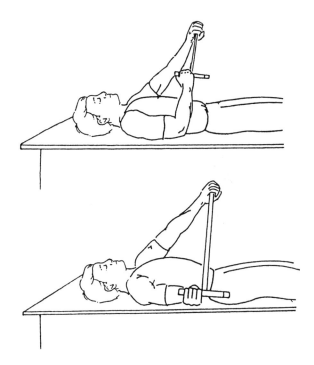

B. Lie on back with involved arm 45° from body and elbow bent at 90°. Grip T-bar in hand of involved arm and keep elbow in flexed position. Using opposite arm, push involved arm into external rotation. Hold for 5 seconds, return to starting position and repeat.

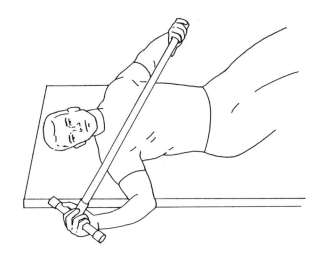

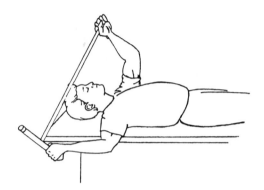

C. Lie on back with involved arm 90° from body and elbow bent at 90°. Grip T-bar in hand of involved arm and keep elbow in a fixed position. Using opposite arm, push involved arm into external rotation. Hold for 5 seconds, return to starting position and repeat.

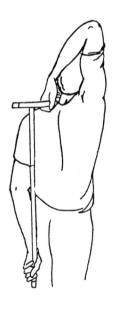

D. Involved arm overhead, standing. Hold T-bar handle behind neck and with uninvolved arm, hold the other end of T-bar and pull down. Hold for 15 seconds.

## 5. Internal Rotation

A. Supine:

Lie on back with involved arm out to side of body at 90° and elbow bent to 90°. Gripping T-bar in hand of involved arm and keeping elbow in a fixed position, use uninvolved arm to push involved shoulder into internal rotation. Hold for 5 seconds and repeat.

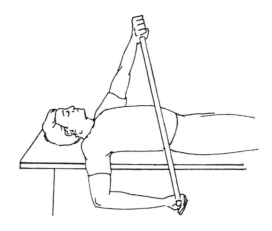

B. Standing:

Involved arm behind back holding T-bar handle. Other arm overhead and pulling bar upwards, further rotating the shoulder inwards. Hold for 5 seconds and repeat.

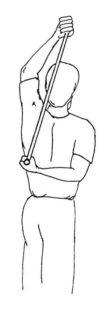

C. Standing with involved shoulder abducted to 90°, elbow at 90°. With bar over top of arm, grip T-bar handle with involved hand. Gripping the other end of the bar, gently pull the shoulder into internal rotation. Hold 5 seconds. Repeat.

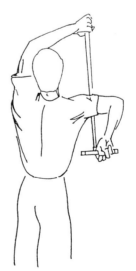

695

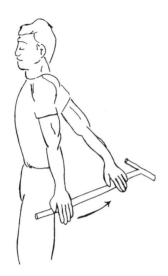

6.  **Standing Shoulder Extension**
    Standing with arms at sides, thumbs facing forward and holding T-bar between thumbs and index fingers. Keeping trunk upright, raise arms behind as far as possible. Hold 5 seconds and repeat.

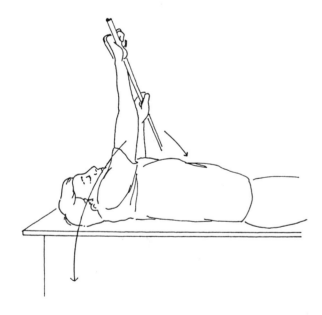

7.  **Horizontal Abduction/Adduction**
    Lie on your back and hold T-bar in front with thumbs up. Keeping your arms straight, take arms to one side of your body as far as possible, hold for 5 seconds and then take arms to other side as far as possible. Hold for 5 seconds and repeat. Perform _____ sets of _____; _____ daily, _____ weekly.

# Self Stretching of Shoulder Capsule

1. **Inferior Capsular Stretch**
   Hold involved arm overhead with elbow bent and arm straight ahead. Using uninvolved arm, stretch arm further overhead. When stretching sensation felt, hold for 5 seconds and repeat.

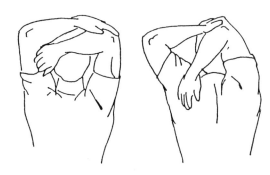

2. **Posterior Capsular Stretch**
   With uninvolved arm, grasp elbow of involved arm. Pull involved arm across chest to stretch the back of involved shoulder. Hold at end point 5 seconds and repeat.

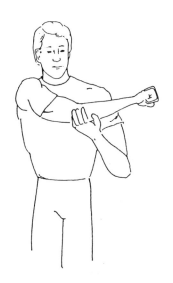

3. **Anterior Capsular Stretch**
   Standing in doorway, elbow straight, shoulder abducted to 90° and externally rotated. With pressure on arm, force arm back to stretch the front of the shoulder. Hold 5 seconds and repeat.

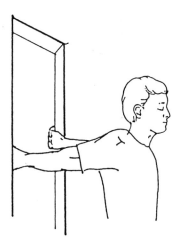

697

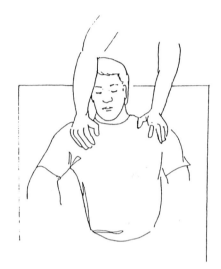

**4. Pectoralis Minor Stretch**
Lie on back, push shoulders towards ceiling with partner giving resistance. Relax, and have partner stretch shoulder down. Hold stretch for 5 seconds.

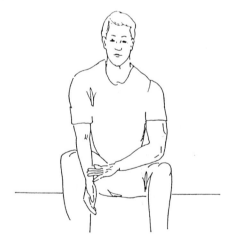

**5. Biceps Stretch**
Seated with elbow extended and resting on leg. With uninvolved arm pushing on forearm, straighten elbow and hold stretch for 5 seconds.

# Strengthening Exercises

## Isometrics

1. **External Rotation**
   Standing against a wall or in a doorway with arm at side and elbow bent to 90°, press back of forearm into surface. Hold a sub-maximal force for 8 seconds and repeat.

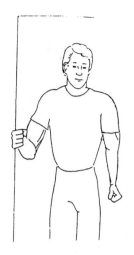

2. **Internal Rotation**
   Standing against a wall or in a doorway with arm at side and elbow bent to 90°, press front of forearm into surface. Hold a sub-maximal force for 8 seconds and repeat.

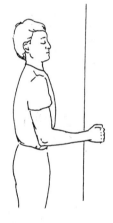

3. **Flexion**
   Standing in doorway facing out the doorway, place involved arm in front of you, place forearm and hand on doorframe and push as if to raise arm overhead. Hold sub-maximal force for 8 seconds and repeat.

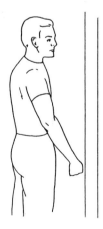

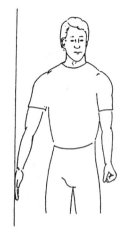

**4. Abduction**
Standing against a wall or in a doorway with involved arm at side, press back of forearm into surface. Keep arm at side with elbow straight. Hold a submaximal force for 8·seconds and repeat.

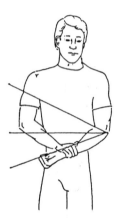

**5. Elbow Flexion**
Use uninvolved arm to hold involved elbow at angles of 45, 90 and 135°. Flex elbow into uninvolved hand keeping elbow still. Hold a submaximal force for 8 seconds and repeat. Perform _____ repetitions at each angle. Perform _____ sets of _____ repetitions; _____ daily, _____ weekly.

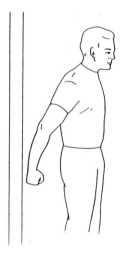

**6. Extension**
Standing in doorway, and in front of doorframe, place involved arm behind you slightly, push backward into doorframe. Hold submaximal force for 8 seconds and repeat.

# Strengthening Exercises

## Isotonics

1. **Side-Lying External Rotation**
   Lie on uninvolved side, with involved arm at side of body and elbow bent to 90°. Keeping the elbow of involved arm fixed to side, raise arm. Hold 2 seconds and lower slowly. Perform _____ sets of _____ repetitions _____ daily.

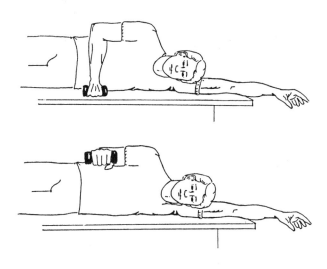

2. **Side-Lying Internal Rotation**
   Lie on involved side with arm against side and elbow bent to 90°. Keeping the elbow fixed against side, lower forearm first to comfort, then raise forearm to trunk. Hold 2 seconds and lower slowly. Perform _____ sets of _____ repetitions _____ daily.

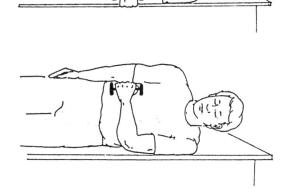

**Weight Progression:**
Begin all exercises with _____ pounds, perform _____ sets of 10 repetitions. All exercises should be performed raising and lowering the arm *slowly*. Progress gradually at your tolerance to _____ sets of _____ repetitions. Weight may be added to your exercises at week _____, increasing by _____ pound(s) and lowering your sets to _____ sets of 10 repetitions. Progress back up to _____ sets of 10 repetitions. Once this level is attained repeat this process up to a maximum of _____ pounds to ensure rotator cuff musculature isolation.

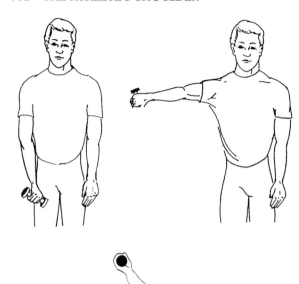

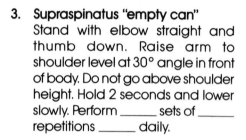

3. **Supraspinatus "empty can"**
Stand with elbow straight and thumb down. Raise arm to shoulder level at 30° angle in front of body. Do not go above shoulder height. Hold 2 seconds and lower slowly. Perform _____ sets of _____ repetitions _____ daily.

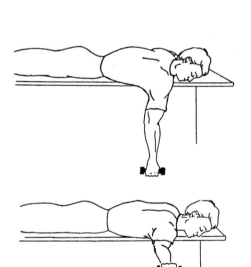

4. **Prone Horizontal Abduction**
Lie on table, face down, with involved arm hanging straight to the floor, and palm facing down. Raise arm out to the side, parallel to the floor. Hold 2 seconds and lower slowly. Perform _____ sets of _____ repetitions _____ daily.

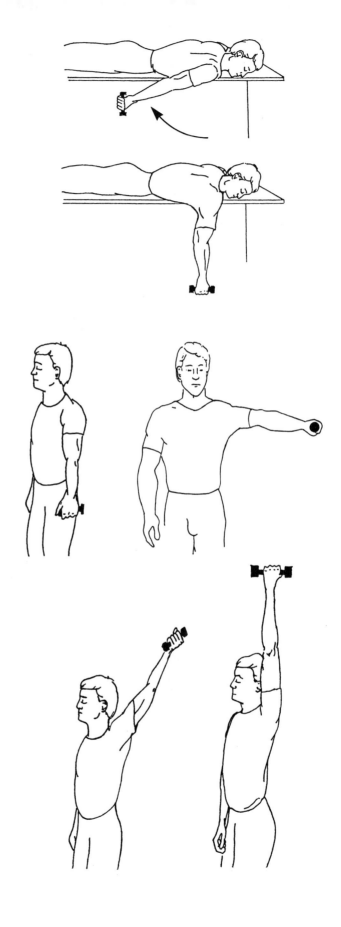

5. **Prone Extension**
   Lie on table, face down, with involved arm hanging straight to the floor, and palm facing in and thumb down. Raise arm straight back as far as possible. Hold 2 seconds and lower slowly. Perform _____ sets of _____ repetitions _____ daily.

6. **Standing Abduction**
   Stand with arm at side, elbow straight, and palm against side. Raise arm to the side, rotating palm up as arm reaches 90°. Continue to raise arm to _____ height, lower slowly. Perform _____ sets of _____ repetitions _____ daily.

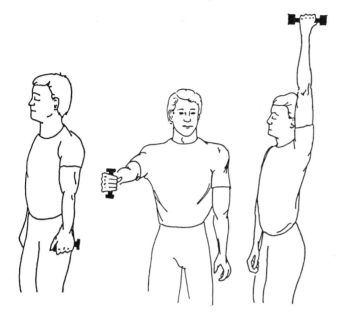

### 7. Standing Flexion
Stand with arm at side, elbow straight, and palm against side. Raise arm in front with thumb up. Continue overhead as far as possible. Lower slowly in reverse. Perform _____ sets of _____ repetitions _____ daily.

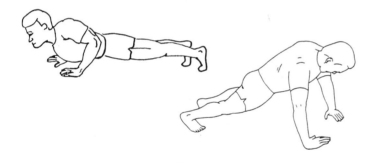

### 8. Progressive Push-ups - Serratus Anterior
Start with push-up into wall. Gradually progress to table top and eventually to floor as tolerable. Perform _____ sets of _____ repetitions _____ daily.

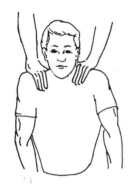

### 9. Shoulder Shrugs
With a partner, have partner resist you as you shrug shoulders upwards. Perform _____ sets of _____ repetitions _____ daily.

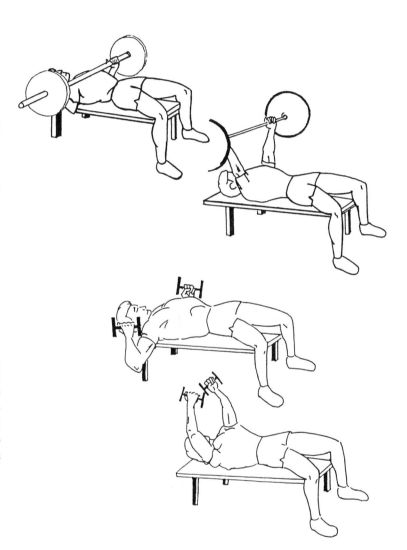

## 10. Bench Press

Lying on bench face up with hands lined up with shoulders on weight bar. Press weight straight up and lower bar to chest. Perform _____ sets of _____ repetitions _____ daily.

## 11. Pectoral Flies

Lying on back, on bench with weight held in each hand, hold weights together in front with arms straight. Slowly lower weights, keeping arms away from body and shoulders abducted 90°. Raise arms to repeat. Perform _____ sets of _____ repetitions _____ daily.

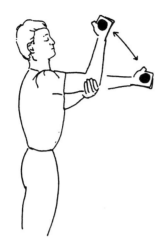

### 12. Biceps Curls
Standing with arm out and palm facing upwards. Support involved arm with opposite hand. Bend elbow to full flexion, hold 2 seconds, then extend arm completely. Extend arm in count of four. Perform _____ sets of _____ repetitions _____ daily.

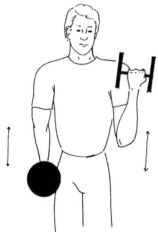

### 13. Biceps Curls
Standing with arm against side and palm facing inwards, bend elbow upward turning palm up as you progress. Return in a count of four. Perform _____ sets of _____ repetitions _____ daily.

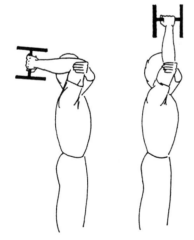

### 14. Triceps Curls
Raise involved arm overhead. Provide support at elbow from uninvolved hand. Straighten arm overhead. Hold 2 seconds and lower slowly. Perform _____ sets of _____ repetitions _____ daily.

**Seated Rowing:**
In a seated position, legs straight and knees locked, grip the handles of the pulleys or grips of the rubber tubing, slowly pull toward your chest, hold for several seconds and repeat.

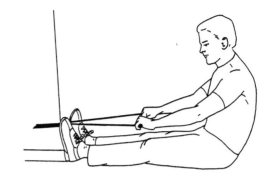

### 15. Wrist Flexion
Supporting the forearm and with palm facing upward, lower a weight in hand as far as possible and then curl it up as high as possible. Hold for 2 counts. Perform _____ sets of _____ repetitions _____ daily.

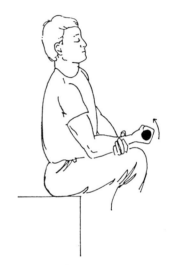

### 16. Wrist Extension
Supporting the forearm and with palm facing downward, raise weight in hand as far as possible and lower slowly as far as you can. Perform _____ sets of _____ repetitions _____ daily.

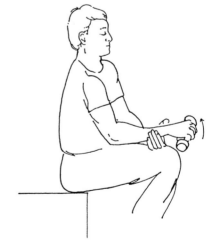

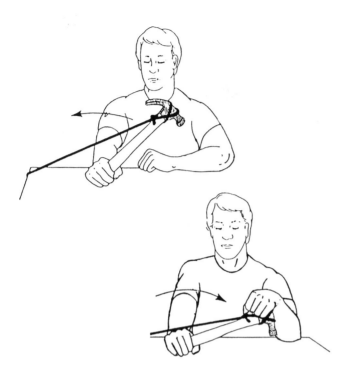

## Trunk Exercises

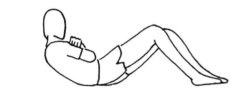

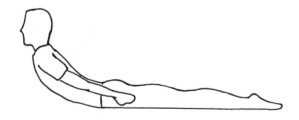

17. **Pronation**
Forearm should be supported on a table with wrist in neutral position. Using a weight or hammer held in a normal hammering position, roll wrist and bring hammer into pronation as far as possible. Hold for a 2 count. Raise to starting position. Perform _____ sets of _____ repetitions _____ daily.

18. **Supination**
Forearm supported on table with wrist in neutral position. Using a hammer or a weight, roll wrist taking palm up. Hold for a 2 count and raise back to starting position. Perform _____ sets of _____ repetitions _____ daily.

19. **Abdominal Curls**
Lie on back with knees bent and arms across chest. Curl trunk upwards towards knees, continuing until shoulders are off surface. Hold for _____ seconds and lower slowly. Perform _____ sets of _____ repetitions _____ daily.

20. **Back Extension**
Lie on floor face down and arms at sides. Lift chest and shoulders off floor, arching the low back. Hold for _____ seconds and lower slowly. Perform _____ sets of _____ repetitions _____ daily.

# Advanced Strengthening Exercises

## Tubing Exercises

1. **External Rotation at 0° Abduction**
Standing with involved elbow fixed at side, elbow at 90° and involved arm across front of body. Grip tubing handle while the other end of tubing is fixed. Pull out with arm, keeping elbow at side. Return tubing slowly and controlled. Perform _____ sets of _____ repetitions _____ daily.

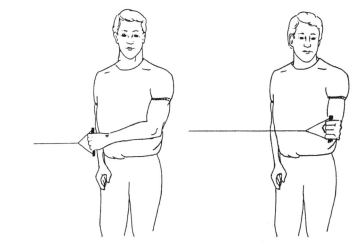

2. **Internal Rotation at 0° Abduction**
Standing with elbow at side fixed at 90° and shoulder rotated out. Grip tubing handle while other end of tubing is fixed. Pull arm across body keeping elbow at side. Return tubing slowly and controlled. Perform _____ sets of _____ repetitions _____ daily.

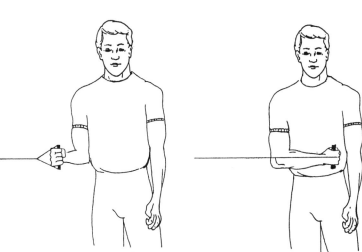

3. **External Rotation at 90° Abduction - Slow**
Stand with shoulder abducted 90° and elbow flexed 90°. Grip tubing handle while the other end is fixed straight ahead. Keeping shoulder abducted, rotate shoulder back keeping elbow at 90°. Return tubing and hand to start position slowly and controlled. Perform _____ sets of _____ repetitions _____ daily.

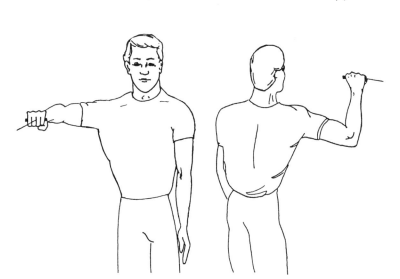

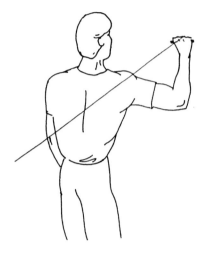

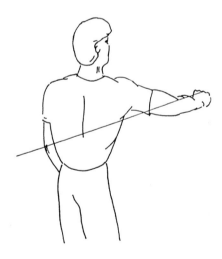

4. **Internal Rotation at 90° Abduction - Slow**

   Stand with shoulder abducted to 90°, externally rotated 90°, and elbow flexed 90°. Grip tubing handle with other end of tubing fixed straight behind. Keeping shoulder abducted, rotate shoulder forward, keeping elbow at 90°. Return tubing and hand to start position slowly and controlled. Perform _____ sets of _____ repetitions _____ daily.

5. **External Rotation at 90° Abduction - Fast**

   Position self as in "3". Rotate shoulder back quickly, keeping elbow at 90°. Return tubing and hand to start position quickly and controlled. Perform _____ sets of _____ repetitions _____ daily.

6. **Internal Rotation at 90° Abduction - Fast**

   Position self as in "4". Rotate shoulder forward quickly keeping elbow at 90°. Return tubing and hand to start position quickly and controlled. Perform _____ sets of _____ repetitions _____ daily.

7. **External Rotation Plyometrics**
Position self as in "3". Pull tubing back into external rotation with maximal tension and hold an isometric contraction in external rotation for 3 seconds. Relax isometric hold allowing fast but controlled motion. When hand hits horizontal, as fast as possible, reverse motion into external rotation then repeat isometric hold. Perform _____ sets of _____ repetitions _____ daily.

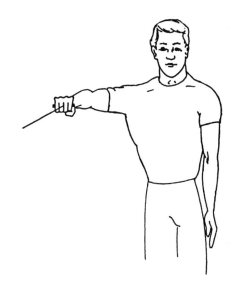

8. **Internal Rotation Plyometrics**
Position self as in "4". Pull tubing down into internal rotation with maximal tension and hold isometric position for 3 seconds. Relax isometric hold allowing fast but controlled motion. When hand reaches vertical, as fast as possible reverse motion into internal rotation then repeat isometric hold. Perform _____ sets of _____ repetitions _____ daily.

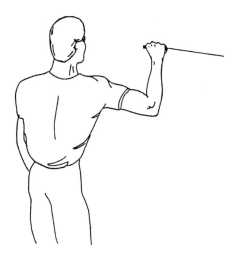

9. **Diagonal Pattern (D1) Flexion**
Gripping tubing handle in hand of involved arm, begin with arm out from side 45° and palm facing backward. After turning palm forward, proceed to flex elbow and bring arm up and over uninvolved shoulder. Turn palm down and reverse to take arm to starting position. Exercise should be performed in controlled manner. Perform _____ sets of _____ repetitions _____ daily.

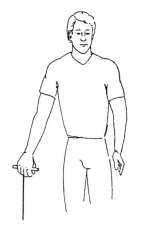
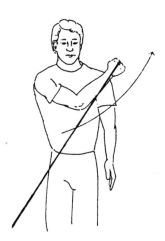

711

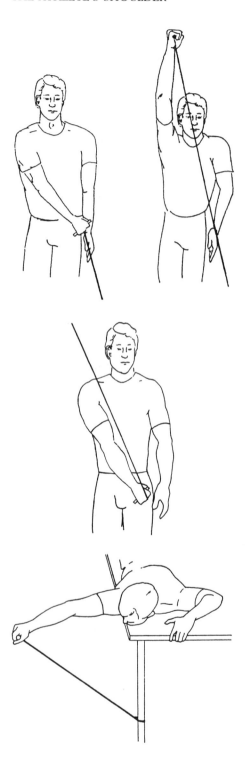

## 10. Diagonal Pattern (D2) Flexion

Involved hand will grip tubing handle across body and against thigh of opposite side leg. Starting with palm down, rotate palm up to begin. Proceed to flex elbow and bring arm up and over involved shoulder with palm facing inward. Turn palm down and reverse to take arm to starting position. Exercise should be performed in a controlled manner. Perform _____ sets of _____ repetitions _____ daily.

## 11. Diagonal Pattern (D2) Extension

Involved hand will grip tubing handle overhead and out to the side. Pull tubing down and across your body to the opposite side of leg. During the motion lead with your thumb. Perform _____ sets of _____ repetitions _____ daily

## 12. Prone Shoulder Abduction Rhomboids/Posterior Deltoid

Lie face down and arm hanging straight to floor. With one end of tubing fastened to table leg, grip handle on other end. Raise arm out of the side with palm facing down. Slowly return to starting position. Perform _____ sets of _____ repetitions _____ daily.

# Throwers Ten Exercise Program

The Throwers Ten Program is designed to exercise the major muscles necessary for throwing. The program's goal is to be an organized and concise exercise program. In addition, all exercises included are specific to the thrower and are designed to improve strength, power and endurance of the shoulder complex musculature.

1. **Diagonal Pattern D2 Extension:**
   Involved hand will grip tubing handle overhead and out to the side. Pull tubing down and across your body to the opposite side of leg. During the motion lead with your thumb. Perform _____ sets of _____ repetitions _____ daily.

   **Diagonal Pattern D2 Flexion:**
   Gripping tubing handle in hand of involved arm, begin wtih arm out from side 45° and palm facing backward. After turning palm forward, proceed to flex elbow and bring arm up and over uninvolved shoulder. Turn palm down and reverse to take arm to starting position. Exercise should be performed in controlled manner. Perform _____ sets of _____ repetitions _____ daily.

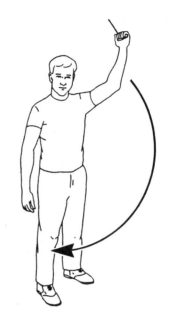

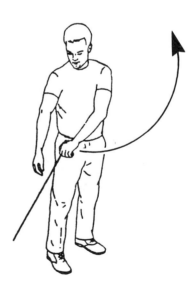

713

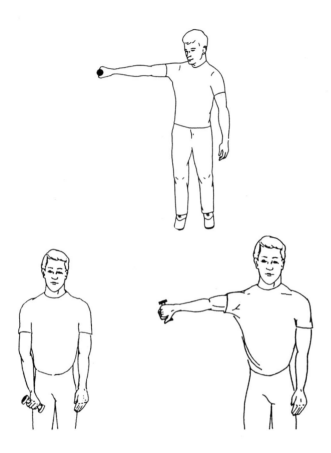

2. **Dumbbell Exercises for Deltoid and Supraspinatus**
   **Deltoid Strengthening:**
   Stand with arm at side, elbow straight, and palm against side. Raise arm to the side, palm down, until arm reaches 90°. Perform _____ sets of _____ repetitions _____ daily.

   **Supraspinatus Strengthening**
   Stand with elbow straight and thumb down. Raise arm to shoulder level at 30° angle in front of body. Do not go above shoulder height. Hold 2 seconds and lower slowly. Perform _____ sets of _____ repetitions _____ daily.

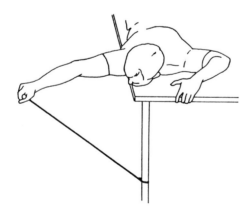

3. **Prone Shoulder Abduction For Rhomboids**
   **Diagonal Pattern D2 Flexion**
   Involved hand will grip tubing handle across body and against thigh of opposite side leg. Starting with palm down, rotate palm up to begin. Proceed to flex elbow and bring arm up and over involved shoulder with palm facing inward. Turn palm down and reverse to take arm to starting position. Exercise should be performed in a controlled manner. Perform _____ sets of _____ repetitions _____ daily.

4. **Prone Shoulder Extension For Latissimus Dorsi**

Lie on table, face down, with involved arm hanging straight to the floor, and palm facing down. Raise arm straight back as far as possible. Hold 2 seconds and lower slowly. Perform _____ sets of _____ repetitions _____ daily.

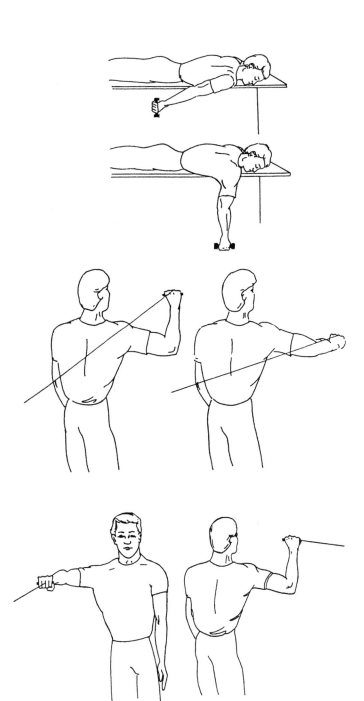

5. **Internal Rotation at 90° Abduction**

Stand with shoulder abducted to 90°, externally rotated 90° and elbow bent to 90°. Keeping shoulder abducted rotate shoulder forward, keeping elbow bent at 90°. Return tubing and hand to start position slowly and controlled.

a. Slow Speed Sets
   Perform _____ sets of _____ repetitions _____ daily.

b. Fast Speed Sets
   Perform _____ sets of _____ repetitions _____ daily.

**External Rotation at 90° Abduction**

Stand with shoulder abducted 90° and elbow flexed 90°. Grip tubing handle while the other end is fixed straight ahead. Keeping shoulder abducted, rotate shoulder back keeping elbow at 90°. Return tubing and hand to start position slowly and controlled.

a. Slow Speed Sets
   Perform _____ sets of _____ repetitions _____ daily.

b. Fast Speed Sets
   Perform _____ sets of _____ repetitions _____ daily.

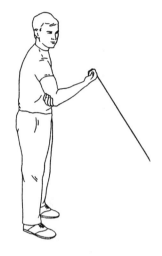

**6. Biceps Strengthening With Tubing**
Stand with tubing securely in hand and opposite end under the same foot of the involved side, controlling tension. Assist with opposite hand flexing arm through full range of motion. Return to starting position within a slow 5 count. Repeat 3 - 5 sets of 10 repetitions.

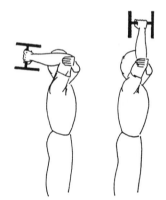

**7. Dumbbell Exercises for Triceps & Wrist Ext/Flexors**

**Triceps Curls**
Raise involved arm overhead. Provide support at elbow from uninvolved hand. Straighten arm overhead. Hold 2 seconds and lower slowly. Perform _____ sets of _____ repetitions _____ daily.

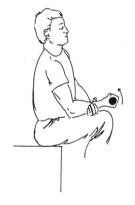

**Wrist Flexion**
The forearm should be supported on a table with hand off edge; palm should face upward. Using a weight or hammer, lower that hand as far as possible and then curl it up as high as possible. Hold for a 2 count. Perform _____ sets of _____ repetitions _____ daily.

### Wrist Extension

The forearm should be supported on a table with hand off edge; palm should face downward. Using a weight or hammer, lower the hand as far as possible then curl wrist up as high as possible. Hold for a 2 count. Perform _____ sets of _____ repetitions _____ daily.

### Forearm Pronation

Forearm should be supported on a table with wrist in neutral position. Using a weight or hammer held in a normal hammering position, roll wrist and bring hammer into pronation as far as possible. Hold for a 2 count. Raise to starting position. Perform _____ sets of _____ repetitions _____ daily.

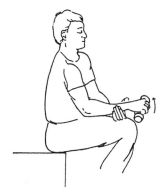

### Forearm Supination

Forearm should be supported on table with wrist in neutral position. Using a weight or hammer held in a normal hammering position, roll wrist bringing hammer into full supination. Hold for a 2 count. Raise back to starting position. Perform _____ sets of _____ repetitions _____ daily.

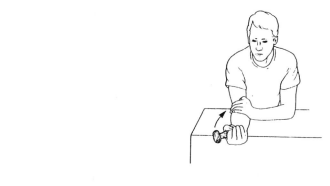

8. **Serratus Anterior Strengthening Program**

   Start with push-up into wall. Gradually progress to table top and eventually to floor as tolerable. Perform _____ sets of _____ repetitions _____ daily.

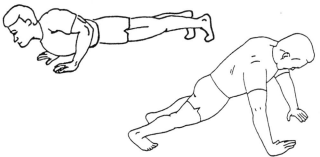

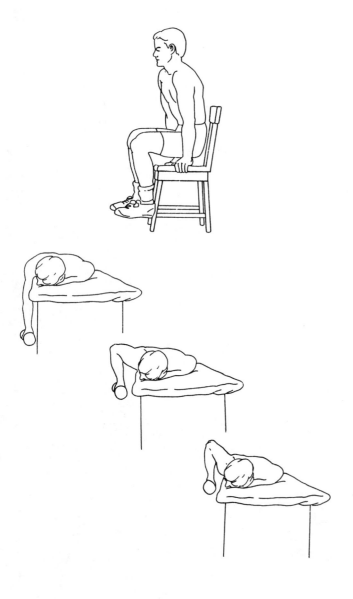

### 9.  Press-Ups

Seated on a chair or on a table, place both hands firmly on the sides of the chair or table, palm down and fingers pointed outward. Hands should be placed equal with shoulders. Slowly push downward through the hands to elevate your body. Hold the elevated position for 2 seconds. Repeat. Perform _____ sets of _____ repetitions _____ daily.

### 10. Rowing

Lying on your stomach with your involved arm hanging over the side of the table, dumbbell in hand and elbow straight. Slowly raise arm, bending elbow, and bring dumbbell as high as possible. Hold at the top for 2 seconds, then slowly lower. Repeat. Perform _____ sets of _____ repetitions _____ daily.

# Index

*Note: Page numbers followed by* f *represent figures; those followed by* t *represent tables.*